Textbook of
VETERINARY ANESTHESIA

*Dedicated to
my Wife and Sons*

Textbook of
VETERINARY ANESTHESIA

edited by

LAWRENCE R. SOMA, V.M.D.

Associate Professor of Anesthesia
Department of Clinical Studies
School of Veterinary Medicine
University of Pennsylvania
Philadelphia, Pennsylvania

The Williams & Wilkins Company BALTIMORE 1971

Made in the United States of America

Reprinted November, 1972
Reprinted June, 1974
Reprinted June, 1977
Reprinted August 1979

Library of Congress Catalog Card Number 79-130473
SBN 683-07845-3

Composed and printed at the
WAVERLY PRESS, INC.
Mt. Royal and Guilford Aves.
Baltimore, Md. 21202, U.S.A.

Contents

v

Introduction

This *Textbook of Veterinary Anesthesia* fills a number of needs. For the student and practitioner up to date techniques for use in clinical practice are described. For the research worker using animals much information is provided on anesthetic management of many species of animal. This applies to investigators wherever they are based, be it in a medical or veterinary school, college, research institute, military, pharmaceutical, or other industrial unit. For the teacher of veterinary medicine, particularly of anesthesia, areas requiring further exploration are suggested.

The chapters have different authors, many of whom are extraordinarily well known in the fields on which they are reporting. A significant number come from faculties of schools of medicine. This broadens the scope of the book and begins a liaison between veterinary and human medicine which must be encouraged to develop even more than at present. Such multiple authorship offers the reader interesting comparisons of the similarities (and there are many) as well as the differences between veterinary anesthesia and anesthesia in man.

The book is intended as a general text and achieves this purpose admirably. There is available in addition sufficient detail for the knowledgable reader.

A bit of history about the Editor may be of interest. Dr. Soma obtained much of his training in human anesthesia, serving as a Special Fellow, supported by the National Institutes of Health, in the Department of Anesthesia of the University of Pennsylvania School of Medicine. He has conducted collaborative research with individuals on the faculty of the School of Medicine at Pennsylvania and is currently working full-time on a special project in the laboratories of the Department of Anesthesia of that School. The relationship has been a long and fruitful one of benefit to all.

Elsewhere I have recorded remarks which I believe pertinent to an introduction to this kind of book. I quote the following: "A large part of the research on living systems has been carried out on anesthetized animals. The disruption of function caused by anesthesia has been identified only relatively recently by persons conducting such research, and there remain many who ignore this disruption completely. These facts give cause for concern, raising as they must the question of how much the anesthetic state has contributed to misinterpretation of experimental results. In the present volume an attempt has been made to describe the changes consequent to anesthesia.

"There is no question that infinitely greater attention must be paid in the future to maintenance of such parameters as normal gas exchange, tissue perfusion, and hepatic or renal function, to mention a few, if studies are not to be conducted on abnormal preparations. This is not to say that even if one prevents hypoxia and respiratory or metabolic acidosis all will be well. The anesthetic drugs under the most favorable circumstances still cause profound changes. The more one learns about these, the more accurately their influence on investigations and observations can be assessed."

It is a personal pleasure to endorse the contribution of Dr. Soma and his distinguished collaborators. But more importantly I am pleased that the specialty of anesthesia is growing in stature in veterinary medicine, for well it should.

ROBERT D. DRIPPS, M.D.
Professor and Chairman
Department of Anesthesia
University of Pennsylvania
Philadelphia, Pennsylvania

Preface

The advances in techniques in veterinary anesthesia have been extensive in the latter part of the 1960's. A most gratifying aspect of this change has been the greater focus on anesthesia as an important part of animal management and care. The attention has shifted from anesthesia as being only a necessary part of a surgical procedure to a greater overall awareness of the part of the clinician of its importance in the management of the animal from the preoperative through to the postoperative period.

The development of newer surgical techniques and diagnostic methods in all phases of veterinary practice and their extension to the older more chronically ill veterinary patient has demanded of the clinician more sophistication in his anesthetic approach. This change has been reflected in a shift from the predominant use of barbiturates, as a sole anesthetic agent, to the use of barbiturates in combination with an inhalation anesthetic or inhalation anesthetics alone. A variety of newer drugs has also been added to the veterinary armamentarium, allowing the safer management of an increasing number of species of animals. Along with this has been a need for more basic information on the clinical pharmacological actions of these drugs and their interaction with other agents.

Along with the use by the practicing veterinarian of newer anesthetic techniques and agents has been a greater interest on the part of the researcher on more up to date methods for the anesthetization of animals. There has also been more concern for the impact of depressant drugs and anesthetic agents on experimental results. Unfortunately, herein lies one of the greatest deficiencies of our knowledge of drug actions, especially when studying respiratory and cardiovascular changes. The rapid development of the field of biomedical engineering has given the researcher the means for the development of more sophisticated chronic models, thereby bypassing acute studies in some instances. This has placed more of a demand on the researcher for the use of better anesthetic techniques and improvement in animal care.

Another area of interest, for both its ecological and comparative pharmacological interest, is the effect of various drugs and anesthetic agents in wild captive and free ranging animals. The study and preservation of our wild life, one of the great gifts of nature to mankind, and the health management of wild animals in captivity have added great impetus to the interest of depressant drugs in a wide variety of wild species, this out of necessity for the management of the recalcitrant animal.

With these many needs in mind, a wide range of authors and topics has been selected in an attempt to be as complete as possible. The sections in the texts by colleagues in the medical and allied professions attest to their contribution to the development of veterinary anesthesia. Veterinary anesthesia as a discipline in American veterinary institutions is only in its developing stages and many owe initial training and encouragement from teachers in the medical profession.

It has been hoped that a volume has been presented which will be a stimulating first encounter for the veterinary student, who is for the first time inquiring into the field of veterinary anesthesia. Chapters and sections of chapters are included which pursue topics in greater detail in an attempt to present the broad scope of anesthesia and encourage the inquiring mind. The needs of the practicing veterinarian and those in related areas have been of prime consideration in the development of the text. Information is provided to aid in the daily management of a variety of species and an in depth coverage of the many phases of anesthetic practices. Also in mind were the researcher and others who are involved in animal management.

My gratitude is extended to the many authors who have contributed their expertise to this text, and to Mrs. Kathleen Gallagher and Miss Gwen Evans, secretaries on whose shoulders the bulk of typing fell. I would also like to thank Mrs. Bernice Cohn for her many contributions. Finally I would like to express my gratitude to my family for hours stolen which are irreplaceable.

LAWRENCE R. SOMA
Philadelphia,   Pennsylvania

Contributors

S. CRAIGHEAD ALEXANDER, M.D., Professor and Chairman, Department of Anesthesiology, University of Connecticut Health Center, Hartford, Connecticut

BURTON M. ALTURA, PH.D., Associate Professor of Anesthesiology and Physiology, Departments of Anesthesiology and Physiology, Albert Einstein College of Medicine, Yeshiva University, Bronx, New York

EMIL BLAIR, M.D., Professor of Surgery, University of Colorado Medical Center, Denver, Colorado

PETER H. BYLES, M.B., M.R.C.S., L.R.C.P., Associate Professor of Anesthesia, State University of New York, Upstate Medical Center, Syracuse, New York

DONALD H. CLIFFORD, D.V.M., PH.D., Chief, Research in Laboratory Animal Medicine, Science and Technology, Veterans Administration Hospital, Houston, Texas

PETER J. COHEN, M.D., Professor and Chairman, Department of Anesthesia, University of Colorado Medical Center, Denver, Colorado

STANLEY DEUTSCH, PH.D., M.D., Professor of Anesthesiology, Pritzker School of Medicine, University of Chicago and Chairman, Department of Anesthesiology, Michael Reese Hospital and Medical Center, Chicago, Illinois

ALLEN B. DOBKIN, M.D., Professor of Anesthesiology, State University of New York, Upstate Medical Center, Syracuse, New York

ROBERT D. DRIPPS, M.D., Professor and Chairman, Department of Anesthesia, School of Medicine, University of Pennsylvania, Philadelphia, Pennsylvania

BENJAMIN E. ETSTEN, M.D., Chairman and Professor, Department of Anesthesiology, Tufts University School of Medicine and Anesthetist-in-Chief, New England Medical Center Hospitals, Boston, Massachusetts

LOREN H. EVANS, D.V.M., Assistant Professor of Surgery, School of Veterinary Medicine, University of Pennsylvania, Philadelphia, Pennsylvania

KARL L. GABRIEL, V.M.D., PH.D., Visiting Associate Professor of Pharmacology, Medical College of Pennsylvania, Philadelphia, Pennsylvania

KIRK N. GELATT, V.M.D., Assistant Professor of Ophthalmology, Section of Comparative Ophthalmology, College of Veterinary Medicine, University of Minnesota, St. Paul, Minnesota

L. W. HALL, PH.D., D.V.A., M.R.C.V.S., University Lecturer in the Department of Veterinary Clinical Studies, University of Minnesota, St. Paul, Minnesota

A. M. HARTHOORN, PH.D., D.V.Sc., D.M.V., F.R.C.V.S., Head, Department of Physiology and Biochemistry, University College, Nairobi, Kenya

S. G. HERSHEY, M.D., Professor of Anesthesiology, Albert Einstein College of Medicine Yeshiva University, Bronx, New York

SYDNEY JENNINGS, M.R.C.V.S., D.V.A., Project Manager, United Nations Project Veterinary Education, Mexico City, Mexico

ALAN M. KLIDE, V.M.D., Assistant Professor of Anesthesia, Department of Clinical Studies, School of Veterinary Medicine, University of Pennsylvania, Philadelphia, Pennsylvania

HARRY W. LINDE, PH.D., Associate Professor of Anesthesia, Northwestern University Medical School, Chicago, Illinois

JAMES G. McCORMICK, PH.D., Research Assistant Professor of Otolaryngology, Department of Surgery, Bowman Gray School of Medicine, Winston-Salem, North Carolina

HENRY L. PRICE, M.D., Professor of Anesthesia, Department of Anesthesia, Temple University Health Science Center, Philadelphia, Pennsylvania

SAM H. RIDGWAY, D.V.M., Research Veterinarian, Naval Undersea Research and Development Center, San Diego, California

LIONEL F. RUBIN, V.M.D., M.MED.SC., Associate Professor of Ophthalmology, Department of Clinical Studies, University of Pennsylvania, School of Veterinary Medicine, Philadelphia, Pennsylvania

JOHN SANFORD, PH.D., M.R.C.V.S., Senior Lecturer, Department of Veterinary Pharmacology, University of Glasgow, Glasgow, Scotland

SHIRO SHIMOSATO, M.D., Associate Professor of Anesthesiology, Tufts University School of Medicine, Boston, Massachusetts

THEODORE C. SMITH, M.D., Associate Professor, Department of Anesthesia, University of Pennsylvania, School of Medicine, Philadelphia, Pennsylvania

J. F. SMITHCORS, D.V.M., PH.D., Technical Editor, American Veterinary Publications, Inc., Santa Barbara, California

LAWRENCE R. SOMA, V.M.D., Associate Professor of Anesthesia, Department of Clinical Studies, School of Veterinary Medicine, University of Pennsylvania, Philadelphia, Pennsylvania

W. DEREK TAVERNOR, PH.D., F.R.C.V.S., Senior Lecturer, Department of Surgery, The Royal Veterinary College, University of London, London, England

RHEA J. WHITE, D.V.M., Resident and Postdoctoral Research Fellow, Department of Clinical Studies, School of Veterinary Medicine, University of Pennsylvania, Philadelphia, Pennsylvania

1
History of Veterinary Anesthesia

J. F. SMITHCORS

The story of anesthesia offers mute testimony to the regrettable fact that medical men, sometimes, have been loathe to heed the lessons of history. While a bit of healthy skepticism is essential in most matters, to ignore deliberately, *i.e.*, not to put to test, what is demonstrated as an apparent fact is to flout the basic tenets of science. However, until recent times, medicine was more art than science. Thus, the potentially anesthetic property of ether was demonstrated three centuries before its clinical use was realized. For nitrous oxide the time lag—following a wholly adequate demonstration of its clinical use—was more than a half-century of needless pain. The latent period for chloroform was considerably less, but was sufficient to cause a pharmacist to observe, regarding this agent, in 1847, "These facts may be noticed as a remarkable instance of how long men may stand on the brink of a discovery without reaching it, to which subsequent reflection may shew them that many circumstances have pointed." [51]

No branch of medicine is exempt from censure in this matter. The anesthetic effects of carbon dioxide, for example, were demonstrated (and publicized) by a British physician in 1824, and were promptly ignored by contemporary medical men. Although small amounts of carbon dioxide have been incorporated in anesthetic mixtures for several decades, its use *per se* was reported in 1964 by a veterinarian, who apparently was unaware that it had been used in an almost identical manner 140 years earlier. [31] Curare offers a reverse example of inadequate communication between the medical professions as well as a lack of historical awareness by both physicians and veterinarians. [44] British veterinarians demonstrated the apparently successful use of curare as a muscle relaxant in tetanus in 1835, but this drug was not used in human medicine until 1858. In 1956, however, a veterinary report on the use of a purified curare compound failed to acknowledge this early work of British veterinarians. [5]

In many respects, the history of anesthesia is a disturbing account of "what might have been"—at least much sooner than was realized, had medical men, including veterinarians, been more aware of history and more willing to verify earlier work. [45] Veterinary surgeons, in particular, relied on heavy handed restraint much longer than was necessary. However, in this regard, human surgery is not exempt from criticism. As recently as 1942 the eminent anesthesiologist R. M. Waters noted that clinical practice was handicapped by failure to correlate and utilize existing knowledge and that "Permanent improvement will develop in the future, as it has come in the past, mainly through consideration of scientific facts—laborious learning, imaginative insight and accumulative application." [54]

Anesthesia in Ancient Times

Relief from pain has been one of the most persistent pursuits of mankind from ancient times, but for only little more than a century has there been anything approaching the clinical use of anesthesia. There are sporadic references to anesthetic agents, real or fancied, in the early literature of most civilizations, and, although few of these relate to animals, some account of their use is appropriate here. For more details of these, and for the fascinating and complete story relating to the development of human anesthesia, the reader is referred to the semipopular works of Robinson[43] and Fullöp-Miller[21] and the excellent history by Keys.[30] Much of the undocumented material presented here is contained in these works.

The first crude applications of anesthetic principles are undoubtedly not recorded. The thousands of prehistoric human skulls showing evidence of precise trephining offer silent testimony to the probability that some form of sense dulling may have been employed. At least it seems unlikely that men would have held still for such intervention. Perhaps it was only a club over the head or, as a refinement, a blow to the jaw or solar plexus. The ancient Greeks knew that carotid pressure would induce unconsciousness, and Aristotle, in his *History of Animals*, says that if the jugular veins are compressed men become insensible and fall to the ground. Trephined animal skulls have been found, but it seems improbable that the ills of animals were ministered to at so early a time; a more likely suggestion is that the purpose was to increase the supply of trephine buttons, in demand as amulets.

Practically all civilizations have known the secret of fermentation, and alcohol has long been recognized as the poor man's anesthetic, at least for the stresses and pain of everyday living. Strangely enough, however, early medical men have rather consistently eschewed its use (for analgesia)—unless this was considered too commonplace to be recorded—and surgeons relied primarily on speedy technique and heavy handed assistants. This concept lingered in veterinary medicine for longer than was warranted after effective anesthetics were readily available.

Although many of the early references to sleep-producing agents are mythological, their prescience suggests more than wishful thinking, and much of our current terminology relevant to anesthesia stems from these tales. Thus, Hypnos, the god of sleep, was the twin brother of Thanatos (whence euthanasia), the god of death, and the father of Morpheus, god of dreams. Lethe was a stream of forgetfulness in the land of Oblivion. More pertinent are the numerous allusions to narcosis by classical writers of ancient times. In the *Odyssey*, Homer states that Helen "cast into the wine a drug to quiet all pain," and in the *Illiad* he speaks of "a bitter root that slayeth pain." Ovid says, "There are drugs which induce deep slumber," and he describes the specific nature of opium. In Virgil's *Aeneid* there is perhaps the first reference to "veterinary" anesthesia when Cerberus, the three-headed dog that guarded the entrance to Hades, is given a drugged meal, "then relaxes and sinks to earth, [and] succumbs to sleep." Aristotle relates that goats on Crete, "when wounded by arrows, are said to go in search of dittany," also used to allay the pain of similar wounds in man. Plato is the first writer to use the term anesthesia, although not with specific reference to its induction; the latter honor usually goes to Oliver Wendell Holmes, although the term was used during the 18th century to denote loss of sensation, as by freezing.

Various specific drugs known today to have narcotic properties were mentioned by early medical writers, but their very number suggests that none was found entirely adequate for the purpose. Hemlock, of Socratic fame, was said by the natural historian Pliny to "have a soothing effect on every variety of pain." The Greek physician and herbalist Dioscorides wrote of opium as "a pain-easer and a sleep-producer," and of decoctions of henbane seed "prepared for lotions to take away pain."

The Roman physician Celsus mentions the poppy, lettuce, mandrake, and hyoscyamus, among other agents, for producing sleep.

Medieval and Renaissance Developments

In the fourth century, St. Hilary distinguished between anesthesia due to disease, as in a withered limb, and that produced by drugs, as "when through some grave necessity part of the body must be cut away, the soul can be lulled to sleep by drugs." Then, and for long afterward, principal reliance was placed upon mandrake (mandragora), but its doubtful efficacy is suggested by its more popular use as an aphrodisiac. The favorite anesthetic of the Middle Ages was the "sleeping sponge," produced by soaking a sponge in extracts of opium, hemlock, hyoscyamus, lettuce, etc. and holding it over the patient's nostrils. Although the presumed potency of this sponge was such that surgeons gave directions how to awaken deeply slumbering patients: "Know that it is well to tweak the nose, to pinch the cheeks or to pluck the beard of such a sleeper," it is perhaps significant that they also employed adequate physical restraint for major surgery. It was not until the purified alkaloids contained in these substances were available that true anesthesia could be produced by them.

The Renaissance promised much but delivered little in the field of anesthesia. Shakespeare, being a major writer on the subject, refers to the poppy, mandragora, and drowsy syrups; in *Romeo and Juliet* the friar assures Juliet that she can, by taking "this distilling liquor . . . appear like death . . . two and forty hours, and then awake as from a pleasant sleep." Medical men, however, became suspicious of drugs in general, and the famous surgeon Pare adopted from the ancient Greeks the method of carotid pressure for producing anesthesia. The unfulfilled promise of the times was ether, discovered in the 16th century, but it was unused as anesthetic for another three centuries. This, despite the fact that the renowned Paracelsus reported: "It has associated with it such a sweetness that it is taken even by chickens, and they fall asleep from it for a while but awaken later without harm . . . . In diseases which need to be treated with anodynes it quiets all suffering without any harm, and relieves all pain." [42] It is useless to speculate on "what might have been," of course, for Paracelsus was neither the first nor last medical genius to suffer such ignominy.

So thoroughly had narcotic drugs been discredited by the mid-17th century that a barber surgeon was fined as a practitioner of witchcraft for administering such a potion. Although refrigeration anesthesia was described at this time, Severino of Naples having advocated that surgeons "apply snow to dull the sensation," it was not until World War II that the technique was exploited.

Similarly, the potential of rectal anesthesia remained dormant long after its discovery in 1847. As reported in the Medical Gazette for that year: "M. Pirogoff [of Russia] has been trying some experiments on the effects produced by the injection of ether vapour into the rectum. Having cleared out the rectum by an enema, M. Pirogoff introduces the ether by means of a catheter attached to a syringe . . . . It was found that in from two to four minutes the odour of the vapour was perceptible in the breath; and the usual effect is produced in from three to five minutes . . . . No injurious symptoms have followed its use in this way, and the most troublesome operations have been performed with great facility." [38]

In reporting this development, however, Braithwaite states: "Professor Pirogoff's employment of ether-vapour enemata was anticipated in India, by Mr. Crawford, who narcotized a dog by ether contained in a bladder with an ivory glyster-pipe." [7] This occurred in March 1847, a month prior to Pirogoff's announcement, and Crawford's superior, writing in the *Madras Spectator*, describes its use "by way of experiment, on three dogs, with the effect of producing symptoms of drunkenness, attended by vomiting and apparent diminution of sensibility in each case." He tried it on a man on April 1, but the patient objected to the discomfort, its principal effect apparently being to cause the expulsion of numerous ascarids.[32]

Rectal anesthesia was reintroduced in France in 1884, but was abandoned promptly because of unfavorable experiences, and was revived in 1903. With the employment of an ether-oil mixture and quinine, the technique was highly popular during the 1920's in obstetrics. Tribromethanol was introduced as a rectal anesthetic in 1927, and during the 1930's was widely used in Britain for cats before the barbiturates were discovered.

Intravenous Anesthesia

In 1665, the British architect and inveterate experimenter Christopher Wren, together with Robert Boyle, induced narcosis in a dog by injecting opium intravenously. The dog was stupefied and, although a crude extract of opium was used, the animal survived. Wren proposed to ligate the femoral veins,

and then opening them on the side of the Ligature towards the Heart, and by putting into them slender Syringes or Quills, fastened to Bladders (in the manner of Clysterpipes) containing the matter to be injected; performing that Operation upon pretty big and lean doggs, that the Vessels might be large enough and easily accessible.

This proposition being made, M. *Boyle* soon gave order for an *Apparatus*, to put it to Experiment; wherein at several times, upon several Doggs, *Opium* & the Infusion of *Crocus Metallorum* were injected into that part of the hindlegs of those Animals, whence the larger Vessels, that carry the Blood, are most easy to be taken hold of: whereof the success was, that the *Opium*, being soon circulated into the Brain, did within a short time stupify, though not kill the Dog; but a large Dose of the *Crocus Metallorum*, made another Dog vomit up Life and all.[6]

In 1665, in what was perhaps the first deliberate attempt at intravenous anesthesia, the physician Elsholz used a solution of opium to produce unconsciousness in a patient. About the same time, however, success in transfusing blood from one animal to another led to excesses in medical practice—including the transfusion of animal blood to man—and the practice fell into disfavor because of the numerous unfortunate accidents. One result of this, apparently, was that further experimentation with intravenous anesthesia was halted for another two centuries.

After experimenting with animals, Pierre-Cyprien Oré used chloral hydrate intravenously to produce anesthesia in human subjects in 1872. But the aftereffects of chloral were too slow in dissipating and its margin of safety too narrow for clinical use. By 1875, chloral was being used as a narcotic and anesthetic in the horse, in doses of 30 to 70 g, by mouth or rectum or, occasionally, by intraperitoneal injection. In 1908, its use intravenously in horses was reported by a Belgian, who found that a 20% solution, at a rate of 10 g/kg of body weight, produced complete general anesthesia in 1 to 2 minutes, "but it has been followed by several accidents which put its value in doubt."[57]

The next drug to receive serious consideration was barbital, synthesized in 1902, but it proved useful only as a sedative. Thirty years later, sodium hexobarbital was the first drug of the barbiturate series for which good qualities as an intravenous anesthetic were demonstrated, and within a decade it had been used in some 4,000,000 anesthesias in Germany alone. In 1934, 2 years after sodium hexobarbital was introduced in Europe, sodium thiopental was discovered in the United States. It was first used orally or by intraperitoneal injection but rapidly became the drug of choice for intravenous use.

Administration of a barbiturate to dogs by intravenous injection was first employed by Auchterlonie in England, using sodium hexobarbital for anesthesia. The excitability characteristic of the recovery period, however, caused this agent to be discarded in favor of pentobarbital and thiopental, the early research on which was done at the Royal Veterinary College, and which, Wright notes, "marked a distinct advance in veterinary anesthesiology." [57]

Nitrous Oxide

Nitrous oxide was discovered by Joseph Priestly in 1776 and, curiously, was almost immediately seized upon by the American arbiter of science, Samuel Mitchill, as the principle of contagion. Dire results would occur if the gas were inhaled by animals or respired by plants in the minutest quantities and, Mitchill claimed, this was the direct cause of cancer, scurvy, and leprosy. This warning notwithstanding, the brash young Britisher, Humphry Davy—he was then barely 17—inhaled nitrous oxide and found it produced euphoria and mirth. Later he found that by inhaling the gas he could relieve the pains of toothache and, on two occasions, nearly died from overdoses.

Undaunted, Davy experimented on a cat, and his report in 1779 is probably the first detailed description of the effects of any anesthetic. He says:

A stout and healthy young cat, of four or five months old, was introduced into a large jar of nitrous oxide. For ten or twelve moments he remained perfectly quiet, and then began to make violent motions, throwing himself round the jar in every direction. In two minutes he appeared quite exhausted, and sunk quietly to the bottom of the jar. On applying my hand to the thorax, I found that the heart beat with extreme violence; on feeling about the neck, I could distinctly perceive a strong and quick pulsation of the carotids. In about three minutes the animal revived, and panted very much; but still continued to lie on his side. [15]

Davy then experimented with kittens, dogs, rabbits, and other animals, some of which died and were examined by him in an effort to determine the cause of death. Apparently satisfied with the safety of nitrous oxide, he tried it on several persons and concluded: "As nitrous oxide in its extensive operation appears capable of destroying physical pain, it may probably be used with advantage during surgical operations in which no great effusion of blood takes place." Here, certainly, was a clear identification of nitrous oxide as an anesthetic agent, documented by adequate animal experimentation. However, for various reasons, medical men ignored Davy's discovery, and surgeons continued their savage ways for another half-century.

Surgeons can be excused for not ferreting out the obscure observations of Paracelsus relative to the potential of ether as an anesthetic. Ether was being used as a remedy for various ills, and it is somewhat surprising that its anesthetic property was not discovered by pure chance. However, surgeons themselves did little experimenting, and there was a wide chasm between them and the more theoretical physicians. The medical fraternity as a whole can be censured for ignoring not only Davy's adequately reported observations on nitrous oxide but his vigrous attempts to bring his discovery to their attention by more direct means. Although surgery continued to be unnecessarily cruel, surgeons were not heartless, despite their unwillingness to utilize this potential boon to mankind. One surgeon wrote: "Before the days of anesthetics [but after Davy's discovery] a patient preparing for an operation was like a condemned criminal preparing for execution. He counted the days till the appointed day came . . . . And then he surrendered his liberty and, revolting at the necessity, submitted to be held or bound, and helplessly gave himself up to the cruel knife." [1] Earlier the famous surgeon John Hunter had said that a surgeon was "a savage armed with a knife."

Paradoxically, it was the mirth-provoking qualities of nitrous oxide that were seized upon—and these to charm the gullible at traveling side shows. It was at one such demonstration in the early 1840's that the Connecticut dentist Horace Wells conceived the idea that nitrous oxide might be used for painless extraction of teeth. He demonstrated this in 1844, but kept it secret and later became embroiled in a bitter controversy with the proponents of ether—with regard to priority of discovery—and committed suicide at the age of 31, before the potential of nitrous oxide had been adequately explored.

With ether gaining the ascendency as a surgical anesthetic, nitrous oxide was virtually forgotten until the late 1860's when another Connecticut dentist, J. H. Smith, saw the light. Interestingly enough, Smith attended a show put on by the same entrepreneur, Gardner Colton, who, two decades earlier, had given Wells his inspiration. Smith took Colton as a senior partner and in 23 days the two were reputed to have extracted nearly 4000 teeth under nitrous oxide anesthesia.

The first surgical operation under nitrous oxide anesthesia occurred in 1868, but its transient effect remained a disadvantage until it was discovered that prolonged narcosis without fear of asphyxia could be achieved by using a nitrous oxide-oxygen mixture. For a time during the 1880's, this anesthetic almost replaced ether and chloroform in obstetrical practice. About the time of World War I, the death rate from nitrous oxide anesthesia was calculated at 1/1,000,000—far safer than ether and, especially, chloroform—but its unpredictability for surgical depths of anesthesia caused it to be relegated almost entirely to the dental profession.

Carbon Dioxide

Following Davy's demonstration of nitrous oxide anesthesia, the British physician and surgeon, Henry Hickman, conducted a series of successful animal experiments with it. Like Davy, he made a strenuous but unsuccessful effort to interest the medical profession of England and France. In retrospect, it is evident that medicine was not ready for so epochal an advance, and perhaps its failure to recognize an apparent fact is more a matter for regret than reproach.

Hickman is noted for his experiments with carbon dioxide, which antedated his use of nitrous oxide. In 1824, he wrote:

I took a puppy a month old and placed it on a piece of wood, surrounded by water, over which I put a glass cover so as to prevent the access of atmospheric air; in ten minutes he showed great marks of uneasiness, in twelve minutes respiration became difficult, and in seventeen minutes ceased altogether; at eighteen minutes I took off one of the ears, which was not followed by hemorrhage; respiration soon returned and the animal did not appear to be the least sensible of pain; in three days the ear was perfectly healed.... Later I took a fully grown dog and plunged him into an atmosphere of the same gas. Within twelve minutes he was completely insensible. He remained so for seventeen minutes. Meanwhile I amputated a leg without his giving any sign of pain.[25]

Hickman apparently realized that the anesthesia produced was the result of asphyxia, and he turned to using nitrous oxide. Confident that this latter method was both safe and effective, he wrote to a friend: "Having made experiments on various animals, I feel perfectly satisfied that any surgical operation might be performed with quite as much safety in an insensible state.... I certainly should not hesitate a moment to become the subject of such an experiment." He petitioned the Royal Society of London and the Paris Academy for a hearing but was refused the opportunity to demonstrate his technique. Disappointed, he continued his work until he died prematurely a few years later, at the age of 29.

Ether

Until its anesthetic property was discovered, ether was used locally as an anodyne for toothache and internally as a remedy for headache, whooping cough, hysteria, and other conditions, perhaps because it was aromatic. In veterinary medicine its use was more limited. Boardman's *Dictionary of the Veterinary Art* (1805) states: "How far this active remedy is suitable for veterinary purposes is left to the inquisitive practitioner to ascertain."[4] In his *Outlines of the Veterinary Art* (1817), Blaine says, "The volatility as well as the value of sulfuric ether will prevent its coming into general use."[3] Later it was used as a stimulant and more or less as a specific in spasmodic colic. Although as early as 1813 Orfila observed that an oral dose of half an ounce of ether would render a dog insensible, there is no evidence that any attempt was made to exploit the anesthetic potential of ether until the late 1840's.

Benjamin Brodie did demonstrate the anesthetic properties of ether in 1821, a fact which seems to have escaped historiographers, but he failed to realize the importance of his discovery and did not report it until 1851. According to a recent biographer:

A guinea pig under a bell jar was made to inhale ether vapour blown over by heating sulphuretted ether over a flame. The animal first appeared intoxicated, then became insensible, and in eight minutes respirations had ceased. The heart continued beating, and on removal from the jar, after the application of artificial respiration through a tracheotomy, he recovered in a few moments. Thus did Brodie demonstrate the anesthetic effect of ether, and the fact that it is reversible. The date on the lecture note is 5 February 1821—that is, 25 years before ether was introduced as an anesthetic agent. What a pity Brodie did not follow up this line![16]

Laughing gas parties were popular in the United States during the 1830's and by about 1840 "ether frolics" became a similar attraction. Noting that persons often hurt themselves without knowing it while under the influence of ether, Crawford Long, a young Georgia physician, administered ether as an anesthetic in removing a tumor from the neck of a friend in 1842. His succinct ledger entry, "James Venable, 1842. Ether and excising tumor, $2.00," later became the basis for acknowledging Long as the first man to use an anesthetic for a surgical operation. Long himself wrote: "I was anxious, before my publication, to try etherization in a sufficient number of cases to fully satisfy my mind that anesthesia was produced by the ether, and was not the effect of the imagination .... I determined to wait to see whether any surgeon would present a claim to having used ether by inhalation in surgical operations prior to the time it was used by me."[36]

Long performed seven more minor operations using ether, satisfying himself that ether was a true anesthetic. But a suspicious backwoods populace forced him to give up the practice, and others claimed the honor of discovery. Had he published his observations promptly, Long might have been accorded the credit due him and averted the acid controversy that developed. Although now recognized as the first to use anesthesia, Long had no influence on its momentous development a few years later, and he remained largely out of the acrimonious debate. After losing his personal fortune during the Civil War, he died as he lived—while administering ether to a woman in childbirth in 1878.

The events surrounding the demonstration of ether as a general anesthetic by Thomas Morton at the Massachusetts General Hospital in 1846 were for many years shrouded in confusion, doubt, and deceit, and many books have been written on the subject. As noted heretofore, Wells had extracted teeth using nitrous oxide as an anesthetic in 1844. Shortly afterward, he had an opportunity to demonstrate his discovery at Harvard Medical School but, apparently as a practical joke, his student subject howled as if in pain, and Wells was laughed out of the arena. When Morton's demonstration was made public, Wells belatedly published his claims to priority, and in 1848 he succeeded in having several major operations performed by the eminent surgeon Henry Bigelow, using nitrous oxide anesthesia. However, the state of near asphyxia produced by the pure gas convinced Bigelow and, through him, others, that ether was the superior anesthetic. Conspicuously unsuccessful in contesting Morton's all-encompassing claim, Wells committed suicide just before losing consciousness while inhaling chloroform.

Although it is incontestable that Morton was the first to demonstrate ether anesthesia publicly, his seemingly singular role in the remarkable event at Massachusetts General in 1846 is open to amplification. Morton, a shrewd Boston dentist, had been a partner of Wells and had observed his erstwhile partner's success with nitrous oxide. Morton consulted with the chemist, Charles Jackson, concerning a substitute for nitrous oxide, and Jackson suggested ether. On September 30, 1846, Morton extracted a tooth from a patient, using ether, and the following day an account of the event appeared in the newspaper. The same day, Morton applied for a patent on his discovery. He then proceeded to arrange with John C. Warren, the surgeon before whose class Wells had failed, to demonstrate the use of ether as a surgical anesthetic, with only the assurance gained from a few tooth extractions that it would work. It was still less than 2 weeks after Morton's first experience with ether and, having been refused by several other surgeons who were unwilling to risk their reputations, it is evident that Morton had far less to lose than Warren if something went wrong. As senior surgeon at the Massachusetts General, however, Warren had seen, and caused, his share of suffering, and he apparently accepted Morton's proposal with alacrity, even though Morton refused to divulge the nature of his preparation. The inhaler to be used had not been constructed, and delay in its completion almost caused Warren to proceed without Morton on that fateful day October 16, 1846.

That the ether anesthesia was a success was announced in Warren's now famous phrase: "Gentlemen, this is no humbug." He later wrote:

A new era has opened on the operating surgeon. His visitations on the most delicate parts are performed, not only without the agonizing screams he has been accustomed to hear, but sometimes in a state of perfect insensibility and, occasionally, even with an expression of pleasure on the part of the patient .... As philanthropists we may well rejoice that we have had an agency, however slight, in conferring on poor suffering humanity so precious a gift.[53]

Morton, however, became embroiled in a bitter controversy with Jackson and spent most of his remaining years trying to establish a clear claim to the discovery of anesthesia. Apparently deranged by his obsession, he died shortly after plunging into a lake while in a frenzy.

Except for his suggestion to Morton concerning the use of ether, Jackson was finally discredited as an outright pretender and he died in an insane asylum. His first act after Morton's demonstration was to consider demanding $500 in return for renouncing his claim, but his friends persuaded him that he was due at least a 10% share in Morton's patent. He then presented his claim to Dr. Warren, who called his bluff by offering him the opportunity to demonstrate his prowess—apparently being sure that Jackson would refuse, as he did. A cunning man, however, he came close to achieving his objective—that of discrediting Morton—and he drove his adversary to an untimely death.

One of Jackson's strategems was to publish accounts purporting to prove that his professed work with ether antedated even Long's now undisputed claim to priority. One such account, of particular interest because it describes his "experiments" with domestic animals, appears in the *Report of the Commissioner of Patents for the Year 1853*. Jackson claims:

In the winter of 1841–'42, I discovered that the nerves of sensation could be temporarily paralyzed to all sensation by the pulmonary inhalation of the vapor of pure sulphuric ether mixed with air, and that while the human body was thus affected, any surgical operation could be performed upon the etherized patient without producing any pain. In 1846, I caused this discovery to be practically exemplified, by applying it in surgical operations .... I also indicated its use in preventing all sensation of pain in domestic animals, upon which surgical operations were to be performed, either for the cure of diseases, or for rendering them more serviceable to man.

In many cases, fractured or dislocated limbs of valuable animals could be cured if they were rendered manageable during the operation, so that the proper adjustments could be made, and the dressings applied. This may readily be accomplished by rendering the animal insensible to pain, and unconscious by the administration of ether vapor. Severe surgical operations—such as the division of nerves, the application of the actual cautery, the removal of tumors, and the castration of domestic animals—may also be rendered entirely painless by this method.[27]

Jackson states that he has never known of a fatal accident from the use of ether, but that, in domestic animals in particular, a mixture of 4 or 5 parts of ether and 1 of chloroform produces the best results. This, incidentally, is one of the earliest recommendations for this mixture, but it seems likely that Jackson's information was lifted from the writings of the veterinary practitioner George Dadd. Jackson's account is at least correct in most of its details and is quoted at length as one of the earliest publications in the area of veterinary anesthesia.

So anxious was Charles Jackson to claim the discovery of anesthesia that he did not hesitate to issue spurious reports concerning work he could not possibly have done himself. One such account appearing in the *Report of the Commissioner of Patents for the Year 1853* is an obvious attempt to get official recognition, and the appearance of the same fraudulent claims in the *Country Gentleman* for 1855 might be construed as an effort to gain popular support for his contentions. Although only the unwary would be deceived at this date, at the time he evidently made a good case for himself. Moreover, his is probably the best account of veterinary anesthesia in America to that time and thus is worth quoting at length. He states:

In the more usual surgical operations on animals, particularly in that of castration of the bull, stallion, hog and ram, we should always apply the ether vapor by the lungs. There is no danger in administering the ether to any animal that has sensible perspiration; but to those which do not sweat, we must apply it more cautiously; thus the ram and bull will bear a very high dose without the least danger to life, while the *cat* is readily killed by a full dose of chloroform. I have not seen death produced by the use of pure ether vapor mixed with air, in any case, nor in any animal, and yet I can conceive how an animal having no free perspiration should retain for a longer time the absorbed vapor of that liquid, as well as of chloroform. Dogs have a perspiration mainly from the tongue, and hence they do not get rid of the absorbed vapor so readily as those animals having a free cutaneous perspiration, and are therefore more likely to suffer ill effects from retained chloroform. All animals excrete the absorbed vapor by the skin, lungs, and kidneys, in their perspiration, breath, and urine; and thus, after the effects of the anaesthetic agent is over, the system clears itself very soon of all traces of it by the above named channels.

In administering ether and chloroform to animals, I make use of a wire muzzle, or basket, which is fastened round the nose and mouth, and fixed in its place by proper straps. On the horse or ox, a head-stall is all that is required to fix the wire basket in its proper position. Into this basket I first put a very coarse open-textured sponge, which has been soaked in water so as to soften and swell it, and then it is squeezed dry. The basket and sponge being put in the proper position, I take this mixture—pure sulphuric ether, one pint; pure chloroform, one gill—and mix them in a bottle; then I pour upon the sponge, from time to time as needed, this fluid, an ounce at a time; renewing it as it evaporates. The animal breaths it freely into the lungs, and soon gently falls down in a deep sleep of insensibility and unconsciousness, and is entirely passive, so that any operation may be performed, and without any struggle of the animal, or any signs of pain. A very refractory horse may, by this means, be made to submit to the farrier in being shod, and will soon learn to submit afterwards, and probably without the repetition of the ether.

The apparatus for etherizing a bull, will, of course, be fitted to the form of his nose, and should be in other respects like that for the horse. He will bear the ether perfectly well in full doses.

The hog I have not seen under etherization, but I doubt not he will readily come under its influence; but I do not think he will bear so well a high dose as a horse or an ox.

Sheep bear it perfectly well; at least they do the breathing of pure ether. I do not know how chloroform may affect them, and should be a little more careful in the administration of that agent. It is probable, however, that the admixture of chloroform with ether will prove safe and efficient. Sheep have been operated upon under ether in England successfully, since the publication of my discovery.

It must be kept in view, that air must be freely admitted in administering all anaesthetical agents; then there is little if any danger to be feared.[27]

Chloroform

In 1831, chloroform was isolated by three investigators working independently in three countries: Liebig in Germany, Soubeiran in France, and Guthrie in America. Guthrie, whose original communication apparently antedated by a few months those of his co-discoverers, found this new compound to be an agreeable drink when mixed with equal parts of water and states that "a great number of persons had drunk of the solution . . . not only very freely but frequently to the point of intoxication . . . leaving, after its operation, little of that depression consequent to the use of ardent spirits." [23] Unless his *post hoc* testimony can be taken at face value, however, it appears that Guthrie failed to realize the potential of his pleasant decoction. Years later, his granddaughter wrote that her mother used to play around the tubs he used in manufacturing chloroform and to taste the product, and "one day she got too much and fell over and he ran to her and picked her up and then found that the liquid in this tub put her to sleep, hence his accidental discovery what chloroform would do." Guthrie himself recalled the event in 1848, after Simpson in Britain had popularized chloroform as an anesthetic.

The anesthetic property of chloroform was discovered in 1847 by the Scottish surgeon James Simpson, who was dissatisfied with ether, especially in obstetric cases. First used in November 1847, in January 1848 the first chloroform fatality was recorded—that of a 15-year-old girl being treated for an ingrown toenail.

Largely through Simpson's advocacy, however, chloroform practically supplanted ether both in Britain and the United States. Simpson himself went so far as to ignore ether altogether and to consider himself the discoverer of anesthesia. Other surgeons were less enthusiastic, however, one stating in 1848 his preference for using ice in local anesthesia whenever possible, despite the common opinion that "a fatal result now and then from the use of chloroform may not be thought a sufficient objection to its use."

Veterinary Experiments

There was no veterinary periodical literature in America at the time, so there is little indication as to just how soon veterinarians around Boston utilized general anesthesia after its demonstration in 1846. As indicated by reports in the *Veterinarian* (London), however, it is evident that British veterinary surgeons were quick to seize upon this discovery. The first report was by the eminent practitioner Edward Mayhew, in January 1847, in which he detailed his experiments on dogs and cats. He placed ether in a flask, to the neck of which a large bladder was attached, and the animal's head was place in the bladder. Breathing pure ether in this manner, cats were completely anesthetized in as little as 10 seconds, and dogs required 13 to 45 seconds to lose consciousness.

Mayhew was able to perform minor operations without evidence of pain, but the excitatory stage of the anesthetic left him disturbed and doubtful over the propriety of using ether. He says:

The results of these trials are not calculated to inspire any very sanguine hopes. We cannot tell whether the crie emitted are evidence of pain or not; but they are suggestive of agony to the listener, and, without testimony to the contrary, must be regarded as indicative of suffering. The process, therefore, is not calculated to attain the object for which in veterinary practice it would be most generally employed, namely, to relieve the owner from the impression that his animal was subjected to torture .... There has been yet no experiment that I know of made to ascertain the action of the vapour on the horse; but I cannot anticipate that it will be found of much service to that animal.[49]

Enough of a humanitarian himself to conduct these early experiments, Mayhew realistically concedes that owners witnessing etherization of their animals would not believe what he had demonstrated—although perhaps not wholly to his own satisfaction—that surgical intervention itself did not elicit pain while the animal was anesthetized. It is perhaps unfortunate that he conveyed the idea that the principal use of anesthesia in veterinary

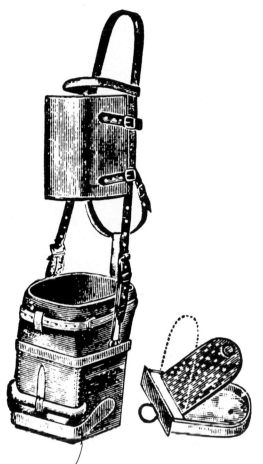

Carlisle's Chloroform Inhaler.

FIG. 1.2. This British inhaler, with a separate container for chloroform, was an improvement over earlier models without blinders and only a solid leather boot with a sponge in the bottom. These types were superseded by others having a canvas bag. (From Liautard, A.: *Manual of Operative Veterinary Surgery.* Sabiston & Murray, New York, 1892.)

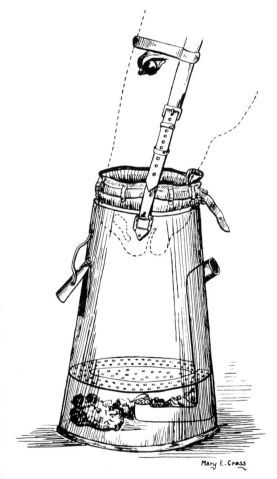

Mary E. Cross

FIG. 1.1. An early British design (*ca.* 1860) for an equine "anesthetic machine." Drawn from contemporary descriptions.

practice would be to relieve the owner's pain.

Ether was used in 1847 in the amputation of a cow's leg at the hock, 4 oz of ether and 17 minutes being required to produce unconsciousness. The animal evidenced no pain and it recovered. Later experiments at the London Veterinary College, in which pure ether rendered horses unconscious in less than 2 minutes, proved the necessity of using an admixture of air and ether, and efficient inhalers were developed as early as 1848. Ether accidents, apparently from use of the pure gas, occurred earlier in veterinary practice than are recorded in human surgery. These led William Percivall, editor of the *Veterinarian*, to urge practitioners "to lose no time in bestirring themselves to ascertain what may or may not be done, so far as their patients are concerned, by the ethereal stifler of pain and sensibility .... It is now notorious enough that both men and horses have succumbed, under the influence of ether, to rise no more, and, as post-mortem examinations of their bodies has shewn, *in consequence* of such influence." [50]

Due in part, perhaps, to the interest already engendered by ether, and partly to the proximity of the discovery of chloroform anesthesia, British veterinarians recorded the results of experiments with this new agent only 2 months after it had been demonstrated by Simpson. As reported in the *Veterinarian* for January 1848, 2 oz of chloroform on a sponge produced complete anesthesia in a horse in 5 minutes and "the usually painful operation of cutting the nerves of sensation in both its front feet [was performed] without a quiver. In twenty-five minutes from the commencement the animal was again on its legs, now perfectly sound." However, another practitioner who had experimented in 1848 with chloroform for neurotomy concluded: "It is, in my opinion, very doubtful whether chloroform will ever become an efficient agent in veterinary practice on the horse, as I believe these two bad-conditioned animals suffered more in being reduced to a state of insensibility, and in recovering from the state, than they did from the operation performed." [51]

In a similar vein, editor Percivall suggests that experiments on dogs and cats "in the days when ether had so great a name as an anaesthetic," did not hold much promise of utility in practice. "Time," he says, "has pretty well verified this prediction in the case of ether; nor, as yet, in the case of chloroform ... has

much better success followed .... There exists the greatest danger of the horse in his delerious moments, throwing himself headlong upon the ground, and doing himself irreparable injury .... The eminent William Field, from a conviction of the risk ... very properly refuses, on his own responsibility, at least, to subject any horse on whom he may have to operate to the influence of chloroform." [51]

Together with an awareness of numerous unfortunate anesthetic accidents, such editorial urging undoubtedly led British veterinarians to become disenchanted with the prospects of anesthesia about as quickly as they had adopted this new technique. The *Veterinarian* for 1847 carried 17 articles on the use of ether and three on chloroform; in 1848 there were three articles on ether and 13 on chloroform; in 1849 but one article on ether and two on chloroform appeared, all three being on the use of these agents in tetanus rather than surgical anesthesia. Other early uses for ether and chloroform were for gastric and intestinal inflammation, spasm, congestion of the lungs and brain, and spasmodic colic. As early as 1818 the American veterinarian James Carver, a graduate of the London school, used a drench of opium, ether, ginger, and camphor for equine tetanus, but he states that ether was too expensive to be used much in veterinary practice.[8]

Local and Regional Anesthesia

Although ice was used as a form of regional anesthesia for limb amputations and for excising pedunculated tumors in the 1850's, true local anesthesia had its inception with the ether spray discovered by Benjamin Richardson in 1867. This method remained in general use for two decades or longer. In 1884 Carl Koller discovered the properties of cocaine in his search for an anesthetic suitable in ophthalmological operations. After experimenting on various animals, including dogs, he demonstrated its action upon himself, thereby revolutionizing ophthalmic practice. Within a year, the brilliant American surgeon William Halstead found that, by injecting cocaine around the nerves, almost any part of the body could be selectively anesthetized, and he reported having used such regional anesthesia in more than 1000 operations. By this time, however, he had, through experiments upon himself, become an addict and was forced to go into seclusion for a time; his work went largely unnoticed until revived in 1900 by Rudolf Matas, also a pioneer in spinal anesthesia. The full development of local anesthesia awaited the discovery of procaine (Novocaine) in 1904 and its clinical application by Braun in 1905. The later use of an oil adjuvant to prolong its action greatly extended the value of procaine, a development which more than compensated for the fact that, unlike cocaine, it had little value for topical application.

In veterinary use, Alexandre Liautard, in 1892, noted that Bouley in France had "long ago" recommended local anesthesia for diagnosis of obscure lameness in horses, and that the method had been introduced recently by several American veterinarians. Methods included ether vaporization, although Liautard preferred subcutaneous injection of ether or chloroform and, as a superior technique, injection of cocaine.[34]

August Bier is generally credited with being the first to employ spinal anesthesia using cocaine in 1898, although the American surgeon James Corning had injected a human spine (not for surgical anesthesia) in about 1885. Following its demonstration in Paris in 1899, spinal anesthesia was used enthusiastically by American surgeons until, in the same year, so many untoward reactions had occurred that the method fell into disfavor. This was due both to the use of cocaine and a technique involving meningeal puncture, nor did the substitution of procaine in 1905 greatly alter the number of accidents. It remained for the veterinarians Retzgen of Berlin in 1925 and Franz Benesch of Austria in 1926 to demonstrate in horses and cattle, respectively, that epidural anesthesia, with the needle introduced distal to the spinal cord proper, was

a safe technique. Since then, spinal and epidural anesthesia have been widely used in both human and veterinary surgery. Later developments in regional anesthesia include the paravertebral nerve block,[19] introduced by James Farquharson in 1940, and the pudendal block[33] (introduced by Larson in 1953), among others, as refinements of simpler techniques used on the limbs since the 1880's.

Morphine

The sense-dulling and temporarily gratifying properties of opium and its related compounds were well known to the ancients. Physicians prescribed it to be taken in food or drink, inhaled as snuff, smoked, or used locally, to produce a soporific state, and during the 17th and 18th centuries some noted medical men, among them Boerhaave of Leyden and Sassard of Paris, administered it as a surgical anesthetic. Others observed the untoward effects of its administration and used it only on persons already addicted, while many more surgeons eschewed its use altogether. Following isolation of morphine in 1806, the pure drug was applied by scarification with a lancet point for various painful conditions.

In Germany, Setürner crystallized morphine from opium and, after proving its efficacy as a pain killer in dogs, demonstrated its effect on man, with himself as the prime subject. Honored in 1831 for his discovery, but later castigated as a scoundrel when the undesirable sequelae of morphine in excess became known, he bent his energies to more potent ways for destroying mankind—guns and gunpowder. Although again honored by his government for his work in this latter field, he became a recluse and died a morphine addict only 10 years after the French had bestowed upon him the title of "benefactor of mankind." Many later investigators were to become addicts, and it is something of a paradox that so many of the men honored as pioneers in anesthesiology should have come to premature and unseemly ends.

Although opium had long been used in

veterinary as in human medicine, there is little evidence that morphine was used to any great extent until after development of the hypodermic syringe by Rynd in 1845 and its refinement in 1851 by the French veterinarian Tabourin and the more prominent physician Pravaz, whose name is still generally applied to the syringe in Europe.

Muscle Relaxants

Although not anesthetics, the use, and sometimes misuse, of muscle relaxants as an adjunct to or substitute for anesthesia makes it pertinent to include them here. Long known to the South American Indians as the prey-immobilizing arrow poison, woorara or woorali, the drug fascinated early naturalists, some of whom learned of its properties first hand. The active principle of arrow poison, curare, was first used (unsuccessfully) to treat tetanus in man in 1858, after which it was employed with indifferent results until the early 1880's and then virtually dropped for nearly 50 years. The physician McIntyre states that the early reports of its use "may be summarized very readily; they do not, either singly or collectively, present proof of the drug's value in this disease." [37]

As a result of the finding in 1944 that prolonged complete curarization in dogs resulted in death even though respiration was artificially maintained, McIntyre recommended that curare be used only to control spasm, although "heroic doses and artificial respiration should be used in those desperate cases that are otherwise almost certain to die."

Less well known than the early medical use of curare is the fact that it was first used, some two decades earlier, to treat tetanus in the horse. In 1835, William Sewell, professor at the London Veterinary College, treated two cases of equine tetanus but his findings were not reported in the veterinary press until 1858, after its demonstration in man. An account of Sewell's first case appears in Watson's *Principles and Practice of Physic* (1845), an extensive series of lectures by the physician Thomas Watson, who states:

A horse, suffering from a severe attack of tetanus and locked-jaw, the mouth being too firmly closed to admit the introduction of either food or medicine, was inoculated on the fleshy part of the shoulder with an arrow point coated with wourali poison [curare]. In ten minutes apparent death was produced. Artificial respiration was immediately commenced, and kept up about four hours, when reanimation took place. The animal rose up, apparently perfectly recovered, and eagerly partook of corn and hay. He was unluckily too abundantly supplied with food during the night. The consequence was over-distension of the stomach, of which the animal died the following day, without, however, having the slightest recurrence of tetanic symptoms. [55]

As reported in the *Veterinarian* for 1858, Sewell's second case was that of an ass "labouring under an attack of the severest form of tetanus." The report continues: "The animal was in a very emaciated state ... and being unable to walk, he was conveyed in a barrow. The Wourali was employed as in the former case, with the same effect, and artificial respiration produced reanimation in about the same time .... [There was not] a sufficient recovery of strength to enable the animal to rise; nevertheless the disease had entirely disappeared, and for twenty-seven hours he was enabled to take a little food; at the end of that time he died without having shown a single symptom of tetanus subsequent to the inoculation of the poison." [52]

Concerning Sewell's work, McIntyre states: "If the original observation of Sewell was correct, the curare used ... seems to have differed considerably from those employed later; for, though convulsions can be interrupted by the curares recently used, convulsions may return when the curare concentration falls, whereas in Sewell's experiences the convulsions did not return after the animal had been resuscitated." [37]

Although it was proposed in 1871 that curare be used as a remedy in hydrophobia, tetanus, and other nervous disorders, and as an antidote to strychnine poisoning, McIntyre states that it was first used for epilepsy in 1860, for chorea in 1878, and for strychnine poisoning in 1905, but that there is no evidence that the drug was ever actually used in rabies. Buried in the body of an extensive article by the veterinary surgeon William Youatt, however, the following appeared in the *Veterinarian* for 1838:

Mr. Morgan having kindly given me some of the Ticunas (arrow) poison, I inoculated a rabid dog with it, in order to see what effect one poison might have in weakening or destroying another. Although not ferocious, the animal had been in a considerable state of excitation. An incision through the integument was made on the inside of the arm, and a pointed bit of wood that had been dipped in the poison was rubbed on the exposed fasciae. No effect being produced, the same bit of wood was introduced into an incision more deeply made. In less than two minutes the dog was more tranquil, and at the expiration of five minutes he dropped motionless, the only indication of his life being a regular and not laborious breathing. In this state he continued eight hours, when I left him for the night. On the following morning I found him dead." [47]

In an article on rabies the following year, Youatt describes several experiments, conducted before a group of veterinarians and medical men, in which dogs and horses were given curare. One ass recovered from the drug after seven hours of artificial respiration, and: "The result of these experiments was extremely gratifying, and the gentlemen who conducted them resolved to avail themselves of the first opportunity to try them in tetanus or rabies." [48] There is no evidence that such attempts were made, however, and when veterinarians essayed using curare for equine tetanus during the late 19th century, they administered the drug orally, apparently unaware of the superior results claimed for parenteral administration, and its undependability caused it to lose favor.

With the advent of pure alkaloid curare, new interest in its potential was stimulated, but the treatment of tetanus remains in an unsatisfactory state. When safer muscle relaxants were introduced in recent times, interest in curare waned, but,

as occurs with so many new drugs, not all of these newer compounds appear to have delivered the promise that they seemed to offer. In particular, many equine practitioners have become disenchanted with the use of succinylcholine chloride. The development of the projectile syringe, however, has stimulated search for a truly safe muscle relaxant for use in capturing wild game.

Although surgeons long wished for a means of securing adequate muscle relaxation in surgical patients and curare was isolated in 1828, curarization as an adjunct to anesthesia was not employed until 1942 when Griffith and Johnson reported satisfactory results in 25 patients. Only light, instead of deep, cyclopropane anesthesia was required to produce proper relaxation when a suitable dose of curare was given.

The warning sounded by Claude Bernard was based on his experiments with curare, but anyone who uses muscle relaxants—especially if unwittingly as a substitute for proper anesthesia—would do well to read Bernard's description of the action of curare:

Within the motionless body behind the staring eye, with all the appearance of death—feeling and intelligence persist in all their force. Can we conceive of a suffering more horrible than that of intelligence present after the succumbing, one by one, of all the organs which are destined to find themselves imprisoned alive within a cadaver? In all times, poetic fiction endeavoring to move us to pity, drew before our eyes sensitive beings imprisoned in motionless bodies. The torture which the poet's imagination invented is produced by Nature by the action of the American poison. Only here we may say that reality surpasses fiction. [2]

Endotracheal Anesthesia

The first administration of anesthesia by way of the trachea appears to have been done by the master of early British anesthetists, John Snow (who died in 1858), who chloroformed a rabbit by opening the trachea and inserting a breathing tube. This technique, *i.e.*, *via* tracheotomy, was employed clinically in 1869 by the German surgeon Trendelenburg, who added the refinement of an inflatable cuff. In 1880, the Scottish surgeon William MacEwen devised a curved metal tube which he passed through the larynx. A semirigid tube which could be passed through the nose was invented in 1911 by Franz Kühn of Germany, who demonstrated the possibility of controlling lung inflation during open chest surgery, an idea refined and applied by the American surgeon Rudolph Matas.

The Magill tube was devised during World War I to facilitate facial surgery and, with introduction of the carbon dioxide absorption technique by Waters—who revived use of the inflatable cuff—endotracheal anesthesia became standard practice. Guedel and Waters proved the efficacy of such a closed system by submerging an anesthetized dog for 1 hour, after which it "stood up, shook the water off, and lay down for a nap."

In conjunction with the newer anesthetics, the endotracheal tube has been hailed as the greatest safety device possessed by the anesthesiologist. Veterinarians, however, adopted its use somewhat belatedly. The technique is not mentioned in French's *Surgery of the Dog* (1936), and some practitioners still use it rarely—if at all—although intubation is now a routine practice in many veterinary hospitals.

In 1927, Hardenbergh and Mann stated that an autoinhalation technique of anesthesia, utilizing an endotracheal tube, had been used in experimental canine surgery at the Mayo Clinic for some 15 years. A rubber tracheal tube was attached to the top of an ether can by means of a three-way valve to permit a current of air to pass through the ether vapor, with the concentration of anesthetic gas being regulated by an opening in one arm of the valve. Later, rigid endotracheal tubes were substituted.[24] A refinement of this technique, utilizing a portable machine used in minor surgery in man, was employed by J. D. Gadd in private practice some time prior to 1939.[22] A comprehensive article on the subject by

J. R. Dinsmore[16] appeared in 1947 and, for the first time in a major textbook, *Canine Surgery*, in 1949.[17] Relatively few practitioners, however, employed the technique routinely until well into the 1950's.

The Beginning of Veterinary Anesthesia

Considering the few graduate veterinarians in the United States at the mid-18th century (said to be only 15 in 1847), it is not surprising that anesthesia for animals had but few advocates. George H. Dadd appears to have been the first veterinary practitioner to use ether or chloroform for surgical operations. Dadd was a nongraduate physician of Boston who had turned to veterinary medicine about the time that ether anesthesia had been demonstrated. Although his proximity made it convenient for him to adopt this new technique, it was undoubtedly his concern for the welfare of his patients that caused him to use it, perhaps to a greater extent than any other practitioner of his time. He had used ether as early as 1852, and in his *The Modern Horse Doctor* (1854) urged its use in all painful operations. For neurotomy he says:

We recommend that, in all operations of this kind, the subject be etherized, not only in view of preventing pain, but that we may, in the absence of all struggling on the part of our patient, perform the operation satisfactorily, and in much less time after etherization has taken place than otherwise. So soon as the patient is under the influence of that valuable agent, we have nothing to fear from his struggles, provided we have the assistance of one experienced to administer it. We generally use a mixture of chloroform and chloric ether in our operations, and consider it far preferable, so far as the life of our patient is concerned, to pure chloroform.[9]

Despite the opprobrious title, Dadd's was the first native American work to call for humane treatment and the application of scientific principles in veterinary practice. While his works sold widely, it would appear that the chief interest was in his cures; few practitioners exhibited the curiosity requisite for scientific practice. Horses continued to be bled and purged with vehemence and operated on without benefit of anesthesia. Dadd used a large sponge, and states, "In all cases of etherization at the Massachusetts Hospital, a simple sponge is used. The complicated and expensive breathing machines are dispensed with."

In his *American Veterinary Journal*, published during the 1850's, Dadd and several of his colleagues make mention of anesthesia several times. In 1856, Dadd states, "Ether is a very excellent remedy in spasmodic colic... it will generally mitigate abdominal pain, and tranquilize the nervous system." [10] (The latter phrase has a modern ring!) For colic, Dadd employed an ether and chloroform mixture, administered by an inhaler composed of "an old sheet and a sponge," to the point of complete anesthesia. [11] In addition to making the patient more manageable, and reducing the likelihood of the animal's damaging itself, Dadd considered that the anesthesia had a direct beneficial effect upon the course of the disease. In 1858 he used ether "to diminish the reflex excitability of the nervous system," in a case of puerpural convulsions in a cow. [12]

In the same year, Robert Jennings reports on "Experiments with Chloroform and Chloric Ether in Veterinary Surgery." He mentions several cases in the practices of John Scott and W. W. Fraley in which chloroform was used to anesthetize horses with fractured limbs, whereupon some experimental surgery was performed and the horses were destroyed. In another instance he assisted G. W. Bowler in an operation for umbilical hernia, and one for removal of a tumor, both under chloroform. In his own practice he had used chloroform anesthesia in removing a tumor, and ether for neurotomy, noting: "Not having an assistant in this case, I found it extremely difficult to administer the anesthetic, and operate myself." [28] This article indicates that a number of practitioners, influenced by Dadd, were using anesthesia at this early date.

In writing on the "Caesarean Operation on Sows," in 1858, Dadd states:

Humanity would suggest that the subject be etherized, when performing so formidable an operation, yet our experience in the use of anesthesial agents on swine, will not warrant us in recommending its universal application." [13] In the same year, Robert Wood used ether in operating for scrotal hernia in pigs, noting: "Of all the animals I have etherized, the pig is the most susceptible and the quickest brought under its influence.[14]

Jennings, founder of the ill-fated Veterinary College of Philadelphia (1855), in his book on *The Horse and His Diseases* (1860), states:

In severe operations, humanity dictates the use of some anesthetic agent to render the animal insensible to pain. Chloroform is the most powerful of this class, and may be administered with perfect safety, provided a moderate quantity of atmospheric air is inhaled during its administration. Sulphuric ether acts very feebly upon the horse, and cannot therefore be successfully used.[29]

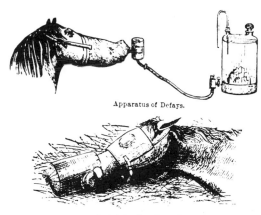

Apparatus of Defays.

Cox's Chloroform Bag in Position.

FIG. 1.3. Late 19th century anesthetic inhalers. The separate canister type had the advantage of more precise regulation of the gas mixture but was vulnerable if the animal struggled. A similar nosepiece was used for small animals. The canvas nosecap was considered superior to those of impervious leather. (From Liautard, A.: *Manual of Operative Veterinary Surgery*. Sabiston & Murray, New York, 1892.)

The only operation for which Jennings specifies the use of anesthesia, however, is that for hernia. On the other hand, Williams, in his *Principles and Practice of Veterinary Surgery* (American edition, 1882), says nothing of the use of anesthesia for hernia operations, specifying instead, "a powerful internal sedative."[56] The only mention of anesthetics by Williams is "full chloroform anesthesia" for lithotomy, and for amputation of the penis. As a matter of passing interest, Jennings states that all that is required in the latter operation is "one swift bold stroke of a sharp knife."

In his *Explanatory Horse Doctor* (1873), Navin states, concerning chloroform:

It is much used in human practice, in performing surgical operation.... Chloroform may be administered to the horse for the same purpose as it is given to man. An experienced

A

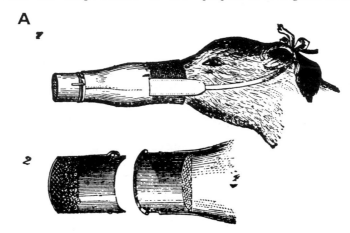

1. Perten's Method of Administering Anaesthetics to Dogs. 2. The Apparatus Taken Apart.

B

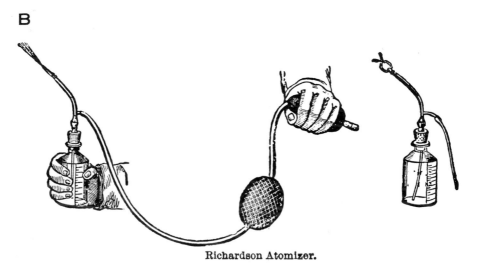

Richardson Atomizer.

FIG. 1.4. *A*, early 20th century method for administering anesthetics, usually various alcohol-ether-chloroform mixtures, to dogs. (From Merillat, L. A.: *Principles of Veterinary Surgery*. Alexander Eger, Chicago, 1906.) *B*, the first practical application of local anesthesia by ether spray (1867) was adopted from human medicine for veterinary use. (From Liautard, A.: *Manual of Operative Veterinary Surgery*. Sabiston & Murray, New York, 1892.)

finger should be on the pulse while the horse is breathing, and if the pulse should be about to stop, the chloroform should be removed from the nose, and a handkerchief wet with aqua ammonia held close to it. The quantity required to get the horse under its influence will vary from one to four ounces. I would not recommend its use in any but the more important operations.[41]

This information appears in a "list of medicines," and Navin does not refer to the use of chloroform as an adjunct to any operation; inasmuch as his book was "intended for the use of the farmer, and not for the professional horse doctor or veterinary surgeon," this omission may have been a fortunate one for the horse.

Professional veterinary writings during the last quarter of the 19th century, however, demonstrate a conspicuous lack of interest in anesthesia on the part of veterinarians. In the first volume of the *American Veterinary Review* (1877), for example, there is but one reference to anesthetics, and none in volume 2. It is a curious fact that many of the early advocates of anesthesia, mainly Dadd and his colleagues, worked outside the pale of organized veterinary medicine. Perhaps one had to be a maverick to stray far from conventional practice.

With the publication of American editions of Dun's *Veterinary Medicines* in the 1880's, veterinarians at least had the opportunity to become acquainted with the properties of chloroform and ether. The 1886 edition devoted some 15 pages to these two agents. While the actions and uses of both are given in great detail, Dun states, however:

Chloroform is not so extensively used in veterinary as in human medicine. It is occasionally given to horses to procure insensibility during castration, firing, and other painful operations but it is wise to warn the owner of the risk attending its administration . . . . Ether closely resembles chloroform . . . . In veterinary practice anesthesia, however, is not always so rapidly and successfully effected; some well-bred horses require to be cast before they can be got to inhale the anesthetic; the

preliminary stage of excitement is occasionally prolonged for some minutes; whilst, for many hours, and even for a couple of days, some patients continue dull and off their feed.[18]

Veterinary Anesthesiology Comes of Age

The development of veterinary anesthesiology in America to the 1890's is epitomized by Alexandre Liautard in his *Manual of Operative Veterinary Surgery* (1892). Liautard, a Frenchman, was a founder and long time guiding hand of the United States Veterinary Medical Association and a leading educator and veterinary surgeon who, as head of the American Veterinary College (1875 to 1900), regularly taught the use of anesthesia. He says:

In veterinary surgery, the indication for anesthesia has not, to the same extent as in human, the avoidance of pain in the patient for its object, and though the duties of the veterinarian include that of avoiding the infliction of *unnecessary* pain as much as possible, the administration of anesthetic compounds aims principally to facilitate the performance of the operation for its own sake, by depriving the patient of the power of obstructing, and perhaps even frustrating its execution, to his own detriment, by the violence of his struggles, and the persistency of his resistance. To prevent these, with their disastrous consequences, is the prime motive in the induction of the anesthetic state.[35]

He considers anesthesia essential in such operations as fracture reduction, hernia, neurotomy, quittor, etc., and often indicated for dentistry, prolapse, parturition, castration, and firing, among other conditions.

Liautard recommends chloroform or chloral hydrate (introduced in 1872) for large animals and ether or chloral for small animals, mentioning that chloroform had been almost totally discarded for the latter because of its danger. Although veterinarians had advocated an ether-chloroform mixture some 20 years before this was widely adopted in human surgery, Liautard states that for large animals, on the basis of experimental work, "Chloroform used singly has proved itself to be the most effective and safest of all," when used with any of a number of inhalers to provide an admixture of air. Chloral injected intravenously, he says, "has been shown to be the best of all modes of obtaining anesthesia . . . but unfortunately it is a method of introducing it into the system which will scarcely ever become sufficiently practicable to be available outside of the laboratory." He mentions the use of morphine as a preanesthetic (introduced in 1881) followed by rectal injection of chloral, but does not indicate whether he employed this technique. He had used chloral balls, "as commonly practised by many veterinarians," with benefit in short, painful operations.

Regarding local anesthesia, Liautard states: "The special indications for this are so numerous that they may almost be considered as general, if not universal, and its application is so simple and easy a process, and its effects usually so certain, that it would become the practitioners of our day to utilize it more frequently and extensively than they do." [35] He recommends it for such operations as urethrotomy, caudal myotomy, tail amputation, mammary tumor removal in dogs, and differential diagnosis of lameness in horses. He mentions the ether spray (introduced in 1867) and freezing mixtures (1852), but prefers the hypodermic use of cocaine (introduced in 1884). Although a number of reports appeared in the veterinary literature about this time, it is evident that local anesthesia was not being used to the extent warranted.

In the most popular canine work of the time, by Müller and Glass, *Diseases of the Dog* (1896), rather less is said concerning anesthesia. Thus, while for fractures: "In cases where there is extreme pain and in order to keep the animal from struggling, it is advisable to etherize," all that is said concerning hernial section is that "under the influence of ether or a narcotic, the reduction is easier"; although, "herniotomy is, as a rule, a rather easy operation in the dog." [40] Cocaine is recommended

for some eye conditions, in conjunction with general anesthesia for lens extraction; otherwise, general anesthesia—a short section on which is included with the discussion on tumor removal—is recommended: "In very serious operations, accompanied by great pain, it is advisable to place the animal under the influence of some anaesthetic." Chloral is used as a clyster, and ether, chloroform, or bromoether as inhalants, preferably following morphine.

As the first American veterinary surgeon to give anesthesia the full attention (30 pages) it warranted, L. A. Merillat in his *Principles of Veterinary Surgery* (1906) says:

In veterinary surgery, anesthesia has no history. It is used in a kind of desultory fashion that reflects no great credit to the present generation of veterinarians . . . . Many veterinarians of rather wide experience have never in a whole lifetime administered a general anesthetic in performing their operations. It reflects greatly to the credit of the canine specialist, however, that he alone had adopted anesthesia to any considerable extent . . . . Anesthesia in veterinary surgery today is a means of restraint and not an expedient to relieve pain. So long as an operation can be performed by forcible restraint . . . the thought of anesthesia does not enter into the proposition . . . . There is, however, some evidence of a change in the proper direction . . . and at the present there is some indication that the practitioner of the near future will take advantage of the expedient that made the rapid advancement of human surgery possible. [39]

Merillat devotes 30 pages to anesthesia and anesthetics, a more thorough treatment than many succeeding texts provided. He divides the phenomenon into three stages: excitement, narcosis, and anesthesia, and describes each adequately, together with minute directions for judging the depth of anesthesia. Concerning the modes of administration, he says none is more practical and satisfactory than the plain rubber or oilcloth sheet and sponge, the adjustable nosebags being "rather treacherous and always somewhat difficult to manage." He recommends

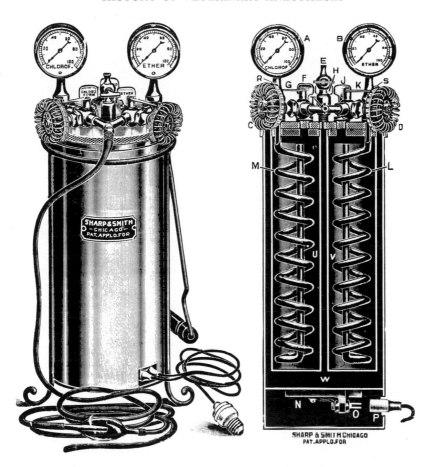

FIG 1.5. Merillat-Christiansen apparatus for administering ether and/or chloroform intrapharyngeally or intratracheally (note endotracheal tube, *lower left*). A water jacket transmitted heat to the chambers containing the anesthetics. However, Merillat himself preferred an oilcloth sheet and sponge as "most practical and satisfactory," and considered the nosebags "treacherous." (From Merillat, L. A.: *Principles of Veterinary Surgery*. Alexander Eger, Chicago, 1906.)

chloroform for large animals and ether for the dog and cat, although 2 to 6 grains of morphine injected hypodermically will often suffice for dogs (and cats!) without using ether. These agents, he says, "will give results that leave but little room for improvement," although he admits chloral hydrate may have some utility in large animals as do alcohol-chloroform-ether mixtures in small animals.

Merillat lists fatalities from inhalation anesthetics as resulting from toxic asphyxia, reflex syncope, direct syncope, or postanesthetic complications, principally pneumonia. He states that equine mortality from chloroform is about 1/800 and with ether in dogs about 1/400; his results

with chloroform in dogs "have been disastrous."

Local anesthetics in general veterinary use he lists as cocaine hydrochlorate, 4 to 10%; eucaine hydrochlorate, 5 to 10%; ethyl chloride; morphine sulfate, 10% with 5% cocaine; chloretone, 1% with 0.01% adrenaline chloride; stovane; and mixtures of cocaine, morphine, carbolic acid, and sodium chloride. Concerning spinal cocainization, he doubts its utility in small animals and, "In the large animals it must not be thought of." Except for the substitution of procaine and development of nerve blocking to a fine art, large animal anesthesia changed little until barbiturate-chloral-magnesium sulfate mixtures were introduced for intravenous use, nor does French in his *Surgical Diseases and Surgery of the Dog* (1936) indicate that much progress was made in small animal anesthesia during the 30 years following Merillat's work.[20]

Hobday, in his *Surgical Diseases of the Dog and Cat* (1906), offers a convenient companion piece, with regard to small animal anesthesia, to the primarily large animal considerations presented by Merillat. To the local anesthetics mentioned by Merillat, Hobday adds holocaine and orthoform, the latter being especially useful as a wound dressing when mixed with 8 parts of collodion. Chloroform, he says, "is the ideal anaesthetic to choose for the average adult dog . . . if given slowly in a proper manner and sufficiently diluted . . . the secret of success is to allow plenty of air." Unskilled anesthetists, however, should use ether or alcohol-chloroform-ether mixture.[26]

Progress in anesthesia, especially as met with in the average veterinary practice, was relatively slow prior to World War II. Developments since then portend a bright future.

REFERENCES

1. Anonymous: Quoted in Robinson,[43] p. 215.
2. Bernard, C.: Quoted in Robinson,[43] p. 312.
3. Blaine, D.: *Outlines of the Veterinary Art*, 5th ed., p. 641. Longman, Orne & Company, London, 1841.
4. Boardman, T.: *Dictionary of the Veterinary Art*, George Kearsley, London, 1805.
5. Booth, N. D., and Pierson, R. E.: Treatment of tetanus with D-tubocurarine chloride. J. Amer. Vet. Med. Ass. *128:* 257, 1956.
6. Boyle, R.: An account of the rise and attempts, of a way to conveigh liquors immediately into the mass of blood. Philos. Trans. 128, 1665.
7. Braithwaite, W.: *Retrospect of Medicine*, vol. 16, p. 409. Simpkins, Marshall & Company, London, 1847.
8. Carver, J.: Farrier's Magazine. Philadelphia, 1818.
9. Dadd, G. H.: *The Modern Horse Doctor*, p. 252. Jewett & Company, Boston, 1854.
10. Dadd, G. H.: Amer. Vet. J. *1:* 150, 1856.
11. Dadd, G. H.: Amer. Vet. J. *1:* 315, 1856.
12. Dadd, G. H.: Amer. Vet. J. *3:* 362, 1858.
13. Dadd, G. H.: Caesarian operation on sows. Amer. Vet. J. *3:* 46, 1858.
14. Dadd, G. H.: Amer. Vet. J. *3:* 70, 1858.
15. Davy, H.: *Researches, Chiefly Concerning Nitrous Oxide*, London, 1800. Quoted in Robinson,[43] p. 51.
16. Dinsmore, J. R.: Intratracheal anesthesia. N. Amer. Vet. *28(12):* 819, 1947.
17. Dinsmore, J. R.: Intratracheal anesthesia. In *Canine Surgery*, edited by H. P. Hoskins and J. V. Lacroix, p. 115. American Veterinary Publications, Evanston, Ill., 1949.
18. Dun, F.: *Veterinary Medicines: Their Actions and Uses*, pp. 265 and 313. W. R. Jenkins, New York, 1886.
19. Farquharson, J.: Paravertebral lumbar anesthesia in the bovine species. J. Amer. Vet. Med. Ass. *97:* 54, 1940.
20. French, C.: *Surgical Diseases and Surgery of the Dog*, p. 10. Alexander Eger, Chicago, 1936.
21. Fullöp-Miller, R.: *Triumph Over Pain*, Literary Guild, New York, 1938.
22. Gadd, J. D.: Intratracheal anesthesia. N. Amer. Vet. *20(5):* 65, 1939.
23. Guthrie, S.: New mode of preparing a spirtious solution of chloric ether. Silliman's J., Art. VI, 1831.
24. Hardenbergh, J. G., and Mann, F. C.: The auto-inhalation method of anesthesia in canine surgery. J. Amer. Vet. Med. Ass. *71:* 493, 1927.
25. Hickman, H.: Quoted in Fullöp-Miller,[21] p. 84.
26. Hobday, F. T. G.: *Surgical Diseases of the Dog and Cat*, p. 23. Bailliere, Tindall & Cox, London, 1906.
27. Jackson, C. T.: Etherization of animals. In *Report of the Commissioner of Patents for the Year 1853—Agriculture*, p. 59. Washington, D.C., 1854.
28. Jennings, R.: Experiments with chloroform and chloric ether in veterinary surgery. Amer. Vet. J. *1:* 315, 1856.
29. Jennings, R.: *The Horse and His Diseases*, p. 342. J. E. Potter & Co., Philadelphia, 1860.
30. Keys, T. E.: *The History of Surgical Anesthesia*. Schuman's, New York, 1945.
31. Klemm, W. R.: Carbon dioxide anesthesia in cats. Amer. J. Vet. Res. *25:* 1201, 1964.
32. Lancet: July 10, 1847, p. 60.
33. Larson, L. L.: The internal pudendal (pudic) nerve block for anesthesia of the penis and relaxation of the retractor penis muscle. J. Amer. Vet. Med. Ass. *123:* 18, 1953.
34. Liautard, A.: *Manual of Operative Veterinary Surgery*, chap. I. Sabiston & Murray, New York, 1892.
35. Liautard, A.: *Manual of Operative Veterinary Surgery*, Sabiston & Murray, New York, 1892.
36. (Long, C. W.): Crawford W. Long, the pioneer in ether anesthesia. Bull. Hist. Med. *12:* 191, 1942.
37. McIntyre, A. R.: *Curare, Its History, Nature, and Clinical Use*, p. 183. University of Chicago Press, Chicago, 1947.
38. Medical Gazette: May 14, 1847, p. 842.
39. Merillat, L. A.: *Principles of Veterinary Surgery*, p. 223. Alexander Eger, Chicago, 1906.
40. Müller, G., and Glass, A.: *Diseases of the Dog*

and *Their Treatment*. Alexander Eger, Chicago, 1896.

41. Navin, J. N.: *Navin's Veterinary Practice: or Explanatory Horse Doctor*, p. 458. J. B. Hann, Cincinnati, 1873.
42. (Paracelsus): Quoted in Robinson,[43] p. 35.
43. Robinson, V.: *Victory Over Pain*. Henry Schuman, New York, 1946.
44. Smithcors, J. F.: The treatment of tetanus with curare—a little known chapter in veterinary history. J. Amer. Vet. Med. Ass. *129:* 303, 1956.
45. Smithcors, J. F.: The early use of anesthesia in veterinary practice. Brit. Vet. J. *113:* 284, 1957.
46. Thomas, K. B.: Benjamin Brodie, physiologist. Med. Hist. *8:* 286, 1964.
47. Veterinarian *11:* 1838.
48. Veterinarian *12:* 1839.
49. Veterinarian *20:* (January) 1847.
50. Veterinarian *20:* (February) 1847.
51. Veterinarian *21:* 1848.
52. Veterinarian *31:* 1858.
53. Warren. J. C.: *Etherization, with Surgical Remarks*. Boston, 1848. Quoted in Fullöp-Miller,[21] p. 161.
54. Waters, R. M.: Quoted in Keys,[30] p. 92.
55. Watson, T.: *Principles and Practice of Physic*, 2nd American ed., p. 365. Lea & Blanchard, Philadelphia, 1845.
56. Williams, W.: *Principles and Practice of Veterinary Surgery*, pp. 627 and 635. W. R. Jenkins, New York, 1882.
57. Wright, J. G.: Anaesthesia in animals: a review. Vet. Rec. *76:* 710, 1964.

2
Theories of Anesthetic Action*

PETER J. COHEN

It is natural that those who use a drug should wish to understand its mode of action. This has been possible for such agents as the antimetabolites, some of the antibiotics, and the neuromuscular blockers. Drugs that exert their effect upon as complex a system as that involved in anesthesia are far more difficult to attack. The many proposed theories of narcosis have been reviewed by a number of authors.[8, 18, 33, 38] In this chapter I summarize and interpret a variety of approaches, as well as elaborate some new information.

Let us first examine some of the problems involved in formulating a general theory of narcosis. Such a theory must gather together a vast number of observations pertaining to a heterogeneous group of substances and synthesize them into a unified concept. It must both have a predictive value and set forth conditions *necessary* and sufficient to explain drug actions that are already known.

The anesthetics exert their effect not only upon the central nervous system, but throughout the organism, on cardiac and skeletal muscle, renal and hepatic function, and even upon the hematopoietic system. These agents have no common chemical structure; some are hydrocarbons, others are ethers, some are halogenated, and some are noble gases. Until recently, it was assumed that the anesthet-ics were biologically inert (with the exception of trichloroethylene); *i.e.*, they were excreted by the lung without undergoing any metabolic changes. It is now established that these drugs normally undergo considerable biodegradation.[39a, 45] Furthermore, some are capable of inducing increased activity in the enzyme systems responsible for their degradation.[13]

In spite of extensive knowledge of neurophysiology, there is no complete understanding of the state of *consciousness*. It is difficult, therefore, to develop a theory on the *unconscious* state. Many "theories" are, in fact, only descriptions, while others deal with the *effects* of anesthesia rather than the *mechanism* by which these effects are produced. For these reasons, it is not difficult to see why no proposed theory of narcosis has met with general acceptance.

Colloid Theory

This theory represents an early attempt to deal with the mechanisms of anesthesia and is of only historic interest. It was claimed that a reversible aggregation of cell colloids causes or accompanies anesthesia. Changes have been observed in the physical and biological properties of simple life forms (*e.g.*, slime mold and ameba) following exposure to anesthet-ics.[7, 42] The mechanisms involved are unclear, and it cannot be concluded that the same effects occur in cells of other species. Furthermore, this is a description of a

---

*This review represents a survey of the literature through 1968.

nonspecific action of many substances, only some of which are anesthetics.

Lipid Theory

Since nerve cells and membranes contain lipids, it has been proposed that there is a direct relationship between the affinity of an anesthetic for a lipid and its anesthetic action. Recently, excellent correlation has been shown between the potency of numerous agents and their fat solubility.[16] It is reasonable to assume that an agent must enter the central nervous system in order to produce central nervous system depression, and that its ease of entrance may be dependent on fat solubility. Fat solubility alone, however, does not guarantee cerebral depression; moreover, some fat-soluble drugs may produce convulsions.[27] Furthermore, simple lipids comprise but a small fraction of the brain constituents. Thus, this approach disregards the presence of phospholipids (the solubility of anesthetics in phospholipids is dissimilar to that in olive oil), proteins, and water. Finally, this "theory," while having considerable merit in showing a common factor involved in anesthesia, does not offer an explanation of how the anesthetic effect is produced once the drug has entered the brain.

In focusing attention on the relationship between anesthetics and lipids, the ability of the so-called "inert" gases to interact with protein molecules should not be overlooked.[19, 40, 41] Free amino and carboxyl groups of proteins can induce areas of partial negativity or positivity (i.e., a dipole) in a gas molecule which otherwise would be electrically neutral. This results in binding of the anesthetic molecule at the protein surface. It is also possible that the anesthetic molecule actually penetrates the interior of the protein. In either case, conformational changes are induced in the *protein* molecule which could conceivably be related to the anesthetic state.

Cell Permeability Theory

General anesthetics may be capable of altering cell permeability, thus interfering with normal membrane depolarization.[47] Ether and chloroform partially prevent the normal decrease in membrane resistance which occurs during excitation.[50] The inhalation agents are also capable of exerting profound effects on sodium transport across membranes.[4, 22] The entry of glucose into human erythrocytes is normally stimulated by carbon dioxide. Increased permeability is inhibited by therapeutic concentrations of halothane, methoxyflurane, and diethyl ether.[23] The mechanism of this inhibition has not yet been clarified. Although both the inhalation and local anesthetics affect the membrane state, it has not been determined whether or not this is the only cause of anesthesia. In addition, the manner in which the anesthetic affects membrane function is not at all certain. Finally, such drugs as digitalis and d-tubocurarine influence membrane physiology but do not cause anesthesia.

Biochemical Theories

Energy is stored in the form of adenosine triphosphate. This compound in turn is formed by the phosphorylation of adenosine diphosphate, a chemical reaction which requires energy input. This energy is provided by the transfer of electrons from substrate (*e.g.*, glutamate or succinate) to molecular oxygen. The process of electron transfer (respiration or oxygen uptake) is linked or coupled to the phosphorylation of adenosine diphosphate (oxidative phosphorylation). These events normally occur in the mitochondria.

Drugs may affect cellular metabolism in a number of ways. They may interfere with oxygen uptake by blocking the transfer of electrons within the mitochondrion. They may dissociate adenosine triphosphate production (energy storage) from oxygen consumption by preventing the normal phosphorylation of adenosine diphosphate (uncoupling of oxidative phosphorylation). A change in oxygen uptake may reflect decreased tissue energy requirements rather than an abnormally low rate of energy production.

Exposure of brain slices to barbiturates results in a considerable decrease in the rate of oxygen utilization.[31, 39, 46] The ability of barbiturates to uncouple oxidative phosphorylation has also been demonstrated in vitro.[3,6] The effect of thiobarbiturates (e.g., thiopental) is irreversible. The concentration of the drug required to produce these changes is at least 10 times that needed for anesthesia in the intact organism. In addition, substances such as 2,4-dinitrophenol, a potent uncoupler of oxidative phosphorylation, have no anesthetic properties whatsoever.

Some[30,37] but not all[25] investigators have found anesthetic concentrations of nitrous oxide to be without effect on tissue respiration. Both nitrous oxide and xenon leave oxidative phosphorylation unaltered. High concentrations of diethyl ether produce a 20% decrease in oxidative phosphorylation but do not affect oxygen uptake.[26] Halothane (1%) inhibits oxygen uptake of rat brain and liver slices.[24]

There are a number of criticisms which apply to the experiments which form the basis of this hypothesis. Often, the dose of anesthetic to which the preparation was exposed far exceeded that found during the actual state of anesthesia. In addition, in many instances the investigators failed to determine whether the reported changes were completely reversed when the anesthetic was removed. Furthermore, in some instances in which this has been determined, reversibility was not always found.

Recent studies on the effects of halothane on mitochondrial metabolism indicate the ability of anesthetic concentrations of halothane to reduce mitochondrial oxygen uptake markedly,[10,11] and these effects are totally reversible. The drug appears to act upon mitochondrial electron transfer at a point between nicotinamide adenine dinucleotide and flavine adenine dinucleotide.

There is a good deal of information pertaining to anesthetic action in the intact organism. The effects of anesthetics on cerebral metabolism have been studied in detail. Large doses of thiopental decrease cerebral oxygen uptake in the normal human.[36] The inhalation agents also affect cerebral oxygen uptake in man.[2,12,48] It is certainly possible that the site of action responsible for these findings is the same

in vivo as it is in vitro. This would indicate that the block of normal metabolism produces both anesthesia and decreased oxygen uptake. However, decreased oxygen uptake may only represent a decrease in metabolic needs which accompanies anesthesia. Thus, it has been shown that brain content of high energy phosphate does not decrease when the intact organism is subject to anesthesia.[31]

Neurophysiological Theories

In 1952 Larrabee demonstrated that anesthetics selectively inhibit synaptic transmission.[28,29] Concentrations of the inhalation agents which did not alter axonal function were able to block propagation of an impulse across the synapse.

Painful impulses from the periphery normally gain access to the brain via two pathways. One, the so-called lemniscal pathway, rapidly conducts impulses through the thalamus and then to the sensory cortex. The second pathway, or extralemniscal system, conducts synapses more slowly in a number of subcortical structures, and radiates to the cerebral cortex through the reticular formation. It is possible to stimulate an experimental subject repeatedly (e.g., with a flash of light, a noise, or electrical stimulation of a peripheral nerve) and, by means of electroencephalographic recording and computer averaging of the evoked response, obtain information about both paths of sensory transmission. It has long been felt that the ascending reticular formation is important in the maintenance of consciousness. It also has been proposed that the extralemniscal system is sensitive to the inhalation anesthetics and barbiturates.[1,14,15,21] Thus, the state of anesthesia represents a situation in which painful impulses are rapidly and directly transmitted to the sensory cortex, while blockage of extralemniscal pathways abolishes consciousness and awareness.

The neurophysiologist's approach to this problem aids our understanding of cerebral function. However, none of the investigators have proposed mechanisms by which this selective inhibition is obtained. In a sense, this "theory" simply says that anesthetics act by causing anesthesia. We are presented with a description, albeit sophisticated, of another facet of the anesthetic state. We can easily see that there are many levels of explanation. The neurophysiological approach "explains" anesthesia by showing what sensory pathways have been interrupted. It does not "explain" anesthesia by detailing the mechanism of this interruption.

Recent investigations have demonstrated that the classic separation of sensory transmission into lemniscal and extralemniscal pathways may not be completely valid. When low concentrations of cyclopropane are administered to man, unconsciousness does not result. He remains able to inform the investigator when electrical stimulation is applied to his ulnar nerve; thus, he is "aware" of the stimulus. At the same time, however, electroencephalographic recording demonstrates inhibition of both lemniscal and extralemniscal transmission. Clearly, if the subject remains conscious of stimulation while cortical potentials are no longer evoked by this stimulation, a good deal of further investigation into both normal neurophysiology and the effect of drugs upon the central nervous system is in order.

Physical Theories

Numerous investigators have attempted to relate anesthetic potency to certain physical characteristics of a drug. Among the earlier examples of this approach have been the attempts to relate anesthesia to lipid solubility. Other investigators have correlated anesthetic action with thermodynamic activity as evidenced by molecular volume, intermolecular attraction, heat of absorption, the ratio of the partial pressure producing anesthesia to the saturated vapor pressure of the drug, and the drug's effect upon surface tension.[5,9,17,20,33,49] There is a considerable body of information regarding the relationship between structure and physical, chemical, and pharmacological properties of the anesthetic drugs.[43] However, there are no known physical properties which can guarantee that a compound will be an effective anesthetic. In addition, all of the above mentioned factors are not independent, for they are all concerned with the relationship between drug molecules' attraction to each other and their attraction to molecules of the central nervous system. It is not unreasonable that anesthesia may occur when a definite fraction of the cell's constituents is bound to the anesthetic. Thus, good correlations between one physical property and anesthetic potency do not necessarily result in being able to demonstrate a reasonable relationship between all other physical properties and drug effect. These approaches are all based upon correlations and by no means are able to predict the characteristics of a drug of an entirely new structure.

In recent years, a number of investigators have sought to explain anesthetic action on a molecular level. The ability of drugs to bind to protein molecules has already been discussed. The chemical properties of anesthetics preclude their being able to produce narcosis through chemical reactions involving formation and breaking of ordinary covalent chemical bonds. Many anesthetic drugs are also incapable of forming hydrogen bonds. Although xenon is a noble gas, and nearly completely unreactive chemically, it is a true anesthetic. For these reasons, Pauling chose to focus his attention on water rather than to examine protein or lipid molecules.[34, 35] The ability of one water molecule to form a weak hydrogen bond with another is responsible for water's expanding on freezing. The attraction of water molecules to each other also explains the observation that both the melting and boiling points of water are higher than would be predicted. For the same reason, water molecules are able to form polyhedrons or hydrate crystals. Pauling[34] has stated that "the only chemical property that it (xenon) has is that of taking part in the formation of clathrate (Lat. Clathri = lattice) crystals. In these crystals the xenon atoms occupy chambers in a frame-work formed by molecules that interact with one another by the formation of hydrogen bonds. The crystal of this sort of greatest interest to us is xenon hydrate, $(Xe \cdot 5\,{}^{3}/_{4}H_2O.)$" Hydrate crystals are formed in a similar manner by the interaction of other anesthetic agents with water to form a polyhydron in which the anesthetic occupies the center. Miller[32] has proposed a similar theory in which the anesthetic agent is able to stabilize water in the form of "icebergs." It has been postulated that these stabilized water crystals are able to interfere with function of the central nervous system and thus produce anesthesia. Fairly good agreement has been demonstrated between hydrate dissociation pressure and anesthetic potency. However, although clathrates have been produced in the test tube,[44] all available evidence indicated that such crystals are unstable at the temperature and pressure normally present within the central nervous system. Furthermore, although the theory is provocative, there is no experimental evidence that such phenomena take place during anesthesia.

REFERENCES

1. Abrahamian, H. A., Allison, T., Goff, W. R., and Rosner, B. S.: Effects of thiopental on human cerebral evoked responses. Anesthesiology 24: 650, 1963.
2. Alexander, S. C., Cohen, P. J., Wollman, H., Smith, T. C., Reivich, M., and Van der Molen, R. A.: Cerebral carbohydrate metabolism during hypocarbia in man. Studies during nitrous oxide anesthesia. Anesthesiology 26: 624, 1965.
3. Aldridge, W. N., and Parker, V. H.: Barbiturate and oxidative phosphorylation. Biochem. J. 76: 47, 1960.
4. Andersen, N. B.: Effect of general anesthetics on sodium transport in the isolated toad bladder. Anesthesiology 27:304, 1966.
5. Brink, F., and Posternak, J. M.: Thermodynamic analysis of the relative effectiveness of narcotics. J. Cell. Physiol. 32: 211, 1948.
6. Brody, T. M., and Bain, J. A.: Barbiturates and oxidative phosphorylation. J. Pharmacol. Exp. Ther. 110: 148, 1954.
7. Bruce, D., and Christiansen, R.: Morphologic changes in the giant amoeba Chaos chaos induced by halothane and ether. Exp. Cell Res. 40: 544, 1965.
8. Bunker, J. P., and Vandam, L. D. (editors): Effects of anesthesia on metabolism and cellular functions. Pharmacol. Rev. 17: 183, 1965.
9. Clements, J. A., and Wilson, K. M.: The affinity of narcotic agents for interfacial films. Proc. Nat. Acad. of Sci., U. S. A. 48: 1008, 1962.
10. Cohen, P. J., and Marshall, B. E.: Effects of halothane on respiratory control and oxygen consumption of rat liver mitochondria. In Toxicity of Anesthetics, edited by B. R. Fink, pp. 24–36. The Williams & Wilkins Company, Baltimore, 1968.
11. Cohen, P. J., Marshall, B. E., Harris, J. E., Lecky, J. H., and Rosner, B. S.: Halothane-induced changes in mitochondrial oxygen uptake and respiratory control. Fed. Proc. 27: 705, 1968.
12. Cohen, P. J., Wollman, H., Alexander, S. C., Chase, P. E., and Behar, M. G.: Cerebral carbohydrate metabolism in man during halothane anesthesia. Effects of $PaCO_2$ on some aspects of carbohydrate utilization. Anesthesiology 25: 185, 1964.
13. Conney, A. H.: Pharmacological implications of microsomal enzyme induction. Pharmacol. Rev. 19: 317, 1967.
14. Davis, H. S., Collins, W. F., Randt, C. T., and Dillon, W. H.: Effects of anesthetic agents on evoked central nervous system responses: gaseous agents. Anesthesiology 18: 634, 1957.
15. Davis, H. S., Dillon, W. H., Collins, W. F., Randt, C. T.: The effect of anesthetic agents on evoked central nervous system responses: muscle relaxants and volatile agents. Anesthesiology 19: 441, 1958.
16. Eger, E. I., Brandstater, B., Saidman, L. J., Regan, M. J., Severinghaus, J. W., and Munson, E. S.: Equipotent alveolar concentrations of methoxyflurane, halothane, diethyl ether, fluroxene, cyclopropane, xenon, and nitrous oxide in the dog. Anesthesiology 26: 771, 1965.
17. Eger, E. I., Saidman, L. J., and Brandstater, B.: Temperature dependence of halothane and cyclopropane anesthesia in dogs: correlation with some theories of anesthetic action. Anesthesiology 26: 764, 1965.
18. Featherstone, R. M., and Muehlbaecher, C. A.: The current role of inert gases in the search for anesthesia mechanisms. Pharmacol. Rev. 15: 97, 1963.
19. Featherstone, R. M., Muehlbaecher, C. A., DeBon, F. L., and Forsaith, J. A.: Interactions of inert anesthetic gases with proteins. Anesthesiology 22: 977, 1961.
20. Ferguson, J.: The use of chemical potentials as indices of toxicity. Proc. Roy. Soc. [Biol.] 127: 387, 1939.
21. French, J. D., Verzeano, M., and Magoun, H. W.: A neural basis of the anesthetic state. Arch. Neurol. Psychiat. 69: 519, 1953.
22. Gottlieb, S. F., and Savran, S. V.: Nitrous oxide inhibition of sodium transport. Anesthesiology 28: 324, 1967.
23. Greene, N. M., and Cervenko, F. W.: Inhalational anesthetics, carbon dioxide, and glucose transport across red cell membranes. Acta Anaesth. Scand. (suppl.) 28: 1, 1967.
24. Hoech, G. P., Jr., Matteo, R. F., and Fink, B. R.: Effect of halothane on oxygen consump-

tion of rat brain, liver, and heart, and anaerobic glycolysis of rat brain. Anesthesiology 27: 770, 1966.

25. Hosein, E. A., Stachiewicz, E., Bourne, W., and Denstedt, O. F.: The influence of nitrous oxide on the metabolic activity of brain tissue. Anesthesiology 16: 708, 1955.

26. Hulme, N. A., and Krantz, J. C., Jr.: Anesthesia. XLV. Effect of ethyl ether on oxidative phosphorylation in the brain. Anesthesiology 16: 627, 1955.

27. Krantz, J. C., Jr., Esquibel, A., Truitt, E. B., Jr., Ling, A. S. C., and Kurland, A. A.: Hexafluorodiethyl ether (Indoklon)—an inhalant convulsant. Its use in psychiatric treatment. J. A. M. A. 166: 1555, 1958.

28. Larrabee, M. G., and Holiday; D. A.: Depression of transmission through sympathetic ganglia during general anesthesia. J. Pharmacol. Exp. Ther. 105: 400, 1952.

29. Larrabee, M. G., and Posternak, J. M.: Selective action of anesthetics on synapses and axons in mammalian sympathetic ganglia. J. Neurophysiol. 15: 91, 1952.

30. Levy, L., and Featherstone, R. M.: The effect of xenon and nitrous oxide on in vitro guinea pig brain respiration and oxidative phosphorylation. J. Pharmacol. Exp. Ther. 110: 221, 1954.

31. McIlwain, H.: Biochemistry and the Central Nervous System, 2nd ed., pp. 229–243. Little, Brown, and Company, Boston, 1959.

32. Miller, S. L.: A theory of gaseous anesthetics. Proc. Nat. Acad. Sci. U. S. A. 47: 1515, 1961.

33. Mullins, L. J.: Some physical mechanisms in narcosis. Chem. Rev. 54: 289, 1954.

34. Pauling, L.: A molecular theory of general anesthesia. Science 134: 15, 1961.

35. Pauling, L.: The hydrate microcrystal theory of general anesthesia. Curr. Res. Anesth. Analg. 43: 1, 1964.

36. Pierce, E. C., Jr., Lambertsen, C. J., Deutsch, S., Chase, P. E., Linde, H. W., Dripps, R. D., and Price, H. L.: Cerebral circulation and metabolism during thiopental anesthesia and hyperventilation in man. J. Clin. Invest. 41: 1664, 1962.

37. Pittinger, C. B., Featherstone, R. M., Cullen,

S. C., and Gross, E. G.: Comparative in vitro study of guinea pig brain oxidations as influenced by xenon and nitrous oxide. J. Lab. Clin. Med. 38: 384, 1951.

38. Pittinger, C. B., and Keasling, H. H.: Theories of narcosis. Anesthesiology 20: 204, 1959.

39. Quastel, J. H.: Biochemical aspects of narcosis. Curr. Res. Anesth. Analg. 31: 151. 1952.

39a. Rehder, K., Forbes, J., Alter, H., Hessler, O., and Stier, A.: Halothane biotransformation in man: a quantitative study. Anesthesiology 28: 711, 1967.

40. Schoenborn, B. P.: Binding of cyclopropane to sperm whale myoglobin. Nature (London) 214: 1120, 1967.

41. Schoenborn, B. P., and Nobbs, C. L.: The binding of xenon to sperm whale deoxymyoglobin. Molec. Pharmacol 2: 491, 1966.

42. Seifritz, W.: The effects of various anesthetic agents on protoplasm. Anesthesiology 11: 24, 1950.

43. Suckling, C. W.: Some chemical and physical factors in the development of fluothane. Brit. J. Anaesth. 29: 466, 1957.

44. Van der Heem, P.: Preparation of a solid hydrate of halothane. Anesthesiology 27: 84, 1966.

45. Van Dyke, R. A., and Chenoweth, M. E.: Metabolism of volatile anesthetics. Anesthesiology 26: 348, 1965.

46. Webb, J. L., and Elliott, K. A. C.: Effects of narcotics and convulsants on tissue glycolysis and respiration. J. Pharmacol. Exp. Ther. 103: 24, 1951.

47. Winterstein, H.: Die Narkose, 2nd ed. Springer-Verlag, Berlin, 1926.

48. Wollman, H., Alexander, S. C., and Cohen, P. J.: Cerebral circulation and metabolism in anesthetized man. In Clinical Anesthesia Series, vol. 3. F. A. Davis, Philadelphia, 1967.

49. Wulf, R. J., and Featherstone, R. M.: A correlation of van der Waals' constants with anesthetic potency. Anesthesiology 18: 97, 1957.

50. Yamaguchi, T., and Okumura, H.: Effects of anesthetics on the electrical properties of the cell membrane of the frog muscle fiber. Annot. Zool. Jap. 36: 109, 1963.

3
The Physics and Chemistry of General Anesthetics

HARRY W. LINDE

Many aspects of the specialty of anesthesia are based upon the principles of the physical sciences. For example, the administration of an inhalation anesthetic involves the physical laws governing the behavior of gases as well as the chemistry of anesthetic and respiratory gases.[4] For this reason, a knowledge of physics and chemistry as it pertains to anesthesia is important to the thoughtful anesthetist. Not only does a knowledge of fundamental principles permit more intelligent use of currently available agents and techniques, but it also provides for a rational evaluation of new agents and methods.

None of the currently available anesthetic agents are ideal in all respects; each has its drawbacks. Recognizing this, many pharmaceutical companies have their research laboratories searching for new anesthetic compounds. The decade of the 1960's has seen many new general anesthetic agents brought to clinical trial but, so far none of these agents have shown a clear-cut superiority over currently available drugs and none of the inhalation agents have been approved by the United States Food and Drug Administration for general distribution. Almost all of the inhalation agents studied have been fluorinated or mixed halogenated hydrocarbons or related compounds. Nonflammability is an important criterion and the halogenated compounds often possess this property. It is hoped that the 1970's will show continued research activity for new anesthetics.

Physics

PRESSURE, VOLUME, AND TEMPERATURE (THE GAS LAWS)

Inhalation anesthesia involves the transfer of a chemical substance from its container to the central nervous system; in the process, the anesthetic agent must be diluted to an appropriate concentration and supplied in a gas mixture that contains enough oxygen to support life. The mixed gases are then drawn into the lung, dissolved by the blood bathing the alveoli, and carried to all tissues, including the nervous system. This chain of events involves many of the physical properties of gases and vapors that are quantitatively described by the various gas laws. For example, a compressed gas expands to a new volume at a lower pressure according to Boyle's law; gases and vapors mix and behave as described by the laws of partial pressure; and gases dissolve in blood and body fluids according to their partition coefficient as described by Henry's law.

Unlike a liquid or solid, the volume of a gas is defined only by the container which confines it. The amount or number of molecules of a gas held in the container is determined by the temperature and pressure. When more gas is forced into a rigid container, the pressure is increased as is the number of molecules in the container. The converse is also true. The pressure that a given weight of gas exerts is inversely proportional to the volume in which it is confined—if the temperature is constant. This relationship is known as Boyle's law. It may be stated mathematically as:

$$\text{Volume varies as } \frac{1}{\text{Pressure}}$$

or

$$V \times P = \text{A constant}$$

If a fixed quantity (weight) of gas is allowed to expand from a high pressure to a lower pressure (or the reverse), the above relationship is valid at both pressures

$$P_1 V_1 = P_2 V_2$$

that is, the product of pressure times volume at one pressure will be numerically equal to the product of the smaller pressure times the larger volume occupied at this new pressure. For example, a size D cylinder of oxygen contains 4.2 liters of gas at a pressure of 2200 psi. When this gas is allowed to escape from the cylinder and expand to 1 atm (14.7 psi) it will occupy 630 liters of volume:

$$2200 \times 4.2 = 14.7 \times 630$$

If the volume of a gas is held constant, its pressure will increase as its temperature is increased. This relationship, known as Charles' law, may be stated as follows: the volume of a gas is directly proportional to its absolute temperature. Mathematically,

$$\text{volume varies as temperature}$$

or

$$V = \text{(a constant)} \times T$$

and for the same amount of gas at two conditions of temperature and pressure,

$$\frac{V_1}{V_2} = \frac{T_1}{T_2}$$

Charles' law calculations are all based on the absolute or Kelvin temperature scale. On this scale the freezing point of water, which is 0 C (Celsius or centigrade) is 273 K (Kelvin). Zero on the Kelvin scale or absolute zero is -273 C. Celsius temperatures may be converted to absolute temperatures by adding 273.

A simple experiment may be used to demonstrate Charles' law. If 5 ml of air are drawn into a syringe at room temperature (22 C), the syringe capped, and the barrel heated with boiling water (100 C), the plunger will move out as the volume of the gas increases to 6.3 ml.

$$\frac{5 \text{ ml}}{V_2} = \frac{(22 + 273)}{(100 + 273)}$$

$$V_2 = \frac{5 \times 373}{295} = 6.3 \text{ ml}$$

Similar observations and calculations may be made for cooling the syringe below room temperature.

If the pressure of a gas is kept constant and its temperature increased, it will expand. The molecules of the gas have gained thermal (heat) energy and thus move about more rapidly, requiring more space. The converse is also true; i.e., gas cooled at constant pressure requires less space. The mathematical relationship between pressure and temperature for a constant volume of gas is Gay-Lussac's law

$$P = \text{(a constant)} \times T,$$

or, for two sets of conditions for the same amount of gas,

$$\frac{P_1}{P_2} = \frac{T_1}{T_2}$$

Again, the absolute temperature must be used in calculations.

It is convenient for many gas law calculations to combine these laws into a single equation, the general gas law, which may be written:

$$\frac{P_1 \times V_1}{T_1} = \frac{P_2 \times V_2}{T_2}$$

If the pressure, volume, and temperature of a gas are known, the pressure, volume, or temperature at any other set of conditions may be calculated.

In gas law calculations, the mole is of particular significance. Avogadro's law states that 1 mole of any one substance contains the same number of molecules as 1 mole of any other substance. In the metric system, a mole is the molecular weight in grams. In the case of gases, 1 mole of any gas occupies the same volume as 1 mole of any other gas at the same temperature and pressure. The molar volume of solids and liquids varies widely and does not have the same significance as the gaseous molar volume. At "standard" conditions, 760 torr and 0 C, 1 mole of any ideal gas occupies 22.4 liters. At ordinary ambient conditions, 22 C and 760 torr, the molar volume is about 24 liters.

Another form of the gas law may be derived from the relations given above using n moles of gas at standard conditions as the basis:

$$\frac{PV}{T} = n \frac{(1 \text{ atm}) (22.4 \text{ liters})}{273 \text{ K}}$$

or

$$PV = nRT$$

where

$$R = 0.08206 \text{ liter-atm/degrees Kelvin}$$

For this numerical value or R, P must be in atmospheres, V in liters, n in gram moles, and T in degrees Kelvin.

The law of partial pressures states that in mixtures of gases, for example, air, which consists of about 21% oxygen and 78% nitrogen,* each gas exerts the same pressure that it would exert if it alone occupied the same volume at the same temperature. The pressure that each gas exerts is called its partial pressure. In anesthesia, the partial pressure of a gas is often referred to as its tension. If the partial pressures of all of the gases in a mixture are added together, their sum is equal to the total pressure in the system. For example, the partial pressure of oxygen in dry air at 760 torr is 159 torr, and

---

* Argon (0.93%) and small amounts of other gases make up the remainder of air.

that of nitrogen is 594 torr. If the oxygen in a closed container of air was removed chemically, the total pressure would drop to 601 torr, the partial pressures of nitrogen plus argon in air.

All of the foregoing statements and gas laws apply strictly only to so-called ideal gases—that is, the gases which obey these laws. The closer the temperature of a gas gets to its boiling point or the higher its pressure, the less ideal its behavior is; however, all gases and anesthetic vapors (e.g., ether, halothane) may be considered to behave as ideal gases in the range of pressures and concentrations ordinarily encountered in clinical anesthesia.

Temperature, volume, and pressure may be measured in a variety of units, but the metric system is usually used. Some common units and their relationships to one another are given in Table 3.1.

TABLE 3.1
Units and conversion factors

Measurement	Units and Conversion Factors	
Temperature	°C	= °K + 273
Volume	1 liter	= 1000 ml
	1 cubic foot	= 28.3 liters
Pressure	1 atm	= 760 torr
		= 760 mm Hg
		= 14.7 psi*
	1 mm Hg	= 13.5 cm of water
Length	1 m	= 100 cm
		= 1000 mm
	1 inch	= 2.54 cm

* Most pressure gauges read 0 at atmospheric pressure. Consequently, pressures may be given as pounds per square inch gauge (psig) (i.e., pressure above atmospheric pressure) or in pounds per square inch absolute (psia). Pressures given in length units such as millimeters of mercury or centimeters of water refer to the height of a column of the liquid which would be supported by that pressure. A mercury barometer is an 800-cm tube sealed at the top and filled with mercury with its lower end immersed in a dish of mercury. The upper portion of the tube over the mercury is a complete vacuum. The atmosphere pressing on the mercury in the dish causes it to rise in the tube to a height related to the existing atmospheric pressure.

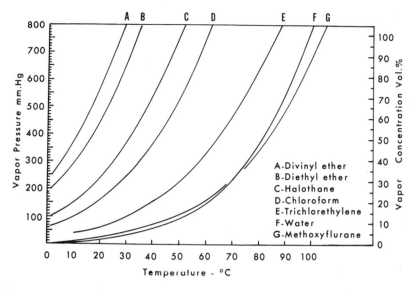

FIG. 3.1. Vapor pressure and vapor concentration—temperature curves for anesthetic agents and water. *Left hand ordinate*, vapor pressure in millimeters of mercury; *right hand ordinate*, vapor concentration as a percentage of the total pressure, assuming a barometric pressure of 760 mmHg. This percentage by pressure is equal to percent by volume. Note that the temperature at which the vapor pressure is 760 mmHg is the normal boiling point of the liquid.

VAPORS AND VAPORIZATION

When a liquid is left in an open vessel, it will evaporate; when heated, it will evaporate more rapidly. If heat is not added, it will cool as evaporation takes place. The tendency for a liquid to evaporate is related to its vapor pressure, and the amount of heat required for its evaporation is called its heat of vaporization. Both of these quantities vary from liquid to liquid and also with temperature.

The molecules of a liquid are in continuous motion, just as are the molecules of a gas; however, liquid molecules influence one another more strongly and, because of this, are much more restricted in their motion. When a moving liquid molecule approaches the surface with sufficient velocity, it will escape from the liquid phase and become a vapor molecule in the gas phase. Some of the vapor molecules above a liquid in a partially filled closed container will also strike the surface of the liquid and re-enter it. With any liquid-vapor system this is a dynamic process; molecules are continually entering and leaving the liquid phase. When the liquid

and its vapor are in equilibrium,† the partial pressure which the vapor exerts is called its vapor pressure. At a higher temperature, there are more molecules in the vapor phase and the vapor pressure is higher. The numerical value of the vapor pressure is determined by the specific liquid and its temperature. Each liquid, whether it be liquid oxygen at −180 C, nitrous oxide in a cylinder, or ether at room temperature, has a specific vapor pressure for each temperature. Curves such as those shown in Figure 3.1 are obtained when the values of vapor pressure and temperature are plotted.

The vapor pressure of an anesthetic agent and its heat of vaporization (see below) determine its ability to vaporize. The marked difference in the ease of vaporizing ether as compared to methoxyflurane is reflected in their vapor pressures at room temperature (Fig. 3.1).

Vapors may be treated in a similar manner to gases with one exception.

---

† That is, when the number of molecules entering the gas phase are equal to the number leaving the gas phase in a given time period.

When using the gas law and the law of partial pressures with vapors, it must be remembered that a vapor cannot exist at partial pressures above its vapor pressure. The volume percent of a saturated vapor may be calculated from its vapor pressure and the total pressure. For example, ether has a vapor pressure of 442 torr at 20 C, and if the total pressure is 760 torr then:

$$\frac{442}{760} \times 100 = 58.1 \text{ vol } \% \text{ ether}$$

If the only other gas present is oxygen, its partial pressure is 760 less 442 torr (the vapor pressure of ether at 20 C); therefore its volume percent is:

$$\frac{318}{760} \times 100 = 41.9 \text{ vol } \% \text{ oxygen}$$

The boiling point of a liquid is defined as that temperature at which its vapor pressure is equal to the prevailing atmospheric pressure. Customarily, the boiling point is stated for the standard pressure of 760 torr. At the boiling point, the vapor pressure is equal to the ambient pressure and bubbles of vapor form within the liquid.

When a liquid is confined in a strong vessel and heated, its vapor pressure will continue to rise with temperature even though this pressure may rise far above atmospheric pressure. At some point, known as the critical temperature, the liquid phase will cease to exist and the contents of the vessel will consist only of vapor. The pressure in the vessel at this critical temperature is known as the critical pressure. At any temperature above the critical temperature, a liquid phase cannot exist, no matter how high the pressure may be. Critical temperatures vary widely; for oxygen it is −119 C; for nitrous oxide, 36.5 C; and for ether, 194 C. When a confined liquid is heated above its critical temperature, the pressure of its vapor increases according to the general gas law—although vapors under these conditions rarely behave as ideal gases.

The volume of gas which will be produced by the evaporation of a liquid may be readily calculated from the gas laws.

One mole of a liquid will evaporate to 1 mole of gas. For example, the volume of ether vapor at 20 C and 1 atm formed upon evaporation of 1 g of ether will be:

$$PV = nRT = \left(\frac{\text{weight}}{\text{molecular weight}}\right) RT$$

$$(1.0)(V) = \frac{1 \text{ g}}{74} \times 0.082 \times (273 + 20) \text{ K}$$

$$V = \frac{0.082 \times 293}{74}$$

$$V = 0.324 \text{ l} = 324 \text{ ml of ether vapor}$$

The molecular weight of ether, 74, is the sum of the atomic weight of all of the atoms in the ether molecule. To simplify the calculation, it is nearly correct to assume that 1 mole of any vapor will occupy 24 liters under ordinary room conditions, thus:

$$V = \frac{1}{74} \times 24$$

$$V = 308 \text{ ml of ether vapor}$$

Ordinarily, volumes rather than weights of liquids are measured. Liquid volume may be converted to weight by multiplying the volume in milliliters by the density in grams per milliliter:

(Volume, ml) × (density, g/ml)
$$= \text{grams of liquid}$$

To calculate the percent composition of the gas flowing from an efficient vaporizer, that is, one that produces complete saturation of the carrier gas with the volatilized agent, it is necessary only to know the temperature of the liquid and its vapor pressure at that temperature.‡ The volume of gas plus vapor leaving the vaporizer will be equal to the volume of gas entering plus the volume of vapor generated by evaporation. Since the concentration of an anesthetic vapor leaving an efficient vaporizer is ordinarily far in excess of that required, this effluent is diluted with oxygen and then delivered to the

‡ The degree of vapor saturation produced by wick and simple bubbler vaporizers varies widely with the rate of gas flow and other factors, and complete vapor saturation may not occur.

anesthetic circuit. What is the concentration of halothane being delivered from the machine if a flow of 120 ml/minute of oxygen through a Copper Kettle (Foregger Company) filled with halothane and at 20 C is diluted with 1 liter/minute of oxygen? The barometric pressure is 755 torr. The vapor pressure of halothane at 20 C is 243 torr.

1. The vapor concentration of halothane in the vaporizer and leaving it will be equal to the partial pressure of halothane divided by the total pressure:

$$\text{Percent halothane} = \frac{243}{755} \times 100 = 32.2\%$$

2. The volume of gas plus vapor leaving the vaporizer will be the original volume of oxygen flowing into the vaporizer plus the volume of halothane vapor added to it. Since the vapor concentration is known from Step 1 and the volume of oxygen is given, the volume of halothane may be calculated from the equation relating percent concentration of halothane and the flow of oxygen through the vaporizer:

$$\text{Percent halothane} = \frac{V_h}{V_h + V_o} \times 100$$

$$32.2\% = \frac{V_h}{V_h + 120} \times 100$$

$$32.2(V_h + 120) = V_h(100)$$

$$32.2V_h + 3864 = 100V_h$$

$$67.8V_h = 3864$$

$$V_h = 56.9 \text{ ml}$$

3. Dilution with oxygen:

$$V_t = V_h + V_o + V_o'$$

$$= 57 + 120 + 1000$$

$$= 1177 \text{ ml}$$

4. Final halothane concentration:

$$\text{Percent halothane} = \frac{V_h}{V_t} \times 100$$

$$= \frac{57}{1177} \times 100 = 4.8\%$$

where V_h = volume of halothane vapor; V_o = volume of oxygen through vaporizer; V_o' = volume of diluting oxygen; and V_t = total delivered volume. Similar calculations may be made for the vaporization and dilution of any volatile agent.

The evaporation of a liquid requires heat, and the amount of heat needed varies with the liquid. This is related to the forces that attract the molecules to one another and hold them together as a liquid. If a liquid evaporates without the absorption of heat from its surroundings, it will use its own heat and thus cool. The amount of heat necessary to evaporate a quantity of liquid to its vapor state without any change in temperature is called its latent heat of vaporization. The latent heat of vaporization is usually expressed as calories per gram of liquid. This heat is not lost when the liquid evaporates, but is stored in the vapor as latent heat. If the vapor is condensed to liquid, the same amount of heat will be given up. The values usually given for the heat of vaporization are those for the normal boiling point. At temperatures below the boiling point, a larger amount of heat is required for vaporization. The additional heat is equal to that needed to raise the liquid to its boiling point less the heat that would be given up by cooling the vapor from the boiling point to the lower temperature. These two quantities of heat are not the same, since the specific heat (the amount of heat required to heat or cool 1 g of the substance) of the vapor is less than that of the liquid.

SOLUBILITY OF GASES IN LIQUIDS

Gases and vapors dissolve in liquids just as solids do. The amount of gas which will dissolve depends on the identity and partial pressure of the gas, the nature of the liquid, and the temperature. Henry's law states that the amount of gas which dissolves in a liquid is directly proportional to the partial pressure of the gas, or

$$V = \alpha P$$

where V is the volume of gas dissolved, P is the partial pressure of that gas, and α is the solubility coefficient for a gas in a particular liquid at a given temperature. A different value of α is needed for each gas-liquid combination and temperature. Ta-

TABLE 3.2
Solubility coefficients at 38 C

Gas	Water	Plasma*	Blood*
Oxygen	2.32	2.09	2.30
Carbon dioxide	55.5	54.1	54.1
Nitrogen	1.27	1.17	1.33

* Human.

ble 3.2 gives some values of α for gases in water, in blood plasma, and whole blood at 37 C. These coefficients are for physical solubility only and do not include solubility due to a chemical reaction such as the combination of oxygen with hemoglobin or the formation of bicarbonate from carbon dioxide and water.

Henry's law applies individually to each gas in a gas mixture. Each gas will dissolve in the liquid according to its partial pressure, as though it alone were present. For example, human blood plasma at 38 C in equilibrium with alveolar air will contain:§

$$V = \frac{\text{partial pressure of gas}}{\alpha \text{ barometric pressure}}$$

$$V = 2.30 \times \frac{100}{760}$$

$$= 0.30 \text{ ml } O_2/100 \text{ ml of plasma}$$

$$V = 1.33 \times \frac{573}{760}$$

$$= 1.0 \text{ ml } N_2/100 \text{ ml of plasma}$$

If an anesthetic agent were also present in the alveoli, it too would dissolve in the blood according to its partial pressure and solubility coefficient.

The solubility of a gas or vapor in a liquid and its α value vary with temperature. Solubility decreases as temperatures increase. The value of α will have a smaller numerical value at higher temperatures.

The solubility coefficient of a gas dissolved in a liquid may be expressed in several different ways. The Bunsen ab-

sorption coefficient is the amount of gas, expressed as its volume reduced to standard temperature and pressure, which will dissolve in 1 volume of liquid when the partial pressure of the gas above the liquid is 1 atm (760 torr). The Ostwald solubility coefficient is the volume of gas absorbed by a unit volume of liquid when the partial pressure of the gas is 1 atm, the volume of gas being expressed at the temperature of the experiment. The partition coefficient is the ratio of concentrations of the gas in the gas phase and in the liquid phase. Any concentration units may be used (volume percent, milligram percent, milligrams per milliliter, etc.) as long as the same units are used for both phases. As with the other coefficients, the partition (distribution) coefficient varies with temperature. Partition coefficients may also be used to relate the ratios of concentrations in any two phases which are in equilibrium, such as liquid-liquid (*e.g.*, oil/water), liquid-solid, or gas-solid.

Another important method of expressing the presence of a gas in a liquid is the so-called "partial pressure" of the gas in the liquid. There is no actual gas pressure in the liquid; however, the partial pressure of a gas in a liquid expresses the pressure in the gas phase which would be in equilibrium with the liquid. The chemical or biological activity of a gas in a tissue is often more closely related to its partial pressure than to its concentration. Partial pressure also is a convenient concept to use, since, at equilibrium, the partial pressure in all phases—for instance, alveolar air, blood, watery tissue, and lipoid tissue—is the same, while concentrations in these spaces may vary widely according to the solubility in that tissue.

The rate of induction of inhalation anesthesia is related to the magnitude of the blood-gas partition coefficient (often referred to as the "solubility") of an anesthetic agent.

The potency of anesthetics has been related to the distribution of the agents between aqueous and lipid phases. The blood-gas distribution of an agent may be considered in the same manner as the dis-

§ The partial pressures of atmospheric gases in the alveoli are reduced by dilution with water vapor and carbon dioxide. The partial pressure of oxygen is 100 torr and that of nitrogen, 573 torr.

tribution of any gas in any liquid. Anesthetic agents vary widely in their distributions between gas and blood and between aqueous and lipid phases. Table 3.3 presents values of the blood/gas, brain/blood, and oil/water ratios for some common agents. The values are approximately correct, but the exact values vary somewhat from animal to animal even within a given species.

PHYSICAL PROPERTIES OF ANESTHETIC AGENTS

A knowledge of the physical properties of anesthetic agents serves a number of

TABLE 3.3

Ostwald solubility coefficients of some anesthetic gases at 37 C and 760 Torr*

Agent	Solubility Coefficients in		
	Blood/gas	Brain/blood	Oil/water
Cyclopropane	0.42		34
Nitrous oxide	0.49	1.1	3
Halothane	2.3	2.6	330
Trichlorethylene	9.2		
Chloroform	10.3	1.0	70
Diethyl ether	15.2	1.1	3
Methoxyflurane	13.0	22.1 (gray)	400
		30.9 (white)	
Divinyl ether	1		41

* Data from Adriani,[1] Larson,[5] Larson et al.,[6] and Abbott Laboratories, North Chicago, Ill.

purposes. They form the basis for quantitative calculations relating to vapor concentrations, amounts dissolved in body fluids, gas volumes, etc. They also allow for comparisons between agents regarding such things as speed of induction and ease of vaporization. Table 3.4 lists some of the important physical properties of common agents. Solubility data have been given in Table 3.3.

Anesthetic Agents and Their Properties

Inhalation anesthetic agents are a diverse group of chemicals, ranging from the monatomic noble gas xenon and the simple triatomic nitrous oxide to the relatively complex methoxyflurane with its 12 atoms of five chemical elements. These substances appear to have little in common chemically. For many years it was believed that the one common factor that united the inhalation agents was their chemical inertness within the body. These drugs were believed to enter and leave the body completely unchanged and to exert their effects in a purely physical manner. However, recent work with radioactive tracers has shown that cyclopropane, ether, fluoroxene, halothane, and methoxyflurane, among others, are metabolized *in vivo* to urinary metabolites and carbon dioxide.[3, 10] At the present time, it is not

TABLE 3.4

Physical properties of anesthetic agents

Agent	Formula	Molecular Weight	Boiling Point	Vapor Pressure at 20 C	Heat of Vaporization*	Specific Gravity of	
						Liquid (water, 1.0 at 20 C)	Vapor (air, 1.0)
			°C	torr	cal/g		
Nitrous oxide	N_2O	44	−89	39,500	41	1.23*	1.5
Ethylene	C_2H_4	28	−102	†		†	0.97
Cyclopropane	C_3H_6	42	−33	4,800	114	0.68*	1.4
Divinyl ether	$(C_2H_3)_2O$	70	28	550	89	0.77	2.4
Diethyl ether	$(C_2H_5)_2O$	74	35	442	84	0.71	2.6
Chloroform	$CHCl_3$	119	61	160	59	1.48	4.1
Ethyl chloride	C_2H_5Cl	64	12	1000	92‡	0.92	2.2
Trichlorethylene	$CHCl=CCl_2$	131	87	60	58	1.47	4.5
Methoxyflurane	$CH_3—O—CF_2CHCl_2$	165	105	23	59	1.42	5.7
Halothane	$CF_3CHBrCl$	197	50	243	35	1.86	6.8

* At the normal boiling point.
† Critical temperature is below 20 C.
‡ At 20 C.

known whether the physical or biochemical properties of the agents are responsible for the production of the anesthetic state.

An important consideration with the use of anesthetic agents is their flammability. Many commonly used agents form flammable or explosive mixtures with air, oxygen, or oxygen-nitrous oxide throughout the concentration range useful for anesthesia. For an explosion or fire to occur, three things are necessary: an oxidizer, a fuel, and a source of ignition. Since an oxidizer, oxygen, is required when giving an anesthetic, and the anesthetic agent is often a flammable fuel, it is important to remove sources of ignition from anesthetizing locations. The sources of ignition may be a static spark, an electrical arc or spark, an open flame, or a hot surface. To protect against these ignition sources, floors, tables, anesthesia equipment, and personnel are made electrically conductive to drain off static charges before they accumulate to the point where they can produce a spark. Electrical equipment is housed in sealed "explosion-proof" containers or kept high above the floor. (All flammable anesthetic vapors except ethylene are heavier than air and will tend to remain in the lower portion of the room.) Hot cautery is not used with flammable agents. High relative humidity (>50%) is recommended for the air in anesthetizing locations. While explosions are a very rare complication of anesthesia, their serious nature along with the complexity of the steps necessary to prevent their occurrence makes nonflammable agents very desirable.

For a fire or explosion to occur, not only must a fuel and an oxidizer be present, but also they must be present in the proper proportions. If too little fuel or too little oxidizer is present, combustion will not occur. These concentrations, which vary with the agent and the oxidizer, are called the lower explosive limit and the upper explosive limit and are expressed in terms of concentrations of the fuel. When the fuel concentration is less than the lower explosive limit, combustion cannot occur; when the fuel concentration is above the upper explosive limit, and thus the concentration of oxidizer is small, combustion cannot occur. The explosive limits are usually given for the concentration of the fuel in air and in oxygen. For practical purposes, all of the flammable anesthetic agents except trichlorethylene and methoxyflurane are used in the explosive range during clinical anesthesia. The explosive limits for a number of anesthetic agents are given in Table 3.5.

The distinction between an explosion and a fire is one of degree. A fire is a more controlled process and less destructive. The combustion of gas and air in a Bunsen burner is an example. If the same proportions of gas and air are mixed in a large volume and then ignited, the combustion reaction will propagate rapidly throughout the volume, causing a sudden increase in temperature and thus pressure in the gas, and an explosion will occur. The most destructive form of explosion is a detonation in which the reaction takes place throughout the whole volume essentially instantaneously (*i.e.*, in milliseconds) with an extremely rapid release of energy.

The flammability of an anesthetic agent is related to its chemical structure. In general, any substance which is capable of reacting with oxygen or another oxidizer will burn or explode when ignited in the presence of the oxidizer. In this connection, nitrous oxide, although itself nonflammable, will supply oxygen for combustion.

TABLE 3.5
Lower explosive limits of anesthetic drugs

Agent	Lower Explosive Limits in	
	Air	Oxygen
	volume percent	
Cyclopropane	2.4	2.5
Ether	1.8	2.1
Vinyl ether	1.7	1.8
Chloroform	Nonflammable	
Trichlorethylene		10.3
Halothane	Nonflammable	
Methoxyflurane	7.0*	5.4*

* Greater concentrations than used clinically.

With the exception of nitrous oxide, all clinically used inhalation agents are organic compounds containing carbon and hydrogen with or without other elements. To date, the only method of producing a useful, nonflammable agent has been by the replacement of hydrogen atoms by halogen atoms. If the halogen is chlorine, the anesthetic potency (and often the toxicity) is also increased. When three of the hydrogens of the highly flammable, nonanesthetic methane, CH_4, are replaced with chlorine, the potent, toxic, nonflammable chloroform, $CHCl_3$, is produced. The introduction of three fluorine atoms into ethyl vinyl ether forms fluoroxene (CF_3CH_2—O—CH$=CH_2$), a compound of lessened flammability. Halothane ($CF_3CHBrCl$) is perhaps the most successful example of a highly halogenated, nonflammable anesthetic agent. It may be looked upon as ethyl chloride (CH_3CH_2Cl, flammable), in which four of the five hydrogens have been replaced with fluorine or bromine.[9] We can summarize by saying that, if the percentage of hydrogen in an organic molecule is kept low, it will not be flammable.

While the volatile anesthetic agents in general are quite stable and unreactive chemically under ordinary conditions, all of them will undergo slight decomposition over relatively long periods of time. The amount of decomposition is usually quite small; however, even small amounts of certain decomposition products may be deleterious. Decomposition is usually initiated or accelerated by light (especially ultraviolet) and by oxygen. Storage in dark bottles and the addition of stabilizers reduce decomposition to a negligible point. Some agents, however, should be discarded after they have been exposed to air for periods of time.

In years past, the anesthetist, as well as other users of drugs, were often concerned over the presence of harmful impurities. Pharmacology texts went into some detail on testing for impurities. Modern methods of manufacture and quality control and the supervision by regulatory agencies have essentially eliminated this problem for the clinician. It is rarely, if ever, necessary to test freshly opened drugs for impurities. Those interested in tests for impurities should consult Adriani[1] or the current U.S. Pharmacopeia.

NITROUS OXIDE

Nitrous oxide, N_2O, is the only inorganic compound which is used as an inhalation anesthetic agent although other inorganic substances such as xenon can produce general anesthesia. Nitrous oxide is prepared by thermal decomposition of ammonium nitrate

$$NH_4NO_3 + heat \rightarrow N_2O + H_2O$$

The principal impurities of manufacture are nitrogen (N_2) and the higher oxides, nitric oxide (NO) and nitrogen dioxide (NO_2). Both of the latter compounds, which are toxic, are removed by scrubbing with alkaline potassium permanganate. Nitrogen is removed by liquefying the nitrous oxide and allowing the lower boiling nitrogen to distill out. Nitrous oxide, which is a gas at ambient conditions, is sold as a liquified gas under pressure in cylinders. It is extremely stable and does not undergo any chemical reactions under ordinary conditions. Like air or oxygen, it will support combustion if sufficient energy such as a flame or spark is present to initiate combustion. It will not, however, supply oxygen for lower temperature reactions such as metabolism.

CYCLOPROPANE

Cyclopropane, $\overline{CH_2—CH_2—CH_2}$, is the only hydrocarbon which enjoys much clinical use as an anesthetic agent, although ethylene ($CH_2=CH_2$) and acetylene (CH$=$CH) are occasionally used. A great many other hydrocarbons will produce anesthesia with varying degrees of potency and side effects. Cyclopropane is synthesized by reductive ring closure of a liquid 1,3-dihalogenated propane in a water dispersion:

$$ClCH_2—CH_2—CH_2Cl + Zn \rightarrow$$

$$
\begin{array}{c}
H_2 \\
C \\
\diagup \diagdown \\
H_2C———CH_2
\end{array}
+ ZnCl_2
$$

Since cyclopropane boils at a much lower temperature than the halogenated propane, it is readily separated from the reaction mixture. The principal impurities are propylene ($CH_3CH=CH_2$), halogenated propylenes and propanes (*e.g.*, $Cl \cdot CH_2CH_2CH_3$), and hydrogen from reaction of zinc with water. The unsaturated compounds are removed by chlorination of the double bond which yields much less volatile substances:

$$CH_2 = CH_2CH_3 + Cl_2 \rightarrow CH_2ClCHClCH_3$$

Hydrogen is removed by liquefying the cyclopropane and allowing the hydrogen to escape. Small amounts of propylene (less than 1%) are not harmful; however, pure propylene causes serious cardiac arrhythmias.[1]

Cyclopropane is highly flammable in mixtures with air, oxygen, or nitrous oxide. Cyclopropane is sold in cylinders as a liquefied gas under pressure.

DIETHYL ETHER

Diethyl ether (ethyl ether or ether), $CH_3CH_2—O—CH_2CH_3$, has been used clinically for over 100 years as an anesthetic agent. While it has certain disadvantages, it still has much to recommend it, not the least of which is the considerable background of experience with this drug. Chemically, the name ether connotes two hydrocarbon or substituted hydrocarbon groups linked through an oxygen which may be looked on as water, H—O—H, with the two hydrogens replaced with organic radicals.

Methyl propyl ether (Metopryl, $CH_3—O—CH_2CH_2CH_3$), which is an isomer (that is, it has the same number and kind of atoms in its molecule but arranged differently) of diethyl ether, and ethyl propyl ether, $CH_3CH_2OCH_2CH_2CH_3$, have been studied as anesthetic agents. They have little or no advantage to offer over ethyl ether and are rarely used. The only two

ethers other than ethyl which have any current popularity are divinyl ether and methoxyflurane.

The most important method of synthesizing diethyl ether is the dehydration of ethyl alcohol with sulfuric acid at temperatures below 130 C. The reaction proceeds through the formation of ethylsulfuric acid with the net effect of removal of a molecule of water from two molecules of alcohol.

$$C_2H_5OH + H_2SO_4 \rightarrow$$
$$C_2H_5HSO_4 + H_2O$$

$$C_2H_5HSO_4 + C_2H_5OH \rightarrow$$
$$C_2H_5—O—C_2H_5 + H_2SO_4$$

$$2C_2H_5OH \rightarrow$$
$$C_2H_5—O—C_2H_5 + H_2O$$

When concentrated sulfuric acid, which is a powerful dehydrating agent, becomes sufficiently diluted with water, the reaction stops. Ethyl ether is more volatile than the water, acid, or alcohol and is readily separated by distillation. A small amount of ethyl alcohol which remains with the distillate is desirable and is not removed from anesthetic ether.

Diethyl ether, especially when dry, will form peroxides which are extremely sensitive to shock and are violently explosive. The addition of up to 2% of ethyl alcohol and water to anesthetic ether inhibits the formation of peroxides. Certain metals, especially copper and iron, react preferentially with oxygen and thus also inhibit peroxide formation. Some commercial ether cans are internally copper-plated for this reason.

Ether should be drained periodically from vaporizers and discarded. The U.S. Pharmacopeia XVII requires ether to be discarded if it has been removed from the original container for more than 24 hours. While this is probably unduly conservative, ether should be removed from clear glass jar vaporizers every several days. Ether in metal (especially copper) vaporizers can be used safely for longer periods; however, periodic drainings are advisable.

The alcohol in the ether serves the additional function of lessening the formation of ice on open drop masks. The ice is formed by moisture in the exhaled air being cooled by the evaporating ether.

DIVINYL ETHER

Vinyl ether, $CH_2=CH-O-CH=CH_2$, was synthesized in an attempt to combine the anesthetic properties of two chemical configurations occurring in molecules known to possess anesthetic potency: the ether structure and unsaturation, as exemplified in ethyl ether and ethylene.[7] Whereas, in the light of present concepts, this approach of combining chemical functional groups is less valid, it nonetheless represented a rational approach to the discovery of a new anesthetic agent.

Divinyl ether is prepared by chlorinating diethyl ether to form dichlorodiethyl ether which is reacted with molten potassium hydroxide to form the unsaturated compound

$$ClCH_2CH_2-O-CH_2CH_2Cl + 2KOH \rightarrow$$
$$CH_2=CH-O-CH=CH_2 + 2KCl$$

A number of side reactions reduces the overall yield of these two steps. Impurities are removed by washing, absorption, and distillation, the usual procedures for purification of organic chemicals.

Vinyl ether is much more reactive chemically than ethyl ether because of its double bonds. It does not form peroxides but may be oxidized to form aldehydes or organic acids or may polymerize, especially in the presence of strong mineral acids, to a tacky resin. An inhibitor, N-phenyl-1-naphthylamine (0.01%), is added to retard the polymerization and oxidation reactions. (This inhibitor also causes a purplish fluorescence.) Ethyl alcohol (3.5%) is added to lessen frosting on open drop masks. The U.S. Pharmacopeia XVI requires that divinyl ether be discarded after the container has been opened for 48 hours; however, a well stoppered bottle stored in a cool place is suitable for use for at least 10 days.[1]

CHLOROFORM

Chloroform, $CHCl_3$, like ether and nitrous oxide, was used initially as a general anesthetic agent over 100 years ago. Its potential hepatotoxic and cardiotoxic properties limit its use as a clinical anesthetic.

Chloroform may be prepared by the chlorination of acetone (CH_3COCH_3) or ethyl alcohol in the presence of calcium hydroxide or by the reduction of carbon tetrachloride with iron

$$CCl_4 + H_2O + Fe \rightarrow CHCl_3 + Fe(OH)Cl$$

In the presence of heat, light, and air, chloroform will slowly oxidize to form phosgene ($COCl_2$), a highly toxic gas. Ethyl alcohol (1%) is added to anesthetic chloroform to react with any phosgene formed to produce the nontoxic ethyl carbonate $C_2H_5-O-CO-OC_2H_5$. Chloroform should be kept in tightly stoppered dark bottles in a cool place.

Liquid chloroform cannot be ignited by flame or spark, and its vapor is nonflammable in any concentration in air. Chloroform vapors, however, may form phosgene in the presence of oxygen and a flame or hot surface; thus it should be used cautiously with cautery.

Chloroform does not react to an appreciable degree with soda lime and is safe for use in rebreathing systems. The small amount of reaction which does take place yields nonvolatile products which remain with the soda lime.

TRICHLORETHYLENE

Trichlorethylene, $CHCl=CCl_2$, is a widely used industrial solvent; its analgesic properties were accidentally discovered during commercial use. It is prepared by dechlorination of symmetrical tetrachloroethylene by boiling with lime:

$$2CHCl_2-CHCl_2 + Ca(OH)_2 \rightarrow$$

$$2CH=C\begin{array}{c} Cl \\ \diagup \\ \diagdown \\ Cl \end{array} + CaCl_2$$

Tetrachloroethane may be prepared directly from chlorine and acetylene ($CH\equiv CH$). Like other unsaturated and halogenated compounds, trichlorethylene tends to decompose slowly in the presence of light, oxygen, and moisture. A small amount of thymol (0.01%) is added to retard this decomposition.

Industrial trichlorethylene is stabilized with substances such as amines or cresol which may be toxic and it should not be used clinically. A blue dye is added to anesthetic trichlorethylene to distinguish it from chloroform and other drugs with similar odors.

A unique hazard with trichlorethylene is its reactivity with alkaline substances (such as carbon dioxide absorbents) to form the toxic dichloroacetylene $CCl \equiv CCl$). For this reason, trichlorethylene must never be used in closed circle anesthesia, and equipment used for trichlorethylene anesthesia must be thoroughly freed of this drug before being used in a closed circle. Trichlorethylene can dissolve in rubber and persist for some time. When trichlorethylene has been administered to an animal, the animal should not be put on a rebreathing circuit containing soda lime for several hours. If a rebreathing circuit has been inadvertently contaminated with trichlorethylene, the soda lime should be discarded, the canister washed, the system ventilated, and the rubber and plastic goods allowed to air for a day or so.

Trichlorethylene is metabolized to a significant extent in the body. While it is difficult to ascertain precisely, it appears that as much as one-quarter of the drug which is absorbed by the body may be metabolized to trichloroacetic acid ($Cl_3 \cdot CCOOH$) or trichloroethanol ($Cl_3CCH_2 \cdot OH$). The metabolites are excreted principally in the urine in free or conjugated form for a number of days after administration. There is no evidence that the metabolites are harmful or that they play any part in the mechanism of anesthesia.

Trichlorethylene presents only a slight flammability hazard in oxygen and is nonflammable in air. The temperature of liquid trichlorethylene must be at least 25.5 C in order for its vapor pressure to be great enough to form a flammable mixture.

HALOTHANE

The molecule of halothane, 1,1,1-trifluoro-2-bromo-2-chloroethane ($CF_3CH \cdot$

BrCl), was synthesized as a potent, stable, nontoxic, and nonflammable anesthetic agent. An interesting discussion of its development is given by Suckling.[9]

Starting with trichlorethylene, halothane may be prepared through the series of reactions which include hydrochlorination, fluorination, and bromination:

$$CHCl = CCl_2 + HCl \rightarrow$$
$$CH_2ClCCl_3$$

$$CH_2Cl - CCl_3 + 3HF \rightarrow$$
$$CH_2Cl - CF_3 + 3HCl$$

$$CH_2Cl - CF_3 + Br_2 \rightarrow$$
$$CHBrCl - CF_3 + HBr$$

All reactions are carried out in the vapor phase at elevated temperatures. Antimony pentachloride ($SbCl_5$) is used to catalyze the reaction. The products of the final reaction are washed with dilute sodium hydroxide, dried, and fractionally distilled to yield pure halothane.

The introduction of multiple fluorine atoms into organic molecules conveys unusual properties to the resulting compounds. When two or more fluorine atoms are attached to a single carbon atom, the combination becomes very stable. While other halogens, e.g., chlorine or bromine, are readily removed from groups such as $-CCl_3$, extreme conditions, such as boiling in sodium metal, must be used to break down the $-CF_3$ group. In halothane, the presence of the $-CF_3$ group also stabilizes the bromine and chlorine on the adjacent carbon. Without this stabilization, these atoms would be labile. It should be noted here that, although fluorine is a halogen, neither its organic nor its inorganic chemical compounds react as those of the other halogens. When considering the properties of "halogenated" anesthetics, a distinction should be made between such groupings as $-CF_3$ and $-CF_2$ and carbon-chlorine or bromine compounds. In this respect, fluorine behaves more like a nonflammable hydrogen in the organic molecule.

Like most halogenated anesthetic agents, halothane does have a tendency to decompose in the presence of light and oxygen. This decomposition is inhibited by the addition of thymol (0.01%) and by storage in brown bottles. Long periods of usage of halothane in copper vaporizers do not appear to cause decomposition or an accumulation of impurities. Halothane examined after long use in Copper Kettle vaporizers contained the same quantities of trace impurities as found in freshly opened halothane and an accumulation of thymol and its reaction products.[2] It is unlikely that these thymol compounds present any toxic hazards because of their low volatility, but they do impart a yellow color to the halothane.

Halothane exerts a solvent action on some polymers and will swell rubber and some other plastics. Vapor deposited with moisture slowly decomposes to form halogen acids which will corrode many metals. The reactive metals such as aluminum, zinc, and iron are attacked. Copper is not attacked, but brass may have zinc removed from it.

Liquid halothane will not burn and its vapor is nonflammable in all proportions of air or oxygen.

METHOXYFLURANE

Methoxyflurane, 2,2-dichloro,1,1-difluoroethyl methyl ether ($CHCl_2CF_2$—O—CH_3), is a recently introduced, potent, halogenated anesthetic agent which is nonflammable under ordinary conditions of use. Chemically, it is a chlorinated and fluorinated ether which owes its low flammability to the large proportion of fluorine and chlorine in its molecule. Its vapor is flammable only when the vapor concentration reaches 7% in air, 5.4% in oxygen, or 3.6% in 80% nitrous oxide in oxygen. In order to achieve a flammable concentration in air or oxygen, the liquid and the vapor must be above ordinary room temperatures, about 32 and 37 C respectively; however, the vapor pressure at 23 C in 80% nitrous oxide-oxygen will form a flammable mixture. The concentrations of methoxyflurane available for induction or maintenance of anesthesia with air or oxygen are well below the flammable concentrations. During the induction of anesthesia with 80% nitrous oxide in oxygen, a flammable concentration may be attained if a high efficiency vaporizer such as a Copper Kettle is used and if the temperature of the vaporizer is 23 C or above. Summer temperatures even in temperate zones go well above 23 C, so suitable precautions should be taken when high concentrations of methoxyflurane are used with high concentrations of nitrous oxide.

Methoxyflurane has the highest boiling point of any of the volatile liquids in current use in anesthesia (105 C), and the lowest vapor pressure. The vapor pressure-temperature curve (Fig. 3.1) is similar to that of water. At room temperature, a maximum vapor concentration of about 3.5% can be achieved. It is only because of the high potency of this agent that a sufficient gas concentration is reached to produce anesthesia. Even so, induction of anesthesia with methoxyflurane alone is prolonged because of its low vapor pressure and its high blood/gas partition coefficient. Anesthesia is ordinarily induced with an intravenous barbiturate or other drug.

Methoxyflurane is supplied in dark bottles with an antioxidant, 0.01% butylated hydroxytoluene. The antioxidant gradually becomes discolored and gives a yellow-brown color to the liquid. The manufacturer suggests that vaporizers be drained every day, with the drug being returned to its original container. Methoxyflurane is reported not to harm metal even after prolonged use. The vapor will dissolve in rubber and may revaporize from the rubber parts after discontinuing methoxyflurane.

The aging of rubber parts is accelerated by methoxyflurane. Methoxyflurane will dissolve in and diffuse through many plastics. Plastics such as polyvinylchloride which are softened with plasticizers will have their plasticizers extracted and become hardened.

Information is not available about the synthesis of methoxyflurane.

OXYGEN

Several gases which are not anesthetic agents are important in clinical anesthesia. Oxygen (O_2) is by far the most important. While oxygen may be prepared by the electrolysis of water or by the thermal decomposition of salts such as potassium chlorate ($KClO_3$), the major source of oxygen is the atmosphere. Oxygen is separated from the air by a process which involves compression, cooling, and liquefaction of air. Nitrogen (boiling point, -196 C) and oxygen (boiling point, -183 C) are separated by distillation. Currently, plants are in operation which produce as much as 1000 tons of oxygen a day in the form of gas or liquid. Oxygen gas is handled in steel cylinders at pressures of 2000 to 2400 psi and as a liquid in large vacuum insulated containers at atmospheric pressure. For large scale use, it is often economical to store oxygen as a liquid and vaporize it as it is used, thus avoiding the handling and storage of high pressure cylinders. Commercial oxygen from the major producers is more than 99.5% pure and exceeds the purity requirements of the U.S. Pharmacopeia in all respects. The impurities in oxygen are mainly argon and nitrogen which are physiologically inert in these concentrations. Oxygen sold for medical use is commonly from the same source as commercial oxygen, but may be subject to more rigorous testing. In addition, medical oxygen cylinders are cleaned and painted regularly.

CARBON DIOXIDE

Carbon dioxide (CO_2) is produced by burning carbonaceous fuel in air or as a by-product of fermentation. Pure carbon dioxide is marketed in cylinders as a liquid under pressure or as the solid Dry Ice. Mixtures of 5 to 10% carbon dioxide in oxygen are available as a compressed gas in cylinders.

HELIUM

Helium (He) is used as a diluent gas in anesthetic gas-oxygen mixtures to reduce flammability. Because of its lower density, helium flows through small openings readily. Helium-oxygen mixtures, for this reason, are used in conditions of increased airway resistance such as asthma. The low solubility of helium allows it to remain in an inactive lung for a longer period than a more soluble gas such as oxygen or nitrogen, thus preventing the lung from collapsing.

Helium is an inert elemental gas. It does not enter into any chemical reactions and will not burn or support combustion. The only important sources of helium are natural gas wells in the United States and Canada. It is present in the natural gas (mainly methane, CH_4) to the extent of 0.5% or less. It has the lowest boiling point of any known substance and is separated from the natural gas by distillation.

The Chemistry of Carbon Dioxide Absorption

The removal of metabolic carbon dioxide from anesthetic rebreathing systems is accomplished by chemical absorption by the hydroxide of an alkali or alkaline earth metal, for example:

$$CO_2 + 2NaOH \rightarrow Na_2CO_3 + H_2O$$

$$CO_2 + Ca(OH)_2 \rightarrow CaCO_3 + H_2O$$

$$CO_2 + Ba(OH)_2 \rightarrow BaCO_3 + H_2O$$

The basic reactions in any case are the hydration and ionization of carbon dioxide followed by the neutralization of hydrogen ions by hydroxyl ions:

$$CO_2 + H_2O \rightleftharpoons H_2CO_3 \rightleftharpoons 2H^+ + CO_3^=$$

$$2H^+ + 2OH^- \rightarrow 2H_2O$$

The neutralization reaction liberates a considerable quantity of heat (13.8 kg cal/mole of water formed). Water is necessary to hydrate carbon dioxide and to provide a reaction medium; consequently, absorbents are prepared with water in their composition.

Any alkaline hydroxide could be used to absorb carbon dioxide; however, for the practical reasons of speed of carbon dioxide absorption, freedom from excessive caking or dusting, adequate particle strength, and low cost, only two preparations are widely used. One, soda lime, which was developed for use in World War I gas masks, consists of calcium hydroxide with 5% sodium hydroxide, a small amount of silica (SiO_2) (to give strength to the particles), and 14 to 18% water. The other, barium hydroxide lime, is a mixture of 20% barium hydroxide octahydrate, $Ba(OH)_2 \cdot 8H_2O$, with calcium hydroxide. Water is not added, but is provided by the water of hydration of the barium hydroxide.

Both substances function adequately as carbon dioxide absorbers. Both are strongly alkaline and are corrosive to skin and mucous membranes. Barium hydroxide is also quite toxic if ingested.

Compressed Gases

SUPPLY AND STORAGE

Except in the simplest kind of anesthetic administration, it is necessary to use compressed gases of which oxygen, nitrous oxide, and cyclopropane are the most common, although many other gases including helium, nitrogen, carbon dioxide, ethylene, acetylene, and compressed air may be used in some circumstances. Compressed gases are stored in cylinders made of low alloy steel and dispensed through a valve screwed into the neck. Sizes range (in the United States) from the 10½-inch high A cylinder to the 55-inch G or H cylinder (Table 3.6). In the United States, the construction and testing of compressed gas cylinders is strictly regulated by the Interstate Commerce Commission. Cylinders are stamped near the top to indicate the metal alloy used, allowable working pressure, the owner, and his serial number and dates when the cylinder was retested.

High pressure cylinders must be retested every 5 years by subjecting them to pressures 1.66 times the normal working pressure. Larger gas cylinders such as those for oxygen therapy ordinarily have threaded outlet fittings to which a pressure-reducing valve may be fitted. There are different standard thread and fitting types for the different medical gases

TABLE 3.6

*Compressed gas cylinder specifications**

Agent	A (2.8 × 10.5 inches)	B (3.5 × 16 inches)	D (4 × 20 inches)	E (4 × 30 inches)	M (7 × 47 inches)	G (8 × 55 inches)	H (9 × 55 inches)	Filling Pressure (Nominal)
				liters				*psig†*
Oxygen	76§	151	360	655	3,030	5,290	6,910	2,200
Nitrous oxide‡	190	380	950	1,590	7,570	12,110	14,520	800
Cyclopropane‡	152	380	870	1,440	6,990	12,110		79
Ethylene	114	380	760	1,250	6,060	10,600		1,250
Carbon dioxide‡	151	380	950	1,590	7,570	4,160		800
Helium	57	106	300	500	2,290	4,350	5,930	1,650

* The cylinder sizes and designations are those commonly used in the United States by medical gas manufacturers. Sizes and contents as well as filling pressures may vary slightly. Gases for industrial use may be supplied in cylinders of different sizes, designations, and pressures; however, the volume of gas in the cylinder (at 70 F and 1 atm) is usually specified on the label.

† Pressures given are nominal values and depend on the cylinder test pressure and the manufacturer's practices; for example, oxygen cylinders in common use have test pressures of 1800, 2200, or 2400 psig.

‡ These gases are liquids under pressure in the cylinder. The pressure noted is their vapor pressure at room temperature.

§ Equivalents:

1 liter	= 0.264 gallons	= 0.035 cubic feet
1 cubic foot	= 28.3 liters	= 7.48 gallons
1 gallon	= 3.79 liters	= 0.132 cubic feet

TABLE 3.7

Color code for compressed gas cylinders

Gas	Color
Oxygen	Green (U.S.), white (WHO
Carbon dioxide	Gray
Nitrous oxide	Light blue
Cyclopropane	Orange
Helium	Brown
Ethylene	Red (U.S.), purple (WHO

which do not allow reducing valves to be fitted incorrectly to cylinders in such a manner as to create a hazard.

The smaller cylinders which fit directly on most anesthesia machines have a flush-type medical outlet with pin indexing. The pin index system, designed to prevent the accidental interchange of cylinders, consists of two small holes in the valve body on the arc of a circle concentric with the gas outlet. Pins on the yoke to which the cylinder is fitted match these holes. Each gas or gas mixture for use in anesthesia has a specific location for these holes. For easy identification, cylinders are painted different colors which indicate their contents. Cylinders containing gas mixtures show both colors on the shoulder. The recommended color coding of the U.S. Bureau of Standards and of the World Health Organization are shown in Table 3.7. Industrial gas cylinders, on the other hand, are painted a wide variety of colors depending on the manufacturer's desires. Standardization of cylinder outlet fittings for industrial gases is progressing rapidly (in the United States).

At room temperature, cyclopropane, nitrous oxide, and carbon dioxide are below their critical temperatures and will liquefy under pressure. Cylinders of these gases as sold contain about two-thirds of their volume filled with liquid and one-third with compressed vapor. On the other hand, oxygen, helium, and ethylene are above their critical temperatures and will not liquefy under any amount of pressure. They are marketed as compressed gases. Cylinders containing liquid will be under a pressure equal to the vapor pressure of the liquid at the ambient temperature. At

room temperature (20 C), this is about 78 psig for cyclopropane, 735 psi for nitrous oxide, and 825 psig for carbon dioxide. Cylinders of these gases will exhibit a constant pressure until all of the contained liquid has vaporized. In actual use the liquid may cool appreciably from heat loss from vaporization and cause the pressure to drop. Compressed gas cylinders are usually filled to pressures between 1800 and 2400 psig according to the type of cylinder used.

Compressed and liquefied gases in cylinders present the twin hazards of pressure and combustion. A cylinder of gas at 2000 psig can jet propel itself through a concrete block wall if the valve is broken off at the neck. Gas escaping freely from a cylinder valve can penetrate skin, causing severe trauma. For this reason, a cylinder valve should never be opened unless the outlet is pointed away from people or animals. No comment is necessary on the damages that might be caused by high pressure gases directly entering the trachea. In addition to the hazards of high pressure, which are the same for all gases, there are hazards of oxidation and combustion. Oxygen and nitrous oxide under pressure are strong oxidizing agents and will cause oil, grease, or other combustible matter to explode on contact. Nothing which will come in contact with compressed oxygen or nitrous oxide should be oiled or greased. This includes pressure-reducing valves, needle valves, tubing, fittings, components of anesthesia machines, etc. (Special noncombustible greases and oils are available; however, no lubricant should be used without the assurance of the equipment manufacturer that it is suitable.) Equipment such as reducing valves, tubing, etc. which has been used for combustible gases should never be put in oxygen or nitrous oxide service.

PRESSURE-REDUCING VALVES

Pressure-reducing valves as used in anesthesia machines or directly on compressed gas cylinders serve to reduce the pressure of the gas in the cylinder to some lower value. They also provide a constant pressure at the outlet over a wide range of flows, as long as the cylinder contains adequate gas pressure. This low constant pressure provides three distinct advantages. First, since it applies a constant pressure to the needle valve which controls flow to the flowmeter, the gas flow will not drop as the cylinder pressure falls. The flowmeter will not have to be continuously reset to maintain a constant flow. Second, a large pressure drop across the needle valve, as would result from direct connection to high pressure, would make the flow rate extremely sensitive to even small changes in the needle valve setting. Third, only a small portion of the gas system operates at the more hazardous high pressures.

In addition to the one-stage regulator, two-stage regulators are also available. These regulators give a better control of pressure and are desirable for applications which require close control. Two-stage regulators are, in effect, two one-stage regulators in which the low pressure side of the first stage serves as the high pressure side of the second stage. Externally, a two-stage regulator is often indistinguishable from a one-stage regulator. For a more detailed coverage of the subject, the reader is referred to MacIntosh et al.[8]

FLOWMETERS

The gas flowmeters in current use in anesthesia depend on the fact that the rate of flow through a restriction is dependent on the pressure difference on the two sides of the restriction. Two types of flowmeters are common: the variable and the fixed orifice. In the variable, the orifice is the annular space between a movable float and a tapered transparent tube; in the fixed, the orifice is a small hole drilled in a metal block. In both cases, the rate of flow is altered by changing the pressure upstream to the orifice. The most common type of flowmeter for anesthetic machines is the rotameter, which consists of a bobbin or float moving in a tapered vertical tube (Fig. 3.2). Gas flows into the bottom of the tube, around the float, and

out of the top of the tube. The annular space between the float and the tube may be looked upon as the variable orifice. A gas flowing through this restriction undergoes a drop in pressure. This pressure differential from the bottom to the top of the float lifts the float up in the tapered tube, rising until it reaches a point where the pressure drop across it is just sufficient to support its weight. It remains at that point as long as the gas flow is constant.

The pressure drop is ordinarily quite small, approximately 1 cm of water. The floats in most rotameters are designed so that they rotate (hence the name) in the flowing gas to avoid friction with the wall of the tube. Certain older types of flowmeters are inclined from the vertical, but the effect of wall friction is taken into account in their calibration.

Two physical constants of the gas govern the rate of flow of gas in a rotameter: the viscosity and the density. If the annu-

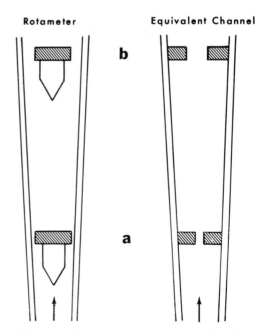

FIG. 3.2. Rotameter flowmeter. a, at low flows, the length of the annulus between the float head and the tube is greater than its width. The equivalent channel (right) is a tube. b, at high flows the width of the annulus between the float head and the tube is greater than its length. The equivalent channel (right) is an orifice.

lar space between the float and the tube approximates a capillary tube (if the length of the annulus is large in relation to its width), the viscosity of the gas is the flow-controlling physical constant. This is the condition that generally prevails at

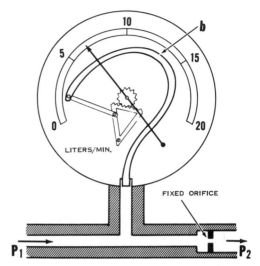

FIG. 3.4. Fixed orifice flowmeter. Gas enters at P_1 at a pressure set by adjustment of the pressure-reducing valve, passes through the orifice. P_1 is measured by the Bourdon tube, b, and indicated on the scale. Since P_2 is a constant pressure (just slightly above atmospheric) the flow through the orifice depends only on P_1 and the rate of flow may be varied by varying P_1. Pressure in the Bourdon tube causes it to expand and to thus increase the radius of its arc, which, through mechanical linkages, rotates the pointer. While the gauge actually measures the pressure, P_1, it indirectly measures flow and is calibrated in flow units. The Bourdon tube principle is also used in most pressure gauges.

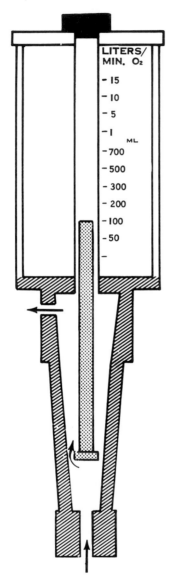

FIG 3.3. Heidbrink flowmeter. The Heidbrink flowmeter is similar to the rotameter, except that the variable orifice is in a metal tube below the scale and the taper of the tube is not uniform. The tube is ground to two tapers to accommodate a wider range of flows while still permitting somewhat accurate measurements at low flows.

low flows when the float is near the bottom of the tube. On the other hand, when the annulus approximates an orifice, that is, when the diameter is large in comparison to its length, the density of the gas assumes a more important role in governing the flow rate. When the float is nearer the top of the tube, the annulus is more like an orifice (Fig. 3.2). Both viscosity and density influence the flow of a gas through a rotameter, thus, the calibration scale on a rotameter is valid only for a single gas. Flowmeters must be recalibrated for use with another gas.

The Heidbrink flowmeter is similar to the rotameter except that the tapered tube is metal and its bore has been machined to a series of tapers. This allows a wide range of flows to be measured on a short scale. The float itself is not visible, but an extension of the float rises into a glass tube with an adjacent flow scale (Fig. 3.3). Because of the wide range of flows, the Heidbrink flowmeter is not as accurate as the rotameter.

A fixed orifice flowmeter is more commonly used in oxygen therapy than in anesthesia. This is a Bourdon tube pressure gauge with a fixed metal orifice (Fig. 3.4). These flowmeters are often mounted as an integral part of a pressure-reducing valve with the low pressure gauge being calibrated in liters per minute rather than in pressure units. The only difference between this flowmeter and a reducing valve is the insertion of a calibrated orifice in the outflow tube.

The Bourdon tube flowmeter is not as accurate as rotameter flowmeters mainly because of the inaccuracies of the pressure gauge. If the orifice becomes plugged or enlarged, the accuracy will be affected. Any back pressure built up on the outflow side will also make the meter inaccurate. This type of flowmeter will indicate flow even if its outlet is occluded. Bourdon tube flowmeters are unsatisfactory for low flows and are ordinarily calibrated for flow rates of 1 or 2 liters/minute and above. The pressure on the higher side of the orifice may reach 50 psig.

REFERENCES

1. Adriani, J.: *The Chemistry and Physics of Anesthesia*, 2nd ed. Charles C. Thomas, Publisher, Springfield, Ill., 1962.
2. Butler, R. A., and Linde, H. W.: Trace compounds in halothane. Anesthesiology *25:* 397, 1964.
3. Greene, N. M.: The metabolism of drugs employed in anesthesia. I and II. Anesthesiology *29:* 127, 1966.
4. Lambertsen, C. J.: Gas exchanges of the atmosphere, lungs and blood. In *Medical Physiology*, edited by P. Bard, p. 574. The C. V. Mosby Company, St. Louis, 1961.
5. Larson, C. P.: Solubility and partition coefficients. In *Uptake and Distribution of Anesthetic Agents*, edited by E. M. Papper and R. J. Kitz, chap. 1. Blakiston Division, McGraw-Hill Book Company, Inc., New York, 1963.
6. Larson, C. P., Eger, E. I. II, and Severinghaus, J. W.: Ostwald solubility coefficients for anesthetic gases in various fluids and tissue. Anesthesiology *28:* 686, 1962.
7. Leake, C. D., and Chen, M.: Anesthetic properties of certain unsaturated ethers. Proc. Soc. Exp. Biol. Med. *28:* 151, 1930.
8. MacIntosh, R., Mushin, W. S., and Epstein, H. G.: *Physics for the Anesthetist*, 3rd ed. Blackwell Scientific Publications, Oxford, 1963.
9. Suckling, C. W.: Some chemical and physical factors in the development of Fluothane. Brit. J. Anaesth. *29:* 466, 1957.
10. Van Dyke, R. A., and Chenoweth, M. B.: Metabolism of volatile anesthetics. Anesthesiology *26:* 348, 1965.

4

Factors Affecting the Alveolar Tension of an Anesthetic Gas

THEODORE C. SMITH

The concept of dose (of deworming tables or penicillin injections) seems unambiguous to most. The dose of inhalation anesthetics is not intuitively clear, since during anesthesia an increasingly large fraction of inhaled drug is immediately exhaled. Several studies in the last decade have put the concept of dosage of anesthetic agents on a pharmacologically rational basis. Two concepts are postulated. The first is that it is the partial pressure within brain tissues of an anesthetic gas or vapor which measures the effect, and hence the dose. The second is that the partial pressure in the brain is directly related to (and nearly equal to) the anesthetic tension within the alveoli. In the following discussion we examine the rise of alveolar concentration of anesthetic agents during induction of inhalation anesthesia. Starting with a simple model of the lung, we increase the complexity of the model in three stages— as aids in understanding basic ideas, pharmacokinetics, and certain special effects in the induction of anesthesia. The first model assumes that negligible quantities of the anesthetic (an inert, insoluble agent) are delivered to or removed from the alveoli, except by process of respiration. The second model considers the fact that anesthetics are moderately or highly soluble in body fluids and, hence, are removed from the alveoli by the pulmonary blood flow and distributed to the rest of the body. The last model stipulates that anesthetic agents are presented to the patient in the inspired gas in varied concentrations, depending on factors involving the breathing circuit, the animal's respiration, and the intentions of the anesthetist.

The Rise of Alveolar Concentration of an Inert, Insoluble Gas

To start, we develop an intuitive idea of an exponential or first order process for a simple model. The phrase "exponential process" or "first order reaction" is used in describing a specific pattern of change which has wide applications in chemistry and biology. The rate of excretion of Bromsulphalein (the BSP liver test), the mixing of an intravenous dose of thiopental with the entire blood volume, and the approach of reacting chemical species to equilibrium are all described by exponential processes. Their common characteristic is that the rate of reaction is proportional to the concentration of reactant. In other words, the more there is of a reactant, the faster the reaction. As the reaction uses up a reactant, the reaction slows down.

THE FIRST MODEL

As an illustration, consider 1 gallon of ink in a punch bowl (Fig. 4.1) which is

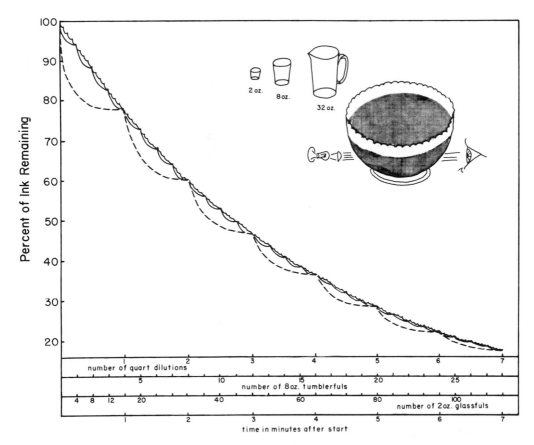

FIG. 4.1. The punch bowl experiment. Ink in a bowl of 1-gallon capacity is diluted by adding clear water, mixing, and emptying. The rate of adding and of emptying is 1 quart/minute, but three different containers are used to do it: a quart pitcher once per minute, a water glass four times per minute, and a shot glass 16 times per minute. The ink remaining decreases in a similar way for all three. As the steps are made smaller (and correspondingly faster) they approach a smooth curve called a decreasing exponential, characterized by a rate (slope) proportional to the amount remaining.

progressively diluted by a quart of clear water. Fill a quart pitcher with water, empty it into a punch bowl, mix, and remove a quart of the resulting mixture. The volume of solution in the bowl is the same as we started with, but the ink is now somewhat diluted. After a minute refill the pitcher with clear water, empty it into the punch bowl, mix, and empty another quart down the drain. The ink is again a little more diluted. As we continue this process, the color of the fluid in the bowl gets progressively lighter. After the first few steps you might be able to see some light transmitted through the solution and after more steps the solution will be obviously transparent although still

darkly colored. However, as we continue the process of diluting, mixing, and emptying, the decrease in color becomes less and less marked. After perhaps 20 repetitions, we find that each quart produces no clear-cut improvement in the clarity of the solution. It now may require 5 or even 10 or more steps before noticable improvement occurs.

MORE RAPID EXCHANGE IN THE FIRST MODEL

If we were to measure the color of ink in the bowl (and assume that intensity of color was proportional to the amount of ink remaining) we could draw a graph which would look like the *dashed line curve* of Figure 4.1. Notice that more ink is removed per step in the early steps than later. In fact, the amount of ink removed in each step is related to how much ink is present at the beginning of each step; the more ink present, the more removed.

Now consider that exactly the same experiment is done with an 8-oz glass instead of the quart pitcher. To make up for the size of the glass, the steps of diluting, mixing, and emptying the glass are carried out 4 times as fast, *i.e.*, one step every 15 seconds. If we now compare the color of the bowl of ink after four water tumblers of water have been mixed into it and emptied, we will find it identical with the color in the bowl after one pitcher of water has been added, mixed, and emptied. Similarly, the color after 8 and 12 glasses of water will be the same as after 2 and 3 pitchers. A graph of this experiment is also shown in Figure 4.1 as the *solid line*. Now imagine what would happen if the size of the mixing steps was made smaller and smaller and correspondingly more

rapid per step. The graph from an experiment with a 2-oz juice glass mixed 16 times per minute is also shown in Figure 4.1. Notice that the resulting records have smaller and smaller steps as the size of the glasses gets smaller. Eventually they approach a smooth line called an exponential curve. Such a curve is generated in our experiment because the amount of dye that can be removed with each step depends on the amount of dye remaining. Obviously, when the dye has become very dilute there are few molecules in each glassful and hence few will be removed. In other words, the rate of removal depends on the concentration of the dye and is therefore a first order process.

RISING RATHER THAN FALLING CONCENTRATIONS

The experiment could be run backwards with results that differ only in one simple way. Consider starting with a bowl full of water and emptying in glassfuls of ink,

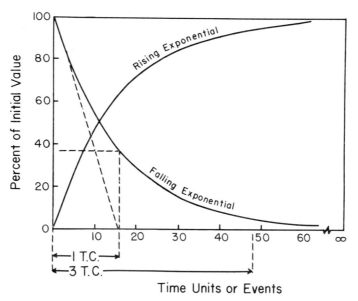

FIG. 4.2. The falling exponential, representing the ink remaining in the punch bowl experiment, is closely related to a second curve, a rising exponential, representing the ink removed in the punch bowl experiment. The maximum amount of ink that can be removed is no more than the amount present at the start of the experiment. A rising exponential curve can be obtained from a falling curve simply by turning it upside down. The time taken to reach 37% of the initial value of a falling curve or to reach 63% of a rising curve is called the time constant (*T.C.*). The initial slope, if extended and unchanged, would reach zero at one time constant. In ventilated systems (lung, for example) the time constant is the quotient of volume and ventilation.

mixing, discarding an equal volume, adding another glassful of ink, etc. The concentration of dye in the mixture will rise rapidly at first. As the dye becomes very concentrated in the bowl, however, its removal rate, *i.e.*, the product of the volume of the glass and the concentration being emptied out after mixing, gets very close to the addition rate (the product of the volume of the glass and the concentration of the dye being added). At this point the rate of increase in dye concentration in the whole punch bowl is very slow compared to the initial rate. A graphic plot of this experiment gives curves that rise steeply at first and level off, rising less and less with time, or with steps of addition, eventually approaching the horizontal line representing the final concentration. This, too, is an exponential process, sometimes referred to as a rising exponential. It is described mathematically by considering not the actual concentration of the dye, but the difference between the eventual concentration of the dye and the actual concentration of the dye. This can be done graphically by taking a falling exponential curve and turning it upside down, as shown in Figure 4.2. With this simple process of turning curves upside down, we can use exponential equations to describe both increasing and decreasing processes.

Certain properties of these curves are worth knowing. The mathematical equation for a first order reaction is:

$$X_t = X_{initial} \, e^{-at} \text{ (falling exponential)}$$

or

$$X_t = X_{final} (1 - e^{-at}) \text{ (rising exponential)}$$

This says that the value of something, X, at time t, is X_t and has a magnitude equal to the initial (or final) value of X, multiplied by e (the base of natural logarithms) raised to the negative power at, where t is elapsed time and α is a constant which describes how fast the value of X changes initially and depends on the size and inflow rate of the system. α is inversely related to a number called the time constant. The time constant of an exponential curve is the time that it takes to reach about 37% of its initial value (or, more precisely, to reach $1/e$ of the initial value). The time constant is also the time that a process would take to reach its final value if its initial rate did not slow progressively, but stayed constant. This is shown by the *steep dashed line* in Figure 4.2, tangent to the falling curve at its origin, and reaching zero at one time constant. As a rule of thumb, three time constants give 95% of the final value and five time constants give about 99%.

When a well mixed system behaves exponentially, the time constant depends on the size of the system and the flow into the system. In the punch bowl, the volume of the bowl (1 gallon) is its size, and the addition of water (32 oz/minute) is its inflow. The time constant is the quotient of the volume and inflow, *i.e.*, 1 gallon divided by 32 oz/minute = 128 oz divided by 32 oz/minute = 4 minutes. Note that a time constant has units of time.

The lungs of normal animals are usually nearly a single well mixed system. Their size, the functional residual capacity and their inflow, and the alveolar ventilation determine their time constant. A dog with a functional residual capacity of 1 liter and alveolar ventilation of 2 liters/minute has a time constant of 30 seconds. If this dog were suddenly to breathe oxygen rather than air, and if ventilation were unchanged, he would exhale 63% of his alveolar nitrogen in $1/2$ minute, 95% in $1\,1/2$ minutes, and 99% in $2\,1/2$ minutes. (This neglects the small volume of nitrogen dissolved in body tissues which would enter the alveoli when oxygen breathing begins. Such consideration is important only when high nitrogen pressure has stored a lot of gas in tissue, as in deep sea diving breathing air.[3])

THE ANESTHETIC APPLICATION OF THE FIRST MODEL

Anesthetic tensions rise within the alveoli of the lung when one begins to breathe an anesthetic mixture. As a first approximation for insoluble agents, alveolar tension rises exponentially as the gas rinses out the functional residual capacity of the lung. Consider for the moment that the anesthetic is so insoluble that almost none of it dissolves in blood, so very little leaves the lung in the pulmonary venous drainage. Also, suppose for the moment that, at some instant in time, once begins inhaling a constant concentration of the anesthetic gas which will eventually produce anesthesia. The size of the tidal volume is like the size of the glass in the ink experiment. The frequency of breathing is like the frequency of repetitively mixing and dumping the mixture in the ink experiment, and the size of the functional residual capacity of the lung is like the size of the punch bowl in the ink experiment. One can now use the idea of the punch bowl experiment to see how alterations in the concentration of inspired anesthetic agent, in the size of the animal and his functional residual capacity, in relation to the tidal volume, and in the respiratory minute volume affect the rate of induction of anesthesia.

The Effects of Removal of Soluble Gases by the Pulmonary Blood

Anesthetic agents are all moderately to markedly soluble in blood and tissues[10] compared with nitrogen or oxygen. Therefore, the pulmonary blood flow removes some of the drug from the alveoli as long as the partial pressure of the agent in venous blood is lower than that in alveoli. This lowers the alveolar concentration and slows the rate of rise of alveolar tension during induction. For a completely insoluble agent (hypothetical), the blood supply to the lung (cardiac output) is immaterial, since it cannot remove any of the agent (insoluble). In this case, the rate of use of alveolar concentration is dependent only on the concentration inspired, the lung volume, and the alveolar ventilation. For a very soluble agent, such as ether or methoxyflurane, the pulmonary blood flow removes a great amount of drug and distributes it to the tissues. In this case, the maximum alveolar concentration for any inspired concentration

depends on the cardiac output until the tissues are saturated with the gas, which may be days to weeks for soluble drugs.

THE SECOND MODEL

Consider the punch bowl experiment where ink was added to the bowl. Imagine that a pump draws water out of the bowl, pushes it through a filter (removing the ink particles), and returns it to the bowl. If the pump has a constant flow and the filter completely removes the ink from that flow, then the actual amount of ink removed in a first order process, since it depends on the concentration of ink in the bowl. This model would follow a decreasing exponential.

If we start with no ink in the bowl and add it exponentially (as along the rising exponential of Fig. 4.2) but have the pump and filter working, the rate of rise will be slower than the curve of Figure 4.2 and will flatten out below 100% at the point where the rate of addition of dye and of removal of dye are equal (Fig. 4.3). In other words, when two first order processes proceed in opposite directions, a steady state is reached, intermediate between the two.

APPLICATION OF THE MODEL TO ANESTHETIZATION

Applying these ideas to the case of induction of anesthesia produces certain obvious conclusions. Blood leaving alveoli has the same *tension* of anesthetic agent as have the aveoli. The amount of the agent in blood (as opposed to the tension or partial pressure) depends on the solubility of the agent in blood. Blood contains 14 times as much methoxyflurane (a very soluble agent) as an equal volume of alveolar gas with the same partial pressure. Therefore, if ventilation delivers 14 volumes of methoxyflurane to alveoli in a certain period, 13 of these will leave in the pulmonary blood flow and the remaining alveolar concentration will be about 7% of what it would have been without loss to the blood. (This simplification assumes a $V_A/\dot{Q}c$ of 1.0 and no venous tension.) Had the anesthetic been ethylene (a less solu-

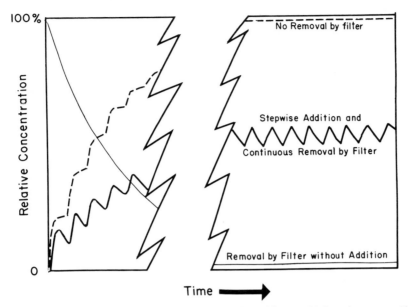

Fig. 4.3. The punch bowl experiment repeated with stepwise addition of ink and constant filtering out of ink. The result is an initial rapid rise (when ink is added faster than the filter removed it) and a later period of slow rise—plateau—when the ink is removed almost as fast as added. If the filter can be considered to eventually load up completely, the plateau would rise eventually to the top.

ble gas with a blood/air partition ratio of 0.14, about 2 parts of 14 brought to the alveoli by ventilation—as compared to 13 parts out of 14 (methoxyflurane)—will be removed by circulation. The alveolar concentration in this case will be more than 85% of that predicted for a totally insoluble gas in the same period of breathing.

In the real animal, the rate of removal of agent is not solely dependent upon the alveolar concentration and blood flow. As the anesthetic-bearing blood is distributed to the tissues, the anesthetic diffuses out, causing a rise in tissue tension. The venous blood draining the tissue contains some anesthetic, however, and, as time passes, contains more and more. Thus, as time passes and the venous content rises, the ability of the blood flow to remove anesthetic from the lungs decreases. The rate of decrease is very slow for the very soluble agents and more rapid for relatively insoluble agents. A "plateau" will appear in the plot of alveolar concentration as a function of time. This plateau is fairly stable for the time period involved in most surgical procedures. However,

eventually, the alveoli, the tissues, and the venous blood anesthetic tension reaches the inspired tension. Thus, the circulatory factors slow the rate of rise of alveolar tension but do not alter the final tension. The sole exception to this statement is the case where the anesthetic drug is metabolized. This would cause a constant removal so that a true plateau would be reached in those tissues metabolizing the drug at a concentration less than inspired. Only trichlorethylene of all commonly used anesthetics is metabolized in appreciable quantities,[14] although the very sensitive methods of radiochemistry have shown some metabolic degradation of most other agents.[16]

The lesson of this section is that the rate of rise of alveolar concentration depends on both ventilatory and circulatory factors. The degree of dependence on these two depends, in turn, on the solubility of the agent in blood. The alveolar concentration of insoluble agents depends mostly on ventilation, while the concentration of soluble agents depends in large part on how much is removed by the pulmonary blood flow, as well as on how much is brought to the alveoli by ventilation.

THE ELECTRICAL ANALOG

In an electrical circuit, the rate of charge of a capacitor through a resistor from a battery is also described by an exponential equation, as is the rate of discharge and the actual charge on the capacitor. For these reasons models are often constructed of resistors and capacitors; such a model is an analogue computer. Usually the battery or source voltage is considered analogous to the partial pressure of inspired gas. The capacitors represent the tissues and store electric charge as tissues store anesthetic. The blood supply to tissue is represented by the conductance to a capacitor (conductance is the reciprocal of a resistor's value). Large resistors are associated with low flow and small resistors permit rapid flow. Different tissues are represented by different capacitors, each with its own resistance. Further details are given by Mapleson.[11]

The Actual Situation where Inspired Concentration Cannot be Kept Constant

In this section we describe the practical application of the previous two sections. The model is complicated by three new concepts. The first is the practical limitation imposed on the inspired concentration by the anesthetic apparatus; the second is the need for the anesthetist to make a decision as to what mixture to supply at various times; and the third is that the anesthetist does not know the partial pressure of anesthetic agent in the various tissues and blood flow but can only judge the result by those observations that he makes (which collectively comprise the signs of depth of anesthesia). This latter complication is discussed in other chapters. The concept of the model (although not its construction) can be simplified by imagining that the various tissues of the body, with their blood flows and capacities to store anesthetic agents, are all enclosed inside a black box. We can see only some reflection of the concen-

tration within the brain (the signs of anesthesia). Furthermore, we cannot feed the model a constant alveolar concentration, but must mix up a concentration with our rotameters and vaporizers and let the model inhale it from some sort of apparatus.

The complexity of any real animal exceeds the model's. This results in the deviation of real anesthetic tensions within the lungs, the blood stream, the brain, and other organs of animals from those predicted by our experimental models. However, models of simple approximations have been described which give predictions that are within a few percent of reality, and which give useful insights into the importance of such factors as the size of the animal's body, the rate of his cardiac output, the size of his functional residual capacity, his tidal volume and respiratory frequency (and their product, the respiratory minute volume), and the apparatus used for inducing anesthesia, as well as the technique in administering the anesthetic agents.[2, 6, 15]

THE LIMITATION OF THE APPARATUS AND AGENTS

Knowledge of exponential processes helps in understanding how the breathing circuits themselves might affect the induction and maintenance of anesthesia. They have an internal volume and a ventilation (the fresh gas inflow) and behave approximately like first order systems.[4] For any given fresh gas inflow rate, circuits with a large volume will require more time for the completion of induction. For any given size breathing circuit, the greater the fresh gas inflow, the more rapid the induction. For any given size breathing circuit and fresh gas inflow, the more rapid the mixing within the circle (generally achieved by ventilation of the animal), the more rapid the induction. The quantitation of these limitations is complicated. When a first order process supplies the input for a second first order input, the second is said to be convoluted by the first. This now states that the rise of the alveolar concentration is also dependent upon the rate of rise of the anesthetic agent in the anesthesia circuit (see Chapter 17). A mathematical discussion has been presented in describing the uptake of inert gas by the brain.[17]

There are certain physical and physiological limitations on the anesthetist's decision as to inspired gas concentration. For example, at ordinary room temperatures the vapor pressure of methoxyflurane limits the inspired concentrations that the anesthetist can choose to those at or below 3%, and even 3% is achieved only with very efficient vaporizers of modern design employing efficient thermodynamic concepts to keep the temperature of the liquid methoxyflurane constant.[12]

No matter how much nitrous oxide the anesthetist might wish to deliver, he is restricted to a total partial pressure equal to the barometric pressure unless he is inducing anesthesia within a hyperbaric chamber. In addition to this physical limitation of nitrous oxide, he is limited by the anesthetic potency of this drug. Even with prior oxygenation of the lungs he can administer 100% nitrous oxide only for a few minutes.

Finally, there is the practical limitation of the irritating concentration. Concentrations of 3 to 4% diethyl ether in air represent minimum alveolar concentrations producing anesthesia and are not irritating, but they will not induce anesthesia in a reasonable period of time. On the other hand, although diethyl ether can be administered in concentrations up to 60 or 65% in air or oxygen, this concentration will not be inhaled by an animal because it is irritating, producing cough, laryngeal spasm, and breath-holding. The concentration which can be inhaled without coughing and laryngospasm depends in part on the concentration of diethyl ether in the animal's brain. As the animal becomes more deeply anesthetized the irritating threshhold rises.

The Need to Alter Inspired Gas Concentration during Induction and Maintenance

Suppose that the inspired concentration of anesthetic gas is just sufficient to produce anesthesia when the alveolar concentration reaches the inspired concentration. Inspection of the curve in Figure 4.4 shows that the patient will be anesthetized only after a very long time, since an exponential approaches its limit very slowly at the end, yet patients may be rapidly anesthetized. How? If the anesthetic concentration inspired was doubled, anesthesia would be induced when the alveolar concentration reaches half of the inspired concentration. Compare this with the time taken for induction when the inspired concentration is 4 times the anesthetizing concentration (and hence anesthesia will be induced when the alveolar concentration is 25% of the inspired concentration—see Fig. 4.4). As the concentration inspired is doubled, the time to anesthesia is more than halved. This technique is used during anesthesia with those agents in which the inspired concentration can freely be increased and is not limited by the need for oxygen. It is exactly analogous to the concept of a loading dose during clinical therapy with sulfonamide or of a loading dose for the kidney function tests of inulin and p-aminohippurate clearance.

Anesthetists may initially administer several times the concentration needed to maintain anesthesia. The patient is then anesthetized rapidly. If the volume of the lung is very large, as in emphysema, the ventilation must be very large also, to keep the duration of induction from becoming extended. On the other hand, especially with very small animals with relatively large ventilatory rates in respect to their size, induction times may be very short and the inspired concentration of the anesthetic must be reduced sooner to maintenance concentrations in order to prevent overdose. Thus, the process of anesthetization involves more than simply offering an anesthetizing concentration to an animal.

SPECIAL EFFECTS OF THE SOLUBILITY OF ANESTHETIC AGENTS

At the start of inhalation of 80% nitrous oxide, the mixed venous tension of nitrous oxide is zero. As nitrous oxide replaces nitrogen in the alveoli, it diffuses

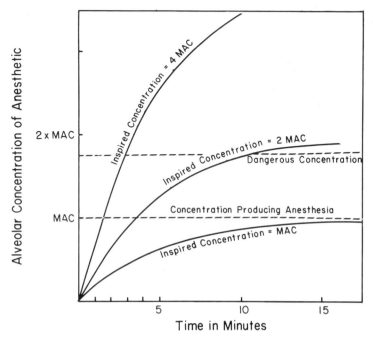

Fig. 4.4. Graph of the rise of alveolar concentration of an ideal insoluble agent when three different concentrations are inspired. *MAC*, minimum alveolar concentration of agent producing anesthesia. If only 1 × minimum alveolar concentration is offered, the alveoli will not reach an anesthetic concentration. To speed induction, 2 × minimum alveolar concentration could be offered. To prevent too deep anesthesia, the inspired concentration must be reduced before about 10 minutes. An inspired concentration of 4 × minimum alveolar concentration would produce a very rapid induction with the danger of rapidly entering too deep a plane.

rapidly into the pulmonary blood, since it is soluble in blood. A large portion of the inspired volume of each breath may be absorbed and carried from the lungs by the pulmonary blood flow. This decreases the total alveolar pressure of nitrous oxide, literally causing further flow of the anesthetic and oxygen toward the alveoli. The extra ventilation (mass flow) speeds the rise in alveolar concentration of nitrous oxide and hence increases the initial uptake rate. If a lower concentration of nitrous oxide were inhaled, the rate at which its concentration rises within the alveoli would not be as greatly augmented by the extra inspiratory ventilation, since less would be absorbed by the blood and less negative pressure created to augment inspiration. The rapid removal of the anesthetic agent from the alveoli produces a concentration difference between the alveoli and the

upper airway in that a flow of gas occurs toward the alveoli. This effect increases more proportionally as the concentration inspired increases. This effect is called the "concentration effect."[5]

The concentration effect results from a marked increase of inspired minute volume (relative to expired minute volume). This extra inspiratory ventilation increases the alveolar tension of any other gas in the inspired mixture. With an abrupt shift from breathing room air to breathing 79% nitrous oxide and 21% oxygen, the alveolar concentration of oxygen may rise from 15 to nearly 25% in the first 3 to 5 minutes even though the inspired oxygen concentration, the alveolar carbon dioxide tension, and the expired volume are unchanged. This concentrating effect of rapid nitrous oxide uptake on alveolar oxygen has been called the "second gas effect."[7] The concentration effect makes the administration of seemingly hypoxic nitrous oxide mixtures safe for brief periods of time during induction (especially after brief prior oxygenation) and may also speed induction with other agents, since the second gas effect will speed the rate of rise of alveolar halothane or ether if these agents are administered with the nitrous oxide-oxygen mixtures.

An analogous but inverse situation occurs during emergence from anesthesia when an insoluble gas such as room air is inspired. Inspired nitrogen dilutes the nitrous oxide content of the alveoli with the first several breaths of air. This creates a large diffusion gradient for nitrous oxide from pulmonary blood to alveoli. Because nitrous oxide is soluble in blood, there is a large quantity of nitrous oxide in the venous blood at the end of anesthesia. It then pours out into the alveoli, diluting the other gases. When an abrupt shift is made from breathing 80% nitrous oxide and 20% oxygen to breathing room air, the alveolar tension may fall from 15 or 16% to 9 or 10%. This process, referred to as diffusion hypoxia,[9] can be prevented from becoming clinically significant by inspiring 100% oxygen for 1 minute or so before allowing air to be inspired. Diffusion hypoxia is in fact a "second gas effect," causing *decrease* in oxygen tension since nitrous oxide is coming *out* of the body (inverse of the case where increased oxygenation is associated with nitrous oxide uptake).

The Composition of Alveolar Gas: the Limiting Cases

The lessons learned in the previous sections may be reinforced by considering the same information from a different point of view, *i.e.*, the oxygen-carbon dioxide diagram (Fig. 4.5). When inspired gas is a mixture of O_2, CO_2, and inert gas having no exchange (*i.e.*, nitrogen), and when the tension of O_2 and CO_2 in the mixed venous blood is specified, $P\bar{v}O_2$ and $P\bar{v}CO_2$, a unique curve may be drawn between the point representing inspired gas and that of mixed venous blood tension, called the ventilation perfusion curve ($\dot{V}/\dot{Q}$ line). This line specifies the only possible mixtures of O_2, CO_2, and inert gas tension that can exist in alveoli receiving the specified mixed venous blood and the specified inspired gas mixture, no matter what the ventilation and perfusion are. Furthermore, on the same diagram, a series of lines describing various respiratory quotients (RQ's) may be drawn which intersect the $\dot{V}/\dot{Q}$ line. For any given alveolus, the intersection of its $\dot{V}/\dot{Q}$ line with its RQ line specifies its unique gas composition. The *center curve* in Figure 4.5 shows the $\dot{V}/\dot{Q}$ line for air breathing, where $P\bar{v}CO_2$ is 43 and $P\bar{v}O_2$ is 40. The light line up from and to the left of the *PI* point is the $RQ = 1.0$ line. Any and all alveoli with an RQ of 1.0 receiving this inspired gas and venous blood must then have an oxygen tension of 106 and a carbon dioxide tension of 38. Further description of this diagram and its construction are given by Rahn and Fenn.[13] Metabolism and ventilation relative to cardiac output are inherently specified if the mixed venous blood tensions, inspired gas composition, and RQ are specified.

When an abrupt change is made from breathing air to breathing nitrous oxide-oxygen mixtures, the usual $\dot{V}/\dot{Q}$ line no longer applies, but a simple modification illustrates the changes in alveolar gas composition. The assumption that the total partial pressure of all four gases (O_2, CO_2, N_2, and N_2O) must add up to barometric pressure is still valid, but not the assumption that those gases other than O_2 and CO_2 are in equilibrium and not exchanged. This has been shown by Farhi and Olszowka[8] to change the $\dot{V}/\dot{Q}$ curve on the O_2-CO_2 diagram in a remarkable way. The $\dot{V}/\dot{Q}$ line at the start of induction of anesthesia is shown by the curve *above* and to the *right* in Figure 4.5. It is clear that there are a number of possible alveolar gas compositions which include oxygen tensions as high or higher than that inspired, and, at the same time, an appreciable CO_2 tension (indicating that blood flow and exchange must be

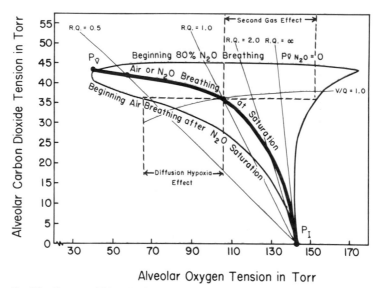

FIG. 4.5. The O_2-CO_2 diagram. If inspired gas composition is specified (P_i on diagram) and mixed venous blood tensions specified ($P\bar{v}$ on diagram) there is a unique line describing all the possible mixtures of oxygen, carbon dioxide, and remaining gas that can exist in an alveolus receiving air and blood, no matter in what proportion. This line (heavy control curve) is called the $\dot{V}_A/\dot{Q}_c$ line. In addition, a fan of straight lines radiating up and to the left from the point P_i can be drawn, a different line for each possible respiratory quotient, RQ. The intersection of the $\dot{V}/\dot{Q}$ and RQ lines describes the *only* possible concentration of gases in an alveolus with the specified $P\bar{v}$, P_i, and RQ. At the start of breathing 80% nitrous oxide, a different $\dot{V}/\dot{Q}$ line applies, due to the rapid uptake of the anesthetic, above and to the right of the normal air-breathing curve. As uptake decreases and venous tension rises, the $\dot{V}/\dot{Q}$ line contracts and falls back on the normal line, becoming essentially superimposed at infinite time. If, then, air rather than nitrous oxide is inspired, the appropriate $\dot{V}/\dot{Q}$ line is the *lower left curve*, which rises toward the normal as nitrous oxide is eliminated from the body. If expired ventilation is kept constant, P_{ACO2} is constant, represented by a horizontal line. This diagram shows that at constant P_{ACO2}, the alveolar oxygen is higher than normal during induction (explaining the second gas effect) and lower than normal during elimination (diffusion hypoxia results).

continuing in the alveoli). This is a graphic illustration of the second gas effect of Epstein, where oxygen is concentrated. As anesthesia progresses, the tension of nitrous oxide in mixed venous blood increases. The curve slowly contracts and falls back upon the normal $\dot{V}/\dot{Q}$ line. At infinite time, 79% nitrous oxide with 21% oxygen would be nearly indistinguishable from air breathing on the O_2-CO_2 diagram. If, after this equilibrium has been attained ($P\bar{v}N_2O$ = P_{AN2O}) the animal suddenly breathes air, a new $\dot{V}/\dot{Q}$ line results, below and to the left of the air-breathing $\dot{V}/\dot{Q}$ line. There are some possible alveolar gas compositions which contain both less oxygen and less carbon dioxide than that in mixed venous blood. Since there is less CO_2

than in mixed venous blood, there must be some ventilation of these alveoli. This ventilation is due to the egress of nitrous oxide from blood, not inspiration of air, and hence the oxygen content is reduced. There is also less oxygen anywhere on this $\dot{V}/\dot{Q}$ line than during air breathing at the same PCO_2. The same PCO_2, by convention, implies the same alveolar ventilation. The reason for the decreased oxygen tension is that the volume of nitrous oxide leaving the pulmonary blood represents a portion of the total ventilation. Thus, during nitrous oxide excretion, the volume of air inspired is less than the total ventilation by an amount equal to the nitrous oxide evolved from the blood and exhaled. Since the inspired air volume is decreased, the volume of oxygen inspired is less during nitrous oxide excretion than during the steady state of air breathing, so alveolar oxygen is necessarily reduced. This is the diffusion hypoxia effect of Fink. As air breathing continues, $P\bar{v}N_2O$ falls and the $\dot{V}/\dot{Q}$ line contracts to the right and up toward the normal air-breathing line.

REFERENCES

1. Andrews, P. M., Minor, G. R., and Eastwood, D. W.: Arterial oxygen saturation and respiratory minute volume: studies during induction with light concentrations of nitrous oxide. (abst.) Anesthesiology 19: 94, 1958.
2. Brown, E. S., Seniff, A. M., and Elam, J. O.: Carbon dioxide elimination and closed system. Anesthesiology 25: 31, 1964.
3. Diving Hazards: U.S. Navy Diving Manual, Chap. 1.6. Navy Department, Washington, D.C., 1963.
4. Eger, E. I., II: Factors affecting the rapidity of alternate of nitrous oxide in a circle system. Anesthesiology 21: 348, 1960.
5. Eger, E. I., II: Effect of inspired anesthetic concentration on the rate of use of alveolar concentration. Anesthesiology 24: 153, 1963.
6. Eger, E. I., II, and Ethans, C. T.: The effects of inflow, overflow, and valve placement on economy of the circle system. Anesthesiology 29: 93, 1968.
7. Epstein, R. M., Rachow, J., Salanitre, E., and Wolf, G. L.: Influence of concentration effect on the uptake of anesthetic mixtures: the second gas effect. Anesthesiology 25: 364, 1964.
8. Farhi, L. E., and Olszowka, A. J.: Analysis of alveolar gas exchange—the presence of soluble inert gases. Resp. Physiol. 5: 53, 1968.
9. Fink, R. B.: Diffusion anoxia. Anesthesiology 16: 511, 1955.
10. Larson, C. P., Eger, E. I., II, and Severinghaus, J. W.: Ostwald solubility coefficients for anesthetic gases in various fluids and tissues. Anesthesiology 23: 686, 1962.
11. Mapleson, W. W.: An electric analogue for uptake and exchange of inert gases and other agents. J. Appl. Physiol. 18: 197, 1963.
12. Morris, L. E., and Feldman, S. A.: Considerations in the design and function of anesthetic vaporizers. Anesthesiology 19: 642, 1958.
13. Rahn, H., and Fenn, W. O.: A graphical analysis of the respiratory gas exchange in the O_2-CO_2 diagram. The American Physiological Society, Washington, D.C., 1955.
14. Powell, J. F.: Trichlorethylene: absorption, elimination, and metabolism. Brit. J. Industr. Med. 2: 142, 1945.
15. Severinghaus, J. W.: Role of lung factors. In Uptake and Distribution of Anesthetic Agents, edited by E. M. Papper and R. J. Kitz. Blakiston Division, McGraw-Hill Book Company, Inc., New York, 1963.
16. Van Dyke, R. A., and Chenoweth, M. E.: Metabolism of volatile anesthetics. Anesthesiology 26: 348, 1965.
17. Wollman, H., Alexander, S. C., Cohen, P. J., Stephen, G. W., and Zeiger, L. S.: Two-compartment analysis of the blood flow in the human brain. Acta Neurol. Scand. (suppl. 14) 41: 79, 1965.

5

The Pharmacodynamics of Diethyl Ether

S. CRAIGHEAD ALEXANDER

Diethyl ether, the first successful inhalation anesthetic, has been in use for over 120 years. Although it has been largely displaced by newer agents, ether is still frequently used when highly trained personnel or elaborate anesthetic equipment is not available and when economy is an important consideration.

Ether is a liquid at room temperature and its vapor is flammable. It is readily vaporized, since its boiling point is only 37 C and its ease of vaporization, together with a wide margin of safety, allows it to be used with simple vaporizers. It is highly soluble in blood, the blood/gas solubility coefficient being approximately 12. This characteristic slows the induction of anesthesia and delays recovery. For the induction of anesthesia, 15 to 20% ether vapor is usually needed. When the desired depth is attained, the inhaled concentration is reduced to about 5%. The administration of ether is discontinued prior to the completion of surgery in order to speed recovery.

Respiratory Effects

LOCAL ACTIONS ON RESPIRATORY TRACT

Ether is irritating to the respiratory tract. During the induction of anesthesia with a mask, the inhaled concentration may produce laryngospasm or severe coughing and breath holding. This effect varies with the species of animal; it is common in man and occurs in the cat, but is generally uncommon during the induction of anesthesia in the horse. Bronchial and salivary secretions in large amounts can be minimized by prior administration of atropine.

Clinical experience has led to the concept that ether relaxes bronchial smooth muscle and increases anatomic dead space. This concept has led to its suggested use for the treatment of bronchospasm during anesthesia. Although it has been demonstrated to dilate bronchi *in vitro*, this effect of ether has not been measured *in vivo*.[1]

PULMONARY VENTILATION DURING ETHER ANESTHESIA

During light planes of anesthesia with diethyl ether, there is a consistent increase in pulmonary ventilation above the awake level. This response is unique for this drug; virtually all other inhalation agents depress minute ventilation. The augmentation of respiratory minute volume during the light planes of ether anesthesia is due to an increased respiratory rate. Tidal volume is usually unchanged or slightly diminished. With deeper planes[3, 4] of anesthesia, tidal volume diminishes and there is a progressive decrease in ventilation until apnea occurs. However, arterial carbon dioxide tensions are not elevated significantly in man until blood ether concentration approaches a level necessary to produce respiratory arrest. Unfortunately, data relating $PaCO_2$ and depth of anesthesia in other species are not readily available.[26] Some measurements of $PaCO_2$ in the dog have indicated a hypocarbia, reflecting the marked respiratory stimulating effect of ether in the dog.

The tachypnea which occurs during ether anesthesia, which can be marked in the dog, has been attributed to a number of reflex, humoral, and chemical mechanisms. These are as follows.

Reflex Mechanisms. Whitteridge and Bülbring[29] noted that the discharge frequencies of both inflation and deflation receptors in the lungs of the cat were increased during the inhalation of ether vapor. They postulated that ether sensitized the pulmonary stretch receptors, thereby shortening the duration of both inspiration and expiration and increasing respiratory rate. However, this mechanism cannot wholly account for the respiratory stimulation which occurs during ether anesthesia, since the increased discharge from pulmonary receptors is only transitory, and tachypnea during ether anesthesia is not abolished by vagotomy.[22]

Irritation of the lower respiratory tract is also known to produce reflex hyperpnea by irritating the bronchial mucosa. However, the reflex response to bronchial irritation rapidly accommodates to continued stimulation, and volatile anesthetics have been hypothesized to paralyze the airway receptors after initially stimulating them. Therefore, the role of this reflex in respiration during ether anesthesia is uncertain.[26]

Stimulation of nonpulmonary receptors has also been suggested as a cause of respiratory tachypnea during ether inhalation. Comroe and Schmidt[9] produced a stimulation of respiration in decerebrate dogs by injecting ether-equilibrated saline into the femoral artery. This effect was abolished by denervation of the limb, and it was hypothesized that the drug acted on peripheral receptors in muscle and joints.

Humoral Mechanisms. Blood concentrations of norepinephrine and epinephrine are elevated during ether anesthesia. In conscious man, intravenous infusion of these substances stimulates respiration primarily by increasing tidal volume;[8, 10] endogenously released catecholamines may stimulate respiration during ether anesthesia. Since the effects of elevated blood catecholamine levels on respiration have apparently not been studied in conscious animals or during general anesthesia in any species, their contribution to the tachypnea of ether can only be inferred from measurements in man.

Chemical Mechanisms. As further described under "Metabolic Effects," acidosis frequently accompanies ether anesthesia, especially in the dog. An increased blood hydrogen ion concentration is also a stimulus to respiration. Thus, metabolic acidosis occurring during ether anesthesia may be partially responsible for the augmentation of respiration.

Although the peripheral actions of ether stimulate respiratory rate and tend to maintain alveolar ventilation at normal levels, ether, like other anesthetic agents, is a depressant of central respiratory centers. Several investigators have measured a depressed respiratory response to inhaled CO_2 during ether anesthesia.[17, 22] The inhalation of this drug by decerebrate cats elevates the intensity of the medullary electrical stimulus required to initiate inspiration.[22] Finally, the respiratory effects of ether are stongly influenced by the prior administration of other drugs. Drugs which are used as premedicants frequently depress respiration. Ether anesthesia following the administration of such substances may be characterized by a progressive depression of pulmonary ventilation.

Circulatory Effects

Ether has long enjoyed a wide use because of its benign actions on the circulation; typically, cardiovascular functions are well maintained, even at depths of anesthesia sufficient to produce respiratory arrest. Early in the administration of this anesthetic little change in blood pressure occurs, cardiac rate is increased, and stroke volume is reduced. In the dog, blood pressure and stroke volume are reduced in a linear fashion with deepening of anesthesia.[3]

Circulatory stability during ether inhalation is due to an increased activity of the sympathetic nervous system and an increase in the blood concentrations of catecholamines.[5] Myocardial contractility, cardiac output, and ventricular end diastolic filling pressures may be increased during light levels of ether anesthesia; such alterations are typical of those which occur during the administration of catecholamines. As the deep planes of anesthesia are attained, contractility and cardiac output are progressively reduced.[14]

Ether is a profound myocardial depressant, as can be demonstrated in the isolated heart preparation. Myocardial function is also severely depressed in the adrenalectomized and sympathectomized dog during ether anesthesia. This depression is largely eliminated by the infusion of epinephrine or norepinephrine.[5, 14] These and other data indicate that increased sympathetic nervous activity is extremely important for maintenance of circulatory stability during ether anesthesia.

Ether does not predispose the heart to cardiac arrhythmias. Consequently, moderate doses of both epinephrine and norepinephrine may be administered during its inhalation without fear of precipitating ventricular arrhythmias. During more profound depths of anesthesia, an atrioventricular nodal rhythm is not uncommon.

Although diethyl ether does not seriously impair the function of the heart and the macrocirculation, during the upper planes of anesthesia its actions on the microcirculation are less benign. During light ether anesthesia the metarterioles have an enhanced sensitivity to topically applied epinephrine, and capillary vasomotion is increased. These changes are

apparently not deleterious. However, vascular reactivity and vasomotion are progressively depressed during moderate and deep anesthesia; arteriolar vasodilatation occurs; and blood flow is a slowed in the capillary bed.[2] After the cessation of ether administration, the recovery of the microcirculation to its normal active state is slow. This agent, like other general anesthetics, inhibits homeostatic peripheral vascular mechanisms and tends to decrease the resistance of the organism to hemorrhage or shock.

Metabolic Effects

Anesthesia with diethyl ether produces alterations of endocrine function, carbohydrate metabolism, and acid-base balance. These changes are more profound than those accompanying the administration of any other anesthetic and are most pronounced in the dog.

ENDOCRINE FUNCTION

Alterations in pituitary and adrenal function occur during ether inhalation. There is both stimulation of adrenocorticotropic hormone production by the anterior pituitary and an increased secretion of 17-hydroxycorticoids by the adrenal cortex.[27] This adrenocortical response is believed to be proportional to the depth of anesthesia.[28] Ether may also increase blood corticoid levels indirectly by depressing hepatic and renal function, thereby slowing hormonal excretion.

The adrenal medulla is stimulated to release catecholamines during ether anesthesia, producing an increased blood level of epinephrine in the dog.[25] This medullary stimulation is believed to contribute to the circulatory stability noted with this agent, as discussed earlier. Finally, ether, like other general anesthetics, causes a secretion of antidiuretic hormone by the posterior pituitary gland. The implications of this phenomenon are considered in the section on renal function.

CARBOHYDRATE METABOLISM

Blood concentrations of glucose, lactate, and pyruvate progressively increase for at least 2 hours during the inhalation of diethyl ether. Glucose concentration frequently increases by 100 mg %, and an 8-fold increase in lactate concentration has been reported.[4, 7] There is a rise in the lactate/pyruvate ratio since the increase in blood pyruvate concentration is less marked than the change in lactate concentration. An elevated "excess lactate" concentration has been demonstrated in man, possibly due to the presence of tissue hypoxia during ether anesthesia.[18] Corroborating evidence of inadequate tissue oxygenation during ether anesthesia has not been found. In addition, "excess lactate" need not be indicative of increased anaerobic metabolism.[23] The elevations of blood glucose, lactate, and pyruvate concentrations have also been interpreted as being a consequence of the sympathoadrenal response to ether inhalation. Blockade of the sympathetic nervous system eliminates this hyperglycemic response and markedly reduces the lactacidemia.[4] A similar elevation of blood glucose and lactate concentrations can be produced by infusion of epinephrine. Thus, the sympathoadrenal response to this anesthetic may be a factor in producing the changes in carbohydrate metabolism.

The hyperglycemia associated with ether anesthesia also has been attributed to either an impairment of tissue glucose utilization or to an "anti-insulin" effect.[12, 19, 20] Recent *in vitro* studies on the mouse diaphragm indicate that ether causes a decrease in tissue glucose utilization and an increased breakdown of glycogen to glucose.[6] Ether does not inhibit the increased uptake of glucose in the presence of insulin. There is thus evidence that ether anesthesia alters carbohydrate metabolism by a direct effect at the subcellular level as well as indirectly through elevation of catecholamine levels.

ACID-BASE BALANCE

Metabolic acidosis is associated with ether anesthesia in the dog. Blood pH may be decreased by 0.1 unit or more despite the presence of a normal level of arterial PCO_2. The increased acidity of the blood is largely due to an increased concentration of lactate, although the concentration of other nonvolatile acids is also increased.[4] These changes result from alterations of carbohydrate metabolism, and they can be almost entirely prevented by blockade of the sympathetic nervous system. The tendency of ether to produce metabolic acidosis reduces its usefulness in animals with pre-existing acidosis from other causes.

Hepatic and Liver Function

Permanent liver damage does not ensue after ether anesthesia. However, this agent, like other general anesthetics, depresses hepatic function. This mild impairment may continue for several days in normal man and is more severe and longer lasting in the presence of pre-existing liver disease.[15, 16] Postoperative studies of liver function have not been reported in animals.

Ether, in common with other general anesthetics, depresses renal function. Urine volume is markedly diminished, and there is retention of sodium. These phenomena are partially explained by a reduction in renal blood flow and glomerular filtration rate. The liberation of antidiuretic hormone is also believed to play a role in reducing urinary volume and sodium excretion during ether anesthesia.[13, 24]

Neuromuscular Effects

The degree of muscular relaxation produced during ether anesthesia is greater than that produced by other inhalation anesthetics. Because of this property, low concentrations of this agent are often administered with other inhalation agents in order to achieve better muscular relaxation.

This drug has been said to resemble *d*-tubocurarine in its mode of action, but recent evidence indicates that this may not be so in all species. The neuromuscular effects of diethyl ether have recently been studied in man and in the cat.[21] Little or no depression of neuromuscular transmission occurs in either species at a time when the abdominal muscles are well relaxed and electromyographic activity is markedly depressed. A neuromuscular blocking action can be elicited in the cat only by the close intra-arterial injection of 2 to 6 ml of 5% ether in saline per kg. With these extreme concentrations there is a poorly sustained tetanus and post-tetanic facilitation, and this block is poorly antagonized by cholinesterase inhibitors. Evidence is accumulating that in man and in the cat, at least, ether produces muscular relaxation by a depression of the central nervous system rather than by a blockade of neuromuscular transmission.[21] Recently, other workers have also obtained evidence that inhalation anesthetics produce muscular relaxation by decreasing the excitability of the spinal motoneuron pool rather than by acting at the myoneural junction.[11]

Ether increases the intensity and duration of action of both d-tubocurarine and succinylcholine in the cat, although the action of succinylcholine is intensified in only 50% of humans studied.[21] For this reason, the dosage of neuromuscular blocking agents should be determined with care during ether anesthesia.

REFERENCES

1. Adriani, J., and Rovenstine, E. A.: The effect of anesthetic drugs upon bronchi and bronchioles of excised lung tissue. Anesthesiology 4: 253, 1943.

2. Baez, S.: Anesthetics and the microcirculation. In Effects of Anesthetics on the Circulation, edited by H. L. Price and P. J. Cohen, p. 182. Charles C Thomas, Publisher, Springfield, Ill., 1964.

3. Bagwell, E. E., Woods, E. F., and Linker, R.: Influence of reserpine on cardiovascular and sympathoadrenal responses to ether anesthesia in the dog. Anesthesiology 25: 15, 1964.

4. Brewster, W. R., Jr., Bunker, J. P., and Beecher, H. K.: Metabolic effects of anesthesia. IV. Mechanism of metabolic acidosis and hyperglycemia during ether anesthesia in the dog. Amer. J. Physiol. 171: 37, 1952.

5. Brewster, W. R., Jr., Isaacs, J. P., and Waino-Andersen, T.: Depressant effects of ether on myocardium of the dog and its modification of reflex release of epinephrine and norepinephrine. Amer. J. Physiol. 175: 399, 1953.

6. Brunner, E. A., and Haugaard, N.: Effects of diethyl ether on carbohydrate metabolism in skeletal muscle. Unpublished data.

7. Bunker, J. P.: Neuroendocrine and other effects on carbohydrate metabolism during anesthesia. Anesthesiology 24: 515, 1963.

8. Coles, D. R., Duff, W. H., Sheperd, W. H. T., and Whelan, R. F.: Effect on respiration of infusion of adrenaline and nonadrenaline into the carotid and vertebral arteries in man. Brit. J. Pharmacol. 11: 346, 1956.

9. Comroe, J. H., Jr., and Schmidt, C. F.: Reflexes from the limbs as a factor in the hyperpnea of exercise. Amer. J. Physiol. 138: 536, 1942.

10. Cunningham, D. J. C., Hey, E. N., Patrick, J. M., and Lloyd, B. B.: Effect of nor-adrenaline infusion on the relation between pulmonary ventilation and the alveolar PO_2 and PCO_2 in man. Ann. N.Y. Acad. Sci. 109: 756, 1963.

11. DeJong, R. H., Hershey, W. N., and Wagman, I. H.: Measurement of a spinal reflex response (H-reflex) during general anesthesia in man. Anesthesiology 28: 382, 1967.

12. Drucker, W. R., Costley, C., Stults, R., Holden, W. D., Craig, J., Miller, M., Hoffman, N., and Woodward, H.: Studies of carbohydrate metabolism during ether anesthesia. I. Effect of ether on glucose and fructose metabolism. Metabolism, 8: 827, 1959.

13. Dudley, H. F., Boling, E. A., LeQuesne, L. P., and Moore, F. D.: Studies on antidiuresis in surgery: effects of anesthesia, surgery, and posterior pituitary antidiuretic hormone on water metabolism in man. Ann. Surg. 140: 354, 1954.

14. Etsten, B., and Li, T. H.: Current concepts of myocardial function during anesthesia. Brit. J. Anaesth. 34: 884, 1962.

15. Fairlie, C. W., Barss, T. P., French, A. B., Jones, C. M., and Beecher, H. K.: Metabolic effects of anesthesia in man. IV. A comparison of the effects of certain anesthetic agents on the normal liver. New Eng. J. Med. 244: 615, 1951.

16. French, A. B., Barss, T. P., Fairlie, C. W., Bengle, A. L., Jr., Jones, C. M., Linton, R. R., and Beecher, H. K.: Metabolic effects of anesthesia in man. V. A comparison of the effects of ether and cyclopropane anesthesia on the abnormal liver. Ann. Surg. 135: 145, 1952.

17. Gordh, T., and Astrom, A.: Respiratory effects of oxygen deficiency and carbon dioxide excess during ether and barbiturate anesthesia in the dog. Anesthesiology 16: 245, 1955.

18. Greene, N. M.: Lactate, pyruvate and excess lactate production in anesthetized man. Anesthesiology 22: 404, 1961.

19. Henneman, D. H., and Bunker, J. P.: Effects of general anesthetic on peripheral blood levels of carbohydrate and fat metabolites and serum inorganic phosphorus. J. Pharmacol. Exp. Ther. 133: 253, 1961

20. Henneman, D. H., and Vandam, L.: Effect of epinephrine, insulin, and tolbutamide on carbohydrate metabolism during ether anesthesia. Clin. Pharmacol. Ther. 1: 694, 1960.

21. Katz, R. L.: Neuromuscular effects of diethyl ether and its interaction with succinylcholine and d-tubocurarine. Anesthesiology 27: 52, 1966.

22. Katz, R. L., and Ngai, S. H.: Respiratory effects of diethyl ether in the cat. J. Pharmacol. Exp. Ther. *138:* 329, 1962.

23. Olsen, R. E.: Excess lactate and anaerobiosis. Ann. Intern. Med. *59:* 960, 1963.

24. Papper, S., and Papper, E. M.: The effects of pre-anesthetic medication, anesthetic and post-operative drugs on renal function. Clin. Pharmacol. Ther. *5:* 205, 1964.

25. Price, H. L.: General anesthesia and circulatory homeostasis. Physiol. Rev. *45:* 187, 1960.

26. Severinghaus, J. W., and Larson, C. P., Jr.: Respiration in anesthesia. In *Handbook of Physiology*, Section 3, Respiration, vol. II, p. 1219, American Physiological Society, Washington, D.C., 1965.

27. Van Brunt, E. E., and Ganong, W. F.: The effects of pre-anesthetic medication, anesthesia and hypothermia on the endocrine response to injury. Anesthesiology *24:* 500, 1963.

28. Vandam, L. D., and Moore, F. D.: Adrenocortical mechanisms related to anesthesia. Anesthesiology *21:* 531, 1960.

29. Whitteridge, D., and Bülbring, E.: Changes in the activity of pulmonary receptors in anesthesia and their influence on respiratory behavior. J. Pharmacol. Exp. Ther. *81:* 340, 1944.

6

The Pharmacodynamics of Halothane

STANLEY DEUTSCH

Halothane is one of a series of halogenated hydrocarbons which have been synthesized in an effort to produce potent, nonexplosive anesthetics. Suckling, in 1951, described its synthesis following the report by Robbins, in 1946,[30] that fluorohydrocarbons had anesthetic properties with therapeutic ratios greater than those of ether and chloroform. Addition of fluorine to a hydrocarbon confers marked stability to the compound and reduces its narcotic activity, toxicity, and flammability. The pharmacology of halothane was first described in animals by Raventos,[28] and, in 1956, Johnstone[16] reported on its clinical use in man.

Source, Chemistry, and Physical Properties

Halothane is synthesized by high thermal reactions (400 to 500 C), either with exchange halogenation of 1,1,1-trifluoro-2-chloro-2,2-dibromoethane and 1,1,1-trifluroro-2-chloroethane, or by direct bromination of 1,1,1-trifluoro-2-chloroethane. In another method, trifluorochloroethylene is reacted with hydrogen bromide and the product is rearranged with aluminum chloride at 90 C or by irradiation with ultraviolet light. Originally hexflurodichlorobutene, in a concentration of 0.01%, was present in the manufactured product, but further distillation has eliminated all traces of butene. This contaminant has been demonstrated to form as a result of interaction with copper in the presence of oxygen[4] and is also thought to concentrate in vaporizers, when not emptied, as a result of differential evaporation. The butene was at one time thought to be responsible for liver toxicity following halothane administration.

The chemical formula for halothane is CF_3—$CHClBr$ (1,1,1-trifluoro-2-bromo-2-chloroethane). It is a clear, colorless liquid with a specific gravity of 1.86 and a boiling point of 50.2 C. Halothane has a sweet, nonirritating, not unpleasant odor and is not flammable or explosive in the ranges of concentration used clinically. It is stable in the presence of soda lime, but is slowly decomposed by light to phosgene, hydrochloric acid, and other free halogens. Thymol, 0.01%, is added to inhibit decomposition, and it is further protected from light by storage in dark brown glass bottles. The blood/gas coefficient is 2.3 in man and in the dog, which results in greater delay in establishing an alveolar and arterial blood level than with nitrous oxide or cyclopropane, but which is more rapid than with diethyl ether. Its solubility in lipids results in deposition within fat-containing tissues which may serve as a reservoir to maintain blood levels of halothane following discontinuation of its administration. Halothane's solubility in fat has been correlated with its potency,[30] as have all anesthetics. Its vapor pressure at 20 C is 243 mm Hg. Halothane forms a constant boiling mixture or azeotrope when mixed with ether in proportions of 68% halothane and 32% ether. This mixture has been employed in clinical practice with the hope of overcoming the cardiovascular and respiratory depressant properties of halothane by addition of ether. Concentrations of the azeotrope greater than 10.7% are flammable, obviating one of the main attributes of halothane.

Halothane reacts with metals including brass, copper, stainless steel, magnesium, aluminum, bronze, and tin, resulting in their corrosion. Nickel and titanium are exceptions. Rubber and most plastics except polyethylene are also attacked by halothane, resulting in their deterioration. The high solubility in rubber reduces concentration in the inhaled mixture if low flow circle techniques are used. This is also true for other anesthetic agents with high rubber solubility such as methoxyflurane.

Action on Organ Systems

CENTRAL NERVOUS SYSTEM

Halothane is a "complete anesthetic" capable of producing 4th-stage anesthesia without oxygen deprivation. Unlike diethyl ether, halothane is not as potent an analgesic in the early period of anesthesia. The minimum alveolar concentration required in the dog and in man to prevent a muscular response to a painful stimulus in 50% of subjects is 0.76, making halothane at equilibrium the second most potent anesthetic used clinically.[31] A 65% reduction in minimum alveolar concentration for halothane is observed when 70% nitrous oxide in oxygen is added.[8]

Changes in the electroencephalogram have been described with halothane and are correlated with increased depth of anesthesia. Seven distinct wave form patterns have been described and are not markedly different from those observed with ether.[12]

Effects of halothane on the reticular activating system have been demonstrated by studies of evoked potentials with electrodes implanted within the brain and spinal cord of animals and by surface electrodes in man. These studies describe some of the neurophysiological mechanisms which occur during the state of altered consciousness and also explain some of the effect of halothane on the cardiovascular system.[38] Direct depressant effects of halothane on central sympathetic nervous system centers have been demonstrated by one series of experiments which imply that the major effect on the cardiovascular system is centrally mediated, while others have suggested that the depression of the cardiovascular system by halothane is the result of an action of peripheral sites rather than central vasomotor depression.[25, 37] Depression of the cardiac response to preganglionic stimulation has been observed at high frequencies of stimulation.[13] Needless to say, the exact location of the major effect of halothane has not been elicited.

Halothane is a mild cerebral vasodilator and, at surgical levels of anesthesia, cerebral blood flow is increased slightly above normal because of this slight dilation of cerebral vessels. The cerebral vessels exhibit a normal response to increased carbon dioxide tensions (vasodilation) and constrict with hypocapnia. A small decrease in the cerebral metabolic rate for oxygen is observed during halothane.[49]

PULMONARY SYSTEM

Halothane, unlike diethyl ether, is nonirritating to the upper and lower respiratory tracts. Bronchial secretions are therefore not stimulated, and the inspired concentration presented may be increased relatively rapidly during induction of anesthesia without producing coughing. Seldom is it necessary to exceed 3%, but, occasionally, 4 to 8% halothane can be used to effect a rapid induction, especially when nitrous oxide is not used.

Depression of respiratory centers has

been reported as evidenced by a decreased ventilatory response to increasing concentration of carbon dioxide which under normal conditions would be a stimulant to the respiratory centers. The ventilatory response is diminished as anesthesia is deepened (see Chapter 14).[20] Unlike ether, there is no stimulation of ventilation during the lighter planes of anesthesia. This is probably due to a lack of stimulation of pulmonary and other peripheral receptors. Respiratory rate increases and tidal volume decreases with increased depth of anesthesia.[7] Increased arterial carbon dioxide tension has been observed with increased depth of anesthesia, indicating reduction in alveolar ventilation.[3] At surgical levels of anesthesia, ventilation should be assisted or controlled to avoid respiratory acidosis.

In the isolated trachea preparation, high concentrations of halothane produce bronchiolar dilation as the result of a direct action on smooth muscle.[11] Increased pulmonary compliance has been observed in man and in animals. Reduced airway resistance has been related to stimulation of β-adrenergic receptors in the airway.[18] These effects form the basis for the use of halothane in the management of anesthesia in patients with asthma. A recent study revealed that halothane administered directly into the airway can reverse the increased airway resistance induced by hypercapnia.[22] Halothane administered systemically via cardiopulmonary bypass had no effect on airway resistance, which suggests a direct effect of halothane. In the cardiopulmonary bypass study, halothane had no effect on airway resistance when administered to the airway or systemically at normal carbon dioxide tensions.

CARDIOVASCULAR SYSTEM

Cardiovascular depression, evidenced by arterial hypotension, reduction in both cardiac output and peripheral resistance, and a decrease in myocardial contractility are observed with halothane at surgical levels of anesthesia.[7] This cardiovascular depression was recognized shortly after introduction of halothane and was largely responsible for the development of precision vaporizers for its administration. The degree of cardiovascular depression increases with increased depth of anesthesia.

Explanations for the depression observed include the following. (a) Direct myocardial depression has been reported in the isolated heart, isolated strips of heart muscle, and heart-lung preparation.[15, 19, 33] Digitalis has been reported to prevent and reverse myocardial depression produced by halothane.[14] Recently, evidence has been presented to indicate that the negative inotropism induced by halothane is the result of a dose-dependent depression of the intensity of energy conversion by the contractile element of heart muscle.[35] (b) Failure of an increase in sympathetic nervous activity during halothane which might overcome the myocardial depression and peripheral vasodilation produced by direct effects of halothane on cardiac and vascular smooth muscle has been reported.[23, 26] Central nervous depression of sympathetic activity has been mentioned previously. Evidence for sympathetic ganglionic blockade by halothane has also been presented.[13] (c) Reduction by halothane of the effect of catecholamines on myocardial and vascular smooth muscle has been reported.[10, 27] (d) Increased parasympathetic nervous activity with resultant reduction in heart rate and myocardial depression has been presented.[19]

Action on the peripheral circulation is predominantly one of vasodilation in both skin and skeletal muscle vessels.[2] Other peripheral actions of halothane rather than central autonomic effects have been mentioned previously. In the presence of reduced blood volume, the reduction in blood pressure may be severe following induction of anesthesia with halothane as a result of vasodilation.

Alterations in cardiac rhythm including bradycardia and atrioventricular nodal rhythm, often the cause of hypotension, can occur during halothane anesthesia at lighter levels of anesthesia, and are indicative of the increased parasympathetic nervous activity. Atropine sulfate administered intravenously will reverse both arrhythmias.[19] The reversal of the bradycardia which can occur in the dog is not always complete after intravenous atropine. If arterial carbon dioxide tension is allowed to increase because of reduced alveolar ventilation, premature ventricular contractions and a multifocal ventricular tachycardia may be observed.[1] Halothane, like the other halogenated hydrocarbon anesthetics, sensitizes the myocardium to the arrhythmic effects of catecholamines. Limiting the quantity of exogenously administered catecholamines by the careful subcutaneous administration of a solution of epinephrine no more concentrated than 1 : 100,000 and not more than 10 ml (100 μg) in any 10-minute period or 30 ml (300 μg)/ hour will result in a very low incidence (1 in 100) of cardiac arrhythmias.[17] Halothane sensitizes the myocardium to catecholamines to a far lesser degree than cyclopropane and only slightly more than trichlorothylene.

Cardiovascular effects of halothane are made use of in the practice of "deliberate hypotension" to reduce arterial pressure during some operations, and, therefore, to reduce bleeding and local edema. Ganglionic blocking drugs are sometimes added to increase the degree of hypotension, and maintenance of positive airway pressure to reduce venous return and, therefore, cardiac output, is also used in this technique.

SKELETAL MUSCLE

Although halothane has some effect on neuromuscular transmission and spinal monosynaptic and polysynaptic pathways, muscular relaxation is not as prominent at light levels of anesthesia as with ether. In animals, abdominal muscle relaxation is more easily achieved because of the smaller abdominal muscle mass. Neuromuscular blocking drugs are therefore used in man to provide satisfactory abdominal muscle relaxation at lighter levels of halothane anesthesia. Gallamine triethiodide has been recommended for use with halothane because of its ability to block the vagal effects of halothane.[34] Administration of curare may be accompanied by further reduction in arterial pressure and peripheral resistance because of the ganglionic blocking effect and is not advised in the dog or cat, but has been used in the horse (see Chapter 12).

LIVER AND KIDNEY

Liver function tests are temporarily abnormal following halothane, as with all anesthetics. Splanchnic blood flow is reduced during halothane on the basis of a reduction in perfusion pressure and not an alteration in splanchnic vascular resistance.[9] No evidence for hypoxia in this regional bed has been observed during halothane anesthesia[24]—as evidenced by no reported changes in lactate/pyruvate ratio or increased arterial-venous "excess lactate" across the liver.

Reports of acute hepatic necrosis following halothane administration prompted a retrospective study of the relationship between halothane and hepatic necrosis by the National Research Council.[20, 36] In a review of more than 10,000 necropsy reports following over 850,000 anesthetic administrations with all agents in 34 institutions, a total of 184 cases of massive or intermediate necrosis were confirmed by means of histological study. Most instances were related to operations with high risk (cardiac) and were explained by circulatory shock, sepsis, or previous hepatic disease. The possible rare occurrence of halothane-induced hepatic necrosis could not be ruled out. The incidence of necrosis with halothane was 1 : 1,200— no greater than the average for all anesthetics. Repeated exposure to halothane has been related to hepatic necrosis on the basis of development of a hypersensitivity which results in hepatic damage. A hepatotoxic metabolite of halothane may also explain this phenomenon, although none has been demonstrated.

With respect to renal function, significant reductions in glomerular filtration rate, renal plasma flow, and water and sodium excretion have been observed during halothane anesthesia.[5] The antidiuresis observed in man may be reversed by ethanol, an inhibitor of antidiuretic hormone, which indicates that the antidiuresis may be in part explained by the liberation of antidiuretic hormone during anesthesia as well as by the hemodynamic changes produced. Hemodynamic changes may be explained by the general hemodynamic effects of halothane that reduce cardiac output and arterial pressure. In addition, changes in renal vascular resistance as evidenced by increased filtration fraction and calculated renal vascular resistance contribute to the observed changes in glomerular filtration rate and renal plasma flow.

Increased plasma renin levels have been observed during halothane anesthesia.[6] The angiotensin produced as a result of this increased renin release may be in part responsible for the increased intrarenal vascular resistance observed during halothane.

MISCELLANEOUS EFFECTS

Halothane at light levels of anesthesia apparently has little effect on uterine tone and motility. At deeper levels, halothane produces relaxation and failure of the uterine smooth muscle to respond to oxytocics. This uterine relaxation has resulted in increased bleeding following placental separation in man. This has not been a problem in the dog. Halothane is an excellent agent for fetal or intrauterine surgery, when surgery is a problem because of excessive uterine tone.

Reduction in basal metabolic rate has been observed during halothane.[32] Adrenal cortical stimulation is not observed with halothane. This and the lack of increase in catecholamine liberation as a result of reduced sympathetic tone explain the absence of hyperglycemia and lactacidemia.

The pulmonary epithelium is the main area of both absorption and excretion of halothane. A small percentage (12 to 20%) of halothane undergoes biotransformation. Trifluoroacetic acid and bromide have been detected as metabolites in the urine.[29] It is not clear whether this biotransformation has any clinical or toxic importance.

Acute toxicity is related to overdose. With reduced blood volume, profound hypotension may be produced early in the induction of anesthesia. With severe cardiac disease and therefore reduced myocardial reserve, severe hypotension may be produced as a result of myocardial depression. This does not preclude the use of halothane for patients with cardiovascular disorders, but it does necessitate care in its administration.

THERAPEUTIC USES

The relative lack of respiratory irritation, flammability, and incidence of postanesthetic nausea and vomiting have made halothane the most popular clinical anesthetic agent in the western world. With control of its administered concentration by precision vaporization, supplementation of its analgesia with nitrous oxide, and addition of neuromuscular blocking drugs, excellent conditions may be provided for all operations.

Unpleasant effects related to its use include postoperative shivering in an attempt to increase body temperature lowered as a result of heat loss during operation. The vasodilation produced by halothane with loss of heat from the skin and losses from the respiratory tract and thoracic and abdominal wounds frequently result in marked lowering of the body temperature during operation.

Its solubility in blood and fat as compared to cyclopropane may result in maintenance of blood levels following extensive surgical periods with prolonged awakening if halothane is not discontinued toward the end of the operation. Thiopental is frequently used to speed the induction of anesthesia followed by maintenance with halothane-oxygen or halothane-nitrous oxide-oxygen.

REFERENCES

1. Black, G. W., Linde, H. W., Dripps, R. D., and Price, H. L.: Circulatory changes accom-

panying respiratory acidosis during halothane (Fluothane) anesthesia in man. Brit. J. Anaesth. *31:* 238, 1959.

2. Black, G. W., and McArdle, L.: The effects of halothane on the peripheral blood vessels. Anaesthesia *17:* 82, 1962.
3. Black, G. W., and McKane, R. V.: Respiratory and metabolic changes during methoxyflurane and halothane anaesthesia. Brit. J. Anaesth. *37:* 409, 1965.
4. Cohen, E. N., and Bellville, J. W.: Impurities in halothane anesthetic. Science *141:* 899, 1963.
5. Deutsch, S., Goldberg, M. L., Stephen, G. W., and Wu, W. H.: Effects of halothane anesthesia on renal function in normal man. Anesthesiology *27:* 793, 1966.
6. Deutsch, S., Hickler, R. B., Pierce, E. C., Jr., and Vandam, L. D.: Changes in renin activity of peripheral venous plasma during general anesthesia. Fed. Proc. *26:* No. 2, 503, 1967.
7. Deutsch, S., Linde, H. W., Dripps, R. D., and Price, H. L.: Circulatory and respiratory actions of halothane in normal man. Anesthesiology *23:* 631, 1962.
8. Eger, E. I., II, Brandstater, B., Saidman, L. J., Regan, M. J., Severinghaus, J. W., and Munson, E. S.: Equipotent alveolar concentrations of methoxyflurane, halothane, diethyl ether, fluroxene, cyclopropane, xenon and nitrous oxide in the dog. Anesthesiology *26:* 771, 1965.
9. Epstein, R. M., Deutsch, S., Cooperman, L. H., Clement, A. J., and Price, H. L.: Splanchnic circulation during halothane and hypercapnia in normal man. Anesthesiology *27:* 654, 1966.
10. Flacke, W., and Alper, M. H.: Actions of halothane and norepinephrine on the isolated mammalian heart. Anesthesiology *23:* 793, 1962.
11. Fletcher, S. W., Flacke, W., and Alper, M. H.: The actions of general anesthetic agents on tracheal smooth muscle. Anesthesiology *29:* 517, 1968.
12. Gain, E. A., and Paletz, S. G.: An attempt to correlate the clinical signs of Fluothane anesthesia with electroencephalographic levels. Canad. Anaesth. Soc. J. *4:* 289, 1957.
13. Garfield, J. M., Alper, M. H., Gillis, R. A., and Flacke, W.: A pharmacological analysis of ganglionic actions of some general anesthetics. Anesthesiology *29:* 79, 1968.
14. Goldberg, A. H., Maling, H. M., and Gaffney, T. E.: The value of prophylactic digitalization in halothane anesthesia. Anesthesiology *23:* 207, 1962.
15. Goldberg, A. H., and Ullrick, W. C.: Effects of halothane on isometric contractions of isolated heart muscle. Anesthesiology *28:* 838, 1967.
16. Johnstone, M.: The human cardiovascular response to Fluothane anaesthesia. Brit. J. Anaesth. *28:* 392, 1956.

17. Katz, R. L., Matteo, R. S., and Papper, E. M.: The injection of epinephrine during general anesthesia. Halothane. Anesthesiology *23:* 597, 1962.
18. Klide, A. M., and Aviado, D. M.: Mechanism for the reduction in pulmonary resistance induced by halothane. J. Pharmacol. Exp. Ther. *158:* 28, 1967.
19. Laver, M. B., and Turndorf, H.: Atrial activity during anesthesia in man. Circulation *28:* 63, 1963.
20. Linenbaum, J., and Leifer, E.: Hepatic necrosis associated with halothane anesthesia. New Eng. J. Med. *268:* 525, 1963.
21. Munson, E. S., Larson, C. P., Babed, A. A., Regan, M. J., Buechel, D. R., and Eger, E. I., II: The effects of halothane, fluroxene, and cyclopropane on ventilation: a comparative study. Anesthesiology *27:* 716, 1966.
22. Patterson, R. W., Sullivan, S. T., Malm, J. R., Bowman, F. O., and Papper, E. M.: The effect of halothane on human airway mechanisms. Anesthesiology *29:* 900, 1968.
23. Price, H. L.: Circulatory actions of general anesthetic agents and the homeostatic role of epinephrine and nor-epinephrine in man. Clin. Pharmacol. Ther. *2:* 163, 1961.
24. Price, H. L., Deutsch, S., Davidson, I. A., Clement, A. J., Behar, M. G., and Epstein, R. M.: Can general anesthetics produce splanchnic visceral hypoxia by reducing regional blood flow? Anesthesiology *27:* 24, 1966.
25. Price, H. L., Linde, W. H., and Morse, H. T.: Central nervous actions of halothane affecting the systemic circulation. Anesthesiology *24:* 770, 1963.
26. Price, H. L., and Price, M. L.: Has halothane a predominant circulatory action? Anesthesiology *27:* 764, 1966.
27. Price, M. L., and Price, H. L.: Effects of general anesthetics on contractile responses of rabbit aortic strips. Anesthesiology *24:* 770, 1963.
28. Raventos, J.: The action of Fluothane—a new volatile anaesthetic. Brit. J. Pharmacol. *11:* 394, 1956.
29. Rehder, K., Forbes, J., Alter, H., Hessler, O., and Stier, A.: Halothane biotransformation in man: a quantitative study. Anesthesiology *28:* 711, 1967.
30. Robbins, B. H.: Preliminary studies of the anesthetic activity of fluorinated hydrocarbons. J. Pharmacol. Exp. Ther. *86:* 197, 1946.
31. Saidman, L. J., Eger, E. I., II, Munson, E. S., Babad, A. A., and Muallem, M.: Minimal alveolar concentrations of methoxyflurane, halothane, ether and cyclopropane in man: correlation with theories of anesthesia. Anesthesiology *28:* 994, 1967.
32. Severinghaus, J. W., and Cullen, S. C.: Depression of myocardium and body oxygen consumption with Fluothane. Anesthesiology *19:* 165, 1958.

33. Shimosato, S., and Etsten, B.: Performance of digitalized heart during halothane anesthesia. Anesthesiology 24: 41, 1963.
34. Smith, N. T., and Whitcher, C. E.: Hemodynamic effects of gallamine and tubocurarine administered during halothane anesthesia. J. A. M. A. 199: 704, 1967.
35. Sugai, N., Shimosato, S., and Etsten, B.: Effect of halothane on force-velocity relations and dynamic stiffness of isolated heart muscle. Anesthesiology 29: 267, 1968.
36. Summary of the National Halothane Study. J. A. M. A. 197: 775, 1966.
37. Wang, H., Epstein, R. A., Markee, S. J., and Bartelstone, H. J.: The effects of halothane on peripheral and central vasomotor control mechanism of the dog. Anesthesiology 29: 877, 1968.
38. Winters, W. D., Mori, K., Spooner, C. E., and Bauer, R. O.: The neurophysiology of anesthesia. Anesthesiology 28: 65, 1967.
39. Wollman, H., Alexander, S. C., Cohen, P. J., Chase, P. E., Melman, E., and Behar, M. G.: Cerebral circulation of man during halothane anesthesia. Anesthesiology 25: 180, 1964.

7

The Pharmacodynamics of Methoxyflurane

PETER H. BYLES AND ALLEN B. DOBKIN

Methoxyflurane was developed as a general inhalation anesthetic agent based on the studies of Artusio and Van Poznak[2] and by Artusio and co-workers.[3] It is a halogenated ether, containing chlorine and fluorine ($CHCl_2CF_2OCH_3$), which is stable in the presence of air, light, alkali, or moisture under all normal conditions, and can safely be used in a closed circuit. It is supplied containing 0.01% butylated hydroxytoluene as an antioxidant and, on exposure to air, the latter slowly darkens to a yellow or brown color over a prolonged period without affecting the potency or safety of the agent. When stored in glass containers, in direct sunlight, there is some discoloration and precipitate formation when in contact with copper, copper alloys, or aluminum. Polyvinylchloride plastics and gum rubber are damaged by methoxyflurane, and the vapor is soluble to an appreciable extent in the usual rubber used in anesthetic apparatus.[15, 16, 17] Methoxyflurane will not burn in air, nitrous oxide, or oxygen at any temperature below 75 C.

The vapor pressure-temperature curve of methoxyflurane quite closely approximates that of water, and, at normal room temperature, the vapor pressure is about 30 torr. Thus, at room temperature (20° C) even the most efficient vaporizer cannot deliver concentrations of vapor above 3%. The blood level of the agent rises slowly during the induction of anesthesia as the anesthetic agent passes rapidly into body tissues, including the fatty deposits of the body. A marked arteriovenous concentration difference is maintained as long as the methoxyflurane administration continues and fat concentration rises steadily during the first 5 hours of anesthesia, even though the inhaled concentration is gradually reduced. At the end of administration, the arterial levels fall to a little below the venous and both fall gradually over a period of hours, while the fat levels continue to rise and take many hours to approach zero.[9] In practice, this means that induction with methoxyflurane alone is somewhat slow, equilibrium or saturation is only reached in procedures lasting many hours, and recovery is equally slow as the poorly perfused fat desaturates itself into the venous blood. Excretion is probably almost all via the lungs, and thus postoperative depression of respiration will further delay recovery. It is thus advisable in most cases to use some other agent, *e.g.*, thiopental, for induction, and to discontinue the administration before the completion of surgery, particularly where the operation has been lengthy. It is possible to turn off the methoxyflurane 30 minutes or more before the end of surgery on human subjects and to continue with nitrous oxide and oxygen alone, without any premature awakening.[12, 14] This method, with or without nitrous oxide, has been used in dogs to hasten recovery. A high flow of gases should be used toward the end of surgery to eliminate rebreathing and to hasten desaturation of both the patient and of the rubber parts of the anesthetic machine.

The arterial concentrations in dogs (35 to 45 mg %) were measured during light to deep anesthesia; the corresponding figures for man were stated to be 9 to 15 mg/100 ml in arterial blood.[5, 8, 9] These figures will, of course, depend to some extent on other factors such as the clinical status of the patient, the drugs used for premedication, etc. In terms of inhaled concentrations, 0.5 to 1.5% v/v is usually sufficient for maintenance, although higher values may be used to hasten induction to the depth required, provided that the vital signs remain stable. The classical eye signs of Guedel are poor guides to the depth of methoxyflurane anesthesia, and the blood pressure, respiratory pattern, and muscle tone should be observed as an index of depth. Hypotension and decrease in heart rate probably are the most useful and imperative signs of overdosage.

Respiration

Although it has a distinctive odor, methoxyflurane, in moderate concentrations, e.g., 0.5 to 1.5%, is not irritating to the respiratory tract, and may be used for induction although the prior use of an intravenous barbiturate is usually more convenient. Excessive increases in salivary or bronchial secretions have not been observed. In light planes of anesthesia, there is little disturbance of the normal pattern of respiration, although in dog experiments methoxyflurane tended to depress both the rate and depth of respiration.[11, 12, 13] There is general agreement that increasing the depth of anesthesia will certainly depress respiration, and assisted or controlled ventilation is required to prevent hypoventilation. It has been suggested that this depression constitutes a "built-in" safety factor against overdose during spontaneous respiration, but it would be unwise to rely upon this; it probably is best to augment ventilation in all but the shortest and most minor operative procedures.[1, 3, 18, 19, 26-29, 32, 33]

Cardiovascular

The effects of methoxyflurane on the heart are summarized in Figure 7.1. In common with most general anesthetic agents, methoxyflurane tends to reduce the blood pressure, depress the myocardium, and reduce cardiac output; these effects are proportional to the depth of anesthesia.[4, 10] The peripheral vascular tone appears to be well maintained and, hence, the blood pressure fall is counteracted quite effectively in most cases. Prolonged deep anesthesia will lead to hypotension and, as with any agent, a reduction in inhaled concentration will usually produce a restoration of blood pressure rapidly, provided that hypovolemia does not exist.[4, 14, 19] This compensating peripheral vasoconstriction is probably responsible for the widely reported occurrence of postoperative pallor in the presence of normal vital signs.[19]

The cardiac rate usually remains stable at a reduced rate and spontaneous arrhythmias are uncommon.[10-13, 18-22] Although some workers have found no hazard in the administration of epinephrine for hemostasis to patients under methoxyflurane anesthesia, experiments on dogs have produced serious and potentially lethal arrhythmias with this combination. Although premedication with appropriate agents can reduce these effects to some extent, it seems wise to limit the dose of epinephrine in a concentration not exceeding 1:200,000, or, preferably, to avoid its use altogether. It appears that methoxyflurane has about the same potentiality for producing cardiac arrhythmias with epinephrine as the halothane-ether azeotrope and light chloroform anesthesia, but less than that of halothane, trichloroethyl-

EFFECT OF METHOXYFLURANE ON THE HEART

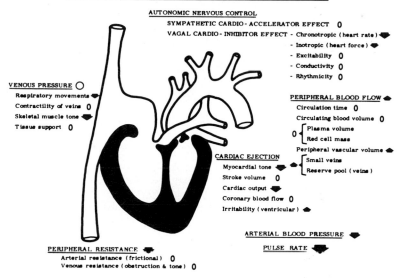

FIG. 7.1. Effect of surgical anesthesia with methoxyflurane on the heart and circulation

ene, and cyclopropane.[6, 13, 20-23] The inter-reaction of methoxyflurane with various other pressor amines has been studied, and only a slight reduction in the normal response was found; ventricular arrhythmias were generally uncommon.[10]

Musculoskeletal

Methoxyflurane is a good hypnotic and a potent analgesic; many workers have remarked on the persistence of a useful degree of analgesia well into the recovery period, reducing the need for narcotics at this time.[3, 24, 30, 31] This may be somewhat related to a generally slower recovery from general anesthesia. It can also produce quite marked muscle relaxation; some consider this to be primarily an action at spinal cord level.[25] Methoxyflurane is compatible with both depolarizing and nondepolarizing relaxants. Since it depresses respiration both centrally and peripherally, facilities should always be available for assisting or controlling ventilation to maintain adequate ventilation. The acid-base studies mentioned below suggest, in any case, that augmented ventilation is advisable in any but the shortest and most superficial procedures.[14]

Metabolic Effects

As would be expected, when respiratory depression is allowed to develop, there is respiratory acidosis with elevation of $PaCO_2$ and a fall in pH, but if ventilation is assisted to an appropriate degree only mild metabolic acidosis may occur[14] (Fig. 7.2). Estimations of arterial blood lactate and pyruvate have shown no significant change even when mild hypoxia or hypercarbia are present.[11] No significant changes in serum levels of sodium, potassium, and chloride were found in the dog.[12]

There is no appreciable change in the blood sugar levels although a slight rise may occur if pulmonary ventilation is inadequate. Serum inorganic phosphorus also rises under similar circumstances. Plasma catecholamines and whole blood histamine and serotonin are not altered under clinical conditions[11, 12] (Fig. 7.3).

Hepatic Function

Artusio has reported extensive liver function investigations on human subjects which revealed no impairment as judged by thymol turbidity, alkaline phospha-

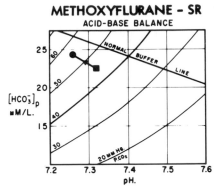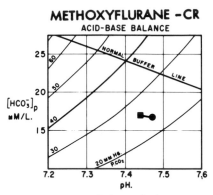

FIG. 7.2. Effect of surgical anesthesia with methoxyflurane on acid-base balance during spontaneous respiration (*SR*) and controlled respiration (*CR*). During spontaneous ventilation, a definite respiratory acidosis can occur; when the respiratory acidosis is reversed by adequate ventilation, a slight metabolic acidosis is noted.

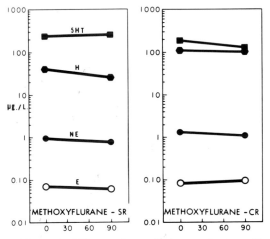

FIG. 7.3. Effect of surgical anesthesia with methoxyflurane on whole blood histamine and serotonin and plasma catecholamines.

tase, and bilirubin tests; the only abnormality found was a transient increase in sulfobromophthalein retention, maximal on the 3rd to 5th postoperative days.[3] The cephalin-cholesterol flocculation test becomes positive in dogs after 90 minutes of anesthesia but returns to normal within a few days, and there are no significant changes in serum glutamic oxalacetic transaminase and serum glutamic pyruvic transaminase estimations.[11, 12] The hepatic impairment appears to be similar in degree to that produced by ether, that is,

slight and transitory, although some clinicians have advised caution in the use of the agent in the presence of pre-existing liver disease.[32] In studies in dogs which were subjected to hypotension, hypoxia, hypercarbia, and deep planes of anesthesia, water vacuolization of the hepatic cells was found at biopsy; this was regarded as nonspecific and reversible.[7] No significant microscopic changes were found in the kidneys.

Renal Function

Urine output is suppressed during methoxyflurane anesthesia as with all strong inhalation agents, and there is prompt resumption of normal output during recovery.[11] However, renal function is not otherwise impaired even after frequent exposure to high concentration and conditions of hypoxia and hypovolemia.[7]

Miscellaneous

Recovery to a full preoperative state of consciousness tends to be lengthy, and some dogs have been sluggish for up to 24 hours after 90 minutes of anesthesia with 1% methoxyflurane, but, if the tapering off of dosage mentioned above is correctly judged, the protective reflexes will have returned very soon after the end of anesthesia.[11, 12] The vital signs usually remain stable in the recovery period without undue instability of the vasomotor system. Delirium is rare and nausea and vomiting are uncommon. There is a reluctance in dogs to take food and fluids for some time after anesthesia, in a few cases necessitating intravenous infusions.[10-12] The agent is compatible with all the usual premedicants, but its respiratory depressant properties should be kept in mind. An anticholinergic, e.g., atropine, is usually indicated for its vagal depressing action as well as to reduce salivation.[14]

REFERENCES

1. Andersen, N., and Andersen, E. W.: Methoxyflurane: a new volatile anaesthetic agent. Acta Anaesth. Scand. 5: 179, 1961.
2. Artusio, J. F., Jr., and Van Poznak, A.: The concept of intermediate potency. Far East J. Anesth. 2: 27, 1958.
3. Artusio, J. F., Jr., Van Poznak, A., Hunt, R. E., Tiers, F. M., and Alexander, M.: A clinical evaluation of methoxyflurane in man. Anesthesiology 21: 512, 1960.
4. Bagwell, E. E., and Woods, E. F.: Cardiovascular effects of methoxyflurane. Anesthesiology 23: 51, 1962.
5. Bagwell, E. E., Woods, E. F., and Gadsden, R. H.: Blood levels and cardiovascular dynamics during methoxyflurane inhalation in dogs. Anesthesiology 23: 243, 1962.
6. Bamforth, B. J., Siebecker, K. L., Kraemer, R., and Orth, O. S.: Effect of epinephrine on the dog heart during methoxyflurane anesthesia. Anesthesiology 22: 169, 1961.
7. Cale, J. O., Parks, C. R., and Jenkins, M. T.: Hepatic and renal effects of methoxyflurane in dogs. Anesthesiology 23: 248, 1962.
8. Chenoweth, M. B., and Hake, C. L.: The smaller halogenated aliphatic hydrocarbons. Ann. Rev. Pharmacol. 2: 363, 1962.
9. Chenoweth, M. B., Robertson, D. N., Erley, D. S., and Golhke, R.: Blood and tissue levels of ether, chloroform, halothane and methoxyflurane in dogs. Anesthesiology 23: 101, 1962.
10. Dobkin, A. B., and Byles, P. H.: The interaction of vasopressor drugs with halogenated anesthetics. In Proceedings of the Third World Congress of Anesthesiology, San Paulo, Brazil, vol. 2, p. 106, 1964.
11. Dobkin, A. B., Byles, P. H., and Neville, J. H., Jr.: Neuroendocrine and metabolic effects of general anaesthesia and graded haemorrhage. Canad. Anaesth. Soc. J. 13: 453, 1966.
12. Dobkin, A. B., and Fedoruk, S.: Comparison of the cardiovascular, respiratory and metabolic effects of methoxyflurane and halothane in dogs. Anesthesiology 22: 355, 1961.
13. Dobkin, A. B., and Israel, J. S.: The effect of SA-97, perphenazine, and hydroxyzine on epinephrine-induced cardiac arrhythmias during methoxyflurane anesthesia in dogs. Canad. Anaesth. Soc. J. 9: 36, 1962.
14. Dobkin, A. B., and Song, Y.: The effect of methoxyflurane-nitrous oxide anesthesia on arterial pH, oxygen saturation, $PaCO_2$ and plasma bicarbonate in man. Anesthesiology 23: 601, 1962.
15. Eger, E. I., and Brandstater, B.: Solubility of methoxyflurane in rubber. Anesthesiology 24: 679, 1963.
16. Eger, E. I., and Shargel, R.: The solubility of methoxyflurane in human blood and tissue homogenates. Anesthesiology 24: 625, 1963.
17. Gadsden, R. H., McCord, W. M., Woods, E. F., and Bagwell, E. E.: Gas chromatographic determination of methoxyflurane in blood. Anesthesiology 23: 831, 1962.
18. Hudon, F.: Methoxyflurane. Canad. Anaesth. Soc. J. 8: 544, 1961.
19. Hudon, F., Jacques, A., Clavet, M., Houde, J. J., Pelletier, J., and Trahan, M.: Symposium on methoxyflurane. Canad. Anaesth. Soc. J. 10: 276, 1963.
20. Israel, J. S., Byles, P. H., and Dobkin, A. B.: The cardiac effect of epinephrine during anaesthesia in hyperthyroid dogs. Canad. Anaesth. Soc. J. 9: 437, 1962.
21. Israel, J. S., Criswick, V. G., and Dobkin, A. B.: Effect of epinephrine on cardiac rhythm during anesthesia with methoxyflurane (Penthrane) and trifluoroethyl vinyl ether (Fluoromar). Acta Anaesth. Scand. 6: 7, 1962.
22. Israel, J. S., Dobkin, A. B., and Robidoux, H. J., Jr.: The effect of sympathetic blockade or hyperventilation on epinephrine-induced cardiac arrhythmias during anaesthesia with halothane and methoxyflurane. Canad. Anaesth. Soc. J. 9: 125, 1962.
23. Jacques, A., and Hudon, F.: Effect of epinephrine on the human heart during methoxyflurane. Canad. Anaesth. Soc. J. 10: 53, 1963.
24. Lambie, R. S.: The analgesia of methoxyflurane. Canad. Anaesth. Soc. J. 10: 469, 1963.
25. Ngai, S. H., and Hanks, E. C.: Effect of methoxyflurane on electromyogram, neuromuscular transmission, and spinal reflex. Anesthesiology 23: 158, 1962.
26. North, W. C., Knox, P. R., Vartanian, V., and Stephen, C. R.: Respiratory, circulatory and hepatic effects of methoxyflurane in dogs. Anesthesiology 22: 138, 1961.
27. Power, D. J.: McGill University experiences with methoxyflurane. Canad. Anaesth. Soc. J. 8: 488, 1961.
28. Romagnoli, A., and Korman, D.: Methoxyflurane in obstetrical anaesthesia and analgesia. Canad. Anaesth. Soc. J. 9: 414, 1962.
29. Siebecker, K. L., Jumes, M., Bamforth, B. J., and Orth, O. S.: The respiratory effect of methoxyflurane in dog and man. Anesthesiology 22: 143, 1961.

30. Torda, T. A. G.: The analgesic effect of methoxyflurane. Anaesthesia *18:* 287, 1963.
31. Van Poznak, A., Ray, B. S., and Artusio, J. F., Jr.: Methoxyflurane as an anesthetic for neurological surgery. J. Neurosurg. *17:* 477, 1960.
32. Wasmuth, C. E., Greig, J. H., Homi, J., Moraca, P. P., Isil, N. H.. Bitte, E. M., and Hale, D. E.: Methoxyflurane, a new anesthetic agent. A clinical evaluation based on 206 cases. Cleveland Clin. Quart. *27:* 174, 1960.
33. Wyant, G. M., Chang, C. A., and Rapicavoli, E.: Methoxyflurane (Penthrane): a laboratory and clinical study. Canad. Anaesth. Soc. J. *8:* 477, 1961.

8
The Pharmacodynamics of Cyclopropane

BENJAMIN E. ETSTEN AND SHIRO SHIMOSATO

Cyclopropane is an exceptional anesthetic agent because of its pharmacodynamics. This agent has been successfully employed in almost every type of surgical procedure, but it is particularly useful in subjects with poor circulatory status (*i.e.*, hypovolemia, anemia, and congenital heart disease), since, in moderate concentration, it tends to support the cardiocirculatory system.

Cyclopropane was first prepared by Freud in 1882 by reducing trimethylene dibromide with sodium in an alcoholic solution. The agent is a stable cyclic hydrocarbon, a colorless, nonirritating, highly flammable gas at room temperature. It has a boiling point of -32.89 C at atmospheric pressure, a density in relationship to air of 1.46, and a molecular weight of 42.05. The blood/gas solubility coefficient is 0.41 at 37 C and 1 atm.[14] The coefficient decreases as hemoglobin concentration of blood decreases (Fig. 8.1). Minimum alveolar concentration required to prevent response to a painful stimulus for cyclopropane is 17.5 vol % at sea level.[8] One of the clinical values of cyclopropane is the ease of induction and rapidity of recovery due to its physical and chemical properties. Cyclopropane has been considered as one of the more potent agents in depressing the amplitude of evoked potentials from the thalamus and midbrain reticular activating system of the cat.[6]

Respiratory System

The administration of cyclopropane frequently causes a progressive depression of tidal volume and respiratory frequency as inspiratory concentrations are increased. Preanesthetic medication, especially with opiates, should be kept minimal, since cyclopropane does not exert any stimulation upon the lower respiratory tract, as is the case with diethyl ether. However, in the patient without narcotic premedication, respiratory depression is usually minimal during the light plane of anesthesia and acid-base balance remains within normal limits. During deep cyclopropane anesthesia, respiratory frequency increases and tidal volume decreases, but the increase in rate is insufficient to compensate for the depression of the tidal volume. Therefore, respiratory acidosis will occur unless assisted or controlled respiration is initiated to maintain adequate alveolar ventilation.

Sensitization of pulmonary stretch receptors occurs during cyclopropane anesthesia as with other anesthetics.[34] The increase of respiratory frequency occurring during the deeper planes of anesthesia may be related to the increased activity of these pulmonary receptors. Recent studies in cats revealed that cyclopropane also caused increased activity of the carotid chemoreceptor as determined by changes

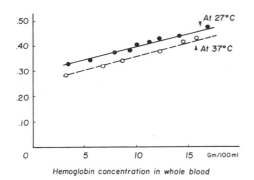

FIG. 8.1. Blood/gas solubility coefficients of cyclopropane plotted against hemoglobin concentrations in whole blood at 27 and 37 C.

in the chemoreceptor response curves for oxygen and carbon dioxide.[2]

Circulatory System

Cyclopropane may be considered a "pressor" agent. This is related to (a) an inotropic influence upon the myocardium; (b) a vasopressor action upon peripheral circulation; and (c) the stimulation of the sympathoadrenal systems.[10]

These effects on the myocardium and the sympathoadrenal system increase heart rate, blood pressure, cardiac output, and sudomotor activity.

This action of cyclopropane in eliciting a strong adrenergic response (i.e., arterial hypertension and increased plasma catecholamine concentrations) has been related to a selective and early depression of the bulbar vasodepressor center (Fig. 8.2).[20, 22] This concept has been challenged by investigators who have studied both single dog preparations and cross-circulation preparations where the anesthetic could be administered solely to the cephalad portion of the circulation.[17] They concluded that the excitatory vasomotor mechanisms appeared more susceptible to depression by the agent than the vasodepressor mechanisms. The effects of cyclopropane on the circulatory mechanisms have been studied in dogs by implanting devices for measuring arterial pressure and blood flow to the hind limb with stimulating electrodes in the hypothalamic and mesencephalic vasoactive areas

and carotid loops.[18] These experiments demonstrated that cyclopropane (inspired concentraton, 20 and 30%) depresses the pressor responses to extrinsic medullary stimulation and carotid occlusion. In the light of these conflicting observations, another group of investigators studied the effects of cyclopropane on cardiovascular reflexes in the cross-perfused dog gracilis muscle preparation.[5] They found that the vasoconstriction produced by cyclopropane may be related to the direct drug effect and not to sympathetic activation.

These conflicting data suggest that cyclopropane may exert a dual effect upon the autonomic nervous system: sympathomimetic and parasympathomimetic.[9] The directional changes in cardiac output and its related hemodynamics may be related to a predominating influence of the agent upon the autonomic nervous system in the experimental animal. In dogs premedicated with morphine (3 mg/kg) 35 minutes before induction of anesthesia, the cardiac output and heart rate are reduced during cyclopropane anesthesia.[12, 28] In contrast, in nonpremedicated trained dogs, cyclopropane causes an increase in cardiac output.[12, 26] Evidently, the preanesthetic medication may condition the agent's dominant effect on the autonomic nervous system. The central venous pressure, pulmonary arterial pressure, mean arterial pressure, and heart rate are increased during cyclopropane anesthesia. These hemodynamic changes have been explained in part by the increase in circulating catecholamines, particularly epinephrine.[7] On the other hand,

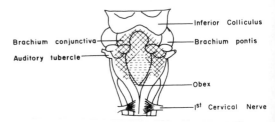

FIG. 8.2. Localization of pressor and depressor centers in the brain stem of the dog. Vasopressor (excitatory) regions indicated by *cross-hatching* and vasodepressor regions by *horizontal hatching*.

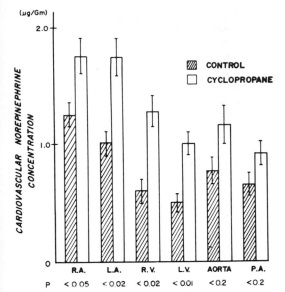

FIG. 8.3. Mean values (±S.E.) of norepineph-rine in cardiovascular tissues of dogs anesthetized with cyclopropane compared with control dogs. *R.A.*, right atrium; *L.A.*, left atrium; *R.V.*, right ventricle; *L.V.*, left ventricle; and *P.A.*, pulmonary arterial tissues.

cyclopropane causes a significant increase in norepinephrine concentrations in the myocardial tissue of dogs with marked reduction of epinephrine concentration (Fig. 8.3).[16] The increase in myocardial norepinephrine concentration during cyclopropane anesthesia is related to the increase in the activity of postganglionic sympathetic nerve endings.[16]

Most of the investigation relating to the direct depressant effect of cyclopropane upon the heart has been based on the studies of an isolated heart or heart-lung preparation.[21, 23] However, when the assessment of myocardial performance is made in terms of ventricular function curves (*i.e.*, relationship between the ventricular end diastolic pressure and stroke work) in dogs with an intact thorax during cyclopropane anesthesia, the left and right ventricular function curves are not significantly altered (Fig. 8.4).[9, 10, 29] Left ventricular stroke power is unaltered at a given end diastolic ventricular pressure with increased mean aortic pressure.[9, 10, 29]

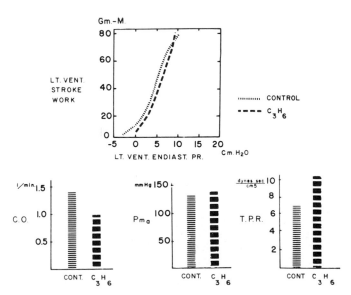

FIG. 8.4. *Top*, left ventricular function curve before and during cyclopropane anesthesia (arterial blood concentration, 30 mg %), showing no change in the left ventricular stroke work at any given left ventricular end diastolic pressure. *Bottom*, hemodynamic changes before and during cyclopropane anesthesia obtained in the same dog. *C.O.*, cardiac output in liters per minute, *Pm_a*, mean aortic pressure in millimeters of mercury; *T.P.R.*, total peripheral resistance in dynes per second per centimeter².

The direct "pressor" effect of cyclopropane upon the vascular bed through the liberation of catecholamines may be responsible for the increased mean aortic pressure. These data suggest that the heart is capable of producing the same amount of external stroke work and power from any given resting fiber length.

Recently, it has been shown that the contractile state of isolated cardiac muscle, like that of skeletal muscle, may be characterized best in terms of the relation between force of contraction and velocity of shortening.[1, 30] Subsequently, it has been demonstrated that the force-velocity relations also apply to the intact heart and that a change in the position of the force-velocity curve reflects a change in the contractile state of the myocardium.[4, 15, 27] In the intact ventricle, the left ventricular end diastolic pressure (LVEDP) is analogous to a preload (*i.e.,* a small load applied before contraction), which determines the fiber length prior to contraction or left ventricular end diastolic volume.[10] The mean aortic pressure is analogous to an afterload (*i.e.,* added load which determines the loading condition during the fiber shortening).[10]

When the mean aortic pressure (afterload) is experimentally elevated during steady state anesthesia, there is an increase in left ventricular stroke work with unchanged stroke power at any given LVEDP (preload).[10] It has been suggested that changes in left ventricular stroke work and power with and without increased mean aortic pressure (afterload) at any given LVEDP may be associated with unaltered force-velocity relationship during cyclopropane anesthesia.[10]

Recently, the effect of cyclopropane on "myocardial contractility" was determined by means of force-velocity relationship in intact dogs. The instantaneous relations between myocardial force and contractile element velocity obtained during the course of single, isovolumic beats in dogs anesthetized with chloralose-urethane solution are not altered during the surgical level of cyclopropane anesthesia (Fig. 8.5). The rate of force development,

manifested by the changes in the first derivative of left ventricular pressure (dP/dt) decreases during cyclopropane anesthesia (Fig. 8.6, *top*). There are accompanying decreases in peak force with increased time to peak force during anesthesia (Fig. 8.6), *bottom*). It has been suggested that the maximum velocity is an experimental measure of the rate of force-generating chemical process of the cardiac muscle, whereas the peak isometric force is a function of the number of active force-generating contractile sites.[3, 19] Changes in the actual performance of the cardiac muscle have been characterized by changes in both intensity and duration of active state, which is the mechanical measure of changes in excitation-contraction coupling and/or in the chemical interactions of the contractile proteins. Recent studies of cat heart muscle demonstrate that the rate of force development reflects the intensity of the active state and the time required to reach peak force reflects the duration of the active state.[31] The unaltered force-velocity relations with the increased time to peak force accompanied by the de-

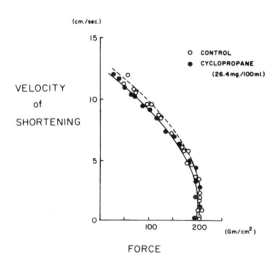

FIG. 8.5. Velocity of shortening of the contractile element of myocardium in centimeters per second plotted against myocardial wall force per unit of circumference in grams per cubic centimeter during isovolumic beats. Two instantaneous force-velocity curves shown were obtained before (O) and during (●) cyclopropane anesthesia (arterial blood concentration, 26.4 mg %) in the intact heart of the dog.

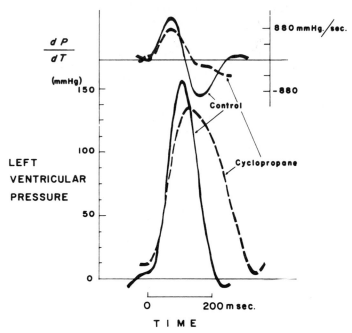

FIG. 8.6. Simultaneous recordings of the left ventricular pressure pulse and the first derivative of the ventricular pressure (rate of changes in the pressure) before (——) and during (– – –) cyclopropane anesthesia during isometric beats in the same dog as in Figure 8.5.

creased rate of force development and peak force observed during the administration of cyclopropane may be related to the fact that decreases in the intensity of active state are counteracted by increases in its duration. The contractile state of the intact heart has been characterized uniquely by the three-dimensional diagram (force-velocity-length relationship, Fig. 8.7).[10, 27] It should be noted that power is portrayed on the vertical plane as the product of force and velocity. The work is shown on the horizontal plane (length-tension relationship) and may be calculated as the product of force (pressure) and the fiber shortening, manifested by the volume change (stroke volume). At a given LVEDP (preload) and mean aortic pressure (afterload), changes in the inotropic state of the heart (i.e., myocardial contractility) are determined characteristically by the change in position and shape of the force-velocity curve.

It has been reported that the ventricular diastolic volume-pressure relationship, which is analogous to the length-tension relationship of the isolated cardiac muscle, was altered during cyclopropane anesthesia.[13] This phenomenon may be related to the change of the length-tension curve (Fig. 8.7), and may be responsible for maintenance of stroke volume when the afterload was further elevated during cyclopropane anesthesia. These findings may be strong evidence that the intrinsic contractile state of the intact heart (i.e., myocardial contractility) is unaltered during cyclopropane anesthesia.

Characteristics of cardiac arrhythmias occurring during cyclopropane anesthesia appear to be ventricular in origin and are usually transitory and purely functional in nature. Most common types of arrhythmias are atrioventricular nodal rhythm and ventricular extra systole. The incidence of cardiac arrhythmia has been related to increases in both arterial cyclopropane concentrations and carbon dioxide tension.[25] Adequate alveolar ventilation, in order to avoid hypoxia and hyper-

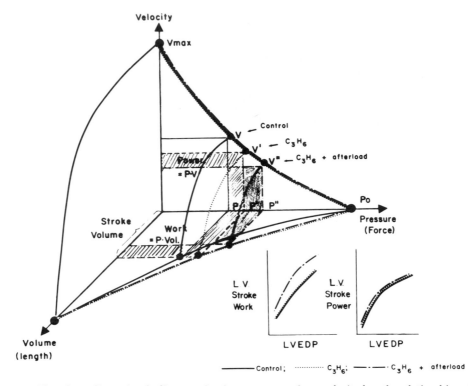

FIG. 8.7. The three-dimensional diagram for instantaneous force-velocity-length relationship of intact left ventricle of dogs. The three coordinates are: mean aortic pressure (force) on the horizontal axis, velocity of shortening on the vertical axis, and the intraventricular volume (length) on the third axis which increases towards the observer. Note that with cyclopropane anesthesia the myocardial contractility as determined by the force-velocity-length relations remains unaltered with unchanged power (vertical plane) and work (horizontal plane). Force-velocity-length relations were unaltered with added afterload (increases in mean aortic pressure) during anesthesia. The effects of cyclopropane with and without added afterload on ventricular performance are shown in the *inset*. *Vmax*, maximum velocity of shortening; *Po*, peak isometric force; *LVEDP*, left ventricular end diastolic pressure.

carbia, is the best preventive and therapeutic measure against cardiac arrhythmia which occurs during cyclopropane anesthesia.

Miscellaneous Effects

Cyclopropane decreases both portal and hepatic artery blood flow.[11] However, it does not produce damage to the normal liver and does not alter the rate of repair of liver injury due to chloroform.[24] Cyclopropane does not exert marked deleterious effects upon the kidney and, in moderate concentration, does not produce significant effect either on the uterine activity or tone in dogs.[13] However, during deep anesthesia, this agent is capable of causing a decrease in tone of the uterine musculature and duration and amplitude of contractions.[33] Cyclopropane tends to enhance intestinal tone. This anesthetic agent (10 to 15% in oxygen) provoked a fall in γ-aminobutyric acid level and a concomitant rise in glutamic acid.[32] This phenomenon may be due to an interference with the formation of γ-aminobutyric acid from glutamic acid or an acceleration in the formation of glutamic acid from the metabolized glucose.

REFERENCES

1. Abbott, B. C., and Mommaerts, W. F. H. M.:
   A study of inotropic mechanism in the papil-

lary muscle preparation. J. Gen. Physiol. *42:* 533, 1959.

2. Biscoe, T. J., and Millar, R. A.: Effects of inhalation anaesthetics on carotid body chemoreceptor activity. Brit. J. Anaesth. *40:* 2, 1968.

3. Buccinco, R. A., Sonnenblick, E. H., Spann, J. F., Friedman, W. F., and Braunwald, E.: Interactions between changes in the intensity and duration of the active state in the characterization of inotropic stimulation on heart muscle. Circ. Res. *21:* 857, 1967.

4. Covell, J. W., Ross, J., Jr., Sonnenblick, E. H., and Braunwald, E.: Comparison of the force-velocity relation and the ventricular function curve as measures of the contractile state of the intact heart. Circ. Res. *19:* 364, 1966.

5. Cristoforo, M. F., and Brodu, M. J.: The effects of halothane and cyclopropane on skeletal muscle vessels and baroreceptor reflexes. Anesthesiology *29:* 36, 1968.

6. Davis, H. S., Collins, W. F., Randt, C. T., and Dillon, W. H.: Effect of anesthetic agents on evoked central nervous system responses: gaseous agents. Anesthesiology *18:* 634, 1957.

7. Deutsch, S., Linde, H. W., and Price, H. L.: Circulatory and sympathoadrenal responses to cyclopropane in the dog. J. Pharmacol. Exp. Ther. *135:* 354, 1962.

8. Eger, E. I., II., Brandstater, B., Saidman, L. J., Regan, M. J., Severinghaus, J. W., and Munson, E. S.: Equipotent alveolar concentrations of methoxyflurane, halothane, diethyl ether, fluroxene, cyclopropane, xenon and nitrous oxide in the dog. Anesthesiology *26:* 771, 1965.

9. Etsten, B., and Li, T. H.: Current concepts of myocardial function during anesthesia. Brit. J. Anaesth. *34:* 884, 1962.

10. Etsten, B., and Shimosato, S.: Myocardial contractility: performance of the heart during anesthesia. In *Anesthesia and the Circulation,* p. 55. F. A. Davis Company, Philadelphia, 1964.

11. Galindo, A.: Hepatic circulation and hepatic function during anaesthesia and surgery. II. The effect of various anaesthetic agents. Canad. Anaesth. Soc. J., *12:* 337, 1965.

12. Greisheimer, E. M., Ellis, D. W., Makarenko, L., and Stewart, G. H.: Effect of morphine and cyclopropane on cardiovascular function in dogs. Anesthesiology *18:* 196, 1957.

13. Hamilton, W. K., Larson, C. P., Bristow, J. D., and Rapaport, E.: Effect of cyclopropane and halothane on ventricular mechanics: a change in ventricular diastolic pressure-volume relationships, J. Pharmacol. Exp. Ther. *154:* 566, 1966.

14. Laasberg, L. H., and Etsten, B. E.: Gas chromatographic analysis of cyclopropane in whole blood. Anesthesiology *26:* 216, 1965.

15. Levine, H. J., and Britman, N. A.: Force-velocity relations in the intact dog heart. J. Clin. Invest. *43:* 1383, 1964.

16. Li, T. H., Laasberg, L. H., and Etsten, B. E.: Effects of anesthetics on myocardial catecholamines. Anesthesiology 25: 641, 1964.

17. Markee, S., Wang, H. H., and Wang, S. C.: Effects of cyclopropane on the central vasomotor mechanisms of the dog. Anesthesiology *27:* 742, 1966.

18. Nagai, S. H., and Bolme, P.: Effects of anesthetics on circulatory mechanisms in the dog. J. Pharmacol. Exp. Ther. *153:* 495, 1966.

19. Podulsky, R. J.: The mechanism of muscular contraction. Amer. J. Med. *39:* 708, 1961.

20. Price, H. L., Cook, W. A., Jr., Deutsch, S., Linde, H. W., Mishalove, R. D., and Morse, H. T.: Hemodynamic and central venous actions of cyclopropane in the dog. Anesthesiology 24: 1, 1963.

21. Price, H. L., and Helrich, M.: Effect of cyclopropane, diethyl ether, nitrous xode, thiopental and hydrogen ion concentration on myocardial function of dog heart-lung preparation. J. Pharmacol. Exp. Ther. *115:* 206, 1955.

22. Price, H. L., Price, M. L., and Morse, H. T.: Effects of cyclopropane, halothane and procaine on the vasomotor "center" of the dog. Anesthesiology *26:* 55, 1965.

23. Prime, F. J., and Gray, T. C.: Effect of certain anesthetics and relaxants on circulatory dynamics. Brit. J. Anaesth. *24:* 101, 1952.

24. Raginsky, B. B., and Baourne, W.: The effect of cyclopropane anesthesia on normal and impaired liver. Canad. Med. Ass. J. *31:* 500, 1934.

25. Robbins, B. H.: *Cyclopropane Anesthesia,* 2nd ed., p. 41. The Williams & Wilkins Company, Baltimore, 1958.

26. Robbins, B. H., and Baxter, J. H.: Cardiac output in dogs under cyclopropane anesthesia. J. Pharmacol. Exp. Ther. *32:* 179, 1938.

27. Ross, J., Jr., Covell, J. W., Sonnenblick, E. H., and Braunwald, E.: Contractile state of the heart characterized by force-velocity relations in variably afterloaded and isovolumic beats. Circ. Res. *18:* 149, 1966.

28. Schull, L. G., Berry, B., Villarreal, R., and Thomas, J.: The effect of morphine on the cardiovascular system of the dog anesthetized with cyclopropane. Anesthesiology *22:* 199, 1961.

29. Shimosato, S.: Ventricular function during anesthesia. In *Effects of Anesthetics on the Circulation,* edited by H. L. Price and P. J. Cohen, p. 135. Charles C Thomas, Publisher, Springfield, Ill., 1964.

30. Sonnenblick, E. H.: Force-velocity relations in mammalian heart muscle. Amer. J. Physiol. *202:* 931, 1962.

31. Sonnenblick, E. H.: Active state in heart muscle. J. Gen. Physiol. *50:* 661, 1967.

32. Tsuji, H., Balagot, R. C., and Sadove, M. S.:

Effect of anesthetic on brain gamma-amino-butyric and glutanic acid levels. J. A. M. A. *183:* 659, 1963.

33. Van Liere, E. J., Mazzocco, T. R., and Northup, D. W.: The effect of cyclopropane, trichlorethylene, and ethyl chloride on the uterus of the dog. Amer. J. Obstet. Gynec. *94:* 861, 1966.

34. Whitteridge, D.: Effect of anesthetics on mechanical receptors. Brit. Med. Bull. *14:* 5, 1958.

9

The Pharmacodynamics of Chloroform

PETER H. BYLES AND ALLEN B. DOBKIN

Chloroform was discovered independently by von Liebig, Soubeiran, and Guthrie in 1831.[1, 12] Its name and chemical properties were described by Dumas in 1835, and Flourens first described its anesthetic properties in 1847.[13] In the same year, following a suggestion from a Liverpool chemist, David Waldie, James Young Simpson used it clinically.[25] It became popular, having the advantages over diethyl ether of being less irritating, more potent, and nonflammable. However, a growing concern with its low safety margin led to its declining use in human medicine and, in 1912, the Committee on Anesthesia of the American Medical Association condemned its use for major surgery. In 1950, re-evaluation of the drug was advocated in the light of modern techniques and research.[29] Since then, new work has demonstrated the limited efficacy of this anesthetic.[5, 8-10]

Chloroform, or trichlormethane ($CHCl_3$), is a colorless, aliphatic, halogenated hydrocarbon. Heat, light, and exposure to air favor the conversion of chloroform to phosgene (carbonyl chloride, $COCl_2$) which is highly poisonous. Thus, it is supplied in dark, sealed bottles with 1% ethyl alcohol added.

In theory, chloroform can react with a strong alkali, producing various toxic substances such as phosgene, dichloracetalde-hyde, carbon monoxide, and formates,[2] but, in fact, very little, if any, of these compounds are formed when chloroform is used with soda lime CO_2 absorbers. It is nonflammable in air, oxygen, or nitrous oxide, but will decompose at high temperatures into phosgene.[27]

Many methods have been devised for estimating the concentrations in gas, blood, and tissue, mostly based on the Fugiwara color reaction of halides with alkaline pyridine, but the development of the gas chromatograph has probably made these techniques obsolete.[29]

Respiration

Chloroform is a potent respiratory depressant at levels of anesthesia adequate for surgical intervention. Induction is usually quite smooth because of its nonirritating properties. It causes minimal salivation and marked relaxation of the bronchial muscles. For safety, it should therefore be administered in a nonrebreathing system, employing artificial respiration and a precision vaporizer capable of accurate regulation at low concentration.[5]

During induction and light anesthesia, the respiratory rate and tidal volume increase, but, in the deeper planes of anesthesia, respiration is progressively depressed. In contrast to many other anesthetic agents, myocardial depression may progress faster than respiratory depression; this constitutes a special hazard. A sudden rise in inspired concentration can provoke laryngeal spasm and breath holding, and rapid fluctuations in the inspired levels can be very dangerous to cardiovascular function.[24-29]

Circulation

Myocardial tone and contractility are reduced in proportion to the depth of anesthesia; the stroke volume and cardiac output tend to fall, and there is bradycardia which is mediated by the vagus and blocked by premedication with atropine (Fig. 9.1). The average fall in cardiac output in dogs given chloroform by open drop mask to a level adequate for surgery is 28%.[3] In other studies in which chloroform was given to the point of apnea, the cardiac output was reduced to a mean of 25% of the control figure.[4] Blood pressure and pulse pressure are reduced due to a central depression of vasomotor tone and peripheral vasodilation. The opinions expressed in the past have been that chloroform anesthesia cannot safely be prolonged beyond 1 hour because of serious cardiovascular depression. Although high concentrations of the drug can reduce

cardiac output to very low levels, careful quantitative administration from a calibrated vaporizer can give adequate surgical levels of anesthesia without excessive hypotension, and there is no longer any good reason to impose an arbitrary time limit as long as the concentration is controlled carefully.[9, 10] In dogs, chloroform has been shown to exceed halothane in potency,[8] and low concentrations can lead to apnea.[6, 9] The relative nonirritability and ease of vaporization increases the danger of overdose. Snow[26] emphasized myocardial depression and was one of the first to use a quantitative method for its administration. For maximum safety a vaporizer should be used which is capable of giving incremental increases in the concentration of chloroform of no more than 0.1%.[29] It is worth noting that a saturated vapor at room temperature contains 15 to 20 times the concentration required for anesthesia.

Much attention has been directed to the effect of chloroform on the cardiac rhythm and the means by which it can produce cardiac arrest.[20] Three mechanisms are suggested: (a) direct myocardial depression from overdose leading to asystole; (b) reflex vagal inhibition often following a sudden rise in the inhaled concentration; and (c) ventricular fibrillation. Adequate

EFFECT OF CHLOROFORM ON THE HEART

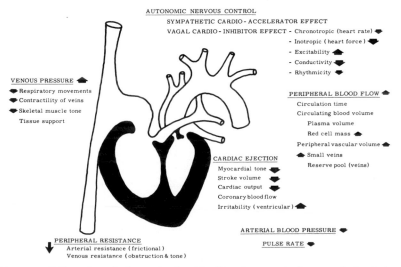

FIG. 9.1. Effect of surgical anesthesia with chloroform on the heart and circulation

premedication with atropine or scopolamine will produce enough of a vagal blockade to protect against reflex inhibition, provided that surgical stimulation is not started until an adequate depth of anesthesia has been reached. Ventricular fibrillation is a comparatively uncommon occurrence compared with direct myocardial depression[11, 18, 19] and it is well established that most arrhythmias occurring during anesthesia are much more common in the presence of suboxygenation and high blood carbon dioxide levels.

Arrhythmias reported in man include a high incidence of ventricular extrasystoles and premature contractions, artrioventricular rhythm and atrioventricular block, and ventricular tachycardia. The sequence of events in the isolated turtle heart as the concentration of chloroform increased was frequently atrioventricular block to atrioventricular nodal rhythm, ventricular rhythm to asystole.[29]

Arrhythmias were uncommon in dogs during chloroform anesthesia when ventilation was well maintained, although with spontaneous respirations there was a tendency towards respiratory acidosis, with $PaCO_2$ readings up to 67 torr.[8] In human beings undergoing surgery, there is the same low incidence of arrhythmias if the patients receive an oxygen-enriched gas mixture and ventilation is controlled with a mechanical ventilator to prevent respiratory acidosis.[10]

Chloroform, in common with other halogenated hydrocarbons and cyclopropane, sensitizes the heart to the arrhythmic effects of catecholamines, whether endogenous in origin, e.g., from preinduction stress and fright or a stormy induction, or exogenous, e.g., administered to facilitate hemostasis. In a study of the comparative tendency of various anesthetic agents to sensitize the heart to epinephrine, 0.5% chloroform was found to be less dangerous in this respect than trichlorethylene, cyclopropane, or halothane.[7]

Hepatic Effects

Chloroform has long had a reputation for producing a significant depression of liver function or causing actual centrilobular hepatic necrosis and liver failure.[15, 23, 30] For a long time it was not fully realized that the preoperative starvation or disease, causing depletion of carbohydrate and protein, hypoxemia, and/or reduced hepatic perfusion during surgery, would all greatly increase the incidence of these complications. Furthermore, it is almost impossible to entirely exclude other factors which might have a deleterious effect on the liver, such as other medications, blood transfusions, and infection.

Dogs may show only slight fatty changes of the liver after repeated surgical anesthesia with chloroform.[29] However, others have concluded that chloroform has a worse effect on the canine liver than either diethyl ether or halothane.[14] Other studies show a tendency of chloroform to cause fatty infiltration of the liver resulting in abnormal hepatic function tests.[16, 22, 28]

Renal Effects

In experimental dogs, there is no significant depression of urea clearance in tests performed 4 to 5 days after chloroform anesthesia.[29] In comparing chloroform with a number of other agents in human subjects, it has been found that all tend to impair renal function (estimated by urea clearance, phenosulphthalein excretion, alkali reserve, and blood nonprotein nitrogen estimations) to a moderate and similar degree for a short time postoperatively, with a rapid reversion to normal. Chloroform usually produces an oliguria followed by compensatory polyuria after cessation of administration.[1, 6] It must be emphasized that many factors other than the anesthetic agent are involved in producing renal function changes after surgery, and that the kidney, like the liver, is sensitive to hypoxia, hypercarbia, and hypotension.

Metabolic Effects

Chloroform anesthesia in dogs which are breathing spontaneously depresses respiration, leading to a progressive respiratory acidosis. With prolonged administration there was also a trend toward metabolic acidosis.[6, 8] However in human subjects undergoing surgery in whom respiration is controlled, there is minimal metabolic acidosis.[10] There is little change in blood electrolytes (Na$^+$, K$^+$, and Cl$^-$). Blood glucose levels rise during spontaneous respiration, a change which is minimized by controlled ventilation.[6, 8] During spontaneous respiration, chloroform causes a slight increase in the serum inorganic phosphorus and a slight increase in whole blood lactate and pyruvate without appreciable changes in excess lactate. There is no change in the whole blood histamine and serotonin or in the plasma catecholamine blood levels. During controlled respiration, similar changes are seen, except that serum inorganic phosphorus does not rise.[6]

Miscellaneous

The hematocrit rises, partly due to contraction of the spleen and partly to increased capillary permeability with fluid translocation.[6] The white blood count increases in the postoperative phase with a relative increase in polymorphonuclear leukocytes, and platelets show no significant change.[1]

The peristalic and secretory activity of the bowel is decreased, and nausea and vomiting are common in man during recovery.[31]

The uterus is well relaxed in the deeper planes and, while this may on occasion be useful in man, as with all general anesthetics, it carries a risk of postpartum hemorrhage. The agent readily crosses the placenta and affects the fetus, but, despite this, chloroform has been used for light obstetrical anesthesia.

Good muscular relaxation can be obtained in planes 2 and 3 of stage 3 anesthesia, but in view of the cardiovascular and respiratory effects of chloroform, it is probably wiser to use a muscle relaxant drug rather than deeper anesthesia if profound relaxation is required.[5]

Potency of Chloroform

Various methods have been used for the estimation of chloroform blood levels, and wide variations have been noted between different species and also within species.[21]

In man, blood levels in stage 3 anesthesia ranged from 7 mg % for plane 1 to 13 mg % for plane 4. When nitrous oxide was used in combination with chloroform, blood concentrations were a little lower, but, in all cases, the scatter was very wide. The concentration of chloroform given in the inspired gas is usually in the range 0.5 to 1.5 vol %.

A large portion of the blood chloroform is transported in the erythrocytes and, probably, some is bound to blood protein.[17] Chloroform, for all practical purposes, is eliminated unchanged by the lungs. Provided that respiration is adequate, elimination is quite rapid, and 30 to 50% is excreted in the first 15 minutes.[29] Recovery is slower than that seen following halothane anesthesia.[8]

Many techniques have been used to vaporize chloroform, but it is desirable that a vaporizer be used that allows incremental changes in vapor concentration. Assisted or controlled respiration is essential in any but a very brief administration, or else a progressive respiratory acidosis will occur, and hypercarbia is known to increase the hazards of chloroform anesthesia.

Conclusions

Following the initial early enthusiasm for chloroform in the latter half of the 19th century, there has been a steady decline in its popularity in both human and veterinary medicine, largely because of its capability of producing rapid cardiac failure and hepatic disease. However, Waters and co-workers, in 1951, called for a re-evaluation of the drug in the light of modern knowledge and methods, and suggested that its bad reputation was ill-deserved. This view has been violently attacked by Sykes,[27] who observed that the number of cases involved in the Wisconsin Study was so small that its conclusions were of questionable value, and that, even so, the incidence of cardiac dysfunction reported was enough to be highly alarming. Further work since 1951, incorporating controlled ventilation and precision control of the administered concentration, has tended to confirm Water's conclusion that chloroform does not deserve to be abandoned, provided that the precautions already suggested are stringently observed. Nevertheless, it remains a potentially dangerous agent in that it is (with fatal results) easy to give badly—in which case disaster may strike almost unheralded; it is the opinion of the writers that other anesthetic techniques are available which offer the advantages of chloroform with a wider margin of safety, albeit at higher cost.

REFERENCES

1. Adriani, J.: *The Chemistry and Physics of Anesthesia*. Charles C Thomas, Publisher, Springfield, Ill., 1962.
2. Bassett, H. L.: Action of soda-lime on chloroform. Lancet 2: 561, 1949.
3. Blalock, A.: The effect of ether, chloroform and ethyl chloride anesthetics on the minute cardiac output and blood pressure. Surg. Gynec. Obstet. 46: 72, 1928.
4. Boniface, K. J., Brown, J. M., and Kronen, P. S.: The influence of some inhalation anesthetic agents on the contractile force of the heart. J. Pharmacol. Exp. Ther. 113: 64, 1955.
5. Dobkin A. B.: The effects of anesthetic agents on the cardiovascular system: a review. Canad. Anaesth. Soc. J. 7: 317, 1960.
6. Dobkin, A. B., Byles, P. H., and Neville, J. H., Jr.: Neuroendocrine and metabolic effects of general anaesthesia. I. Under normal conditions, during spontaneous breathing, controlled breathing, mild hypoxia and mild hypercarbia. Canad. Anaesth. Soc. J. 13: 130, 1966.
7. Dobkin, A. B., Donaldson, H., and Purkin, N.: The effect of perphenazine on epinephrine-induced cardiac arrhythmias in dogs. II. Anaesthesia with cyclopropane, chloroform and trichlorethylene. Canad. Anaesth. Soc. J. 6: 251, 1959.
8. Dobkin, A. B., Harland, J. H., and Fedoruk, S.: Chloroform and halothane in a precision system. Comparison of some cardiovascular, respiratory and metabolic effects in dogs. Brit. J. Anaesth. 33: 239, 1961.
9. Dobkin, A. B., Johnston, H. J., and Skinner, L. C.: A study of chloroform anaesthesia in a precision system. I. The effect on anion-cation balance in man. Canad. Anaesth. Soc. J. 7: 257, 1960.
10. Dobkin, A. B., Skinner, L. C., and Johnston, H. J.: A study of chloroform anaesthesia in a precision system. II. The effect on circulatory dynamics and anesthetic morbidity. Canad. Anaesth. Soc. J. 7: 379, 1960.
11. Embly, E. H.: The causation of death during the administration of chloroform. Brit. Med. J. 1: 817, 1902.
12. Featherstone, H. W.: Chloroform. Anesthesiology 8: 362, 1947.
13. Flourens, M. J. P: Quoted by Sykes. C. R. Acad. Sci. [D] (Paris) 24: 340 and 482, 1847.
14. Green, H. D., Ngai, S. H., Sulak, M. H., Crow, J. B., and Slocum, H. C.: Effect of anesthetic agents on hepatic structure and function in dogs. Anesthesiology 20: 776, 1959.
15. Guthrie, L.: Quoted by Sykes. Lancet 1: (January 27) 193, 1894.
16. Jones, W. M., Margolis, G., and Stephen, C. R.: Hepatotoxicity of inhalation anesthetic drugs. Anesthesiology 19: 715, 1958.
17. Kety, S. S.: The theory and applications of the exchange of inert gas at the lungs and tissues. Pharmacol. Rev. 3: 1, 1951.
18. Levy, A. G.: The genesis of ventricular extrasystoles under chloroform with special reference to consecutive ventricular fibrillation. Heart 5: 299, 1914.
19. Levy, A. G., and Lewis, T.: Heart irregularities resulting from the inhalation of low percentages of chloroform vapor and their relationship to ventricular fibrillation. Heart 3: 99, 1911.
20. Meggison: Quoted by Sykes. Med. Times (February 5) 317, 1848.
21. Pearcy, W. C., Knott, J. R., Pittinger, C. B., and Keasling, H. H.: Encephalographic and circulatory effects of chloroform in dogs. Anesthesiology 18: 88, 1957.
22. Richards, C. C., and Bachman, L.: A study of liver function in dogs after anesthesia with trichlorethylene and chloroform. Anesth. Analg. (Cleveland) 34: 307, 1955.
23. Sheehan, H. L.: Delayed chloroform poisoning. Brit. J. Anaesth. 22: 204, 1950.
24. Siebecher, K. L., and Orth, O. S.: A report of seven administrations of chloroform for open thoracic operations. Anesthesiology 17: 792, 1956.
25. Simpson, J. Y.: Quoted by Sykes. Lancet 2: (November 20) 549, 1847.
26. Snow, J.: *On Chloroform and Other Anaesthetics*. J. & A. Churchill, Ltd., London, 1858.
27. Sykes, W. S.: *Essays on the First Hundred Years of Anaesthesia*. Vol. I, 1960, Vol. II, 1961, E. S. Livingstone, Ltd., Edinburgh, 1961.
28. Virtue, R. W., Payne, K. W., Caranna, L. J., Gordon, G. S., and Rember, R. R.: Observations during experimental and clinical use of fluothane. Anesthesiology 19: 478, 1958.
29. Waters, R. M. (editor): *Chloroform, a Study after 100 Years*. University of Wisconsin Press, 1951.
30. Whipple, G. H., and Sperry, J. A.: Chloroform poisoning, liver necrosis and repair. Bull. Hopkins Hosp. 20: 278, 1909.
31. Whittaker, A. M., and Jones, C. S.: Report of 1500 chloroform anesthetics administered with a precision vaporizer. Anesth. Analg. (Cleveland) 1: 60, 1965.

10

The Pharmacodynamics of Divinyl Ether, Ethyl Chloride, Fluroxene, Nitrous Oxide, and Trichlorethylene

ALLEN B. DOBKIN AND PETER H. BYLES

Divinyl Ether

Divinyl ether $(CH_2=CH)_2$ is an unsaturated ether which is commercially available as Vinethene, to which is added 3.5% dehydrated alcohol and 9.01% N-phenyl-1-naphthylamine to prevent oxidation and polymerization. It is a highly volatile, clear, colorless liquid with a slight purplish fluorescence, with a boiling point of 28.4 C, specific gravity of 0.77, and vapor density of 2.4. To produce a surgical plane of anesthesia, 2 to 3% in air is adequate. The blood concentration with sufficient anesthesia for abdominal relaxation is approximately 15 mg % when given with air and 5 to 10 mg % when given with nitrous oxide and oxygen (2:1). Divinyl ether is as flammable and explosive as diethyl ether, and it decomposes when exposed to light, air, heat, and acids, giving rise to aldehydes, organic oxides, and acids. It is supplied in sealed, dark brown bottles under nitrogen and should be stored in a cool place. It is compatible with soda lime and so may be administered in a closed system.[1]

Semmler first prepared this compound in 1887. Its anesthetic properties were discovered by Leake and Chen[50, 51] in 1930, and its clinical use was first reported by Gelfan and Bell in 1933.[37] It has been widely used for minor surgical and dental operations of short duration and as an induction agent prior to diethyl ether anesthesia.[8, 39] Similar methods have been utilized in cats and small dogs.

RESPIRATION

Divinyl ether is a potent respiratory depressant, causing rapid shallow breathing during light and moderate depths, and slow, shallow, and irregular breathing at excessive depths. Because of its potency and high volatility, it is dangerous to administer with intermittant positive pressure ventilation unless the administered concentration can be greatly reduced and controlled.[53]

CIRCULATION

Divinyl ether depresses the myocardium. Blood pressure is not affected appreciably during moderate depths of anesthesia, but it falls precipitously during deep anesthesia. There is usually no change in the pulse rate. Cardiac arrhythmias of the supraventricular type are common, and atrioventricular nodal rhythm is seen frequently when the anesthetic is administered in a closed circle system for a long period.[46]

MUSCULOSKELETAL

Muscular relaxation can be produced, but not to the same degree as with diethyl ether. Uterine activity during labor is not inhibited when divinyl ether is used for obstetrical analgesia.[8]

METABOLIC

No comprehensive studies have been reported. Divinyl ether is a weak sympathomimetic agent, causing less release of epinephrine from the adrenal gland than diethyl ether, and there is apparently only a slight rise in blood sugar. In general, metabolic effects are similar to those of light ether anesthesia.[53]

HEPATIC EFFECTS

There is danger of severe damage to the liver if it is used for more than 1 hour, particularly if it is administered with air or if it is used to produce a deep plane of anesthesia. Liver toxicity, causing central zonal necrosis, is more likely to occur with divinyl ether than with chloroform.[9]

RENAL EFFECTS

No effect on kidney function after a single administration has been seen. With repeated administrations, progressive decrease in kidney function, as measured by urea clearance and urine excretion, occurs.[53]

MISCELLANEOUS

There is no alteration in coagulation or bleeding time. Twitching, athetoid-like movements have been seen in cats shortly following the induction of anesthesia. These movements and convulsions have occurred during and after its use, especially if induction has been too rapid and without supplementary oxygen.[7]

Induction and emergence are usually very rapid because of the low solubility coefficient of this agent. Salivary secretions can be profuse and preanesthetic medication should include atropine.

Ethyl Chloride

Discovered by Glauber in 1648, ethyl chloride (CH_3CH_2Cl) is a halogenated hydrocarbon whose anesthetic properties were described by Flourens in 1847; it was first used clinically by Carlson in 1894. It is a clear, very volatile, colorless fluid with an ethereal odor. The boiling point is 12.5 C, specific gravity is 0.92 at 20 C, and its vapor density is 2.3. To produce a surgical plane of anesthesia, 3 to 4.5% is required for inhalation. The blood concentration for anesthesia is 20 to 30 mg %. Respiratory failure occurs at 40 mg %. Since ethyl chloride is a gas at room temperature, it is supplied in glass containers in a liquid state under 30 to 40 mm Hg pressure, equipped with a fine nozzle and spring-loaded tight cap. It can also be used in gaseous form by feeding through a cyclopropane flowmeter on an anesthetic machine.[18] Ethyl chloride can burn and is explosive at 4 to 15% in air and 4 to 67% in oxygen. It cannot be used in a circle system because hydrolysis occurs with soda lime to form ethyl alcohol and ethyl chloride.[40]

Pharmacological and toxic properties are similar but less intense than those of chloroform.[42] However, because of its high volatility and low partition coefficient, the danger of overdose is great; therefore, its use has been limited to speed induction of anesthesia with other agents such as diethyl ether, or for use in very brief operations. Induction and emergence from anesthesia are rapid.[20]

RESPIRATION

During the induction of anesthesia, inhalation of ethyl chloride can cause hyperpnea due to local stimulation, followed by respiratory depression which may lead rapidly to apnea. Laryngospasm may occur if it is administered too rapidly, and the development of tachypnea is taken as a sign of overdose.

CIRCULATION

Blood pressure falls during surgical anesthesia because of the depression of the vasomotor centers and peripheral vasodilation of blood vessels. During the induction of anesthesia, an initial strong vagotonic effect can produce a brydycardia. This can be followed by vagal depression during surgical anesthesia, causing a tachycardia. Subsequent bradycardia is a sign of overdose. Myocardial contractility is decreased, causing a 15% reduction in cardiac output during the surgical plane of anesthesia.[5] Overdose causes apnea first, then asystole due to myocardial depression. Ethyl chloride increases the sensitivity of the myocardium to catecholamines.

MUSCULOSKELETAL

Spasticity of skeletal muscles may occur during induction, causing opisthotonus and rigidity of messeter muscles. Deep anesthesia does not relax abdominal muscles well, and, if anesthesia is prolonged, muscular twitching and convulsions may occur.

METABOLIC

No comprehensive studies on its metabolic effects have been done because it is unsafe for prolonged operations. Jaundice and fatty degeneration of the liver has been reported after repeated use, and it is feared that renal damage may occur, but no data have proven such an effect. No data are available as to its effect on blood sugar or blood clotting factors.

MISCELLANEOUS

During induction, salivation is moderate, and then suppressed. Nausea and vomiting occur frequently during recovery. Because of its narrow margin of safety and flammability, ethyl chloride is useful only for rapid induction of inhalation anesthesia and for very brief operations.

Fluroxene

Fluroxene is the fluorinated ether trifluoroethyl vinyl ether (CF_3—CH_2—O—CH=CH_2) known commercially as Fluoromar. This compound is a clear, colorless, volatile liquid with a mild ethereal odor. It is quite stable, but has 0.01% N-phenyl-1-naphthylamine added to ensure that polymerization and hydrolysis will not occur in the presence of moisture and air, with the formation of trifluoroethanol and acetaldehyde.[58] It is supplied in dark brown bottles to prevent the breakdown of the stabilizer by light. The boiling point is 43.2 C, specific gravity is 1.13, vapor density is 4.4, and vapor pressure at 20 C is 286 mm Hg. To produce a surgical plane of anesthesia, 4 to 6% is required in air or oxygen and 3 to 5% in nitrous oxide with oxygen (2:1). The blood concentration for anesthesia is 15 to 40 mg %.[59] When fluroxene vapor is circulated over soda lime with oxygen, carbon dioxide, and water vapor, no free fluoride ion or acetaldehyde is released; thus, it may be used in closed circuit anesthesia.

Fluroxene was first prepared by Shukys in 1951, and its anesthetic properties were discovered by Krantz and co-workers in 1953.[48] It was first used as an anesthetic in 1953 by Sadove, but it has not been accepted widely, although it is effective and safe, because its lower flammability limit (4% fluroxene) is still within the range of concentrations used for clinical anesthesia.[55, 63] It has satisfactory hypnotic, analgesic, and muscle relaxant properties, it is less of a depressant to the cardiorespiratory system than halothane, and it provides much pleasanter anesthesia than diethyl ether.[15, 59, 66] Electroencephalogram (EEG) levels are somewhat different from diethyl ether, giving the impression of lighter anesthesia than in fact occurs.[10] Hypotension is the best sign of overdose.[36]

RESPIRATION

During spontaneous breathing of fluroxene, a marked tachypnea develops along with a progressive decrease in the tidal volume.[26, 31, 66] However, if excessive depth of anesthesia is avoided, pulmonary ventilation remains adequate as reflected by a minimal change in the arterial blood pH and pCO_2, and there is no metabolic acidosis as is seen with diethyl ether anesthesia.[26, 27] Controlled respiration is easily achieved with fluroxene.[26]

CIRCULATION

Fluroxene produces little or no effect on the arterial blood pressure up to a moderate surgical plane, and then there is a progressive rapid fall, particularly when the inhaled concentration is increased too quickly.[59, 66] The myocardium is depressed only during deep anesthesia. Pulse rate usually increases slightly.[27] Arrhythmias are very uncommon. Occasionally, transient displacement of the pacemaker and ventricular arrhythmias may appear during induction or when respiratory depression occurs and breathing is not augmented during deep anesthesia. Serious arrhythmias may develop if epinephrine is injected, but the danger of ventricular fibrillation is remote even in the presence of hyperthyroidism[43, 44] (Fig. 10.1).

MUSCULOSKELETAL

Muscular relaxation is weak during a moderate depth of surgical anesthesia,

but is adequate for abdominal surgery in the dog and cat.

METABOLIC EFFECTS

During fluroxene anesthesia, there is a moderate rise in blood sugar and serum inorganic phosphorus and a marked increase in blood lactate and pyruvate, but the lactate/pyruvate ratio is not appreciably elevated nor is there a significant accumulation of excess lactate (Fig. 10.2). There is also no appreciable rise in plasma catecholamines or whole blood histamine and serotonin (Fig. 10.3). During controlled breathing, the rise in the blood sugar is suppressed. If mild hypoxia is permitted, there is a moderate rise in the plasma catecholamines.[27]

HEPATIC EFFECTS

No appreciable alterations of liver function occur during the administration of fluroxene. Serum transaminase (serum glutamic oxalacetic transaminase and serum glutamic pyruvic transaminase) estimations remain within normal limits, Bromsulphalein retention is slightly elevated for a brief period, and the thymol turbidity test remains normal.[11, 27, 63]

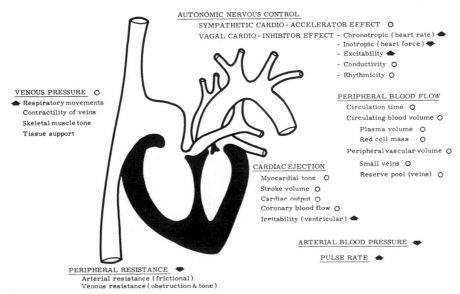

FIG. 10.1. Effect of surgical anesthesia with fluroxene on the heart and circulation

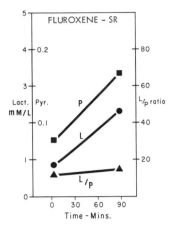
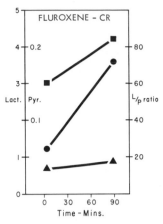

FIG. 10.2. Effect of surgical anesthesia with fluroxene on whole blood lactate (L), pyruvate (P), and L/P ratio during spontaneous (SR) and controlled (CR) respirations.

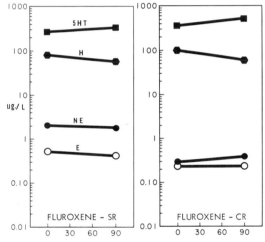

FIG. 10.3. Effect of surgical anesthesia with fluroxene on whole blood histamine (H) and serotonin ($5Ht$) and plasma epinephrine (E) and norepinephrine (NE) during spontaneous (SR) and controlled (CR) respirations.

RENAL EFFECTS

There is a marked suppression of urine excretion, which becomes apparent within 5 to 10 minutes after induction of anesthesia with fluroxene. However, urine output resumes promptly after the anesthetic is eliminated.[27] Urea clearance tests have been essentially normal following fluroxene anesthesia.

MISCELLANEOUS

No alteration in coagulation time has been noted, but bleeding time may be lengthened for a short period. Induction and emergence from anesthesia are relatively rapid. Salivation is not a prominent occurrence, being less than with diethyl ether. The occurrence of nausea and vomiting is also less than with ether.[59]

Nitrous Oxide

Discovered by Priestley in 1772, the analgesic properties of N_2O were mentioned by Davy in 1799, and it was first used deliberately as an anesthetic by Wells in 1844. It is a sweet smelling, non-irritating, inorganic gas. It is supplied in tanks as a liquid at a pressure of 800 psi. Its boiling point is -89 C, and its specific gravity in 1.5. Although it supports combustion, it is not flammable or explosive, and it is quite stable and nonreactive with soda lime.

The anesthetic qualities of this gas have been studied in man.[4, 32] There is no doubt that, in man, complete analgesia for dental work and obstetrics can be obtained,[47, 61] and light general anesthesia can be produced in a concentration that permits adequate oxygenation (20 to 30% O_2). In normal, healthy, calm individuals, 40 to 50% produces good analgesia and 80 to 90% produces light general anesthesia. Nitrous oxide anesthesia is more effective in the presence of a low basal metabolism or debility, whereas it may be virtually ineffective in producing general anesthesia in vigorous healthy patients, and can only be useful when supplemented with drugs or other anesthetics, *e.g.*, halothane, ether, thiopental. It is very difficult to maintain smooth general anesthesia in dogs with nitrous oxide alone, but has been used in a combination with halothane anesthesia. It has been used in cats to facilitate the induction of anesthesia with other inhalation agents.

Nitrous oxide is relatively insoluble in blood and body tissues, and induction and emergence are rapid. Uptake of nitrous oxide by blood is 200 to 500 ml/minute, and 70% is eliminated within 3 minutes. EGG patterns are similar to the early levels observed with diethyl ether.[32] Signs of anesthesia are similar to Guedel planes down to stage 3, plane 1, beyond which the signs of hypoxia supervene when the concentration is increased beyond 80%. Deeper planes of anesthesia cannot be obtained unless supplemented with other anesthetic agents.

RESPIRATION

Nitrous oxide is nonirritating, and protective reflexes are not completely obtunded. During induction of anesthesia, there is progressive depression of the primary senses (smell, hearing, sight, touch, and pain), the nasopharynx becomes insensitive to stimulation, and the rate of breathing increases slightly during light general anesthesia, but it remains regular provided that the airway is clear.[12, 61] If the attempt is made to induce deeper anesthesia with higher concentrations of nitrous oxide, expiration becomes forced and then gasping and irregular due to asphyxia. Bronchial muscles are not affected.

CIRCULATION

If anesthesia is induced smoothly, there is virtually no change in the central venous or arterial blood pressure, pulse rate, or cardiac output, and no electrocardiographic changes appear which might indicate alterations in myocardial conduction or irritability.[74] Slight cardiac dilation may occur. Dilation of peripheral veins occurs during general anesthesia, an effect similar to that of the more potent anesthetic agents.

MUSCULOSKELETAL

Resistive movements are seen during induction of anesthesia, which gives way to quietude during light anesthesia, but without apparent relaxation of skeletal muscle tone. If deeper anesthesia is attempted by increasing the concentration of nitrous oxide and reducing the oxygen concentration, the muscles show signs of hypoxia, rigidity, and twitching, which give way to flaccidity if cardiovascular collapse ensues. Nitrous oxide does not potentiate the effects of muscle relaxant drugs.

METABOLIC, HEPATIC, AND RENAL EFFECTS

No comprehensive studies of nitrous oxide anesthesia alone have been done with respect to hepatic and renal function. Urine output is not suppressed.

Similarly, during smooth nitrous oxide anesthesia with adequate provision of oxygen, there is apparently no release of catecholamines, blood sugar is not increased, and serum inorganic phosphorus, lactate, pyruvate, and serum transaminase levels are not altered appreciably. Oxygen consumption may be decreased in stage 3 anesthesia.[27]

MISCELLANEOUS

There is no significant effect on the autonomic nervous system. Salivation may increase during induction of anesthesia, but it is depressed thereafter. Bleeding and coagulation time are unaffected in adults, but may be prolonged in newborn infants.[64] Induction and emergence of anesthesia are relatively rapid, but may be marked by excitement. Postoperative vomiting occurs relatively frequently, especially if a hypoxic concentration is administered.[6]

Diffusion anoxia can occur at the end of nitrous oxide anesthetia because of its initial rapid elimination from the blood. This transient hypoxia can occur as the oxygen in the lungs is diluted by the outpouring of nitrous oxide from the blood and may cause hypoxia (diffusion anoxia). This can be prevented by the addition of oxygen at high flows during the first 2 to 3 minutes of emergence from nitrous oxide anesthesia.[33]

Trichlorethylene

Trichlorethylene ($CHCl=CCl_2$) is an unsaturated chlorinated hydrocarbon which was discovered by Fischer in 1864.[35] Its analgesic properties were first discovered by Lehmann about 1911, and its propensity for affecting the trigeminal nerve was noted by Plessner in 1915.[22, 23] Not until 1933 was serious investigation undertaken to determine the efficacy of this compound as a general anesthetic.[45]

It is a colorless liquid having a sweet odor like chloroform. The boiling point is high (86.7 C), specific gravity is 1.5, vapor density is 4.53, and vapor pressure is 59 mm Hg. The preparation used for anesthesia contains 0.1% thymol as a stabilizer and 1:200,000 waxoline blue to aid identification. It is unstable to light and heat and with soda lime, forming the toxic products phosgene and hydrochloric acid and dichloracetylene, respectively.[14] It is not flammable below 10% concentration.

Trichlorethylene is a potent analgesic in 0.5% concentration. If general anesthesia is produced with this agent alone, toxic effects occur. It is only used alone to produce analgesia for obstetrics or minor surgical proceedures. If general anesthesia is desired, it should be supplemented with nitrous oxide. A maximum inhaled concentration of 1.5% trichlorethylene should not be exceeded. This corresponds to a blood concentration of approximately 10 mg %.[17] The EEG changes with trichlorethylene, when used with nitrous oxide, show low amplitude high frequency waves during surgical anesthesia. Toxic signs are tachypnea and cardiac arrhythmias, and the EEG loses its rhythmicity, but the pattern alterations are not seen.[19] Trichlorethylene is addicting if exposure is frequent.[49] It is slowly absorbed, and it takes a long period to accomplish saturation. Most of the drug is excreted unchanged in the lung, but some undergoes degradation with formation of trichloracetic acid, monochloracetic acid, and trichloroethanol.[13, 38, 54, 65] Excretion is usually slow, and recovery from anesthesia may be prolonged; thus, the administered concentrations should be reduced progressively during long operations.[62]

RESPIRATION

Analgesic concentrations (0.5%) do not irritate the respiratory tract. Pharyngeal and laryngeal reflexes are obtunded during light anesthesia, and breathing is regular and not depressed; but, when surgical anesthesia is produced without supplementary nitrous oxide, rapid shallow breathing occurs and a respiratory acidosis is likely to occur[30, 31] (Fig. 10.4). The tachypnea is due to the stimulation of the Hering-Breuer reflex.[68] If tachypnea is allowed to persist, cyanosis and respiratory arrest may ensue, accompanied by bradycardia and hypotension.[60] Convulsions have also been reported.[21]

CIRCULATION

Analgesic concentrations (up to 0.5%) have virtually no effect on the blood pressure, pulse rate, and cardiac rhythm (Fig. 10.5). When administered with nitrous oxide for surgical anesthesia, there is no excessive elevation or depression of the blood pressure and only a slight reduction of the heart rate during spontaneous respiration.[24, 27, 67] At high concentration, marked bradycardia, hypotension, and serious ventricular arrhythmias appear. The arrhythmias have been divided into two groups: those developing during induction of anesthesia, comprised of vagus bradycardia, atrioventricular block, and nodal rhythm; and those seen during deep anesthesia, which are atrial and ventricular premature contractions.[3, 52] The combination of trichlorethylene anesthesia with epinephrine is dangerous, causing atrioventricular block, ventricular extrasystoles which can progress to ventricular fibrillation, or asystole.[24, 28, 57] Chlorpromazine and perphenazine protect the heart against epinephrine-induced arrhythmias but should not be relied upon if more than

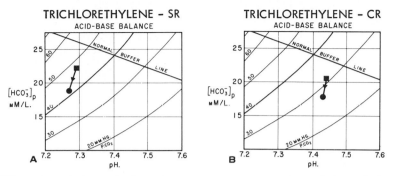

Fig. 10.4. Effect of surgical anesthesia with trichlorethylene on acid-base balance during spontaneous (*SR*) and controlled respiration (*CR*). Carbon dioxide tensions are high (*A*) and there is a progressive decrease in pH as anesthesia is continued. During controlled ventilation (*B*), carbon dioxide tensions are lowered and pH is within normal range, but there is still a developing metabolic acidosis.

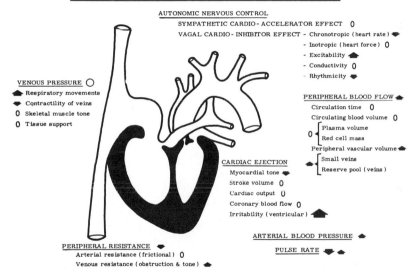

Fig. 10.5. Effect of surgical anesthesia with trichlorethylene on the heart and circulation.

0.5 mg epinephrine is contained in the local anesthetic used for infiltration. Cardiac output does not change appreciably and peripheral vessels are usually constricted; thus, there is no excessive hemorrhagic oozing during trichlorethylene anesthesia.

MUSCULOSKELETAL

There is no marked reduction in muscular tone and, therefore, muscle relaxant drugs should be used if good muscle relaxation is required during trichlorethylene anesthesia.

METABOLIC EFFECTS

During spontaneous breathing, $PaCO_2$ rises if tachypnea is permitted to develop.[25, 30, 31] There is usually no change or there is a slight rise in the blood sugar.[27, 29] Serum inorganic phosphorus usually rises while serum potassium decreases, and there is a slight rise in serum lactate and pyruvate with a subsequent increase in the lactate/pyruvate ratio and excess lactate[27] (Fig. 10.6). Plasma volume decreases somewhat, with an appreciable rise in the hematocrit. There is no change in the blood histamine, serotonin, or cate-

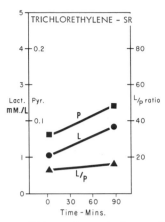

FIG. 10.6. Effect of surgical anesthesia with trichlorethylene on whole blood lactate, pyruvate, and L/P ratio.

cholamines. During controlled breathing, the metabolic effects noted above are less obvious, except for appearance of elevation of blood catecholamines. This effect is also seen with mild hypoxia. Hypercarbia produced by hyperventilation appears to cause an elevation of the blood serotonin.[27] There is no change in the blood urea estimations.[29]

HEPATIC AND RENAL EFFECTS

During clinical anesthesia, there is no significant effect on liver or kidney function, although there is usually a marked suppression of urine output during the period of trichlorethylene administration.[2, 16, 56]

MISCELLANEOUS

No appreciable alterations in the blood constituents have been reported; however, chronic exposure may cause anemia and other toxic signs on the bone marrow. It has minimal effects on the fetus when used for obstetrical analgesia.[41]

REFERENCES

1. Adriani, J.: Stability of vinyl ether (Vinethene). Anesthesiology 2: 191, 1941.
2. Armstrong, D. M.: The assessment of liver damage following trichorethylene and diethyl ether anesthesia. Anaesthesia 2: 45, 1947.
3. Barnes, C. G., and Ives, J.: Electrocardiographic changes during Trilene anaesthesia. Proc. Roy. Soc. Med. 37: 526, 1944.
4. Bennett, J. H., and Seevers, M. H.: The effect

of anoxia on the action of nitrous oxide in the normal human subject. J. Pharmacol. Exp. Ther. 61: 459, 1937.
5. Blalock, A.: The effects of ether, choloroform and ethyl chloride anesthesia on the minute cardiac output and blood pressure. Surg. Gynec. Obstet. 46: 72, 1928.
6. Bodman, R. I., Morton, H. J. V., and Thomas, E. T.: Vomiting by out-patients after nitrous oxide anaesthesia. Brit. Med. J. 1: 1327, 1960.
7. Boston, F. K.: Convulsions under Vinethene anaesthesia. Brit. Med. J. 1: 929, 1940.
8. Bourne, W.: Divinyl oxide anaesthesia in obstetrics. Lancet 1: 566, 1934.
9. Bourne, W., and Raginzky, B. B.: Vinyl ether anaesthesia in dogs: effects upon normal and impaired liver. Brit. J. Anaesth. 12: 62, 1935.
10. Brechner, V. L., and Dornette, W. H. L.: Electroencephalographic patterns under Fluoromar-nitrous oxide anesthesia. Anesthesiology 18: 321, 1957.
11. Brechner, V. L., Watanabe, R. S., and Dornette, W. H. L.: Values of serum glutamic oxalacetic transaminase following anesthesia with Fluoromar. Anesth. Analg. (Cleveland) 37: 257, 1958.
12. Burns, B. D., Robson, J. G., and Welt, P. J. L.: The effects of nitrous oxide upon sensory thresholds. Canad. Anaesth. Soc. J. 7: 411, 1960.
13. Butler, T. C.: Metabolic transformations of trichlorethylene. J. Pharmacol. Exp. Ther. 97: 84, 1949.
14. Carden, S.: Hazards in the use of closed circuit technique for Trilene anaesthesia. Brit. Med. J. 1: 319, 1944.
15. Cavallaro, R. J., and Dornette, W. H. L.: Fluoromar anesthesia in obstetrics. Obstet. Gynec. 17: 447, 1961.
16. Chenoweth, M. B., and Hake, C. L.: The smaller halogenated aliphatic hydrocarbons. Ann. Rev. Pharmacol. 2: 363, 1962.
17. Clayton, J. L., and Parkhouse, J.: Blood trichloroethylene concentrations during anaesthesia under controlled conditions. Brit. J. Anaesth. 34: 141, 1962.
18. Cole, W. H. J.: Ethyl chloride as a gaseous anaesthetic. Anaesthesia 11: 156, 1956.
19. Courtin, R. F.: Electroencephalographic and clinical observations with trichlorethylene and nitrous oxide anesthesia. Dallas Med. J. 41: 613, 1955.
20. Crandell, D. L.: The present status of ethyl ether, vinyl ether and ethyl chloride in anesthesia. North Carolina Med. J. 18: 497, 1957.
21. Culbert, T. D.: Convulsions under trichloroethylene anaesthesia. Brit. Med. J. 2: 679, 1942.
22. Defalque, R. J.: The "specific" analgesic effect of trichlorethylene upon the trigeminal nerve. Anesthesiology 22: 379, 1961.
23. Defalque, R. J.: Pharmacology and toxicology of trichloroethylene. Clin. Pharmacol. Ther. 2: 665, 1961.

24. Dobkin, A. B.: The effects of anaesthetic agents on the cardiovascular system. A review. Canad. Anaesth. Soc. J. 7: 317, 1960.
25. Dobkin, A. B., and Byles, P. H.: The effect of trichloroethylene-nitrous oxide anaesthesia on acid-base balance in man. Brit. J. Anaesth. 34: 797, 1962.
26. Dobkin, A. B., and Byles, P. H.: Effect of fluroxene (Fluoromar) on acid base balance in man. Acta Anaesth. Scand. 6: 115, 1962.
27. Dobkin, A. B., Byles, P. H., and Neville, J. H., Jr.: Neuroendocrine and metabolic effects of general anaesthesia. Canad. Anaesth. Soc. J. 13: 130, 1966.
28. Dobkin, A. B., Donaldson, H., and Purkin, N.: The effects of perphenazine on epinephrine induced cardiac arrhythmias in dogs. 2. Anaesthesia with cyclopropane, chloroform and trichlorethylene. Canad. Anaesth. Soc. J. 6: 251, 1959.
29. Dobkin, A. B., Harland, J. H., and Fedoruk, S.: Trichlorethylene and halothane in a precision system—comparison of some cardiorespiratory and metabolic effects in dogs. Anaesthesiology 23: 58, 1962.
30. Dundee, J. W.: Tachypnoea during administration of trichorethylene. Brit. J. Anaesth. 25: 3, 1953.
31. Dundee, J. W., and Dripps, R. D.: Effects of diethyl ether, trichloroethylene and trifluoroethyl vinyl ether on respiration. Anaesthesiology 18: 282, 1957.
32. Faulconer, A., Pender, J. W., and Bickford, R. G.: The influence of partial pressure of nitrous oxide on the depth of anesthesia and the electroencephalogram in man. Anesthesiology 10: 601, 1949.
33. Fink, B. R.: Diffusion anoxia. Anesthesiology 16: 511, 1955.
34. Fischer, C. W, Bennett, L. L., and Allahwala, A.: The effect of inhalation anesthetic agents on the myocardium of the dog. Anesthesiology 12: 19, 1951.
35. Fischer, E.: Über die Einwirkung von Wasstoff auf Einfach—Chlorkohlenstoff. Jena Z. Med. Naturwiss. 1: 123, 1864.
36. Gainza, E., Heaton, C. W., Willcox, M., and Virtue, R. W.: Physiological measurements during anesthesia with Fluoromar. Brit. J. Anaesth. 28: 412, 1956.
37. Gelfan, G., and Bell, I. R.: The anaesthetic action of divinyl oxide on humans. J. Pharmacol. Exp. Ther. 47: 1, 1933.
38. Gilchrist, E., and Goldschmidt, M. W.: Some observations on the metabolism of trichloroethylene. Anaesthesia 11: 28, 1956.
39. Grogono, E. B.: Divinyl ether anaesthesia. Brit. Med. J. 1: 1068, 1938.
40. Gwathmey, J. J.: Anesthesia. The Macmillan Company, New York, 1929.
41. Helliwell, P. J., and Hutton, A. M.: Trichloroethylene anaesthesia. I. Distribution in the foetal and maternal circulation of pregnant sheep and goats. Anaesthesia 5: 4, 1950.
42. Henderson, V. E., and Kennedy, A. S.: Ethyl chloride. Canad. Med. Ass. J. 23: 226, 1930.
43. Israel, J. S., Byles, P. H., and Dobkin, A. B.: The cardiac effect of epinephrine during anaesthesia in hyperthyroid dogs. Canad. Anaesth. Soc. J. 9: 437, 1962.
44. Israel, J. S., Criswick, V. G., and Dobkin, A. B.: Effect of epinephrine on cardiac rhythm during anesthesia with methoxyflurane (Penthrane) and trifluoroethyl vinyl ether (Fluoromar). Acta Anaesth. Scand. 6: 7, 1962.
45. Jackson, D. E.: Study of analgesia and anaesthesia with special reference to such substances as trichloroethylene and Vinethene (divinyl ether), together with apparatus for their administration. Anesth. Analg. (Cleveland) 13: 198, 1934.
46. Johnstone, M.: The heart during vinyl ether anaesthesia. Anaesthesia 6: 40, 1951.
47. Kinch, A.: Pure nitrous oxide at labour. Acta Obstet. Gynec. Scand. 32: (suppl. 2) 1951.
48. Krantz, J. C., Jr., Carr, C. J., Lu, G., and Bell, F. K.: Anesthesia. XL. The anesthetic action of trifluoroethyl vinyl ether. J. Pharmacol. Exp. Ther. 108: 488, 1953.
49. Lead article: Trilene addiction. Lancet 2: 1205, 1949.
50. Leake, C. D., and Chen, M. Y.: The anaesthetic properties of certain unsaturated ethers. Proc. Soc. Exp. Biol. Med. 28: 151, 1930.
51. Leake, C. D., Knoefel, P. K., and Guedel, A. E.: The anaesthetic action of divinyl oxide in animals. J. Pharmacol. Exp. Ther. 47: 5, 1933.
52. Marquardt, G. H., Mallach, J. F., and Werch, S. C.: Cardiovascular effects of trichlorethylene. Proc. Soc. Exp. Biol. Med. 52: 2, 1943.
53. Martin, S. J., and Rovenstine, E. A.: Vinethene: recent laboratory and clinical evaluation. Anesthesiology 2: 285, 1941.
54. McClelland, M.: Some toxic effects following Trilene decomposition products. Proc. Roy. Soc. Med. 37: 526, 1944.
55. Miller, G. L., and Dornette, W. H. L.: Flammability studies of Fluoromar-oxygen mixtures used in anesthesia. Anesth. Analg. (Cleveland) 40: 232, 1960.
56. Morris, L. E.: Comparison studies of hepatic function following anesthesia with the halogenated agents. Anesthesiology 21: 109, 1960.
57. Morris, L. E., Noltensmeyer, M. H., and White, M. J., Jr.: Epinephrine-induced cardiac irregularities in dogs during anesthesia with trichlorethylene, cyclopropane, ethyl chloride, and chloroform. Anesthesiology 14: 153, 1953.
58. Musser, R. D., Park, C. S., and Krantz, J. C., Jr.: Anesthesia. LVI. Stability of trifluoroethyl vinyl and ethylvinyl ethers in the animal body. Anesthesiology 18: 480, 1957.
59. Orth, O. S., and Dornette, W. H. L.: Fluoromar as an anesthetic agent. Fed. Proc. 14: 376, 1955.
60. Ostlere, G.: Trichlorethylene Anaesthesia. E. S. Livingstone, Ltd., London, 1953.

61. Persson, P. A.: Nitrous oxide hypalgesia in man. Acta Odont. Scand. *9:* (Suppl. 7) 1951.

62. Powell, J. F.: Trichloroethylene: absorption, elimination and metabolism. Brit. J. Industr. Med. *2:* 142, 1945.

63. Sadove, M. S., Balagot, R. C., and Linde, H. W.: Trifluoroethylvinylether (Fluromar). 1. Preliminary clinical and laboratory studies. Anesthesiology *17:* 591, 1956.

64. Sanford, H. N: The effect of gas anesthetics used in labor on bleeding and coagulation time of the newborn. Anesth. Analg. (Cleveland) *5:* 216, 1926.

65. Soucek, B., and Vlachova, D.: Excretion of trichloroethylene metabolites in human urine. Brit. J. Industr. Med. *17:* 60, 1960.

66. Virtue, R. W., Vogel, J. H. K., Press, P., and Grover, R. F.: Respiratory and hemodynamic measurements during anesthesia use of trifluoroethyl vinyl ether and halothane. J. A. M. A. *179:* 224, 1962.

67. Waters, R. M., Orth, O. S., and Gillespie, N. A.: Trichlorethylene anesthesia and cardiac rhythm. Anesthesiology *4:* 1, 1943.

68. Whitteridge, D., and Bülbring, E.: Changes in activity of pulmonary receptors in anesthesia and their influence on respiratory behavior. J. Pharmacol. Exp. Ther. *81:* 340, 1944.

11
The Pharmacodynamics of Thiobarbiturates

HENRY L. PRICE

Chemistry and History

Although attempts at intravenous anesthesia had been made for many years, the method did not become popular in man until the introduction of the short acting barbiturates in the 1930's. Pentobarbital was used for veterinary anesthesia in America in 1931. All bartiturates are modifications of barbituric acid, a compound which results from the condensation of malonic acid and urea. The early barbiturates, like barbituric acid and phenobarbital, were slow in onset and recovery and correspondingly difficult to employ for clinical anesthesia. Both characteristics result from the low lipid solubility of these molecules, which limits their rate of ingress and egress across the lipid-containing membranes of the central nervous system. More rapidly acting barbiturates were prepared by increasing the length and complexity of the hydrocarbon side chains or substituting a sulfur atom for the oxygen attached to the carbon atom of the urea moiety. Both modifications increase lipid solubility, the latter more so than the former. Barbiturates with this sulfur substitution are often called "thiobarbiturates" to distinguish them from the original "oxybarbiturates."

Table 11.1 lists the chemical structures, lipid solubilities (organic phase/water distribution coefficient), delay in onset of anesthetic action (after intravenous injection), and duration of action of four representative barbiturates. It can be seen that acceptable rapidity of anesthetic action is obtained only when lipid solubility is increased about 10-fold above that of barbital or phenobarbital, and that the highest solubility (thiopental) is associated with a rapid onset of narcosis. Effects of each injection are manifested within one circulation time. This barbiturate can be given "to effect" by slow intermittent injections. An excitement phase, as can be seen with pentobarbital in the dog, is extremely rare.

The chemical structure of thiopental provides certain drawbacks as well as advantages. While the paucity of oxygen molecules renders the thiopental molecule lipophilic, it is also hydrophobic and nearly insoluble in water. The water solubility of the molecule is so small that thiopental must be supplied for injection as the sodium salt. This requires the inclusion of a buffer (Na_2CO_3) in all preparations of thiopental, resulting in a strongly alkaline (pH, 11) solution. Such solutions are highly irritating if injected extravascularly. This possible damage to extravascular tissues can be minimized if a 2.5% concentration is used.

TABLE 11.1
Structure-activity relationships of barbiturates
General Formula

Name	R_1	R_2	X	Lipid Solubility	Onset (after Intravenous Injection)	Duration
					min.	
Barbital	Ethyl	Ethyl	Oxygen	1	22	Long
Phenobarbital	Ethyl	Phenyl	Oxygen	3	12	Long
Pentobarbital	Ethyl	1-Methylbutyl	Oxygen	40	~0.2	Intermediate
Thiopental	Ethyl	1-Methylbutyl	Sulfur	600	~0	Short

Pentobarbital, which differs from thiopental only in lacking the sulfur substitution on the urea moiety, is much less lipophilic and hydrophobic than thiopental, and does not require the inclusion of a buffer. Because of its relatively poor lipid solubility, it is less rapidly acting than thiopental, and may be more desirable where prolonged anesthesia is desired. Its peak action is achieved later than thiopental following an intravenous injection. Consequently, overdose may result unless adequate time (usually 40 to 60 seconds) is permitted to assess the effects of *each* intravenous injection of the anesthetic.

Distribution, Metabolism, and Excretion

It is important to recognize that for the ultrashort acting barbiturates the course of anesthesia, from induction to awakening, is largely dependent upon the rate of redistribution of the drug within the body. Metabolism and excretion are unimportant within the temporal range of an ordinary administration. After the drug is injected intravenously, it mixes with blood in a central pool constituting roughly one-fourth of the blood volume, and the concentration of drug which emerges initially from the heart is correspondingly high. Thus, for example, a dose of 20 mg/kg of body weight given as a single dose intravenously results in a peak arterial concen-

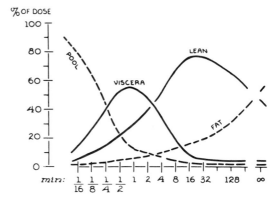

FIG. 11.1. Distribution of thiopental in body tissues at various times following its intravenous injection. (From Price *et al.*[3])

tration which may approximate 1000 mg/liter of blood. This enormous concentration is soon delivered to the rapidly perfused viscera (brain, heart, liver, renal cortex), resulting in profound anesthesia, circulatory depression, and corresponding reductions in hepatic and renal function. However, these viscera comprise only 6% of body weight, with the result that, as the remainder of the body equilibrates with the thiopental present in the circulating blood, the concentrations of the drug in the viscera become rapidly depleted (Fig. 11.1). It can be shown that the rate of redistribution alone is fully sufficient to account for the speed with which consciousness returns following a single intravenous injection of thiopental. Ordinarily, unconsciousness persists substantially less than 1 hour.

During this interval, metabolism of thiopental in the dog is estimated at roughly 5 to 10% of the total dose.[1] The principal metabolite is said to be a carboxylated derivative devoid of anesthetic potency. Urinary excretion of thiopental in the same period is 1 or 2%.

In the case of pentobarbital, the peak concentration in the central nervous system occurs after the blood level of the anesthetic has already fallen substantially; the redistribution process is less important than with thiopental, whereas metabolism is more so. Since metabolism is slow (about 15% per hour in the dog), the duration of action is prolonged.

Under certain conditions (e.g., hemorrhagic shock), the brain may receive an unusually large fraction of the injected dose of barbiturate because of peripheral vasoconstriction and redistribution of blood to the more vital central tissues. Under these circumstances, the barbiturates must be given very carefully. Narcosis may be prolonged because of the lack of subsequent distribution of the barbiturate to peripheral tissues. During apprehension or excitement, on the other

TABLE 11.2
Relation of pH to activity of thiopental

pH	Free	Ionized	Active
	%	%	%
7.6	20	62	8
7.4	25	50	13
7.2	30	38	19

hand, narcosis may be inadequate or brief, since the fraction of the (now greatly increased) cardiac output which goes to the brain is reduced under these conditions (Fig. 11.2).

In the blood stream, the narcotic activity of thiopental is greatly reduced by two mechanisms: binding to serum albumin and ionization. Only free (unbound) and un-ionized thiopental is biologically active. Both of these processes are pH-dependent, and both are increased with increasing acidity. Table 11.2 shows representative data from *in vitro* experiments using human plasma. An almost 3-fold increase in the effective plasma level occurs at the same plasma concentration when the pH is decreased from 7.6 to 7.2. Of course, the situation *in vivo* is more complicated, but the direction of change must be similar. Pentobarbital is less firmly bound to albumin, has a higher pK, and pH-dependent effects are less marked, but do occur.

As is true of thiopental, very little pentobarbital is excreted unchanged in the urine. The very long acting barbiturates, *e.g.*, phenobarbital, are to a much larger extent excreted in the urine. The primary means of drug elimination for drugs such as phenobarbital is renal elimination and not detoxification.

Other Factors which Modify Drug Actions

It was discovered many years ago that *tolerance* to barbiturates develops acutely (*i.e.*, within hours). This implies that the organism in some way generates resistance to the actions of the barbiturate which has been given, and could, theoretically, recover its functions completely while still exposed to a drug concentration which was previously of fully narcotic

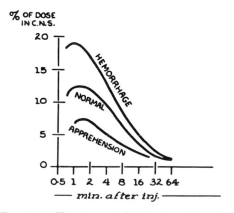

FIG. 11.2. The percent distribution of an intravenous dose of thiopental in central nervous tissue during reduced cardiac output (hemorrhage), normal, and increased cardiac output (apprehension).

potency. For this reason, a single 25 mg/kg dose of thiopental generally does not produce a longer period of anesthesia than a single smaller dose.

If the larger dose is given, tolerance develops to a point where the individual can awaken at a higher blood stream concentration. This concentration at awakening, under normal administration, might have produced profound narcosis had there not been previous exposure to an enormous amount of barbiturate. In addition to acute tolerance to a single barbiturate, there is also cross-tolerance to other barbiturates as well as to other depressants, and vice versa.

There are many conditions which increase the intensity and duration of barbiturate narcosis. Importantly, with barbiturates which depend upon hepatic detoxification, e.g., pentobarbital, for reducing plasma levels, disease which reduces hepatic function will prolong narcosis. Hypothemia, low blood volume, and prolonged and traumatic surgery will all increase the duration of barbiturate narcosis. Uremia and the accompanying electrolyte derangements will increase the intensity and duration of barbiturate narcosis. The underlying mechanism is not clear. Anemia and hypoproteinemia will have a similar effect. Changes occurring during the anesthetic period such as hypoxia, hypercarbia, or excessive blood loss will alter the body's ability to handle barbiturates and other depressants.

Anesthetic Actions and Signs

The mode of action of the barbiturates is believed to involve depression of the central reticular core of the brain stem, sparing the longer, spinothalamic pathways.[2] As practical anesthetics in man, these drugs are without value unless supplemented, but in dogs and cats the intravenous injection of 15 to 25 mg/kg permits performance of many surgical maneuvers. Often smaller doses suffice. The entire dose should never be given rapidly as a single injection.

In dogs, the attainment of adequate anesthesia is marked by absence of lateral canthal reflexes (medial reflexes persist) and full, regular respirations, following an initial sigh. Respiratory minute volume is usually reduced. Corneal reflexes persist almost until death, as do midline, constricted pupils. Airway and salivary secretions are not conspicuous when atropine is given with preanesthetic medication.

The maximal depth of anesthesia is attained in less than 1 minute after an intravenous injection in the case of thiopental but not for a minute or more in the case of pentobarbital. Similarly, the duration of anesthesia is shorter for thiopental than for an equal dose of pentobarbital. Because of its high oil/water partition ratio, thiopental leaves cells without hindrance when the blood stream concentration declines during the redistribution process. Pentobarbital, with a far lower partition ratio, enters and leaves cells more sluggishly and, also, is not concentrated by depot fat. Repeated injections of thiopental (or infusions) may eventually saturate the fat and other tissue with the anesthetic; if this occurs, emergence will depend upon detoxification and will be retarded.

Circulatory Actions

Barbiturates, like the inhalation anesthetics, are myocardial depressants. After rapid intravenous injection, particularly of thiopental, the myocardial content may be large, myocardial depression profound, and circulatory collapse imminent. This is a common cause of death from an anesthetic overdose.

If the anesthetic is given slowly, there is a relatively mild and transient decline in cardiac output and arterial blood pressure. This is promptly antagonized by the increased sympathetic nervous outflow triggered via the barostatic reflexes. As the drug leaves the myocardium, however, the degree of sympathetic nervous activity may be sufficient to *more* than antagonize the existing degree of myocardial depression. When this happens, there is an "overshoot" consisting of increased arterial pressure, increased cardiac output, tachycardia, and occasionally, ventricular arrhythmias. These disturbances of cardiac rhythm (particularly bigeminal rhythm) may persist for some time. Their occurrence is minimized by giving the anesthetic dose slowly.

After the first few minutes of anesthesia, when thiopental and pentobarbital have been substantially redistributed, the level of sympathetic outflow declines toward, or even below, normal. Cardiac output and the various regional blood flows, which have been measured, are restored to normal. Arterial pressure is either normal or elevated. Cardiac rate tends to be elevated and sinus arrhythmia is absent. Total peripheral resistance is usually increased.

Respiration

The central respiratory response to carbon dioxide inhalation is depressed during barbiturate anesthesia, the degree of depression paralleling the depth of narcosis. Responses to peripheral chemoreceptor stimulation persist longer but are also eliminated at a profound depth of anesthesia. At moderate levels of anesthesia, tidal volume is only slightly diminished and respiratory rate is decreased. As anesthesia is deepened, rate and tidal volume both decrease.

Because the respiratory centers may still respond to elevated arterial carbon dioxide tensions and to hypoxia during light anesthesia, this chemical drive can supply the stimulus needed to maintain spontaneous respiration. During moderate levels of anesthesia, hypoventilation will occur, alveolar tension of carbon dioxide will be elevated and (if the animal is breathing air) that of oxygen will be depressed below normal. Marked hypoventilation can occur during profound anesthesia, producing a marked reduction in oxygen tensions. Under these conditions, the hypoxic respiratory drive, through chemoreceptor stimulation from the carotid bodies' chemoreceptors, will sustain respiration. Carbon dioxide tensions will be high and oxygen tensions will be low. When spontaneous respiration is present under such conditions, an increase in the inspired oxygen tension will produce apnea by abolishing the anoxic drive. Respiratory rate may drop to 2 to 3 breaths/minute. Oxygen tensions will be higher after a breath, but this improvement in arterial oxygen tension will be at the expense of a continued increase in arterial carbon dioxide tensions. The proper management of this situation is the institution of controlled ventilation.

Renal and Hepatic Function

Barbiturates depress the transport of p-aminohippurate and the sodium and glucose reabsorptive processes. Urinary volume is reduced, presumably because of an increased liberation of antidiuretic hormone. Renal blood flow and glomerular filtration rate are little altered.

Barbiturates reduce bromsulphalein extraction and clearance without affecting liver blood flow. Barbiturates also stimulate the activity of the enzyme systems which are responsible for their own metabolism. This may, in part, explain the development of tolerance to barbiturates on repeated exposure. The importance of metabolism in terminating the anesthetic actions of the thiobarbiturates is minimal; this is not so for the oxybarbiturates.

Recovery

Recovery from anesthesia is frequently slower than that after an inhalation anesthetic, since most of the barbiturate used to produce unconsciousness is still in the body. Shivering is not uncommon, particularly following long operations in cool operating rooms. Running movements are frequent, particularly in dogs. Marked restlessness is often noted and is frequently intensified by postoperative pain. This reaction may be exaggerated by the fact that rapidly acting barbiturates have an antianalgesic action at low concentrations. Ataxia is nearly always present. Full recovery from the usual anesthetic doses of a barbiturate requires at least 10 hours, and metabolic fragments continue to be excreted for several days.

REFERENCES

1. Brodie, B. B., Mark, L. C., Papper, E. M., Lief, P. A., Bernstein, E., and Rovenstein, E. A.: The fate of thiopental in man and a method for its estimation in biological material. J. Pharmacol. Exp. Ther. *98:* 85, 1950.
2. French, J. D., Verzeano, M., and Magoun, H. W.: A neural basis of the anesthetic state. Arch. Neurol. Psychiat., *69:* 519, 1953.
3. Price, H. L., Kovnat, P. J., Safer, J. N., Conner, E. H., and Price, M. L.: The uptake of thiopental by body tissues and its relation to the duration of narcosis. Clin. Pharmacol. Ther. *1:* 16, 1960.
4. Sharpless, S. K.: The barbiturates. In *The Pharmacological Basis of Therapeutics*, edited by L. S. Goodman and A. Gilman, 3rd ed. The Macmillan Company, New York, 1965.

12
Muscle Relaxants

W. D. TAVERNOR

Our knowledge of muscle relaxants goes back to the 16th century, when travelers returning from the southern hemisphere brought news of the arrow poisons used by the South American natives.

It was not until 1840, however, that Claude Bernard carried out his classical experiments with curare on nerve-muscle preparations and proved that its action was at the myoneural junction. By 1850, he had established the basic facts concerning the physiology of curare.[8] King,[33] in 1935, isolated d-tubocurarine chloride from a sample of crude curare and determined its chemical structure. Although curare had been used in 1835 for treating tetanus in the horse (see Chapter 1), its clinical potential was not realized until 1940 when Bennett used a curare extract to "soften" convulsive shock therapy, and two years later Griffith and Johnson made their important demonstration of the value of curare as a muscle relaxant in anesthesia.[5, 18] This had a revolutionary effect on the practice of anesthesiology and stimulated great interest in the field of muscle relaxants. The literature on curare is immense and is comprehensively reviewed by McIntyre.[40]

Attempts to build molecular models of d-tubocurarine revealed that the actual distance between the two quarternary ammonium groups was relevant to the neuromuscular blocking activity.[32] The neuromuscular blocking properties of the quarternary ammonium compound, decamethonium, was described in 1948.[3, 45] At about the same time, the effects of the synthetic compound gallamine triethiodide, similar in action to tubocurarine, were described in man.[28, 42] Succinylcholine chloride was first reported in 1906,[30] but it was not used as a neuromuscular blocking agent until 1949.[11, 46] Muscle relaxants provide an important instance in the relationship of the chemical structure to the site and mode of action of a drug,[2] and this has led to the investigation of a large number of drugs with neuromuscular blocking properties.

Claude Bernard's fundamental studies in 1850 localized the paralytic action of curare at the myoneural junction, and subsequent studies by Langley in 1909 led to the theory that curare combined with "receptive substances" at the myoneural junction, thus preventing their response to nerve stimuli.[34] From more recent developments in electrophysiology and the chemical theory of neuromuscular transmission, the mode of action of muscle relaxants has been formulated.[16]

The Mechanism of Neuromuscular Transmission

On the arrival of a nerve impulse at the motor nerve ending, acetylcholine molecules are released. It is believed that these molecules are synthesized locally and then stored within the nerve cell. When released, the acetylcholine reacts with a receptor substance on the surface of the motor end plate, which is a specialized region of the muscle fiber. The distance between the nerve membrane and the motor end plate is approximately 1 μ.

Small quantities of acetylcholine are continuously released during periods of nerve cell inactivity but are rapidly hydrolyzed by the enzyme cholinesterase. These small quantities of acetylcholine are not sufficient to alter the electrical potential of the end plate (end plate potential) to enable it to reach the necessary threshold for depolarization. Large quantities of acetycholine are released on the arrival of a nerve impulse and this raises the end plate potential sufficiently to trigger a wave of depolarization which spreads outward along the entire length of the muscle fiber, causing a mechanical contraction.

The majority of the acetylcholine molecules are hydrolyzed at the synaptic junction to acetic acid and choline, the choline being available for resynthesis by the nerve terminal. Some of the acetylcholine diffuses into the interstitial space and is no longer available for resynthesis. Originally, it was thought that all depolarizing drugs produce a similar response at the motor end plate, but it was found that the response varied considerably depending on the species of animals in which a particular drug was used.[64] This finding was of great importance in that it became clear that the results obtained from the muscle of any one mammalian species were valid only for that species.

The Mechanism of Neuromuscular Block

For practical purposes, neuromuscular block can be divided into two types: (a) the block caused by substances that prolong the normal depolarization process produced by the release of acetylcholine at the motor end plate; and (b) the block caused by drugs that occupy the acetylcholine receptors on the membrane of the motor end plate without changing the end plate potential. The former may be referred to as depolarization block and is initiated by drugs such as decamethonium bromide and succinylcholine chloride. The latter type of neuromuscular block is termed nondepolarization block or competitive block, and is exemplified by d-tubocurarine chloride and gallamine triethiodide.

The order of paralysis of muscles following the intravenous injection of a relaxant drug follows a similar course for all species and for all types of relaxant drug. First of all, the eye muscles are affected, followed by the face and limb muscles, then the trunk muscles, and finally the intercostal muscles and diaphragm. Recovery is in the reverse order.

A third group of drugs, the glycerol ethers, have also been used to produce muscular relaxation, although these compounds do not act directly on the motor end plate. These agents diminish reflex activity by depressing conduction across the synapses of the internuncial neurons, and by depressing other spinal and supraspinal polysynaptic pathways.[7] Mephenesin is an example of this type of drug. These drugs are not commonly used for clinical anesthesia.

DEPOLARIZATION BLOCK

Acetylcholine, when released at the motor end plate during normal neuromuscular transmission, produces a transient depolarization of the end plate followed by a wave of depolarization along the length of the muscle fiber. This occupies a fraction of a second followed by a refractory period, during which time a further stimulus will produce no response. After an initial depolarization in the end plate region, repolarization occurs.

Drugs such as decamethonium bromide and succinylcholine chloride produce depolarization at the motor end plate. This depolarization is similar to the transient depolarization produced by acetylcholine, but persists, preventing the passage of further impulses across the neuromuscular junction. There are two divergent views as to the mechanism of the persistent depolarization. One view attributes the persistence of the block to an area of altered sensitivity on the adjacent muscle membrane,[44] while the other attributes the effect to a decrease in the sensitivity of the end plate to the transmitter substance.[61] These differing opinions are probably the result of different experimental techniques in various species.

NONDEPOLARIZATION BLOCK

In this type of block, acetylcholine is produced in the normal manner but is prevented from coming into contact with the receptor sites of the motor end plate. Drugs such as d-tubocurarine chloride are believed to have the same affinity for the protein molecules of the motor end plate as acetylcholine; these drugs do not produce depolarization but prevent acetylcholine from acting upon the receptor. As the concentration of d-tubocurarine in the blood and tissues falls, a point is reached when the number of molecules in the end plate region is insufficient to prevent the acetylcholine from acting upon the end plate. A nondepolarizing block can be reversed by the administration of an anticholinesterase drug such as neostigmine methyl sulfate. This prevents the destruction of acetylcholine by cholinesterase and allows a buildup of acetylcholine. Inasmuch as a competitive (nondepolarizing) block is a quantitative relationship between the available acetylcholine and competitive blocker, the buildup of acetylcholine will lead to the reversal of the block. This will occur if the concentration of d-tubocurarine or gallamine is not excessive.

Drugs Producing Depolarization Block

These drugs initially act like acetylcholine and produce depolarization of the end plate. This is manifested in the animal by visible muscle fasciculations throughout the body. Drugs which inhibit cholinesterase (e.g., neostigmine) do not act as antagonists to this group of drugs;

instead, they prolong their action by slowing down the rate of destruction.

SUCCINYLCHOLINE DICHLORIDE

$$\begin{array}{l} H_3C \\ H_3C - N^+CH_2CH_2OCCH_2CH_2COCH_2CH_2N^+ \\ H_3C \end{array} \quad \begin{array}{l} O \quad O \\ \quad \parallel \quad \parallel \end{array} \quad \begin{array}{l} CH_3 \\ - CH_3 \\ CH_3 \end{array}$$

SUCCINYLCHOLINE

Succinylcholine dichloride (suxamethonium dichloride), a synthetic quaternary ammonium compound, is a white crystalline substance which is unstable in solution unless kept cool. It does not generally have any direct effect on the myocardium or the heart rate, although large doses may produce a temporary rise in blood pressure. This pressor response could be prevented by the prior administration of a ganglion-blocking drug; it was presumed that it was caused mainly by stimulation of the autonomic ganglia.[60] It was suggested that this pressor response was due to temporary inhibition of the activity of true cholinesterase by the drug.[6] It has been shown that the cardiovascular effects of succinylcholine in anesthetized horses can be completely antagonized by the prior administration of hexamethonium bromide and partially antagonized by the administration of the β-adrenergic blocking agent propranolol, or by the application of positive pressure ventilation.[37, 55, 56, 57] It would, therefore, appear that, in the horse, succinylcholine produces an increased sympathetic discharge to the heart.

There is very little evidence to suggest that succinylcholine has any action on the spinal cord or brain, although it has been found to depress the spontaneous activity of the respiratory center in cats.[17] There is no deleterious effect on intestinal motility even in large doses, and it does not appear to cross the placental barrier during normal clinical usage.

In domestic animals there is a wide species variation in the doses of succinylcholine required to produce neuromuscular block. Relatively small doses of the drug produce blockage in dogs, sheep, and cattle, but much higher doses are required in the cat, the pig, and the horse. A correlation between the sensitivity of an animal to this drug and the levels of pseudocholinesterase present in the blood has not been demonstrated,[29] but the injection of a purified pseudocholinesterase preparation in the dog produces a marked increase in resistance to the effect of the drug.[20]

The value of succinylcholine as a short acting muscle relaxant is due to its destruction *in vivo* by pseudocholinesterase. It is hydrolyzed to succinylmonocholine, followed by a slower hydrolysis of succinylmonocholine to succinic acid and choline. Since pseudocholinesterase is formed in the liver, the presence of severe liver damage may result in an increased duration of action.

Clinically, the drug is administered intravenously, and the dosage varies widely with the species under consideration. In the dog, a dose of 0.3 mg/kg produces paralysis for 5 to 10 minutes, whereas in the cat 1.0 mg/kg produces muscle paralysis for only 2 to 3 minutes. The dose in the pig is 2.2 mg/kg, which again causes only 2 to 3 minutes of muscle relaxation. In cattle and sheep, a very small dose (0.02 mg/kg) produces 6 to 8 minutes of paralysis, while in the horse, doses of 0.12 to 0.15 mg/kg will cause paralysis for 5 to 6 minutes. After continuous administration of depolarizing agents by intravenous infusion, a prolonged block can occur. The muscular block bears all the characteristics of a nondepolarizing block and has been reversed by neostigmine. This type of prolonged effect has been designated by various terms: dual block, phase II block, and a desensitization block. No definitive mechanism has been established, and it may be a simple function of an overdose. There is no justification for the use of succinylcholine by continuous infusion when the longer acting, reversible nondepolarizing drugs are available.

The intramuscular administration of succinylcholine has been utilized to immobilize wild animals, the drug being injected by means of a projectile syringe. Once again, there is marked species variation. Doses of 0.66 mg/kg produce paralysis in lions in about 10 minutes, while in ruminants, a very much smaller dose is required; in deer, a dose of 0.068 mg/kg produces paralysis without respiratory arrest.

Drugs Producing Nondepolarization Block

The most commonly used drugs in this group are *d*-tubocurarine and gallamine.

d-TUBOCURARINE CHLORIDE

Although the paralyzing action of *d*-tubocurarine chloride has been known for many years, it was not until 1935 that King isolated the drug in a pure form.[33]

d - TUBOCURARINE

The action of the drug is by competitive inhibition of acetylcholine. The *d*-tubocurarine molecule, by combination with the protein molecule of the motor end plate receptor, prevents the combination of acetylcholine with the motor end plate receptor site.

In dogs, doses 200 times the paralyzing dose can produce cardiac arrest,[28] while small doses well within the relaxant range can produce vagal block in dogs. The drug has an autonomic ganglion-blocking action in animals and also causes the release of significant quantities of histamine. This results in a noticeable fall in blood pressure in both dogs and cats, and for this reason *d*-tubocurarine should be used with caution in these species.

There is no evidence that *d*-tubocurarine has any direct action on the liver or kidneys. It was originally thought that the drug was detoxified by the liver, but subsequent studies indicate that the canine liver does not detoxify *d*-tubocurarine.[49] A total of 20 to 40% is excreted unchanged in the urine, and small quantities are secreted in the saliva and in the gastric juices. The fate of the remainder is uncertain, but the voluntary muscles themselves may well be responsible for a large percentage of the inactivation of the drug.

d-Tubocurarine has been most widely used in the dog at a dose rate of 0.4 mg/kg, but hypotension can occur after intravenous injections. Information on the use of *d*-tubocurarine in other species is limited; but, in pigs, a dose rate of 0.25 mg/kg intravenously produces good relaxation without severe hypotension. In young ruminants, doses of 0.05 mg/kg have been used safely, but in adult cattle, deaths have been recorded following the administration of very small doses.

Reversal of the neuromuscular block produced by *d*-tubocurarine can be achieved by the intravenous administration of an anticholinesterase drug, *e.g.*, neostigmine, but first of all, atropine sulfate should be given intravenously to counteract the muscarinic effect of the neostigmine. The dose of neostigmine for the dog is 0.5 to 1.0 ml intravenously of a 0.05% solution.

GALLAMINE TRIETHIODIDE

Gallamine triethiodide was introduced by Bovet and co-workers in 1947,[12] having been synthetized in a program aimed at the production of compounds based upon the *d*-tubocurarine molecule but of a much simpler structure.

Gallamine is chemically tri(diethylaminoethoxy)benzene triethiodide and has the following structural formula.

$O \cdot CH_2CH_2 \cdot N^+(C_2H_5)_3$
$O \cdot CH_2CH_2 \cdot N^+(C_2H_5)_3$
$O \cdot CH_2CH_2 \cdot N^+(C_2H_5)_3$

GALLAMINE

Gallamine acts at the neuromuscular junction in a manner similar to *d*-tubocurarine. The drug is stable in solution and may be mixed with thiopental.

There does not appear to be any direct action on the myocardium, although there is a marked vagal blocking (vagolytic) action in clinical doses. In dogs, there may be a 10 to 20% rise in heart rate within minutes of the administration of the drug.

Gallamine, like *d*-tubocurarine, does not appear to have any action on the central nervous system and has no direct action on the liver or kidneys. Neither does it appear to affect the contractions of the pregnant uterus but has been shown to cross the placenta in small amounts.[14] The drug is excreted entirely unchanged in the urine, and in cats 30 to 100% of the total dose can be recovered from the urine within 2 hours of injection.[42]

Gallamine would appear to be the nondepolarizing agent of choice in the dog, a dose of 1.0 mg/kg producing complete paralysis within two minutes, the effect lasting from 15 to 20 minutes.[42] Apart from the tachycardia mentioned above, there are no obvious side effects. A similar dose rate is used for cats and may be accompanied by a transient period of hypotension in this species. For pigs, 2 mg/kg are required, but reduced doses are required for young lambs and calves (0.4 mg/kg) and horses (0.5 to 1.0 mg/kg). Respiratory difficulties occur in cattle when the dose exceeds 1.5 mg/kg.[24] Lean subjects required a higher dose rate than fat animals. Neostigmine methylsulfate is an effective antidote for gallamine.

LAUDEXIUM METHYL SULFATE

Laudexium methyl sulfate was synthesized by Taylor and Collier in 1951[59] and appeared to be a very promising nondepolarizing agent. It has about half the potency of *d*-tubocurarine, but its duration of activity is nearly twice that of *d*-tubocurarine. It does not appear to cause the release of histamine or to block transmission of the autonomic ganglia. Because of its long action, there is a danger that the effect of the neostigmine may wear off before that of the relaxant. It is probably for this reason that laudexium has failed to gain wide popularity as a relaxant drug.

STEROIDAL QUATERNARY AMMONIUM COMPOUNDS

In recent years, a number of steroidal bis-quaternary ammonium compounds have been shown to possess neuromuscular blocking actions of the competitive type. Of these compounds, the use of dipyrandium iodide has been reported in man and in the horse[38, 41] and pancuronium bromide has been reported to be used in man.[1] It would not appear, however, that these compounds compare favorably with gallamine or tubocurarine for use in clinical practice.

Interneuronal Blocking Agents

These are compounds which depress polysynaptic spinal reflexes but do not block transmission at the neuromuscular synapse. The site of action of interneuronal blocking agents is in the central nervous system. They do not depress the ability of the muscle to respond to direct stimulation or to stimulation of its motor nerve.

MEPHENESIN

Mephenesin, a glycerol ether, is believed to act on the internuncial neurons of the spinal cord and is capable of diminishing reflex activity in the dog and cat. It will counteract strychnine convulsions and produce paralysis in doses far below toxic levels.[7] Mephenesin is partly detoxified in the liver by conjugation with glycuronic acid and partly excreted unchanged by the kidney.

It was thought that, although mephenesin blocked transmission to the spinal nerves, it had no action on the phrenic nerves, and, therefore, left the diaphragm unaffected. It was found, however, that abdominal relaxation was rarely satisfactory with mephenesin. There is a high incidence of venous thrombosis and hemolysis following the intravenous injection of a 10% solution.

GUAIACOL GLYCERINE ETHER

Guaiacol glycerine ether has also been used for the casting of horses and in combination with other anesthetics.[48, 54, 63] A dose of 4 to 5 g/50 kg in a 5% solution is administrered intravenously. This necessitates the administration of a large volume of solution (1 liter for a horse of 500 kg) and is therefore a slow procedure. Thiopental sodium may be combined with the drug at a dose rate of 5 mg/kg. Stronger solutions may produce hemolysis and are not advocated. The use of this drug at a dose rate of 200 mg/kg has been reported in the dog,[55, 63] but due to its short action and the volume that must be administered, it is unlikely to have any widespread clinical use.

The Clinical Use of Relaxant Drugs

In clinical practice, the relaxant drugs have four main uses. They may be used (a) to produce cessation of spontaneous respiration to facilitate the control of ventilation surgery; (b) to form part of a balanced anesthetic technique and to reduce the amount of anesthetic agents required; (c) to give general muscular relaxation to facilitate surgical access to restricted area; and (d) to facilitate endotracheal intubation.

They are used to facilitate surgery of the diaphragm and thoracic wall, although hyperventilation can be used to cause temporary cessation of respiratory efforts.

In operations of long duration on poor risk patients, light anesthesia may be induced with minimal quantities of short acting barbiturates, and anesthesia may be maintained by minimal doses of inhalation agents; complete muscular relaxation is achieved by the administration of a relaxant drug. Similarly, abdominal operations in the region of the diaphragm as well as the reduction of luxated joints may be facilitated by the judicious use of relaxants.

Although the intubation of the trachea of horses, ruminants, and dogs is compar-

13
Preanesthetic Medication

LAWRENCE R. SOMA

Preanesthetic medication has been well established as an invaluable adjunct in anesthesia, and in many instances it is more essential in animals than in man. Fractious or dangerous animals need preanesthetic sedation to enable their management and to insure a smooth and safe induction of anesthesia. Some classical reasons for administering preanesthetic drugs are as follows: a) to allay fear and apprehension and thus facilitate restraint —this will vary greatly among animals and depends on previous experience of the animal, the species, and the environment; b) to reduce pain or discomfort; c) to facilitate induction of general anesthesia, especially if an intravenous agent is omitted before the induction with a volatile anesthetic agent; d) to serve as an adjunct to regional analgesia; e) to minimize certain untoward effects (salivation) or reflex responses (vagal-vagal) in the patient; and f) to act as pharmacological adjuncts to the general anesthetic agents and thus reduce the amount of the general anesthetic.

There is almost universal agreement about the value of preanesthetic medication, but considerably less unanimity of opinion about the choice of agents. Nearly every clinician favors a particular agent or combination of agents, and habits are established early; in many instances there is little deviation in agents or dosages. Such stereotyped medication, especially in the amount administered, is potentially dangerous because it implies a lack of appre-

ciation for individual variation and variation in response to drugs because of disease and altered physiological state.

There are many drugs that possess desirable preanesthetic properties. The major classes of agents which are in current use are as follows: (a) narcotic analgesics; (b) anticholinergic drugs; (c) sedatives and hypnotics; and (d) tranquilizers. Theoretically this list could be extended to include fluids, blood, antibiotics, insulin, steroids, digitalis preparations, or antihistamines. It is important that the clinician consider the preanesthetic period with a wide focus and not be limited to a few traditional drugs. Other drugs which have been administered before the anesthetic period which may influence the patient's response have to be considered. The preanesthetic agents will be discussed in order of relative importance.

Narcotic Analgesics

The narcotic analgesics are an old and important class of drugs (Fig. 13.1). The sources of the drugs vary from alkaloids of the unripened seed capsule of the opium poppy to synthetic compounds.[129] These drugs depress the respiratory, cardiovascular, and central nervous system. Their addicting properties have stimulated pharmacologists to search for nonaddicting synthetic drugs. The analgesic and sedative properties of narcotics, when needed, are of great benefit to both man and animal, but some of their other prop-

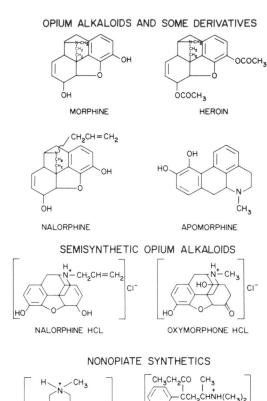

FIG. 13.1. Structure of various narcotic analgesics.

erties are dangerous and have contributed to both the death of man and animals and mental, physical, moral, and social degradation of man. The analgesic and sedative actions of narcotics unfortunately are closely coupled with the addicting, euphoric, respiratory, and cardiovascular depressant effects. In veterinary patients with no "subjective mind" the euphoric aspects which can lead to addiction are not important, but the respiratory and cardiovascular effects have to be considered. This is not to say that addiction and tolerance do not occur in animals, but they are man-made and not due to self-indulgence.

The use of narcotic drugs requires a license which is regulated by the Harrison Act of 1914 and is enforced by the Bureau of Narcotics of the U.S. Treasury Department. The actions of morphine will be discussed in greater detail, because it is the classic drug to which most drugs are compared. Other narcotics will be compared to morphine and their uses discussed.

MORPHINE SULFATE

Morphine was recognized as an effective agent by Claude Bernard.[2] It continues to be commonly administered to dogs, primarily because it produces good sedation, has good analgesic properties, and is inexpensive.

Respiration. The depressing effect of morphine and other narcotics on respiration is a serious disadvantage, and comments on morphine are applicable to other narcotics. The respiratory effects of narcotics are difficult to assess. The casual observation or measurement of tidal volume or rate of ventilation does not completely determine the total effect on alveolar ventilation. More discriminating measurements such as arterial O_2 and CO_2 tensions and CO_2 response curves are necessary (see also Chapter 14). Its actions on ventilation are primarily due to a depression of the respiratory center within the brain stem.

An excellent method of determining the effect of depressants on ventilation is by the use of CO_2 response curve (Fig. 13.2). An increasing concentration of CO_2 in arterial blood will produce an increase in ventilation until a maximal point is reached. At this point a plateau is attained and further increasing the concentration no longer produces a rise. High concentrations (10 to 15%) can produce unconsciousness and subsequent respiratory depression. Narcotics, as well as other depressants, will depress the respiratory center's capability of responding to increasing concentrations of carbon dioxide.[127, 131] The curve is shifted to the right and is dose-related (Figs. 13.2 and 13.3). When narcotics have been administered, the respiratory center is capable of responding to the CO_2 challenge, but higher levels are necessary for a given respiratory minute volume. The alteration in the CO_2 response curve during general anesthesia is greater, and a progressive flattening occurs as anesthesia is deepened (Fig. 13.4). The reduced response to carbon dioxide, whether it is reduction in slope or shift of slope to the right, is indicative of a depression of the respiratory center. Under these conditions the control mechanisms for maintaining arterial CO_2 tensions are less effective.[37, 127] Morphine and other narcotics will progressively depress rate and tidal volume, and toxic doses in many species will produce death through respiratory depression. In some species death is through central nervous system excitement and convulsions.

An important aspect of the depressant effect of narcotics is the reduction of the animal's ventilatory reserve capabilities in maintaining adequate ventilation during stress, pulmonary dysfunction, other diseased states, and subsequent general anesthesia. The additive effect of narcotics and other depressant premedication drugs can also be exemplified by use of the CO_2 response curve (Fig. 13.5).

The administration of narcotics raises the threshold of the respiratory center. The magnitude of ventilatory response is similar when comparing control levels and levels achieved after a narcotic has been given, but higher levels of CO_2 are required. General anesthetics decrease the sensitivity of the respiratory center, and a depression of the CO_2 response slope is produced with increasing concentrations of general anesthetics (Fig. 13.4). The effect of both a narcotic and a general anesthetic is illustrated in Figure 13.5. The narcotic shifts the responsiveness of the center to the right and an equal concentration of the subsequent anesthetic agent produces a greater respiratory effect (Fig. 13.5). This effect on respiration is easily appreciated during the induction of anesthesia with either barbiturates or inhalation agents.

In the animals that pant to control body heat, the thermoregulating mechanisms can alter the respiratory effects of narcotics. After high doses of narcotics in dogs, thermoregulation is disrupted and the dogs will begin panting at a lower body

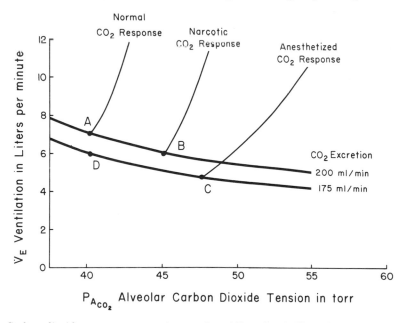

FIG. 13.2. Carbon dioxide response curves in conscious (A), sedated (B), and anesthetized man (C). The sedated and anesthetized man or animal will respond to elevation in CO_2 but at a much reduced level. *Point C* represents a 10 to 15% reduction in metabolic rate due to the anesthetized state. (Courtesy of T. C. Smith. See also Chapter 14.)

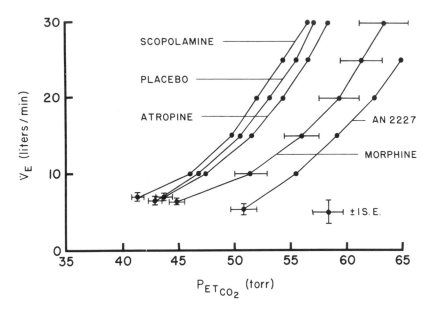

FIG. 13.3. The ventilatory response of 10 normal subjects to rebreathing of carbon dioxide 45 to 60 minutes after the intramuscular injection of scopolamine, saline, atropine, morphine (10 mg), and an experimental narcotic AM-2227 (4 mg). The shift of the curve to the left did occur with scopolamine; however, the slight alteration was not significant. (Courtesy of Smith *et al.*[127])

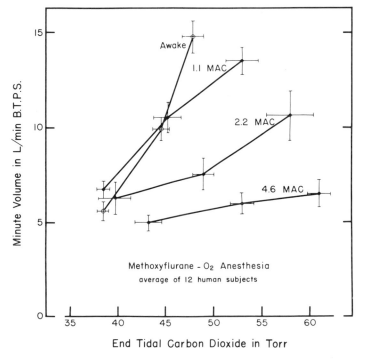

FIG. 13.4. The ventilatory response to increased carbon dioxide tension during the awake state and during increasing levels of methoxyflurane anesthesia. As compared to narcotics, the slope is progressively depressed with no actual shift to the right. The designation *1.1 MAC* indicates the concentration of 1.1 times the minimal alveolar concentration of methoxyflurane. (Courtesy of Dunbar *et al.*[46])

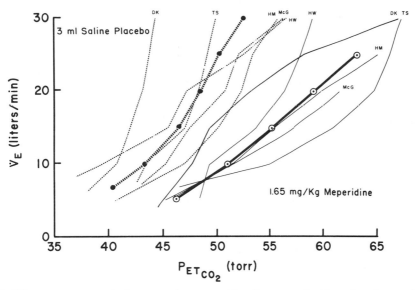

FIG. 13.6. CO_2 response curve in human volunteers with saline controls (*dotted*) and meperidine (*solid*). (Courtesy of Rouge.[118])

disease because it is inactivated by the liver.[142] As with other depressants, meperidine should be used with caution following injury to or loss of function of the central nervous system, during respiratory distress, in toxic animals, in aged or obese animals, and in the very young.

Dosage and Use. A dose of 80 to 100 mg of meperidine is equivalent to 10 mg of morphine when administered to an adult man, although this may not be a sufficient amount for adequate analgesia. The dose for premedication in the dog varies from 2.5 mg/kg to 6.5 mg/kg. The amount used should be determined by the patient's physical status, clinical assessment of the degree of preanesthetic pain, and excitability of the patient (Figs. 13.7 and 13.11). Meperidine, when given in the dose range suggested, produces some sedation, which is one of its beneficial aspects. For postoperative analgesia in dogs, the effective dose is between 5 and 10 mg/kg. Here again the amount selected should be dependent upon the condition of the patient, ventilatory stability, and the overt signs of pain. One of the main advantages of meperidine for premedication is the lack of gastrointestinal stimulation.

Meperidine has been used in the feline species with some success and is one narcotic analgesic which, when used in the correct dosage, may not produce excitement.[21, 26, 28, 29, 98] Compared to man, dog, and the subhuman primate, sedation in the cat is poor and its analgesic properties have not been evaluated. The dosage with or without a tranquilizer should not exceed 11 mg/kg by either the subcutaneous or intramuscular route.[9, 30] Administration of large amounts will produce signs which vary from incoordination and excitement to convulsions and death. These signs may be counteracted with a tranquilizer or barbiturate but not without added depression of the central nervous system and hypoventilation.[141] Occasionally, lower doses will produce mild excitement in cats or a very obvious lack of sedation. This obvious lack of sedation raises doubts on the efficacy of narcotics when used alone in the feline species.

The value of meperidine in cats may be more from its potentiation of barbiturate anesthesia than predictable overt sedation in all animals. More effective than meperidine alone is its combination with a tranquilizer. Meperidine alone or in combination with a tranquilizer potentiates gen-

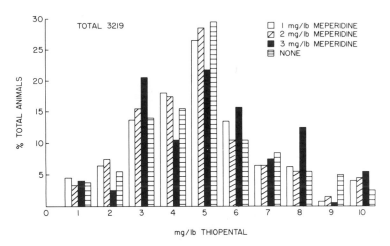

Fig. 13.7. The dose of thiopental sodium for the induction of anesthesia in a large number of clinical cases. The dose of meperidine (Demerol) ranges from 0 to 3 mg/lb. The clinical cases were unselected and ranged from critically ill dogs where no premedication was indicated to healthy patients. The histogram simply illustrates the variation in induction dose of a thiobarbiturate in a clinical situation. The physical status of the animal, its disposition, the time period between the administration of the drug and the induction of anesthesia, and many other variables will influence the induction dose of a barbiturate regardless of the amount of preanesthetic medication.

TABLE 13.1

*Effect of meperidine (11 mg/kg) and promazine (4.4 mg/kg)
on the dose of pentobarbital for the cat**

Number of Cats	Agent	Anesthetic Dose	Lethal Dose
		mg/kg	*mg/kg*
10	Pentobarbital alone	33	72
10	Pentobarbital with merperidine	26	59
10	Pentobarbital with promazine	25	65
	Pentobarbital with merperidine and promazine	18	46

* Courtesy of Clifford, D. H., and Soma, L. R.: *Feline Medicine and Surgery.* American Veterinary Publications, Inc., Santa Barbara, Calif., 1965.

eral anesthesia (Table 13.1), but unfortunately the marked overt signs of sedation, especially in very active cats, is lacking. Irrespective of the overt signs in the cat the subsequent administration of either intravenous or inhalation general anesthesia should be predicated on the knowledge that the effects will be additive. The lack of marked sedation can mislead the clinician into administration of general anesthesia with normal rates and dosages. Meperidine has been used in the horse for pain, especially in colic cases and following orthopedic surgery. The suggested intramuscular dose is 500 to 1000 mg. Intravenous administration can produce hypotension.

METHADONE HYDROCHLORIDE

Many narcotics have been synthesized which have strong analgesic properties, one of which is methadone. Methadone has about twice the potency of morphine with less sedative and addicting properties.[25, 53, 73, 82, 138] Many structural modifications of methadone have been investigated but these do not provide any singular advantages over the parent drug.

Extensive trials have been conducted with methadone in mice, rats, dogs, and man.[6, 122] The initial effects of methadone in dogs are similar to morphine, and vomiting, salivation, defecation, and incoordination are noted. The fact that methadone in equipotent doses produces less sedation in animals may limit its use as a preanesthetic agent.

The pharmacological effects are similar to morphine,[18, 24, 31] with a depressant effect on respiration and a slight decrease in pulse rate and blood pressure. A significant difference is that tolerance develops more slowly and its sedative and addicting properties are less.[34] It is used as a substitute for morphine in the treatment of addicts. The withdrawal symptoms are milder and have a shorter duration.

The dose in dogs is 0.1 to 0.5 mg/kg given subcutaneously or intramuscularly. The higher dose produces a marked effect and is not recommended for routine premedication. Methadone produces excitement in the cat, horse, and other farm animals.

FENTANYL AND DROPERIDOL (INNOVAR-VET)

Neuroleptanalgesia is defined as a state of central nervous system depression and analgesia produced by a neuroleptic (tranquilizer) and narcotic analgesic. States of sedation and analgesia adequate for surgical intervention have been produced in man, dogs, and primates with a combination of the narcotic analgesic fentanyl and the neuroleptic (tranquilizer) droperidol.[130]

The state produced by fentanyl and droperidol is one of analgesia and sedation without total unconsciousness. In man, this can be defined as a state of total indifference or tranquilization and analgesia, whereby man acknowledges verbal commands but is relatively indifferent to pain. This state is manifested in dogs by a responsiveness to auditory stimuli but a reduction or absence of response to painful stimuli.

Up to this time, the search for potent narcotics which do not depress respiration has failed; narcotics generally depress respiration in proportion to the degree of analgesia and sedation. In man, assisted or controlled ventilation is often required. Despite this profound respiratory and central nervous system depression, the circulatory system remains stable. The apnea observed in man is usually not a complicating factor in dogs; in many instances, dogs have an increase in respiratory rate with its reduction in alveolar ventilation because of changes in sensitivity of the thermoregulating center.

These two drugs are currently being used in combination in venterinary medicine, and, because of this, both the pharmacological actions of fentanyl (narcotic) and droperidol (tranquilizer) will be discussed in this section.

Fentanyl. Fentanyl is a potent narcotic analgesic, and its actions are typical of morphine-like drugs. It is approximately 100 times more potent than morphine on a milligram for milligram basis. The rate of onset of action in dogs is very rapid, even following the intramuscular route of injection. Analgesia, sedation, and respiratory depression occur within 5 minutes, with peak intensity occurring within 10 to 15 minutes; on the other hand, the duration of action is short, diminishing considerably within 30 minutes. In pentobarbital-anesthetized dogs, a sharp decrease in rate and tidal volume occurs following the intravenous injection of fentanyl. In the nonanesthetized dog, the effects are not consistent; the respiratory pattern can vary from depression and occasional apnea to panting. The effect of fentanyl on the CO_2 response curve in man is similar to morphine. Morphine in both man and the dog can disrupt the normal function of the heat-regulating centers in the hypothalamus. Because of this, sweating in man and panting in dogs can occur at a lower body temperature. The action of fentanyl, in this respect, is similar to that of morphine when given in high doses.

In the awake or anesthetized dog, bradycardia is a consistent occurrence following either intravenous or intramuscular injection of fentanyl. This distinct change in heart rate is due to an increase in vagal tone. Bradycardia can be prevented by the previous intramuscular administration of atropine; it can also be abolished by intravenous atropine.

Intravenous fentanyl (0.04 mg/kg) given to dogs anesthetized with pentobarbital sodium produces a fall in blood pressure which returns gradually to near normal levels. This fall in blood pressure occurs in both vagotomized and nonvagotomized dogs, indicating that the hypotension is not a function of the changing heart rate.

Unlike morphine, fentanyl does not usually cause vomiting in dogs. Anal sphincter relaxation usually occurs, and there is occasional defecation. The behavioral effects caused by fentanyl are similar to those of other narcotics: analgesia, sedation, decreased motor activity, ataxia, and a decreased response to auditory stimuli.

Droperidol. Droperidol is a butyrophenone derivative. Its action in man can be described as central nervous system depression producing sleepiness and a feeling of detachment. In the dog, the effects are sedation, decreased motor activity, and ataxia. It is classified as a tranquilizer and can be compared in its action to such phenothiazine derivatives as chlorpromazine and promazine. This drug has a wide margin of safety. Tremors, muscle spasticity, and hyperirritability occur only after intravenous administration and at high doses (5 to 10 mg/lb) (see also "Tranquilizers").

Mixtures of Fenanyl and Droperidol. Innovar-Vet for veterinary use contains 0.4 mg/ml of fentanyl and 20 mg/ml of droperidol. The actions of the combined drugs (Innovar-Vet) are primarily those of the narcotic component. The effect of the combination on respiration is variable and primarily due to the narcotic. Panting can occur, but the overall effect is a depression of ventilation, especially if the heat-regulating mechanisms are not superimposed. Fortunately, compared to man, the dog is more resistant to the respiratory depression produced by the narcotic component. However, apnea can occur, and all dogs should be watched carefully when high doses are administered.

Premedication with atropine is essential for prevention of bradycardia produced by the narcotic component. Sedation, ataxia, and some analgesia occur in 3 to 4 minutes after intramuscular injection. Other premonitory signs are bradycardia (with no atropine premedication) and occasional defecation and flatulence. These changes signify cholinergic gastrointestinal stimulation, a characteristic of this mixture. Complete sedation, immobility, and maximum analgesia will be noticed within 10 to 15 minutes.[130]

A slow rhythmic oscillation of the eyeballs may be observed in some dogs; a more consistent finding is persistence of a vigorous eyelid reflex unrelated to the level of sedation. The pupillary constriction which consistently occurred may be used as a guide to the peak effect of the mixture. This effect is not minimized by parenteral atropine. Muscular relaxation is sufficient to enable oral examination and the reduction of many limb fractures. Oropharyngeal and laryngeal reflexes remain. Attempts at endotracheal intubation may evoke swallowing or laryngeal closure. Some oral tone remains in the majority of dogs.

An interesting characteristic of neuroleptic analgesia is the dog's ability to respond to auditory stimuli. A sharp noise such as dropping an object on the floor or the crumpling of paper will evoke a response in many dogs. The movement is slight and consists of lifting the head. This response persists despite the reduction or complete absence of a pedal reflex. It indicates the absence of complete unconsciousness despite deep sedation and analgesia. Unconsciousness is produced by administering nitrous oxide or small amounts of a barbiturate. Spontaneous movements of the head and limbs unrelated to auditory or painful stimulation which resemble a feeble effort to rise occur.

Maximum analgesia is sustained for 30 to 40 minutes. Beyond this period the dog reacts to cutaneous stimulation, although

phosphates), and drugs which have acetyl-choline-like activity (succinylcholine). Anticholinergic drugs are also important in anesthesia and surgery for the suppression of reflex vagotonic activity which can be produced by traction on organs and the direct effect of many anesthetic and preanesthetic drugs.

During the induction and lighter planes of anesthesia, the stimulatory effects of volatile anesthetic agents and secretions can cause reflex closure of the glottis. The laryngeal structures are more responsive to stimuli during this hypersensitive and more reactive phase of anesthesia. Manipulation of the glottic area of the dog with or without concurrent closure can produce an increase in vagal tone, cardiac slowing, and hypotension. These reflexes affecting the cardiovascular system can originate in the trachea, larynx, bronchi, or lungs. The production of complete motor paralysis of the glottis by the injection of muscle relaxants will not prevent the reflex circulatory changes produced by laryngeal manipulation. In the dog and the rabbit, laryngeal or tracheal stimulation produces bradycardia and hypotension; in man and the cat, the predominant response is tachycardia and hypertension.[89] Atropine or scopolamine will block effectively the bradycardia of laryngeal stimulation in the dog.

Barbiturates, particularly the thiobarbiturates used during the induction of anesthesia, increase the sensitivity of the larynx and trachea to vagal stimulation, thereby increasing the likelihood of laryngospasm, bronchospasm, and other undesirable respiratory effects. This has been especially observed in the domestic cat, an effect which is not true in the large undomesticated species. This increased reactivity is probably due to an increase in parasympathetic tone.[47] These intravenous anesthetic drugs do not produce spasms, but only increase the tendency for spasms under lighter planes of anesthesia. Under deeper planes of barbiturate anesthesia, as with other anesthetics, there is central depression of these reflex arcs. Premedication with atropine does not reduce spasm but will minimize the additive effect of secretions on the glottic structures. It will effectively block the vagal bradycardia and hypotension.

There are many drugs and manipulative procedures during surgery which can produce an increase in vagal tone leading to bradycardia and hypotension. An increase in vagal tone can occur as a consequence of pressure or traction on visceral organs, more commonly those in the anterior abdomen and the thorax. This vagovagal reflex may not always be blocked by preanesthetic administration of atropine. When an increase in vagal tone occurs, the manipulative action should stop. If this fails to restore normal heart rhythm, atropine should be administered intravenously. General anesthetic agents, digitalis, hyperkalemia, lowered pH, or the injection of calcium salts all augment these vagal effects.

Halothane and methoxyflurane, like the barbiturates, tend to increase vagal tone, producing a reduction in heart rate. They depress sympathetic outflow and, partially through this action, increase parasympathetic tone. This reduction in heart rate can partially be reversed by the administration of atropine. A complete reversal should not be expected, because part of the decrease, especially in the dog, is through direct negative chronotropic effects and not through the vagal nuclei.[102]

Atropine when administered alone produces little changes in circulation, but will have a marked effect on blood pressure and cardiac output when reversing the effects producing by an increase in vagal tone. It must be emphasized that many drugs administered prior to and during anesthesia can increase vagal tone by central actions, peripheral actions on the heart, and, indirectly, by suppression of sympathetic activity; because of this, atropine is an extremely useful drug.

Respiratory System. Atropine and other belladonna alkaloids reduce glandular secretions of the respiratory tract, gastrointestinal tract, and oral and nasal cavity. This is effective in most species with the exception of the ruminants. Atropine is also a bronchodilator through its relaxation of the bronchial and tracheal smooth muscles. In man, the bronchodilation creates an increase in anatomical and physiological dead space. The subsequent reduction in alveolar ventilation is not accompanied by a decrease in arterial oxygen tension or an increase in carbon dioxide tension. In the awake volunteer there is an increase in minute ventilation which compensates for the increased dead space.[104] The lack of change of blood gases in healthy volunteers would not necessarily hold true for diseased states or following the use of ventilatory depressants. In studies completed in the dog, the physiological dead space was increased less than the anatomical dead space, which, in fact, in this species produced a reduction in alveolar dead space.[123]

Other Systems. Belladonna alkaloids dilate pupils by blocking the response of the iris to cholinergic stimuli. This is a peripheral effect and not centrally mediated.[66] As with the salivary glands, these drugs reduce gastric secretions and gastrointestinal motility and reduce the contraction of the bladder and ureter.

Dosages and Use. The usual subcutaneous or intramuscular dose of atropine sulfate in dogs and cats is 0.02 mg/kg. Larger doses are required in many herbivorous animals because of higher levels of atropinesterase.[65] Suggested dose in the smaller farm animals is 3 to 5 mg, although in the smaller ruminants, as in the cow, salivation still continues but at a somewhat lesser degree. The actions persist for only 1½ to 2 hours. The dose in the horse is 40 to 60 mg. In the large ruminants, atropine is of limited value—the flow of secretions is not appreciably reduced and the thickening of secretions make its removal more difficult.

In general, the effectiveness of atropine in various species of animals is in the following ascending order: rodents, *e.g.*, rabbit, rat; ruminants, *e.g.*, cattle, sheep, goats, swine, horses, dogs, and cats. The toxicity of atropine varies considerably with species, and most herbivores are like the rabbit in that they can feed on the belladonna plant without toxic effects. Swine are more susceptible to the belladonna content of the nightshade plant than horses or cattle.

SCOPOLAMINE

The actions of scopolamine are similar to those of atropine, and it is preferred to atropine by some. Scopolamine has less inhibitory effect on the vagus, although in some species, it is a more potent depressant of the central nervous system and antisialagogue. Central nervous system signs of depression or excitement have been observed following administration of scoplamine to animals.

Scopolamine (0.01 to 0.02 mg/kg) can be used for premedication in dogs and cats.

Tranquilizers

The use of the term tranquilizer or ataractic in veterinary medicine is misleading and does not describe the use and function of these drugs. The term tranquilizer is a clinical term based on the drug's effect on psychomotor function, and the word ataractic is derived from the Greek word meaning without confusion, cool, and collected.[113] This descriptive terminology and others which relate to psychic changes produced in man are not totally applicable in describing the effects in animals. The simple definition that a tranquilizer is a substance that reduces anxiety without clouding consciousness is certainly an oversimplified presentation of its effects.[113] Its use in man is not only limited to the treatment of anxious states, which the definition implies, but the management of various degrees of psychological disorders. The psychomotor effects in man are varied and cannot be categorized by one definition. The end point and final effect depends on the mental state being treated.

Tranquilizers, as opposed to other drugs used for premedication, are considered psychopharmacological agents, a class of compounds which depress many physiological functions, decrease motor activity, can produce mental calming, and increase the threshold to environmental stimulation but do not produce sleep, analgesia, or anesthesia. The sedation produced by tranquilizers differs from the state produced by barbiturates and narcotics in that sedation occurs without hypnosis. The general calming effect produced by the tranquilizers can be reversed with an adequate stimulus. Sedative-hypnotics also decrease motor activity but differ from tranquilizers by their ability to produce depression which leads to sleep, and in higher doses sedatives are potential anesthetics. Tranquilizers are primarily used in man for their neuroleptic effects. Patients do not express anxiety, show little initiative, and exhibit a reduced response to external stimuli. The sedative effect may contribute to this reduced state of activity but it is not necessarily desirable or essential in man.

The desired effect in animals is sedation without marked ataxia. This is especially important in large animals where maintaining the equilibrium is essential. The basic difference in the administration of tranquilizers between man and animals is that in man a psychic disorder or mental disturbance is being treated, whereas in animals no such condition exists. Sedation is not the important aspect of the drug, and lower doses are generally used. In veterinary use, sedation and a tractable animal are the important aspects of the drug and higher amounts are needed.

In animals, adequate doses produce quieting, sedation, ataxia, an increase in the threshold response to environmental stimuli, relaxation of the nictitating membrane, and abolition of conditioned reflexes. Phenothiazine compounds are drugs extensively used, and most congeners have little sedative effect but good antipsychotic effect. Unfortunately, in the development of these drugs the latter aspects of the drugs are the ones sought for, and higher doses are necessary to produce sedation in animals.

Tranquilizers, when used in low doses, impair the ability of animals to perform conditioned responses. Overt sedation may not be observed, but reaction time, avoidance responses, and responses to behavioral training are reduced. This typical inhibitor effect of low doses of neuroleptics has been observed in many species, including the horse.[20] Promazine will reduce the horse's performance in a gallop and cavaletti tests. Tranquilizers also modify the increase in respiratory rate, pulse rate, and body temperature produced by the exercising horse.

The specific mode of action of tranquilizers is not clear but is a combination of reduced activity of the reticular formation and the hypothalamus, plus suppression of the sympathetic nervous system. Chlorpromazine does not deplete the catecholamine stores of the body as with reserpine but depresses the mobilization of these neurohormones both centrally and peripherally. In this mode of action, the reactivity of the organism is reduced by virtue of a central sedation and reduction of sympathetic activity. It must be emphasized that the sedation produced by tranquilizers is reversible and the animal can react in a co-ordinated manner. A horse can still react to painful stimuli and attempts at treatment, and a vicious dog can still bite. The degree of sedation and inactivity produced by the tranquilizers in many instances is dependent on the excitability of the animal being treated. Unlike general anesthetics, additional drug does not necessarily produce a greater degree of sedation and eventually approaches toxic effects.

PHENOTHIAZINE DERIVATIVES

The phenothiazine derivatives have been used extensively for sedation and preanesthetic medication in a variety of animals. The agents commonly used in veterinary medicine are promazine, triflupromazine, and acetylpromazine (Fig. 13.12). The original drug of this large series was the antihistamine promethiazine. The classic tranquilizer chlorpromazine has fallen into general disuse in veterinary medicine because of its hypotensive actions and in many species its inconsistent effect. Inconsistency and a prolonged sedation have been especially noted in the

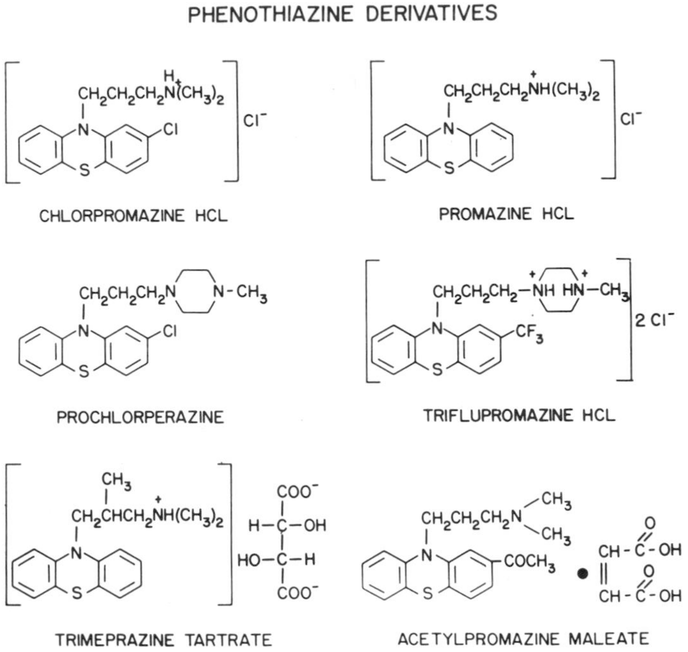

PHENOTHIAZINE DERIVATIVES

CHLORPROMAZINE HCL   PROMAZINE HCL

PROCHLORPERAZINE   TRIFLUPROMAZINE HCL

TRIMEPRAZINE TARTRATE   ACETYLPROMAZINE MALEATE

FIG. 13.12. Structure of various phenothiazine tranquilizers.

horse.[95] It is still used extensively for psychotherapy in humans.

Cardiovascular System. Chlorpromazine and the many analogous phenothiazine derivatives have similar basic structures and actions but vary in potency and intensity of actions (Fig. 13.12). The cardiovascular actions are through its multiple effects on the sympathetic nervous system, the central nervous system, and vascular and cardiovascular smooth muscle. These effects are both central and peripheral. The central manifestation is inhibition of centrally mediated pressor reflexes which reduce both vascular tone and the animal's capabilities of responding by reflex to alterations in the cardiovascular system. The peripheral effects are α-adrenergic receptor blockade, slight ganglionic blocking activity, and direct depression of the myocardium and vascular smooth muscle. The separation of direct effects on vascular smooth muscle from its effects on the autonomic mediation of the vascular system is difficult. Phenothiazines have a negative inotropic action on heart muscle and produce peripheral vasodilation through relaxation of

vascular smooth muscle. The combined actions reduce blood pressure with a usual compensatory increase in heart rate.

In the awake dog hypotension and a tachycardia occur after the administration of phenothiazine tranquilizers. In a comparative study of a group of tranquilizers, chlorpromazine and ethylisobutrazine produced the greatest fall, while promazine produced a moderate change. There was a rise toward control levels within 20 minutes.[72] This tachyphylaxis to the acute cardiovascular effects of tranquilizers may be misleading if measurements are made only during peak sedation. Under these conditions of observation, little change from control may be noted. Chlorpromazine, flupherazine, trifluoperazine, and promazine had similar effects in anesthetized dogs—hypotension followed by a gradual return toward normal.[4, 11, 136]

Studies in the standing horse were similar to the awake dog—a decrease in blood pressure and an increase in heart rate following intravenous promazine. The effect was maximal within 20 minutes. There was a significant increase in cardiac out-

Toxicity. The central effects of chlorpromazine and analogous compounds, which affect behavior, locomotor activity, and the cardiovascular system are extremely diverse, complex, and poorly understood. Part of the neurochemical mechanisms involve the inhibition of catecholamine activity. This adrenergic blockade, both centrally[14] and peripherally at homeopathic doses, is well established and aids somewhat in the explanation of both the sedation and cardiovascular depression produced by tranquilizers. The central sedative effects can be reversed by the administration of d-amphetamine, which is a partial conformation of the central inhibitory action of catecholamine.

The toxic effects of high levels of chlorpromazine have to be separated into chronic and acute manifestations. The toxic effects most commonly described are those of chronic administration and are classed as extrapyramidal and "Parkinson-like." In man, they include tremors, depression, mask-like facial expressions, salivation, rigidity, and involuntary limb and eye movements.[66] Convulsive seizures can also occur. These effects are not generally seen in animals by reason of the method of administration. The chronic toxic effects resemble cholinergic stimulation. Administration of large doses of chlorpromazine in rats has cholinergic stimulatory effects plus the adrenergic blocking actions.[94] Salivation and tremors in rats were signs of this acute overdose, which resembled in part the signs noted in chronic toxicity. The assumption that chronic toxicity is cholinergic is fortified by the suppression of toxic signs by the administration of anticholinergic drugs which can be transferred across the blood-brain barrier. Atropine and scopalamine reduce the cholinergic signs; methylatropine does not. Atropine also reduces the acute toxic cholinergic signs in rats. Daily administration of chlorpromazine can lead to high brain levels due to an intensified localization within the brain.[120] This leads to the inhibition of anticholinesterases with the accumulation of acetylcholine and the manifestation of toxic cholinergic signs.

Most tranquilizers have a high therapeutic ratio. Unlike general anesthetics, tranquilizers produce an optimal effect within a dose range, and increasing amounts do not produce a greater degree of sedation. Large doses in horses may produce muscle weakness and excessive sedation which can give rise to a state of panic. Under these circumstances the animal may be more difficult to control.[71] Orthostatic hypotension can occur in the horse at therapeutic doses. Although rare, it is dramatic and distressing. This does not occur following the intramuscular route which should be the preferred method when time and circumstances permit.

Accidental intracarotid injections of tranquilizers and other drugs have produced disorders ranging from signs of mild disorientation to convulsive seizures and death. The microscopic changes have included endothelial swelling and necrosis.[64] The initial cause of the violent response was probably vascular spasms and tissue ischemia. Drugs which deplete the stores of catecholamines (reserpine) and drugs which reduce the vasoreactivity of vessels (tranquilizers) will partially protect against intracarotid injections.[64]

Common signs of exaggerated effects of tranquilizers usually following intravenous administration are hypotension, hypothermia, recumbency, and deep sedation. Acute administration of high doses can produce the extrapyramidal side effects. These include tremors, muscle spasticity, hyperirritability, spontaneous flexing and extension of forelegs, and convulsions.[86] The treatment is symptomatic and is directed at controlling convulsions and maintaining adequate ventilation.

An interaction between parenteral chlorpromazine and piperazine has been reported in a child and duplicated in experimental dogs and goats.[10] The combination of these two drugs produced the extrapyramidal side effects whereas either drug alone had no observable effects.

Unusual reactions to tranquilizers have

occurred in dogs which include effects completely opposite to the anticipated one. Friendly dogs have become extremely savage[32] and actually attacked the owner. Chlorpromazine has also produced excitement and dissociation in young adults. Personality changes in dogs have also been reported by owners following the use of Innovar-Vet. The animals were unfriendly, growled, and showed aggressive tendencies toward the owner. This effect was noted the day following its use and lasted for 24 hours. This personality change has been produced following the reversal of the narcotic component of Innovar-Vet. The unusual aspect of this reaction to a tranquilizer is that in the case of chlorpromazine[32] and droperidol, the tranquilizer portion of Innovar-Vet, it could not be duplicated in the same dog.

These observations and some of the known cholinergic actions of tranquilizers, plus recent studies on the carbochol-induced killings in rats[126] are worth some speculation as to a possible connection. Stimulation of the lateral hypothalamus with carbochol, a drug which mimics the actions of acetylcholine, triggered aggressive behavioral changes in rats. The produced aggressive reaction could be blocked with atropine methylnitrate, also injected into the hypothalamus. Whether these isolated observations are related is only speculative, but certainly interesting.

Sedatives and Hypnotics

The separation of the effects of drugs into degrees of sedation or depression produced by many-chemically unrelated and related compounds is extremely difficult. Despite this difficulty, there is some value in attempting to categorize effects.[117] For example, sedation implies a mild depression, and hypnosis indicates a stronger degree of depression leading to sleep. Anesthesia is a progression of the state of depression from which arousal cannot be produced even with painful stimuli. The sedation and hypnosis produced by barbiturates are mere gradations of the state of general anesthesia, inasmuch as high doses of these agents can produce excite-

ment followed by general anesthesia. Animals sedated or depressed by these drugs, as compared to tranquilizers, are not as easily aroused and are not as well co-ordinated once aroused. An important distinction in comparing the sedative-hypnotic drugs with the narcotics and the tranquilizers is that increasing doses will produce states of anesthesia. The most important class of compounds in this group of drugs is the barbiturates.

BARBITURATES

Administration of subanesthetic amounts of oxybarbiturates (pentobarbital, secobarbital) orally or parenterally for preanesthetic medication is commonly used in man, but rarely used in animals. Barbiturates have been used in horses for preanesthetic sedation in combination with a tranquilizer. Barbiturates are not commonly employed in animals for preanesthetic medication because of the following. (a) Pentobarbital is still a common intravenous and general anesthetic, and the resultant general anesthesia can be prolonged and difficult to control. (b) Larger doses are necessary in animals to produce sedation.[100] (c) With high doses there is a risk that the animal might pass into the excitatory stage and be more difficult to handle.

In very excitable animals, e.g., horses, the intravenous administration of an oxybarbiturate (pentobarbital) or chloral hydrate following a tranquilizer has clinical application. The dose of a barbiturate for sedation is approximately one-fifth of that required to produce anesthesia. In large animals pentobarbital (0.5 to 2 g) can be used to produce sedation and hypnosis. One gram of pentobarbital intravenously following the recommended dose of promazine or acetylpromazine has been useful in sedating an excitable horse without the danger of casting.

With the use of inhalation anesthetics on the increase, barbiturates in combination with lower doses of tranquilizers should be considered for preanesthetic medication in small and large animals.

CHLORAL HYDRATE, PARALDEHYDE,
TRIBROMETHANOL, AND GLUTETHIMIDE

Chloral hydrate has been used as a sedative hypnotic in large animals and occasionally in other species. Many surgical procedures have been completed using chloral hydrate for deep sedation and a local anesthetic for regional analgesia. It can be used, as the barbiturates are, in combination with a tranquilizer for sedation in the standing horse. The drug should be administered to effect, the dose range being 4 to 5 g/50 kg. It must be appreciated that the peak effect, even following intravenous administration, is manifested within 2 to 3 minutes.

Paraldehyde has been used rectally and by other routes to produce basal narcosis. The response is variable, the margin of safety is poor, and hemoglobinuria may result.[15, 16, 17] In many respects its properties are similar to those of chloral hydrate. It has poor analgesic properties and consequently greater degrees of respiratory and circulatory depression are produced before adequate analgesia or anesthesia is achieved. It irritates the mucous membranes of the digestive tract and has an unpleasant odor. Paraldehyde has been administered intravenously at doses as high as 850 mg/kg.[99, 100]

Tribromethanol has been used as a preanesthetic and basal anesthetic in man and animals. It produced unconsciousness within 20 to 30 minutes after rectal administration, with a duration of approximately 1 hour. Tribromethanol also has a depressant effect on respiration and circulation which, together with its general unpredictability, has discouraged its use by this route. Sedation in dogs is evident 5 to 10 minutes after its rectal administration and lasts for more than an hour; in cats, the depressant effects can last as long as 24 hours. The anesthetic dose by rectal injection for cats is 300 mg/kg, and at this dose level the margin of safety between the lethal and anesthetic doses narrows. Prior to the barbiturates, tribromethanol was the first nonvolatile anesthetic used in cats and had wide application. It has been administered orally to mammals, reptiles, and birds.[103] Its usefulness in anesthesia at the present time is limited.

Glutethimide is a non-narcotic, nonbarbiturate sedative which has been used as a preanesthetic drug in man and animals.[12, 48, 56] Oral doses of 200 and 500 mg/kg in dogs and rabbits, respectively, produced sedation. The intravenous anesthetic dose in dogs is approximately 110 mg/kg, and by this route, it resembles the thiobarbiturates in its duration of effect.[48] Hemolysis, local vascular irritation, and cardiovascular depression have been observed following intravenous administration. One of the most important limiting factors of this drug by parenteral route is its inherent insolubility in water.

Cyclohexamines (Dissociogenic Agents)

Cyclohexamines are a group of related compounds of which phencyclidine has had widespread usage in subhuman primates and wild animals (Fig. 13.13). The state produced by the cyclohexamines has been termed "dissociative." These drugs are analgesic and in high doses produce a state which resembles anesthesia. The analgesia is not accompanied by central nervous system depression and hypnosis, but what appears to be a state of catalepsy. The specific effects will vary with species of animals but generally ocular,

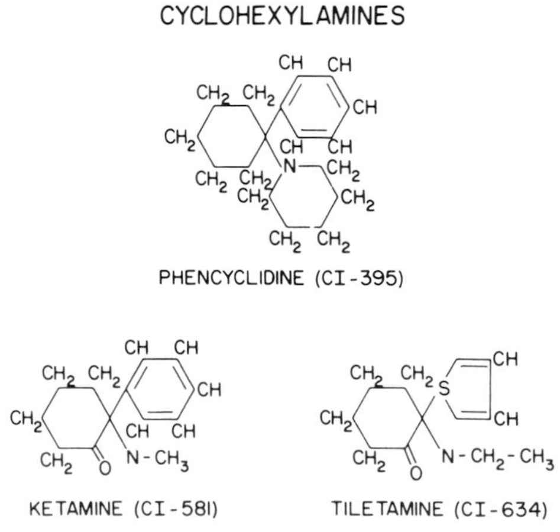

FIG. 13.13. Structure of various cyclohexamines.

oral, and swallowing reflexes are present, eyes remain open, and muscle tone increases. Increasing doses produce tremors and convulsions. In man, visual and some esthetic impulses can reach cortical levels.[37] Psychomimetic effects, such as hallucinations, confusion, agitation, and fear have occurred in man, and this raises questions on the possible dangers of these compounds.[37, 97]

Phencyclidine has had its greatest use in subhuman primates; it was abandoned in man because of its hallucinogenic tendencies. In many species tremors, oculogyric movements, tonic spasticity and convulsions occur. Immobilizing or "subanesthetic" doses are particularly valuable in subhuman primates and other animals which are difficult to handle.[75, 76] Its use as a total anesthetic should be questioned because of the tremors and poor muscle relaxation. In many instances barbiturates are necessary to produce muscle relaxation. Its adverse effects in species other than primates has reduced its value in most animals. The adverse effects could be minimized by the administration of tranquilizers. For the capture of the undomesticated feline and zoo animals, the marked tremors and convulsive activity could be justified on the basis of complete restraint with relative safety to patient and clinician. The recovery period in both the primate and the feline species is prolonged.

Two congeners of phencyclidine, tiletamine and ketamine, have been developed, and these exhibit fewer of the undesirable properties. Tiletamine has shown taming and immobilizing effects in a number of species of animals.[7, 22, 23] Both drugs have an induction time of between 2 and 3 minutes following intramuscular injections. The duration of peak effect is approximately 60 minutes for tiletamine and 20 minutes for ketamine. This is followed by a variable but longer period of ataxia and sedation.

Both drugs have been used in cats for restraint and minor surgical procedures. Cats lose their righting reflexes within 2 to 3 minutes after intramuscular injection. They lie quietly with their eyes open, maintaining palpebral, conjunctival, corneal, and swallowing reflexes. Lachrymal secretions persist and all cats salivate. Atropine is recommended. Extensor rigidity of the forelegs with caudal deflection is observed with both drugs (Fig. 13.14). The rigidity remains during the peak effect of the drug, with gradual subsidence during the recovery period. Hyper-responsiveness to tactile stimuli (Fig. 13.15) and ataxia were noted during the recovery period.

The cardiovascular effects are a drop in heart rate and blood pressure which de-

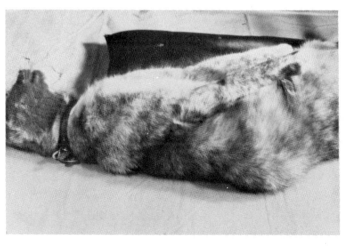

Fig. 13.14. The extensor ridigity of the forelegs with caudal deflection produced by cyclohexamines in the cat.

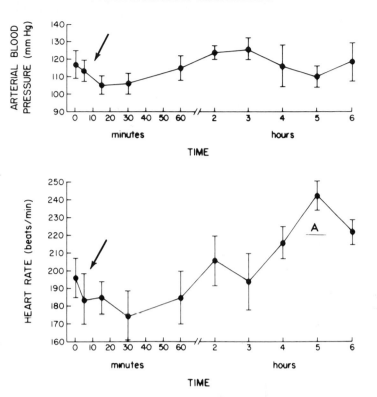

FIG. 13.15. The hyper-responsiveness to tactile stimulation during the tiletamine (CI 634) recovery period is reflected in the stimulation of the autonomic nervous system during handling (A). The drop in blood pressure and heart rate from awake controls occurs within 5 minutes following intramuscular injection (*arrow*).

creases to its maximum within 20 to 30 minutes, with a gradual return toward control (Fig. 13.15). As compared to intramuscular injections, intravenous administration produced a rise in blood pressure and heart rate. Arrhythmias were common with intravenous injections. They included coupled premature ventricular beats which appeared as a bigeminal and trigeminal rhythm. There were fused ventricular beats and an increase in P wave amplitude. Tiletamine produces an irregular respiratory pattern which is apneustic in character, with the animal breath holding during the inspiratory period. The consequence of this abnormal pattern is a respiratory acidosis. There was an increase in carbon dioxide tension and a decrease in pH (Fig. 13.16). These alterations in arterial values occurred within the first 5 minutes and remained significantly different from the awake control during the 1st hour. Oxygen tensions were reduced and remained so for at least 30 minutes (Fig. 13.17).

The persistence of this apneustic pattern with lower doses of tiletamine greatly reduced its usefulness as a preanesthetic agent. The induction of anesthesia with an inhalation agent was irregular and prolonged. Its would-be expected respiratory depression was more pronounced. General anesthesia could be adequately maintained only with controlled ventilation.

Ketamine is a recent derivative of phencyclidine, with further reduction in some of the undesirable effects of phencyclidine and tiletamine. It has been used in man and subhuman primates.[13, 37, 43, 97, 137] Ketamine in man has been used as the sole anesthetic agent and has been used for the induction of anesthesia. Preanesthetic medication was considered necessary with this drug in man to reduce the fre-

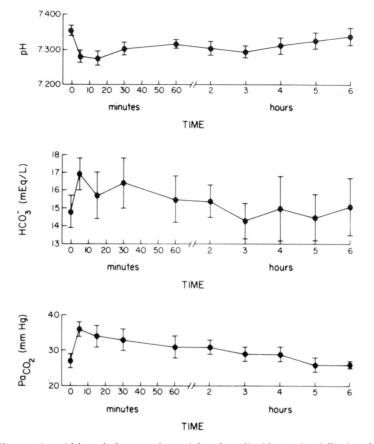

FIG. 13.16. Changes in acid-base balance and arterial carbon dioxide tension following the intramuscular injection of 5 mg/lb (11 mg/kg) of tiletamine (CI 634). The control level is the awake cat.

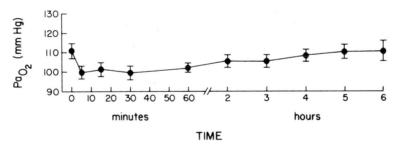

FIG. 13.17. Changes in arterial oxygen tension following intramuscular tiletamine.

quency of temporary psychiatric disturbances.[97] Analgesia appears very early and is present shortly following loss of consciousness. Movements of limbs were observed and were apparently produced in response to pain.[97] Muscle relaxation in man was moderate compared to cats where tremors and stiffness occur. Clinical observations in human use have shown a constant elevation of heart rate and blood pressure. This seems to be related to psychological or organic distress and was minimized with previous sedation.[97] Arterial blood pH and P_{CO_2} were not appreciably affected in man; similar studies in cats have not been reported.

Ketamine is currently on experimental clinical trial in cats. The neuromuscular effects in cats are similar to tiletamine but not as pronounced. This includes the apneustic respiratory pattern. The duration of the peak effect and recovery period are shorter. The question of mechanisms of apneusis has not been settled.[79, 87] One area in dispute is the facilitation or inhibition of the reticular activating system on eupneic respiration. Neurons from the reticular activating system influence both inspiratory and expiratory neurons of the medulla in a facilitory or inhibitory manner simultaneously. Experimental work in cats with ketamine showed some degree of suppression of the reticular formation.[101] The most prominent findings were an alternating pattern of hypersynchronous δ wave bursts and low voltage, fast wave activity in the neocortex and thalamus. This was synonymous with a θ-"arousal" pattern in the limbic system. Similar work with tiletamine showed more of a suppression of the reticular formation,[19] which might explain the greater degree of respiratory depression with this drug.

Use. Phencyclidine has been primarily used in the subhuman primate and wild *Felidae*. The primary disadvantage is the long recovery period. This can be minimized by the reduction in the dose of phencyclidine and the simultaneous intramuscular injection of a tranquilizer. The dose in primates ranges from 0.5 to 2 mg/kg,[133] depending upon the state desired, reduced reactivity, and catalepsis to analgesia and "anesthesia." The dose in the undomesticated feline is 1 to 2 mg/kg. This should be administered with a tranquilizer to reduce the tremors and oculogyric movements. Atropine should be given to reduce salivation. The combination of phencyclidine, a tranquilizer, and atropine has been effective orally in both domesticated and undomesticated cats.

Tiletamine has been used in a gorilla (2.2 mg/kg) and other primates for restraint. The trachea can be intubated and anesthesia induced through the endotracheal tube. Tiletamine can be used in the cat for restraint and minor surgical procedures. The dose is 5 mg/kg. The extensor rigidity of the forelegs and tremors can be eliminated with intravenous diazepam (0.5 mg/kg). The apneustic ventilatory pattern is not altered with diazepam.

The use of ketamine in humans for minor surgical procedures is still in the evaluation stages because of the psychomimetic properties of these drugs. Its use in veterinary anesthesia has not been completely clarified. The muscle tremors and stiffness produced by these drugs certainly minimize their usefulness for abdominal and orthopedic surgery, both from a functional and esthetic point of view. The combination with a muscle-relaxing tranquilizer (diazepam) minimizes some of the objectionable aspects of ketamine. Its combination with other anesthetics has not been evaluated, and its potential use as a restraining agent prior to anesthesia needs further study. At the current stage of development, ketamine has been used in man, subhuman primates, and rats. The dose range for veterinary use is 10 to 20 mg/kg.

REFERENCES

1. Adamson, D. W., and Green, A. F.: New series of analgesics. Nature (London) *165:* 122, 1950.
2. Adriani, J., and Yarberry, O. H., Jr.: Preanesthetic medication. Old and new concepts. Arch. Surg. (Chicago) *79:* 976, 1959.
3. Anonymous: Morphine-apomorphine analgesia. A clinical review. J. Small Anim. Med. *1:* 220, 1952.
4. Bahga, H. S., and Link, R. P.: Cardiovascular effects of two phenothiazines: fluphenazine and trifluoperazine. Amer. J. Vet. Res. *27:* 81, 1966.
5. Bastos, M. L., Tavares, L., and De Oliveira, O.: Chlorpromazine and promazine metabolism in horses. 19th proceedings of the Association of Official Racing Chemists, p. 234, 1965.
6. Batterman, R. C., and Oshlag, A. M.: The effectiveness and toxicity of methadon, new analgesic agent. Anesthesiology *10:* 214, 1949.
7. Bennett, R. R.: The clinical use of 2-(ethylamino)-2-(2-thienyl)cyclohexanone HCl (CI 634) as an anesthetic for the cat. Amer. J. Vet. Res. *30:* 1469, 1969.
8. Bizzari, D., Fierro, F. E., Latteri, F. S., Guiffrida, J., Schmookler, A., and Berger, H. C.: Preanesthetic medication with intravenous hydroxyzine. A double blind. Anesth. Analg. (Cleveland) *40:* 378, 1961.

9. Booth, N. H., and Rankin, A. D.: Evaluation of meperidine hydrochloride in the cat. Vet. Med. 49: 249, 1954.

10. Boulos, B. M., and Davis, L. W.: Hazard of simultaneous administration of phenothiazine and piperazine. New Eng. J. Med. 280: 1245, 1969.

11. Bourgeois-Gavardin, M., Nowill, W. K., Margolis, G., and Stephen, C. R.: Chlorpromazine, a laboratory and clinical investigation. Anesthesiology 16: 829, 1955.

12. Branch, D. R., and Pastorello, R. R.: Use of glutethimide for preoperative medication in children. New Eng. J. Med. 257: 125, 1957.

13. Bree, M. M., Feller, I., and Corssen, G.: Safety and tolerance of repeated anesthesia with CI 581 (ketamine) in monkeys. Anesth. Analg. (Cleveland) 46: 596, 1967.

14. Brodie, B. B., Spector, S., and Shore, P. A.: Interaction of drugs with norepinephrine in the brain. Pharmacol. Rev. 11: 548, 1959.

15. Buckley, J. L., and Bergstrom, W. H.: Paraldehyde as an aid to handling mammals. J. Wildlife Manage. 15: 112, 1951.

16. Burnstein, C. L.: The hazard of paraldehyde administration; clinical and laboratory studies. J. A. M. A. 121: 187, 1943.

17. Burnstein, C. L., and Rovenstine, E. A.: Toxicity of intravenous paraldehyde. Proc. Soc. Exp. Biol. Med. 48: 669, 1941.

18. Burroughs, H. E.: Methadone narcosis in dogs, a clinical report. J. Small Anim. Med. 1: 301, 1953.

19. Butler, R. A.: Department of Anesthesia, University of Pennsylvania School of Medicine, 1969. Personal communication.

20. Carey, F. M., and Sanford, J.: A method of assessing the effect of drugs on the performance in the horse. Proc. Brit. Equine Ass. 52, 1965.

21. Carlson, W. D.: A clinical evaluation of meperidine hydrochloride as a preanesthetic agent in the cat. Vet. Med. 50: 229, 1955.

22. Chen, G., and Ensor, C. R.: 2-(ethylamino)-2-(2-thienyl)cyclohexanone HCl (CI 634): a taming, incapacitating, and anesthetic agent for the cat. Amer. J. Vet. Res. 29: 863, 1968.

23. Chen, G., Ensor, C., Russell, D., and Bohner, B.: The pharmacology of 1-(1-phencylcyclohexyl)piperidine HCl. J. Pharmacol. Exp. Ther. 127: 241, 1959.

24. Chen, K. K.: Pharmacology of methadon and related compounds. Ann. N.Y. Acad. Sci. 51: 83, 1948.

25. Christensen, E. M., and Gross, E. G.: Analgesic effects in human subjects of morphine, meperidine and methadon. J. A. M. A. 137: 594, 1948.

26. Clifford, D. H.: Effect of preanesthetic medication with chlorpromazine, meperidine and promazine on pentobarbital anesthesia in the cat. J. Amer. Vet. Med. Ass. 113: 415, 1957.

27. Clifford, D. H.: Observations on effect of preanesthetic medication with meperidine and promazine on barbiturate anesthesia in an ocelot and a leopard. J. Amer. Vet. Med. Ass. 133: 459, 1958.

28. Clifford, D. H.: Effect of preanesthetic medication on barbiturate anesthesia, hypothermia, traumatic shock and lethal dose of pentobarbital in the feline species. Doctoral thesis. University of Minnesota, Minneapolis, 1959.

29. Clifford, D. H., and Soma, L. R.: Anesthesiology. In Feline Medicine and Surgery. American Veterinary Publications, Inc., Santa Barbara, Calif., 1964.

30. Clifford, D. H., Stowe, C. M., and Good, A. L.: Pentobarbital anesthesia in lions with special reference to preanesthetic medication. J. Amer. Vet. Med. Ass. 139: 111, 1961.

31. Cochin, J., Gruhzit, C. C., Woods, L. A., and Seevers, M. H.: Further observations on addiction to methadon in monkey. Proc. Soc. Exp. Biol. Med. 69: 430, 1948.

32. Collard, J. A.: Unusual reaction to chlorpromazine hydrochloride in a bitch. Aust. Vet. J. 34: 90, 1958.

33. Collette, W. L., and Meriwether, W. F.: Some changes in the peripheral blood of dogs after administration of certain tranquilizers and narcotics. Vet. Med. 60: 1223, 1965.

34. Collins, R. J.: Potency of dihydromorphinone, methadone and codeine compared to morphine in self-maintained addict rats. Fed. Proc. 22: 248, 1963.

35. Conaghan, J. P., Jacobsen, M., Rae, L., and Ward-McQuaid, J. N.: Pentazocine and phenazocine. A double blind comparison of two benzomorphane derivatives in postoperative pain. Brit. J. Anaesth. 38: 345, 1966.

36. Cornbleet, T.: Use of intravenous given hydroxyzine for simple pain producing office procedures. J. A. M. A. 172: 56, 1960.

37. Corssen, G., and Domino, E. F.: Dissociative anesthesia: further pharmacologic studies and first clinical experience with the phencyclidine derivative CI-581. Anesth. Analg. (Cleveland) 45: 29, 1966.

38. Culright, E. G.: The effects of chlorpromazine premedication on anesthesia and post-anesthetic symptoms. J. Amer. Med. Wom. Ass. 11: 45, 1956.

39. Dobkin, A. B.: Efficiency of ataractic drugs in clinical anaesthesia: a review. Canad. Anaesth. Soc. J. 5: 176, 1958.

40. Dobkin, A. B.: Potentiation of thiopental by derivatives and analogues of phenothiazine. Anesthesiology 21: 292, 1960.

41. Dobkin, A. B.: Potentiation of thiopental anaesthesia with Tigan®, Panectyl®, Benadryl®, Gravol®, Marzine®, Histadyl®, Librium®, Haloperidol (R 1625). Canad. Anaesth. Soc. J. 8: 265, 1961.

42. Dobkin, A. B., Lee, P. K. Y., Byles, P. H., and Israel, J. S.: Neuroleptanalgesics: a comparison of the cardiovascular respiratory and metabolic effects of Innovar® and thio-

pentone plus methotrineprazine. Brit. J. Anaesth. *35:* 694, 1963.

43. Domino, E. F., Chodoff, P., and Corssen, G.: Pharmacologic effects of CI-581, a new dissociative anesthetic in man. Clin. Pharmacol. Ther. *6:* 279, 1965.

44. Dripps, R. D., Eckenhoff, J. E., and Vandam, L. D.: *Introduction to Anesthesia*, 3rd ed. W. B. Saunders Company, Philadelphia, 1967.

45. Dripps, R. D., Vandam, L. D., Pierce, E. C., Oech, S. R., and Lurrie, A. A.: Use of chlorpromazine in anesthesia and surgery. Ann. Surg. *142:* 774, 1955.

46. Dunbar, B., Ovassapian, A., and Smith, T. C.: The effects of methoxyflurane on ventilation in man. Anesthesiology *28:* 1020, 1967.

47. Dundee, J. W.: *Thiopentone and Other Thiobarbiturates*. E. S. Livingstone, Ltd., Edinburgh, 1956.

48. Earl, A. E.: Glutethimide (Doriden®): an oral sedative-hypnotic and injectible anesthetic. Ciba Pharmaceutical Company, Summit, N.J., 1965. Personal communication.

49. Eckenhoff, J. E., Elder, J. D., and King, B. D.: N-allyl-normorphine in the treatment of morphine and Demerol narcosis. Amer. J. Med. Sci. *223:* 191, 1952.

50. Eckenhoff, J. E., Helrich, M., and Rolph, D. W.: Effects of promethazine upon respiration and criculation of man. Anesthesiology *18:* 703, 1957.

51. Eckenhoff, J. E., and Oech, S. R.: The effects of narcotics and antagonists upon respiration and circulation of man. *Clin. Pharmacol. Ther. 1:* 483, 1960.

52. Eggers, G. W. M., Jr., Corssen, G., and Allen, G. R.: Comparison of varopressor responses in the presence of phenothiazine derivatives. Anesthesiology *20:* 261, 1959.

53. Eisleb, O., and Schaumann, O.: Dolantin ein neuartiges Spasmolytikum und Analgetileim (chemisches und pharmakologisches). Deutsch. Med. Wschr. *65:* 967, 1939.

54. Epling, G. P., and Rankin, A. D.: Metopon analgesia in the dog. Amer. J. Vet. Res. *15:* 338, 1954.

55. Essig, C. F.: Withdrawal convulsions in dogs following chronic meprobamate intoxication. Arch. Neurol. Psychiat. (Chicago) *80:* 414, 1958.

56. Fastier, F. N.: A comparison of the hypnotics: Doriden and Nembutal. New Zeal. Med. J. *57:* 171, 1958.

57. Feinberg, A. R., Pruzansky, J. J., Feinberg, S. M., and Fisherman, E. W.: Hydroxyzine (Atarax®) in chronic articaria and in allergic manifestations. J. Allerg. *29:* 358, 1958.

58. Feldberg, W., and Paton, W. D. M: Release of histamine by morphine alkaloids. J. Physiol. (London) *111:* 19, 1950.

59. Flyger, V.: Handling wild mammals with new tranquilizer. Transactions of the 26th North American Wildlife and Natural Resources Conference, p. 230, 1961.

60. Foldes, F., Severdlon, M., Siken, E. S., and Eddy, N. B.: *Narcotics and Narcotic Antagonists*. Charles C Thomas, Publisher, Springfield, Ill., 1964.

61. Fowler, W. S.: Lung function studies, respiratory dead space. Amer. J. Physiol. *154:* 405, 1948.

62. Fraser, H. F., and Rosenberg, D. E.: Observations on the human pharmacology and addictiveness of methotrimeprazine. Clin. Pharmacol. Ther. *4:* 596, 1963.

63. Gabel, A. A., Hamlin, R., and Smith, C. R.: Effects of promazine and chloral hydrate on the cardiovascular system of the horse. Amer. J. Vet. Res. *25:* 1151, 1964.

64. Gabel, A. A., and Koestner, A.: The effects of intracarotid artery injection of drugs in animals. J. Amer. Vet. Med. Ass. *142:* 1397, 1963.

65. Godeaux, J., and Tnnesen, M.: Investigations into atropine metabolism in animal organism. Acta Pharmacol. (Kobenhavn) *5:* 95, 1949.

66. Goodman, L. S., and Gilman, A.: *The Pharmacological Basis of Therapeutics*, 3rd ed. The Macmillan Company, New York, 1965.

67. Graham-Jones, O.: Tranquilizer and paralytic drugs. An international survey of animal restraint techniques. Int. Zoo Year Book *2:* 300, 1960.

68. Graham-Jones, O.: Restraint and anaesthesia of some captive wild mammals. Vet. Rec. *76:* 1216, 1964.

69. Graham-Jones, O.: Discussion of Smits.[128]

70. Grinne, L. M.: The excretion of noradrenaline and adrenaline in the urine of rats during chronic morphine administration and during abstinence. Psychopharmacologia (Berlin) *2:* 214, 1961.

71. Hall, L. W.: *Wright's Veterinary Anesthesia and Analgesia*, 6th ed. The Williams & Wilkins Company, Baltimore, 1966.

72. Hall, L. W., and Stevenson, D. F.: Effects of ataractic drugs on the blood pressure and heart rate of dogs. Nature (London) *187:* 696, 1960.

73. Hand, L. V.: Discussion following analgesic effects in human subjects of morphine, meperidine and methadon. J. A. M. A. *137:* 594, 1948.

74. Harris, L. S., and Pierson, A. K.: Some narcotic antagonists in the benzomorphan series. J. Pharm. Pharmacol. *143:* 141, 1964.

75. Harthoorn, A. M.: On the use of phencyclidine for narcosis in the larger animals. Vet. Rec. *74:* 410, 1962.

76. Harthoorn, A. M.: Producing "twilight sleep" in large wild mammals. J. Amer. Vet. Med. Ass. *141:* 1473, 1962.

77. Heavner, J. E.: Morphine for postsurgical use in cats. J. Amer. Vet. Med. Ass. *156:* 1018, 1970.

78. How, C. M., and Wilkinson, J. S.: A diluting effect of chlorpromazine hydrochloride on the circulating blood of dogs. Vet. Rec. 69: 734, 1957.

79. Hori, T.: Facilitation and inhibition of the medullary respiratory neurones, Jap. J. Physiol. 16: 436, 1966.

80. Horst, S. M., Kettlitz, W. K., and Visagie, G. P.: The use of Ro 5-2807 (Roche) as a tranquilizer in wild ungulates. Zool. Afr. 1: 231, 1965.

81. Huebner, R. A.: Meprobamate in canine medicine: summary of 77 cases. Vet. Med. 51: 488, 1956.

82. Isbell, H., Eiseman, A. J., Wikler, A., and Frank, K.: Effects of single doses of 6-dimethylamino-4-4-diphenyl-3-heptanone (amidone, methadone, or "10820") on human subjects. J. Pharmacol. Exp. Ther. 92: 83, 1948.

83. Jansinski, D. R., Martin, W. R., and Heldtke, R.: Evaluation in man of the weak antagonist pentazocine (Pe) for partial morphine (M) against activity. Fed. Proc. 29: 686, 1970.

84. Janssen, P. A., Niemegeers, C. J., and Dony, J. G.: The inhibitory effect of fentanyl and other morphine-like analgesics on the warm water induced tail withdrawal reflex in rats. Arzneimittelforschung. 13: 502, 1963.

85. Johnson, D. W.: Notes on the investigational use of Miltown in veterinary medicine. Lederle Laboratories Division, American Cyanamid Company, Pearl River, N.Y., 1956.

86. Kaelber, W. W., and Toynt, R. J.: Tremor production in cats given chlorpromazine. Proc. Soc. Exp. Biol. Med. 92: 399, 1956.

87. Kahn, N., and Wang, S. C.: Electrophysiologic basis for pontine apneustic center and its role in integration of the Hering-Breuer reflex. J. Neurophysiol. 30: 301, 1967.

88. Khazan, N., Primo, C., Danon, A., Assael, M., Sulman, F. G., and Winnik, H. Z.: The mammotropic effect of tranquilizing drugs. Arch. Int. Pharmacodyn. 136: 291, 1962.

89. King, B. D., Harris, L. C., Jr., Greifenstein, F. E., Elder, J. D., Jr., and Dripps, R. D.: Reflex circulatory responses to direct laryngoscopy and tracheal intubation performed during general anesthesia. Anesthesiology 12: 556, 1951.

90. Kottmeier, C. A., and Gravenstein, J. S.: The parasympathomimetic activity of atropine and atropine methylbromide. Anesthesiology 29: 1125, 1968.

91. Kruegar, H., Eddy, N. B., and Sumwalt, M.: The pharmacology of the opium alkaloids. Public Health Report, suppl. 165. U.S. Government Printing Office, Washington, D.C., (Part I) 1941 and (Part II) 1943.

92. Lasagna, L., and DeKornfeld, T. J.: Methotrimeprazine: a new phenothiazine derivative with analgesic properties. J. A. M. A. 178: 887, 1961.

93. Lowenstein, E., Mallowell, P., Levine, H., Daggett, W. M., Austen, W., and Lavor, M. B.: Cardiovascular response to large doses of intravenous morphine in man. New Eng. J. Med. 281: 1389, 1969.

94. Maichel, R. P.: Diverse central effects of chlorpromazine. Int. J. Neuropharmacol. 7: 23, 1968.

95. Martin, J. E., and Beck, J. D.: Some effects of chlorpromazine in horses. Amer. J. Vet. Res. 17: 678, 1958.

96. Mason, M. M.: Apomorphine in dogs. J. Amer. Vet. Med. Ass. 117: 217, 1950.

97. Matorras, A. A., and Felipe, M. A. N.: Selection of indications on the use of CI-581 and observations on 198 cases. In Progress in Anaesthesiology, Proceedings of the Fourth World Congress of Anaesthesiologists, London, 1968, p. 1000. Excerpta Medica Foundation Amsterdam, 1970.

98. Mayer, K.: Demerol hydrochloride as a sedative for cats. North Amer. Vet. 26: 477, 1945.

99. Maynert, E. W.: The usefulness of clinical signs for the comparison of intravenous anesthetics in dogs. J. Pharmacol. Exp. Ther. 128: 182, 1960.

100. Maynert, E. W., and Klingman, G. I.: Acute tolerance to intravenous anesthetics in dogs. J. Pharmacol. Exp. Ther. 128: 192, 1960.

101. Miyasaka, M., and Domino, E. F.: Neuronal mechanisms of ketamine induced anesthesia. Int. J. Neuropharmacol. 7: 557, 1968.

102. Morrow, D. H., Gaffney, T. E., and Holman, J. E.: The chronotropic and inotropic effects of halothane. Anesthesiology 22: 915, 1961.

103. Mosby, H. S., and Cantner, D. E.: The use of avertin in capturing wild turkeys and as an oral-basal anesthetic for other wild animals. Southwest Vet. 9: 132, 1956.

104. Nunn, J. F., and Bergman, N. A.: The effect of atropine on pulmonary gas exchange. Brit. J. Anaesth. 36: 68, 1964.

105. Nytch, T. F.: Clinical observations on the preanesthetic use of oxymorphine and its antagonist N-allyl-noroxymorphane, in dogs. J. Amer. Vet. Med. Ass. 145: 127, 1964.

106. Orahovats, P. D., Lehman, E. G., and Chapin, E. W.: Pharmacology of ethyl-1-(4-aminophenethyl)-4-phenylisonipecotate, anileridine, a new potent synthetic analgesic. J. Pharmacol. Exp. Ther. 119: 26, 1957.

107. Owen, L. N.: Thiambutene-thiopentone anaesthesia for hysterectomy in pyometra of the bitch. Vet. Rec. 67: 580, 1955.

108. Paradis, B.: Analgesic and anaesthetic properties of levomepromazine (Noziman) (R. P. 704). Canad. Anaesth. Soc. J. 9: 153, 1962.

109. Quentin, J. R. L., and Siry, J. R.: Tranquilizers in veterinary medicine. Agric. Food Chem. 3: 136, 1962.

110. Raker, C. W., and English, B.: Promazine—its pharmacological and clinical effects in horses. J. Amer. Vet. Med. Ass. 132: 19, 1959.

111. Raker, C. W., and Sayres, A. C.: Promazine as a preanesthetic agent in horses. J. Amer. Vet. Med. Ass. 132: 23, 1959.

112. Ratcliffe, H. L.: Diazepam (Tranimal) as a tranquilizer for zoo animals. Report of the

Penrose Research Laboratory of the Zoological Society of Philadelphia, p. 10, 1962.

113. Remmen, E., Cohen, S., Ditman, K. S., and Frantz, J. R.: *Psychochemotherapy, the Physician's manual*, chap. 4. Western Medical Publications, Los Angeles, 1962.

114. Reynolds, A. K., and Randall, L. O.: *Morphine and Allied Drugs*. University of Toronto Press, Toronto, 1957.

115. Robbins, B. H.: Studies on cyclopropane. IX. The effect of premedication with Demerol upon the heart rate, rhythm and blood pressure in dogs under cyclopropane anesthesia. J. Pharmacol. Exp. Ther. *85:* 198, 1945.

116. Roberts, O. J.: The effects of various intravenous agents on the horse. Amer. J. Vet. Res. *4:* 226, 1943.

117. Root, W. S., and Hofmann, F. G. (editors): *Physiological Pharmacology*. Part A, The nervous system, Vol. I, p. 185. Academic Press, New York, 1963.

118. Rouge, J. C.: Levallorphan and meperidine mixtures. ACTA Anaesth. Scand. *13:* 87, 1969.

119. Rubin, A., and Winston, J.: The role of the vestibular apparatus in the production of nausea and vomiting following the administration of morphine to man. J. Clin. Invest. *29:* 1261, 1950.

120. Salzman, N. P., and Brodie, B. B.: Physiological disposition and fat of chlorpromazine and a method for its estimation in biological material. J. Pharmacol. Exp. Ther. *118:* 46, 1956.

121. Sandoval, R. G., and Wang, R. I. H: Naloxone induced withdrawal symptoms of pentazocine. Fed. Proc. *29:* 686, 1970.

122. Scott, C. C., Kohlsteadt, K. G., and Chen, K. K.: Comparison of pharmacologic properties of some new analgesic substances. Anesth. Analg. (Cleveland) *26:* 12, 1947.

123. Severinghaus, J. W., and Stupfel, M. A.: Respiratory dead space increase following atropine in man and atropine, vagal or ganglionic blockade and hypothermia in dogs. J. Appl. Physiol. *8:* 81, 1955.

124. Shemano, I., and Wendel, H.: Effects of meperidine hydrochloride and morphine sulfate on the lung capacity of intact dogs. J. Pharmacol. Exp. Ther. *149:* 379, 1965.

125. Short, C. E., Greenwald, W., and Bendick, F.: Oxygen, carbon dioxide, and pH responses in arterial blood of dogs given analgesic, neuroleptanalgesic and ataractic agents. J. Amer. Vet. Med. Ass. *156:* 1406, 1970.

126. Smith, D. E., King, M. B., and Hoebel, B. G.: Lateral hypothalamic control of killing: evidence for cholinoceptive mechanism. Science *167:* 900, 1970.

127. Smith, T. C., Stephen, G. W., Zeiger, L., and Woolman, H.: Effects of premedicant drugs on respiration and gas exchange in man. Anesthesiology *28:* 883, 1967.

128. Smits, G. M.: Some experiments and experiences with neuroleptic and hypnotic drugs on

ungulates with special regard to Librium. Proceedings of Fifth International Symposium on Diseases of Zoo-Animals. Roy. Neth. Vet. Ass. Tij. Dierg. *89:* 195, 1964.

129. Sollman, T.: *A Manual of Pharmacology and Its Application to Therapeutics and Toxicology*, 8th ed. W. B. Saunders Company, Philadelphia, 1957.

130. Soma, L. R., and Shields, D. R.: Neuroleptanalgesia produced by fentanyl and droperidol. J. Amer. Vet. Med. Ass. *145:* 897, 1964.

131. Stephen, G. W., Banner, M. P., Wollman, H., and Smith, T.: Respiratory pharmacology of mixtures of scopolamine with secobarbital and with fentanyl. Anesthesiology *31:* 237, 1969.

132. Stoeling, V. K.: Analgesic action of pentazocine compared with morphine in postoperative pain. Anesth. Analg. (Cleveland) *44:* 769, 1965.

133. Stoliker, H. E.: The physiological and pharmacological effects of Sernylan® : a review. In *Experimental Animal Anesthesiology*, pp. 148-184. U.S. Air Force School of Aerospace Medicine, Aerospace Medical Division (AFSC), Brooks Air Force Base, San Antonio, Texas, July 1965.

134. Sugioka, K., Boniface, K. J., and Davis, D. A.: The influence of meperidine on myocardial contractility in the intact dog. Anesthesiology *18:* 623, 1957.

135. Talwalker, P. K., Meities, J., Nicoll, C. S., and Hopkins, T. F.: Effects of chlorpromazine on mammary glands of rats. Amer. J. Physiol. *199:* 1073, 1960.

136. Tavernor, W. D.: An assessment of promazine hydrochloride as a sedative in the dog. Vet. Rec. *74:* 779, 1962.

137. Telivuo, L. J., and Vaisanen, R.: Clinical experience with a phencyclidine derivative CI-581. In *Progress in Anaesthesiology*, Proceedings of the Fourth World Congress of Anesthesiologists, London, 1968. Excerpta Medica Foundation Amsterdam, 1970.

138. Troxil, E. B.: Clinical evaluation of analgesic methadon. J. A. M. A. *136:* 920, 1948.

139. Vasko, J. S., Henney, R. P., Browley, R. K., Oldham, H. N., and Morrow, A. G.: Effects of morphine on ventricular function and myocardial contractile force: J. Physiol. *210:* 329, 1966.

140. Wang, S. C., and Barison, H. L.: A new concept of organization of the central emetic mechanism. Gastroenterology *22:* 1, 1952.

141. Way, E. L.: Barbiturate antagonism of isonipecaine convulsions and isonipecaine potentiation of barbiturate depression. J. Pharmacol. Exp. Ther. *87:* 265, 1946.

142. Way, E. L., Swanson, R., and Gimble, A. E.: Studies in vitro and in vivo on the influence of the liver on isonipecaine (Demerol) activity. J. Pharmacol. Exp. Ther. *91:* 178, 1947.

143. Westhues, M., and Fritsch, R.: *Die Narkose der Tiere*, Band I: Lokal Anasthesie. Band II: Allgemein Narkose. Paul Parey, Berlin, 1961.

14
Respiratory Effects of General Anesthesia

THEODORE C. SMITH

Respiration is one of the essential characteristics of living organisms. Higher species have evolved special organs to facilitate the exchange and transportation of oxygen and carbon dioxide between cells and the external environment. These organs comprise the two pumping and distributing systems schematically drawn in Figure 14.1. Muscle contraction (of the chest cage) pumps air into and out of the lungs. Muscle contraction (of the heart) moves blood into the lungs and from the lungs to the rest of the body. The two systems are separated by the semipermeable alveolar capillary membrane across which gases exchange. Sensing and control mechanisms, the chemoreceptors, and respiratory centers of the brain alter the function of both pumps. In normal, unanesthetized mammals, this dual system inspires air with a P_{O_2} of 160 Torr* (mm Hg) of oxygen and less than 1 Torr of carbon dioxide, humidifies it, and equilibrates it with mixed venous blood returning from the tissues. The venous blood has an oxygen tension of 35 to 45 Torr and a carbon dioxide tension of 44 to 48 Torr. The ratio of ventilation to perfusion is

* A Torr is the international unit of pressure, equal to that pressure exerted by a column of mercury 1 mm high at conditions of 0°C and unity gravimetric force.

TABLE 14.1

Symbols used in chapter

Symbol	Definition
P	Indicates a pressure, measured in Torr, at a site identified by subscripts: A, alveolar; B, barometric; a, arterial; pl, pleural. Further subscripts identify chemical species: Pa_{CO_2} is the arterial tension of carbon dioxide.
V	A gas volume, measured in liters, and further identified by subscripts: A, alveolar; D, dead space; E, expired; I, inspired; T, tidal.
F	A concentration, decimally expressed, of a gas. This differs from standard terms only in that the volume is not necessarily that of dry gas.
R	Resistance measured from pressure and flow by assuming Ohm's law, with subscript, aw, to indicate airway.
C	A compliance of the lung, thorax, or both when subscripted L, Th, or L-Th. Otherwise it is the content of gas in blood, modified by subscripts to indicate site and gas: $i.e.$, $C_{v_{O_2}}$ is oxygen content of venous blood.
Q	A volume of blood.
$\dot{V}$, $\dot{Q}$	The dot indicates a time derivative, $i.e.$, a flow rate. Subscripts further identify $\dot{V}_E$ as expired minute volume, $\dot{Q}_{cap}$ a capillary blood flow, $\dot{Q}_S$ as shunt flow, $\dot{Q}_T$ as total flow.

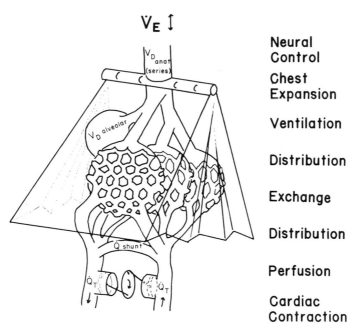

Neural
Control

Chest
Expansion

Ventilation

Distribution

Exchange

Distribution

Perfusion

Cardiac
Contraction

FIG. 14.1. Diagram of the system for external respiration. Neural impulses cause muscle contraction which expands the thoracic cage, indicated by a bellows. Expansion causes ventilation, drawing air through the tracheobronchial tree and distributing it to the alveoli. Oxygen moves by physical diffusion into the pulmonary capillary blood, which has been pumped from systemic veins by the heart and distributed through the pulmonary vasculature. A small portion of the total cardiac output from the right ventricle passes into the pulmonary veins draining the lung, and then into the left ventricle without passing past alveoli. This is indicated in the diagram by a shunt. Some alveoli receive little or no blood supply and act as an air shunt.

roughly 4 parts ventilation to 5 parts of perfusion. The products of the exchange system are arterial blood with an oxygen tension of 90 to 100 Torr and a carbon dioxide tension of approximately 35 to 40 Torr.

Respiration includes all processes involved in transferring useful energy from oxygen and foodstuffs (see Fig. 14.2). General anesthesia has significant effects on cellular respiration and metabolism, and these have recently been described and reviewed.[1, 14, 26, 34]

This chapter will be limited to considerations of external respiration and the effects of general anesthesia on (a) the mechanical aspects of gas transport; (b) the resulting ventilation and its distribution to alveoli; (c) the composition of respired gases and their exchange at the alveolar capillary level; (d) the distribution of blood through the pulmonary arterial capillaries; and (e) the reflex-mediated control of these processes.

Most information on respiratory physiology has been obtained from three animal species: decerebrate cat (neurophysiological investigations of the control of respiration); dog anesthetized with pentobarbital (acute studies); and unanesthetized seated man (able to perform such voluntary acts as breath holding and Valsalva maneuvers). Despite the limited comparative data, the basic physiological principles are applicable over a wide range of anatomical and species variations. Figure 14.3 illustrates the wide variation in the matching of function (oxygen uptake) and size of the organ (lung weight) of mammals. Comprehension of the basic physics and physiology will enable the anesthetist to transfer information obtained in cat, dog, and man to large animals (which have special problems due to the large hydro-

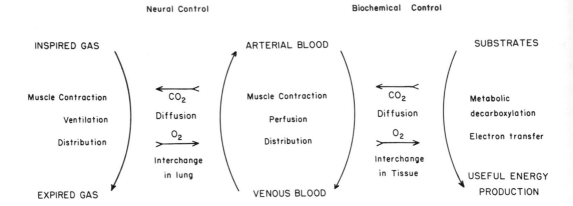

FIG. 14.2. A diagram of the processes involved in respiration. Gases are exchanged across capillary beds by diffusion. The gases reach these capillary beds by transporting mechanisms such as ventilation of gas and circulation of blood. While this chapter concentrates on external respiration, it must be kept in mind that this is just a portion of the total system yielding useful energy production from oxidation of foodstuffs.

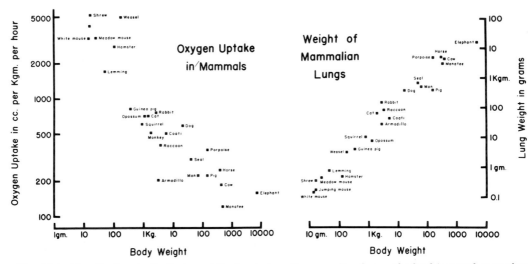

FIG. 14.3. Despite the similarity in architectural plan of mammalian lungs, the load imposed upon them varies considerably. The white mouse uses 20 times as much oxygen per gram of body weight as the elephant, but has only one-third as much lung per gram of body weight. He must use this tissue more effectively and does so by very rapid respiratory rate and high minute volume per gram of tissue.

static pressure differences between ventral and dorsal surfaces of the lung) or to small animals (whose small lungs and rapid respiratory rates create rapid turnover of gases). Knowledge of the abnormalities produced by general anesthesia will permit the anesthetist to anticipate them, minimize the resulting derangements in function, and often compensate for specific stresses.

Mechanical Aspects of Breathing

THE FORCES OF EXPANSION

The lungs are elastic structures analogous to toy balloons which are distended slightly to fill the thorax. Their volume is proportional to the pressure difference across their walls. Increasing the pressure difference increases the volume. Since the unstretched volume of the lungs is smaller

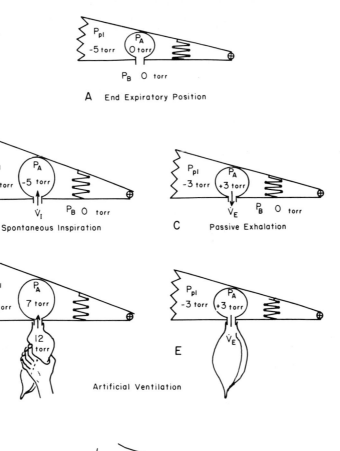

FIG. 14.4. Diagram of the mechanical factors in breathing. The tone of muscles (not shown) tending to open the bellows is opposed by the elastic recoil of the lungs (indicated by coil spring), tending to collapse the bellows. The result is a slightly negative pressure within the pleural space P_{pl}. When alveolar pressure, P_A, is less than the pressure outside the body, P_B, gas flows into the lung, as indicated in Panel B. This is accomplished by muscular effort which lowers the intrapleural pressure. When the muscles causing active inspiration relax, the elastic recoil of the lungs tends to collapse the chest, creating a positive pressure within the alveoli. Since this pressure is higher than ambient, gas flows out of the lungs, as shown in Panel C. The size of the lungs is proportional to the transpulmonary pressure, $P_A - P_{pl}$. Thus, Panels B and D show the same size lung because they have the same transpulmonary pressure, 7 Torr, even though the absolute pleural and alveolar pressures differ. When the chest is opened as in Panel F, the pleural pressure becomes atmospheric and there is nothing to prevent the lungs from collapsing completely.

than the volume of the thorax, the elastic recoil of the lungs tends to pull them away from the chest cage, resulting in a slightly negative pressure in the pleural space (Fig. 14.4A). Contraction of the diaphragm and intercostal muscles further lowers the intrapleural pressure (P_{pl}), and the alveoli expand, lowering intra-alveolar pressure (Fig. 14.4B). When intra-alveolar pressure is less than atmospheric pressure, gas flows down the tracheobronchial tree to the alveoli, completing the processes of inhalation. Exhalation in a rest-ing, unanesthetized animal is usually pas-sive due to the elastic force stored by stretching the lung during inhalation; no muscular activity is required (Fig. 14.4C). If animals are made apneic by anesthesia, a positive pressure must be exerted on the airway to create air flow and distend al-veoli. This is provided by manual com-pression of the anesthesia breathing bag or by a respirator (Fig. 14.4D). Exhala-tion is usually passive, as during quiet, spontaneous breathing.

The muscles of ventilation include the intercostal muscles, the diaphragm, and the muscles of the shoulder girdle, often called the accessory muscles of respira-tion. Since the chest cage covers approxi-mately two-thirds of the lung's surface, and the diaphragm approximately one-third, a given increase in diameter of the chest is twice as effective as a propor-tioned linear descent of the diaphragm.[7] The accessory muscles ordinarily do not contribute directly to gas movement, but do fix the thoracic inlet, keeping the up-per ribs from collapsing during intercostal muscle contraction.

RATE OF INSPIRED GAS FLOW AND AIRWAY
RESISTANCE

Gas flows along the tracheobronchial tree because of the pressure difference between mouth and alveoli. If the flow is smooth (laminar), it follows the hydraulic analogy of Ohm's law. Resistance is the quotient of flow and pressure difference causing the flow. The airway resistance to inflation in the example of Figure 14.4, B and D, is calculated by dividing 5 Torr (atmospheric pressure minus alveolar) by the inspiratory flow rate. Expiratory re-sistance in Figure 14.4, C and E, would be 3 Torr divided by expiratory flow. Resist-ance depends upon the size and geometry of the lungs and on the physical properties of the respired gas.[15] When the ratio be-tween inertial forces and viscous forces causing gas to flow (Reynold's number) exceeds approximately 2000, flow is no longer smooth, but is broken up into eddy currents called turbulence. More energy is

required to sustain turbulent than to sus-tain laminar flow, and the pressure differ-ential must be accordingly larger.[10] If the Ohmic relation is used to calculate resist-ance in this case, it appears to increase rapidly as flow increases. Except for quiet breathing in very large animals, flow in the upper tracheobronchial tree is turbu-lent during part or all of the respiratory cycle. Airway resistance is increased by narrow tubes, abrupt angles, and valves with limited opening. These points should be considered when selecting an anesthe-sia breathing apparatus.

EXTENT OF LUNG EXPANSION

The lungs have inherent elasticity, due to the surface tension at the liquid-air interface of alveolar surfaces, as well as to the elastic tissue. The size of the lungs depends upon the pressure difference across their walls. As the alveolar pleural difference is increased during inspiration, the size of the lungs increases (Fig. 14.5). Over the usual range of tidal volumes, the size and transmural pressure are lin-early proportional to each other.[35] The proportionality constant is termed the lung compliance, and is measured by ob-serving the lung inflation resulting from an increase in pressure. Mathematically:

$$\text{Compliance} = \frac{\Delta V}{\Delta P} = C_L \qquad (1)$$

which states that compliance is the quo-tient of a change in volume (ΔV) induced by an inflating pressure (ΔP). As the lung becomes larger it becomes more difficult to inflate. This is shown in Figure 14.5 by the progressive flattening of the slope of the curve as the total lung capacity is approached. This is appreciated by the anesthetist as requiring more and more pressure to inflate the lung further; the lung feels stiffer. Similarly, it becomes more difficult to deflate the lung past the functional residual capacity; indeed, a negative airway pressure is required to do so. In the latter case, it is thought that some lung units are actually closed, de-creasing the total volume of the lung available. Because surface tension forces

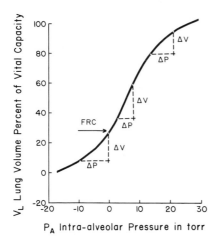

FIG. 14.5. Pressure-volume diagram of the lung. The size of the lung is a function of transpulmonary pressure. As this pressure increases, the lung volume increases as shown by the curved line. In the usual range of tidal volumes, starting from the functional residual capacity (*FRC*), the curve is nearly a straight line. At either extreme, the curve flattens out. The compliance of the lung is the ratio of an increase in volume to an increase in pressure and is the slope of this graph at any given point. The slope, and hence the compliance, is maximal in the range of ordinary tidal exchange and decreases at either extreme of lung volumes. Thus it is harder to inflate a lung if it is nearly empty, or if it is overdistended.

tend to keep collapsed lungs closed, a large pressure is necessary to reopen them.

THE INTERACTION OF RESISTANCE AND COMPLIANCE

The concepts of resistance and compliance are combined in describing the transpleural pressure necessary to generate a flow of gas at a specific lung volume. The total pressure that the animal or anesthetist must generate to inflate the lung has three components. One is used to move gas through the conducting system, one supplies energy for losses resulting from turbulence, and one stretches the lung storing energy which will provide for exhalation. During exhalation, the force causing gas to move is normally that which is supplied solely by the elasticity of the stretched lungs. As gas flows from the

lungs, the remaining volume decreases in a nearly exponential manner, as does the rate of flow itself. An exponential decrease means that in any brief interval of time, the change in volume or flow is a constant fraction of the current volume or flow. The mathematical description of an exponential curve involves two parameters: the initial value and the time constant.[33] The latter is the product of resistance and compliance and gives the number of seconds required for the lungs to empty to 38% of the initial value. A large inflation pressure gives a large initial lung volume. A large resistance or a large compliance (and hence little stored energy) produces a slow flow. Conversely, a low resistance or a low compliance (very stiff lungs) causes a rapid emptying. Increasing either or both R_{aw} or C_L prolongs exhalation—increasing R_{aw} by slowing flow and increasing C_L by giving a larger lung volume to be emptied.

THE EFFECTS OF GENERAL ANESTHESIA ON GAS FLOW

General anesthesia can cause changes in the resistance of the breathing system and the compliance of the lung. The airway resistance is little affected by inhalation agents themselves. To be sure, there is some increase in bronchial caliber following the belladonna drugs used for premedication, but this produces a clinically insignificant change in the airway resistance. Scopolamine has a longer duration of action on bronchial smooth muscle than does atropine.[47] However, considerable resistance to breathing is added by any breathing circuit used during anesthesia.[28, 54] The best modern circle breathing systems, with large bore corregated tubing and low resistance, light weight, one-way valves and jumbo size carbon dioxide canisters, double or triple the overall resistance to breathing. Nonrebreathing circuits with the valves designed for man are only slightly better.

Resistance may be compensated for by either increasing the patient's functional residual capacity or by prolonging the expiratory time. Two warnings are appropriate. First, resistance increases sharply as flow changes from laminar to turbulent. To avoid turbulent flow, sharply angled passages in the breathing system should be minimized and the rebreathing bag must not be allowed to become distended. During intermittent positive pressure ventilation, relatively slow inspiratory flows should be used.

In the spontaneously breathing animal, the chest wall expands actively, but in the apneic animal (whose respirations are controlled by the anesthetist) both the lung parenchyma and the thoracic cage must be stretched by the anesthetist inflating the lung. The total pulmonary compliance (or lung thoracic compliance) is thus of more immediate concern to the anesthetist than lung compliance alone. It varies with the size of the lungs. Pressure of 1 cm of water will produce an inflation of approximately 400 ml in the horse, 30 ml in the dog, and approximately 0.4 ml in the guinea pig. These are the values during general anesthesia. They are approximately half of the normal values in awake, unanesthetized animals in those species where the measurements have been made.[35, 36] The decrease in compliance from the awake state to the anesthetized state may be further augmented by abnormal body positions such as are necessary for some operations and by collapse of the lungs.[32] Alveolar collapse with decreased compliance, associated with increased venous admixture in arterial blood and increased risk of postoperative respiratory complications, is a common event in the spontaneously breathing anesthetized animal, or the animal controlled with shallow, rapid respiration.[5] Inspiration during spontaneous respiration should be slow and deep in order to decrease the effects of turbulence on airway resistance. In order to minimize alveolar collapse, tidal volumes should also be large. The anesthetized animal commonly breathes rapidly and shallowly. These facts constitute a strong argument for assisted or controlled respiration during general anesthetia.

DURATION OF A RESPIRATORY CYCLE

The time of a single respiratory cycle is divided unequally into inspiration (occupying approximately one-third to one-half of the cycle length), and exhalation. As the lungs expand, stretch receptors are stimulated and impulses pass up the vagus nerve which by reflex inhibit respiration (Hering-Breuer reflex). In awake resting animals, the muscles of inspiration relax and the stretched lungs recoil, expelling gas until reflexes initiated by deflation and the inherent rhythmicity of inspiratory neurons in the medulla initiate a new inspiration. During passive exhalation, flow progressively decreases as exhalation continues, and, toward the end of the cycle, becomes so low that it is barely perceptible.

The frequency of breathing, depth of inspiration, and ratio of inspiratory to expiratory times are referred to collectively as the pattern of respiration.

General anesthesia has major effects on this pattern. First, during general anesthesia animals may exhibit active exhalation through contraction of the recti and oblique abdominal muscles. This activity is sometimes spoken of as the abdominal compression reflex, and may, as long as the abdominal wall is intact, assist venous return to the thorax.[25] Second, as anesthesia deepens, there is progressive decrease in inspiratory force in the muscles of respiration, which may be further reduced by the use of neuromuscular blocking agents such as d-tubocurarine. Inhalation anesthetics decrease the efficacy of first the accessory muscles of respiration, then the intercostals, and finally the diaphragm. Thus, deepening of anesthesia is associated with a change of respiratory pattern with eventual passive motion of the chest cage during inspiration and jerky excursion of the diaphragm which now has the entire burden of moving gas and is simultaneously weakened by the state of anesthesia. Recognition of the depth of anesthesia and lightening of anesthesia is the proper treatment in these circumstances.

Finally, the mechanical aspects of ventilation may be impaired by the surgical positioning of the animal or presence of retractors and pads within the abdominal cavity which impede motion of the diaphragm. For these reasons, spontaneous ventilation with air cannot be relied upon in the anesthetized animal to produce normal oxygenation and carbon dioxide removal. In addition, inefficiencies of ventilation and pulmonary circulation (due to alveolar dead space and venous admixture—see below) occur during anesthesia. These are additional reasons for the anesthetist to assume part or all of the mechanical functions of respiration.

MAINTENANCE OF STRUCTURAL INTEGRITY OF THE LUNG

The mammalian lungs with their 300,000,000 air-filled alveoli are somewhat like 300,000,000 soap bubbles packed in a bag. There is a relation among the pressure necessary to distend bubbles, the radii of the bubbles, and the surface tension of the lining of the bubbles. The LaPlace equation describes the ideal case of a single bubble; the pressure within the bubble is inversely proportional to the radius of the bubble ($P = T/r$). The proportionality factor, T, is the surface tension at the interface between gas and fluid. The surface tension of water is very high, 72 dynes/cm. A bubble of air in water with a radius the size of an alveolus would require a large pressure within it to keep it from collapsing. Even the very best bubble pipe cannot blow bubbles of distilled water. However, when soap is added, the surface tension is reduced and bubbles can be blown. There is a material in the watery lining of the alveoli which reduces the surface tension. It is a lipoprotein called surfactant which reduces the surface tension to values as low as 5 dynes/cm. Its remarkable characteristic is that the surface tension is not constant, but decreases as the area of the alveoli is diminished.[13]

As the lung collapses from its expanded volume, the radii of alveoli decrease in diameter. If surface tension remained constant even though low, the transmural pressure necessary to maintain the alveolar structure would increase rapidly. Since the pressure in the alveoli is actually falling, they would become unstable and collapse. However, because of the effects of surfactant, giving smaller surface tension as alveoli decrease in size, when the lung deflates it requires less and less pressure to maintain the structure of the alveoli. Conversely, as the lung is expanded the surface tension increases and it takes more transmural pressure to expand the lung. This gives the effect of elasticity to the alveolar structures and is responsible for more than half of the apparent elasticity (compliance) of normal lung.

Normal awake animals with normal surfactant are just on the verge of alveolar instability.[12] An awake animal has a pattern of respiration which includes occasional yawns or sighs, as well as occasional deep breaths due to exercise or phonation. It is currently believed that these maneuvers are, in part, reflex-stimulated to re-expand collapsed alveolar units. When general anesthesia is induced, respiration becomes shallow and weak and alveolar units begin to collapse. The reflex-induced large breath (yawn or sigh) disappears or is infrequent and ineffective.[21] It is important that the anesthetist maintain the structural integrity of the lung by replacing the yawn with intermittent deep inflations and by augmenting tidal volume. Evidence in dog and man suggests that tidal volumes of 6 ml/kg are probably adequate to prevent the collapse of the lung and the development of atelectasis.[27]

Ventilatory Volume

The volumes of gas inhaled and exhaled are not equal in awake or anesthetized animals breathing relatively insoluble gases. Despite the fact that inspiration is active and exhalation usually passive, it is the exhaled volume of gas that is generally used by physiologists in assessing respiration, for it carries away carbon dioxide. The volume exhaled per breath is called the tidal volume (V_T), and the volume exhaled per minute is the minute volume ($\dot{V}_E$). The use of expired rather than inspired volume is particularly appropriate during anesthesia. The anesthetist can alter the inspired gases at will, providing complete oxygenation of arterial blood in the absence of any ventilation at all if he chooses; ventilation is still required to remove carbon dioxide. The tension of carbon dioxide in blood can be used to measure the efficiency of ventilation. The state of hyperventilation is produced when carbon dioxide is removed from the body at a rate that is greater than it is being produced. The alveolar tension decreases, as do the tensions in arterial blood, tissues, and venous blood, until carbon dioxide excretion falls to the rate of production. Conversely, hypoventilation results from removing carbon dioxide at a rate less than the metabolic production and carbon dioxide tensions in tissue, blood, and alveoli increase.

THE ALVEOLAR VENTILATION

Since carbon dioxide comes only from ventilated alveoli, the carbon dioxide which is excreted in each minute can be calculated by:

$$\dot{V}_{CO_2} = \dot{V}_A \times F_{A_{CO_2}} \times f_{STPD} \qquad (2)$$

This states that the metabolic production of carbon dioxide, $\dot{V}_{CO_2}$, is equal to the alveolar ventilation, $\dot{V}_A$, expressed in liters per minute, corrected to standard conditions by a constant, f_{STPD}, times the fractional concentration of carbon dioxide in the alveoli, $F_{A_{CO_2}}$. The metabolic production of carbon dioxide may be excreted by the lungs when the alveolar ventilation is one-half or one-quarter of normal, but at a cost of doubling or quadrupling the alveolar and arterial concentration of carbon dioxide. This relationship is shown graphically in Figure 14.6, where the horizontal axis is alveolar P_{CO_2}, and the vertical axis is alveolar ventilation. Different curves in the shape of hyperbolas exist for each metabolic rate for CO_2. Points of alveolar tension and ventilation not falling on the hyperbola for a current metabolic rate represent unsteady states. Sup-

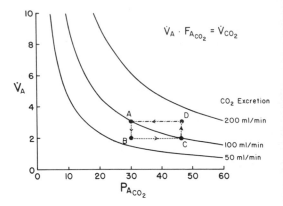

FIG. 14.6. The alveolar ventilation is related to the alveolar carbon dioxide tension by a hyperbolic line representing the carbon dioxide excretion. There is a different hyperbola for each steady state of carbon dioxide excretion. Consider a dog whose metabolic rate is 100 ml of CO_2 per minute, initial P_{CO_2} is 30 Torr, and alveolar ventilation is 3.5 liters/minute (point A on the diagram). If ventilation is decreased by an intraperitoneal barbiturate injection (point B on the diagram), carbon dioxide will not be excreted as rapidly as it is being produced so that the blood tension will rise, eventually reaching point C. If artificial ventilation is imposed on the animal (point D), CO_2 excretion will be restored to normal and the carbon dioxide tension will fall toward point A. Points on the excretion hyperbola represent steady state values for a given metabolic rate. Points not on the line indicate a changing state. If the point is above and to the right of the line, it represents greater CO_2 excretion than production, so that CO_2 will fall, and the point will tend to move to the left. Below and to the left of the line is the area where production exceeds excretion, indicating accumulation of CO_2 in the body, with a tendency for the point to move right and up. The rates of change going from points B to C and from D to A are not constant but are nearly exponential, i.e., rapid at first and slowing as the steady state value is approached.

pose an animal, in steady state at point A of Figure 14.6, is partially paralyzed, reducing his ventilation to point B. He now excretes less carbon dioxide than he produces and so his alveolar tension rises and he moves from point B to point C. If he is manually ventilated (restoring ventilation to point D), he will excrete more carbon dioxide than he produces. Thus, he will move toward point A. The rate of movement from B to C and from D to A is not constant, but is rapid at first and slows as the steady state value is approached.

RESPIRATORY DEAD SPACE

The physiological dead space is another important determinant of the total ventilation necessary to maintain homeostasis. Not all of the gas that an animal exhales comes from the alveoli. The first portion of each exhalation comes from the tracheobronchial tree, contains little or no carbon dioxide, and is referred to as anatomical respiratory dead space gas. Additional gas comes from alveoli which receive little or no pulmonary blood flow and thus contain little or no carbon dioxide except that which they might have inspired. Nonperfused alveoli do not participate in gas exchange. The gas from the tracheobronchial tree (anatomical dead space) and the nonperfused alveoli (alveolar dead space) is referred to as the physiological dead space.[45] The physiological dead space is exhaled with each breath, contributes nothing to respiratory exchange, and is wasted ventilation.

The magnitude of the wasted ventilation is usually given as a ratio of dead space to tidal volume and is calculated from the difference between alveolar and mixed expired carbon dioxide tension, divided by alveolar carbon dioxide tension:[9]

$$\frac{V_D}{V_T} = \frac{P_{A_{CO_2}} \quad P_{E_{CO_2}}}{P_{A_{CO_2}}} \qquad (3)$$

In practice, the dead space may be calculated by using two different estimates of alveolar carbon dioxide tension. If end tidal gas is sampled for carbon dioxide tension and used as an approximation of alveolar gas tension, the resulting dead space is called the anatomical dead space and was originally thought to be the anatomical volume of the conducting passages. If an arterial blood sample is taken and analyzed for arterial P_{CO_2} and this value is substituted in the above equation, the resulting dead space calculation is referred to as the physiological dead space. Notice that the equation alone cannot differentiate between added dead space (in series with the lung) and nonperfused but ventilated alveoli will dilute the carbon dioxide tension of perfused alveoli, resulting in a large difference between end tidal and arterial tension.

A numerical example will show that the equation is sensitive to changes in dead space, but insensitive to changes in right to left blood shunt. Suppose that the mixed venous blood has a normal P_{CO_2} of 46 and the arterial blood has a normal P_{CO_2} of 40 Torr. Suppose 10% of the alveoli are not perfused and hence have a P_{CO_2} of 0, while the others, in equilibrium with arterial blood, have a P_{CO_2} of 40. The end tidal gas will be a mixture of 9 parts of gas with a P_{CO_2} of 40, and 1 part of gas with a P_{CO_2} of 0 for an average tension of 36. Thus, the difference between anatomical and physiological dead space is 40 minus 36 over 40, or $^1/_{10}$; in other words, exactly equal to the proportion of unperfused alveoli. Suppose that 10% of the cardiac output bypasses the lungs so that the arterial blood is now composed of 9 parts of blood with a P_{CO_2} of 40 and 1 part with a P_{CO_2} of 46, which is an average of 40.6 Torr. Thus, an increase in true shunting of 10% is interpreted by the dead space equation as an increase of dead space of (40.6 − 40) divided by 40, or 1.5%. When a difference in gas tension between alveoli and arterial blood exists, it can be considered either as being due entirely to a dead space effect or entirely to a shunt effect. Thus, if one wants to measure the dead space effect and minimize error caused by a true shunt, the use of carbon dioxide is clearly advantageous in the measurement.

THE TOTAL VENTILATION

The minute volume exhaled in the steady state is the sum of the alveolar ventilation ($\dot{V}_A$) necessary to maintain a given carbon dioxide concentration and the dead space ventilation which is equal itself to the product of physiological dead space (V_D) and respiratory frequency (f), i.e.:

$$\dot{V}_E = \dot{V}_A + (V_{D_{phys}} \times f) \qquad (4)$$

The equation given above (Equation 2),

for the metabolic production of carbon dioxide, may be solved for alveolar ventilation, and this expression may be inserted into the equation above:

$$\dot{V}_E = V_{CO_2}/P_{A_{CO_2}} \times K) + V_{D_{phys}} \times f \quad (5)$$

In this equation, K is a constant combining the conversion to STPD and the conversion of fractional concentration to tension and f is respiratory frequency. If ventilation is to be adequate in removing carbon dioxide (and a steady state exists), then the minute volume is seen to depend on the metabolic production of carbon dioxide, the tension of carbon dioxide in the alveoli, the physiological dead space, and the frequency of breathing. Each of these four factors may be affected by anesthetization.

General anesthesia usually decreases the metabolic rate by 5 to 10%, a reduction which may be increased further by very deep anesthesia or by permitting the body temperature of the animal to drop significantly.[22, 23, 37, 51] The rate of fall of metabolic rate with temperature is not linear and is usually expressed as Q_{10}. When the metabolic rate at one temperature is twice the metabolic rate at a temperature 10 C below it, the Q_{10} is said to be 2. Similarly, when the metabolic rate of a given temperature is 3 times the rate at a temperature 10 degrees lower, the Q_{10} is 3. Metabolic processes in animals have Q_{10}'s varying between 2 and 3 generally. Thus, for the CO_2 production to be decreased to half of its normal value, the animal's body temperature must decrease from 37 to 27 C. This is the temperature at which the risk of ventricular fibrillation becomes great.[22]

Anesthetists alter dead space in a number of ways during anesthesia. Atropine premedication may increase the anatomical dead space by 20 to 50%, depending on the state of vagal tone and the dose administered. Narcotic premedication causes a slight decrease in respiratory dead space when given alone, but has negligible effect in counteracting the bronchodilation of atropine. Masks used for induction of anesthesia and other respiratory apparatus constitute variable additions to dead space while the process of tracheal intubation eliminates a large fraction of the anatomical dead space. During general anesthesia, physiological dead space may be increased by factors which tend to alter the ventilation/perfusion ($\dot{V}/\dot{Q}$) ratio in some portions of the lung, or by an increased shunting of blood (see below). When the abnormalities of $\dot{V}/\dot{Q}$ or $\dot{Q}_S$ are considered in their effects on carbon dioxide excretion, their contribution to wasted ventilation is part of the alveolar dead space. Hypotension (due to either depth of anesthesia or blood loss), increased pressure within the alveoli (due to either obstruction to exhalation or positive pressure ventilation), or unusual body position commonly produce major increases in the alveolar dead space. The development of abnormally large alveolar dead space during anesthesia is so frequent that estimates of the volume of dead space during awake conditions are not useful.[3] Generally, the reduction in dead space by tracheal intubation is of the same order as the increase in dead space due to the effects of anesthesia. The respiratory dead space constitutes 30 to 40% of the tidal volume for normal or increased tidal volumes. The effect of general anesthesia on spontaneously breathing animals is usually to decrease the tidal volume, however, and in these circumstances the effective dead space or a wasted ventilation may constitute more than half of the tidal volume.

The alveolar tension of carbon dioxide is, in part, determined by actions of the anesthetist. If the anesthetist is willing to accept a high P_{CO_2}, he needs to provide less ventilation. It is the tension of carbon dioxide and not the content of carbon dioxide in blood that must be considered. The acidosis of severe hypotension or shock decreases the carbon dioxide capacity of blood and elevates the carbon dioxide tension requiring more ventilation. High carbon dioxide results in acidosis which limits both biochemical reactions and physiological compensatory mechanisms. For example, arteriolar constriction with epinephrine is easily impaired by acidosis.[11, 43] Hypocarbia is limited, for practical purposes, to a tension of 20 Torr or more since, within the duration of most operations, it requires such high inflation pressure to reduce carbon dioxide tensions below 20 Torr that pulmonary blood flow and cardiac output may fall.

Respiratory rate, the final of the four factors affecting ventilation, is characteristically increased by anesthesia. Pulmonary compliance is decreased during anesthesia. With stiffer lungs (decrease in compliance), the work of breathing is less at a faster rate. The receptors of inflation and deflation (stretch receptors of the Hering-Breuer reflex) are sensitized by most anesthetics.[53] The dead space ventilation may constitute a very large portion of the minute volume, and what is a normal respiratory minute volume in the awake animal may in these circumstances result in severe hypoventilation.

VENTILATORY STANDARDS

The graphs given in Figure 14.7 represent useful approximations based on currently available data. Given the weight of an intubated, anesthetized animal, the graph shows that the anesthetist is free to choose either a respiratory frequency or a tidal volume, and the graph indicates the other factor. Allowance for hypothermia and hyperthermia, apparatus dead space, or unusual positions or stresses on the animal must be made. If the state of hyperventilation is elected (as may be desirable to decrease brain volume or decrease bleeding), either the rate or tidal volume must be increased; doubling of respiratory frequency or tidal volume will nearly halve the alveolar carbon dioxide in most instances. It is generally better to ventilate at a tidal volume larger than indicated and at a slower respiratory rate than the awake animal selects.

COMPOSITION OF INSPIRED GAS

The composition of gas in a lung unit when breathing ambient air depends only on the gas tension in mixed venous blood (which varies with metabolic rate and cardiac output) and the respiratory exchange quotient, RQ. As far as oxygen is concerned, decreased ventilation can be completely compensated for by an increase in the concentration of inspired oxygen. The extreme case of total paralysis with 100% oxygen supplied at the trachea will provide complete oxygenation of blood passing through the lungs in the absence of any ventilatory motion at all. This process, originally called diffusion respiration, and more correctly referred to as apneic oxygenation or "aventilatory mass flow," will maintain oxygenation of life for a period of many hours.[4] As mixed venous blood from the right heart passes through the lungs and oxygen diffuses into it from the alveoli, the pressure within the alveoli tends to be lowered. The structure of the ribs prevents the lungs from collapsing beyond a level referred to as the functional residual capacity so that a pressure gradient is created between the atmosphere and the alveoli. This causes a flow of gas down the trachea replacing oxygen taken up by hemoglobin. To insure adequate oxygenation of arterial blood, the concentration of oxygen within the lungs must initially be high, and nitrogen (or other gases which are not taken up by the pulmonary blood flow) must not be allowed to enter the trachea. This technique is used in man for brief operations such as bronchoscopy and for brief periods in longer operations when motion of the lungs would be troublesome to the surgeon.

The difficulty is that carbon dioxide elemination decreases to nearly zero with a resulting progressive respiratory acidosis. During complete apnea, carbon dioxide builds up in the arterial blood of dogs and man at an average rate of 3 or 4 Torr/minute.[20] An increase in carbon dioxide of greater than 10 is generally considered undesirable. However, this limitation of 2 to 3 minutes of apnea can be increased to 5 to 10 minutes by a prior period of hyperventilation, reducing the P_{CO_2} to 15 to 20 Torr.

DISTRIBUTION OF VENTILATION

The lungs consist of not one or two balloon-like structures on the end of conducting airways, but 20,000,000 alveolar ducts which terminate in 300,000,000 cup-

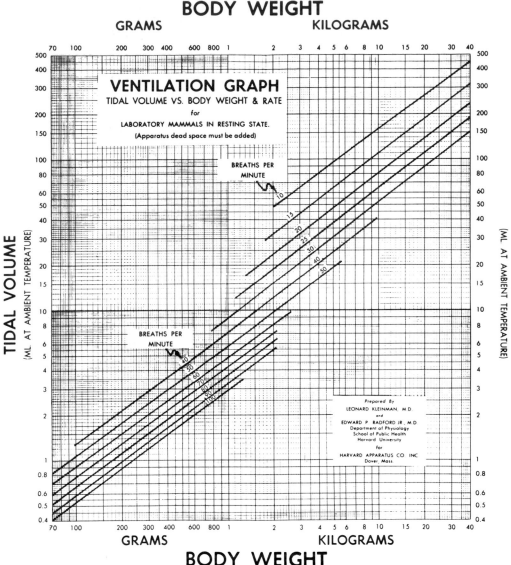

FIG. 14.7. Tidal volume and respiratory frequency in laboratory animals are related to their body weight. This graph is provided through the courtesy of Harvard Apparatus Company (Millis, Mass.) and allows one to choose approximately normal ventilation for intubated, artificially ventilated, anesthetized animals. Any apparatus dead space must be added to the tidal volume.

shaped alveoli. Several respiratory bronchioles arise from one of 200,000 terminal bronchioles which are the last structures of the purely conducting airways. Fundamental lung units consist of a terminal bronchiole, its branching respiratory bronchioles, and related alveolar ducts and alveoli.[49] The gas composition within the lung unit which is supplied by one terminal bronchiole is homogenous. Its blood supply comes from a single branch of the pulmonary artery. The dimensions of this structure are sufficiently small that the gas content is uniformly mixed by diffusion, but when the chest cage expands, creating a negative pressure within the pleural space, each of these 200,000 units does not necessarily expand synchronously and uniformly. Some are further away from the trachea and hence gas encounters a greater resistance in flowing in these units. Some are near inelastic structures of the bronchi and pulmonary vessels, so that less transmural pressure is applied to them and they expand less vigorously. These and other differences in resistance to air flow and resistance to expansion result in a wide distribution of volume of ventilation per volume of lung tissue. In other words, some portions of the lung parenchyma receive a greater portion of the freshly inspired gas than others. During general anesthesia, this distribution of ventilation may be made even more nonuniform by several factors. Some anesthetic agents are irritating and increase the flow of bronchial secretions adding to the airway resistance, particularly in dependent areas of the lung. Some drugs used in anesthesia are bronchoconstrictors such as morphine and d-tubocurarine (through histamine release). When the pattern of respiratory muscle activity changes during anesthesia, the intrapleural pressure generated at the diaphragm is more negative than that generated around the apex of the lung, giving rise to difference in expansion. Finally, there is a tendency toward collapse of the lung during general anesthesia, with small tidal volumes and rapid respiratory rates which further add to the stiffness of the lung and the nonuniformity of gas distribution. In the case of carbon dioxide, hypoventilation in one portion of the lung may be compensated for by hyperventilation in another portion. For example, consider an animal with venous P_{CO_2} of 47 Torr. Each lung initially might receive 1 liter of ventilation. However, if one lung was completely occluded but its blood flow was continued, it would contribute blood with a P_{CO_2} of 47 to the left heart. The ventilation to the other lung, however, would double. The left side of the heart would then receive equal amounts of blood containing 33 and 47 Torr P_{CO_2} so that this grossly abnormal distribution of ventilation would not change the resulting arterial P_{CO_2}.

Such is not the case for oxygenation. A normally ventilated portion of the lung saturates or nearly saturates with oxygen all of the blood it receives. A poorly ventilated portion of the lung may not fully saturate blood, but this cannot be compensated for by hyperventilation of other portions, since no more than fully saturated blood can be produced in those portions. It is necessary to point out here that it is not simply maldistribution of gas within the lung, or maldistribution of perfusion, but a mismatch between the perfusion and ventilation of various areas that causes difficulty.

Gas Exchange

The transfer of oxygen from alveoli to hemoglobin molecules and the release of carbon dioxide from bicarbonate, speeded by carbonic anhydrase, are processes of respiration little affected by general anesthesia. Carbon dioxide diffuses so readily across the thin alveolar capillary membrane that before red blood cells have passed $1/20$ of the way through the capillary bed to the collecting venules, the carbon dioxide tension in alveoli and blood have equilibrated. Oxygen exchange is less rapid because it is less soluble and requires a measurable (although very short) time to react with hemoglobin within the red blood cells.[44] Nonetheless, the diffusion distances are so short that red cells have completely equilibrated their interior oxygen tension with that of alveoli before leaving the alveolar capillary network. When inspired oxygen concentrations are above 21%, as is common during general anesthesia, the driving force for diffusion and oxygenation of venous blood is increased.

Pulmonary Blood Flow

The heart is the sole source of blood perfusing the lung, but neither all of that which goes to the lung via the pulmonary artery goes to functioning pulmonary tissue, nor all of that going to alveolar tissue reaches optimally functioning areas. The results of these deviations from ideal transportation and distribution produce less than the ideal arterialization of blood and can be considered as an admixture of venous blood with "true" arterialized blood (*i.e.*, containing the alveolar tensions of oxygen and carbon dioxide). The components of venous admixture are true or anatomical paths bypassing the lung, alveolar shunt (likely due to atelectasis), and underventilated areas (of $\dot{V}/\dot{Q}$ abnormality).[6] These are considered below. In addition, there are certain differences in function between the right and left ventricles which should be noted.[18]

CARDIAC FACTORS

Both the right and left ventricle comply with certain physiological "laws" which determine (a) their output on the basis of their filling pressure (and hence venous inflow); (b) their work load (product of cardiac output and mean pulmonary or mean aortic pressure); and (c) their capability as pumps (their ventricular function curves). Except over very brief periods, the volumes pumped by the two ventricles are identical. The filling pressures are also similar. The right heart, however, pumps into a lower mean pressure, and consequently does less work. It is accordingly less thick walled and needs less coronary blood flow. The pulmonary circulation responds to an increase in cardiac output (as with exercise) by increasing the caliber and number of perfused arterioles so that pulmonary artery pressure increases very little. The blood supply to one lung may be blocked and the entire cardiac output shunted to the contralateral side, with little or no rise in pulmonary artery pressure.

Anesthesia and anesthetic procedures such as controlled respiration may affect the cardiac output. Most anesthetics are direct myocardial depressants, decreasing cardiac output in proportion to anesthetic concentration.[39] Certain agents, notably cyclopropane and ether, as well as hypercarbia, cause increased sympathetic activity which tends to raise blood pressure

and limit decrease in output.[41] There is some evidence that as anesthesia continues past 1 to 2 hours, there is a slow return of output toward normal despite constant anesthetic concentration. One result of myocardial depression is the need for a higher diastolic filling pressure necessary for any given cardiac output. During positive pressure ventilation, the peripheral venous pressure may become quite higher with enlargement of the venous reservoir and translocation of a considerable fraction of the blood volume to these vessels, decreasing venous return, cardiac output, and hence arterial pressure.[40] This may interfer with the mechanisms controlling distribution of blood flow in the lungs, resulting in a greater venous admixture (see below), possibly through direct effects of altered carbon dioxide tensions as well as through hemodynamic mechanisms.

VENOUS ADMIXTURE OF SHUNTING

In most mammalian species, the pulmonary artery divides dicotomously 12 to 16 times before giving rise to the arterioles that feed the capillaries of a single respiratory unit. There are arteriovenous paths, actual or potential, from the pulmonary artery to the left ventricle which bypass alveolar capillaries. This venous blood entering the left ventricle represents wasted perfusion (right to left shunt). Furthermore, the left ventricle receives venous blood flow from Thebesian, pleural, and bronchial veins which is mixed with the arterialized blood from pulmonary veins, as well as venous blood passing through unventilated (atelectatic) alveoli. Assuming that these sources of venous blood have the same oxygen content as venous blood from the rest of the body, the wasted fraction of circulation may be calculated as the ratio of shunt to total cardiac output:

$$\frac{\dot{Q}_s}{\dot{Q}_T} = \frac{C_{c'} - C_a}{C_{c'} - C_v} \tag{6}$$

This equation says that the ratio of shunt to total pulmonary circulation is equal to the difference between the content of oxygen at the end of capillary blood ($C_{c'}$) and the oxygen content of arterial blood, divided by the difference in oxygen content of blood at the end of the pulmonary capillaries and the mixed venous blood content. This is directly analogous to the dead space (ventilation shunt) equation above, except that it is necessary to use content rather than tensions of blood, since the oxygen content and tension do not bear a linear relation to each other. (The actual relation is the well known hemoglobin dissociation curve.) Only in the special case of hyperbaric oxygenation, when mixed venous blood becomes 100% saturated with oxygen, can tension be used in the shunt equation. Normal values for the oxygen content of pulmonary end capillary blood, arterial blood, and mixed venous blood are 20.0, 19.9, and 15.0 vol %.

While shunts can be calculated from CO_2 data (and dead space from oxygen data) the choice of test gas is dictated by limits of accuracy. An example will show that shunt is more clearly shown by O_2 measurements than is dead space. If 10% of the alveoli are ventilated with air but not perfused (as might be the case during intermittent positive pressure ventilation), their oxygen tension will rise from approximately 100 to nearly 150 and increase the end tidal oxygen tension. This tension, however, if present in all alveoli, would have increased arterial content about 0.1 vol %. When such oxygen measurements are used in the blood shunt equation, these alveoli (which are in fact alveolar dead space) would appear as an increased shunt of only 2%. (When measurements of carbon dioxide are made, the same alveoli cause a calculated 10% increase in V_D/V_T; see above.)

On the other hand, if 10% of the pulmonary blood bypasses the alveoli as a true shunt, the arterial blood oxygen content is now composed of 9 parts of 20 vol % and 1 part of 15 vol %, giving an average of 19.5 vol %, and a calculated shunt of 20 minus 19.5, divided by 5, or 10%. Oxygen, then, is clearly sensitive to shunting changes and insensitive to dead space changes and

is chosen as the gas to measure when dealing with shunts.

Atelectasis as a form of anatomical shunt is usually distinguished from Thebesian and pleural vein shunting because it is (in theory, at least) a correctable lesion. There is a natural tendency for atelectasis to develop during rapid, shallow, monotonous respiration; a tendency normally corrected in the intact animal by sighs, size, phonation, and hyperpnea of exercise. During general anesthesia, the anesthetist must assume the responsibility for preventing or correcting atelectasis.[5] (See above "Maintenance of Structural Integrity of the Lung.")

DISTRIBUTION OF BLOOD

Just as differences in resistance to gas flow and in distensibility (compliance) of the lung give rise to distributions of ventilation within the lung, so do differences in resistance to blood flow and in alveolar vascular capacity give rise to uneven distributions of blood flow within the lung. There is a hydrostatic gradient of pressure within the pulmonary vascular system which tends to keep arterioles and veins in the dependent portion of the lung widely dilated and to permit collapse of blood vessels in the superior portion of the lung. The hydrostatic factor alone gives rise to significant distributional problems in dog and larger animals, but is a factor of little significance in very small animals. When perfusion to a portion of the lung is disproportional to the ventilation of that portion, abnormality of gas exchange results (see below).

NORMAL CONTROL OF $\dot{V}/\dot{Q}$ MATCHING

If the inspired gas is 50% oxygen or greater, the alveolar oxygen tension will be sufficient to nearly completely saturate blood perfusing areas of low ventilation, and only anatomical shunts interfere with oxygenation of blood. However, if inspired oxygen tension is lower, between 15 and 30%, an additional mechanism exists which mimics the effect of shunting. It is due to mismatch of ventilation and perfusion, especially in areas which have large perfusion with respect to ventilation. The alveolar oxygen tension will be lowered below that necessary to fully saturate hemoglobin, and the arterial oxygen content leaving such areas will be intermediate between mixed venous and arterialized blood from well ventilated areas. This difference in oxygen content will not be a linear function of the ventilation because the hemoglobin dissociation curve is not a straight line. Thus, the arterial oxygen content, a mixture of well oxygenated and less well oxygenated blood, will fall below that which results by the exposure of blood to an average alveolar tension. This is interpreted in the shunt equation as an increase in right to left shunt. The increase in apparent or "physiological shunting" with decreased inspired oxygen tension is magnified by abnormalities in ventilation distribution induced during anesthesia[24] and is a strong argument for the use of relatively high inspired oxygen tensions during general anesthesia. It is most marked in elderly animals and species prone to chronic obstructive pulmonary disease such as guinea pig, man, and horse.

Considering the differences in geometry of the various lung portions, it is quite remarkable that more abnormalities in distribution of ventilation and perfusion do not exist. In general, in the awake intact animal the ventilation and perfusion to various portions of the lung are quite well matched. This implies a control mechanism. The matching of ventilation and perfusion is not appreciably disturbed by complete denervation of the lung, so humoral or local rather than nervous factors are generally postulated.

Pulmonary artery and terminal bronchioles travel side by side for some distance before breaking up into alveolar ducts and capillary network meshes. The distances between branches of pulmonary arteries and the accompanying bronchioles are short enough so that some gas exchange of oxygen and carbon dioxide occurs across their walls. Thus, the oxygen and carbon dioxide content of venous blood affects the gas tensions around the smooth muscle of bronchioles by diffusion.[29] Conversely, the bronchiolar oxygen and carbon dioxide content exerts some influence on the gas tension at the smooth muscle of pulmonary artery segments, again by the process of physical diffusion. Carbon dioxide tensions in the two structures are even more likely to influence the environment of smooth muscle within these structures by diffusion, since carbon dioxide diffuses 20 times more readily than oxygen. Thus, an abnormality in the oxygen or carbon dioxide content in either the pulmonary or the bronchioles would be expected to affect the smooth muscle of the other conducting passage. Experiments have shown that the responses to abnormalities of carbon dioxide and oxygen are such that they tend to minimize nonuniformity. Thus, an area of hypoxia in one portion of the lung causes pulmonary artery constriction locally, directing blood flow to other areas.[8, 31, 38, 42] Hypocarbia of pulmonary arterial blood tends to cause bronchoconstriction, diverting gas flow to other areas.[46, 50]

MAGNITUDE OF $\dot{V}/\dot{Q}$ MISMATCH

No single assessment of the extent of $\dot{V}/\dot{Q}$ abnormality is possible since the same disability arises from a small volume of severely mismatched $\dot{V}/\dot{Q}$ or from a larger volume of less abnormal matching. An approximation of the degree of abnormality is derived from assuming the two limiting cases. These extremes are complete perfusion in the absence of ventilation on the one hand, and ventilation in the complete absence of perfusion on the other. Any $\dot{V}/\dot{Q}$ abnormality may be mimicked by a shunt of gas from the inspired to the expired limb of a breathing circle in the case of ventilation and/or by a right to left cardiac shunt in the case of perfusion. When all abnormalities of gas exchange are considered schematically as due to shunting of blood and/or gas, the results are expressed as an increase in physiological dead space and an increase in physiological shunt. Since the difference in carbon dioxide tension between inspired gas and arterial blood is large compared to the difference in tension between arterial blood and mixed venous blood, changes in the amount of blood bypassing the lung (shunted) have little effect on the physiological dead space as computed by carbon dioxide measurements. Conversely, the difference between mixed venous oxygen tension and alveolar oxygen tension is large compared to the difference between inspired oxygen tension and expired oxygen tension, so that changes in the amount of parallel or alveolar dead space (that portion of physiological dead space excluding the anatomical dead space) have little effect on the physiological shunt computed by oxygen measurements.

ANESTHETIC EFFECTS ON BLOOD FLOW AND MATCHING

General anesthesia appears to have three undesirable, disadvantageous effects on the matching of ventilation and perfusion. These effects are not solely due to pharmacological action of general anesthetics themselves, but are related to ventilation and circulation.

a. If the animal is artificially hyperventilated, becoming alkalotic, the pulmonary vasomotor response to hypoxia is abolished.[30]

b. If mean alveolar pressure is raised, by artificial respiration, above the average pressure of the atrium, the pulmonary capillaries act like Starling resistors, impeding the blood flow and hence the cardiac output.[52]

c. Through decrease of myocardial contractile force and reduction of venous return, general anesthesia and mechanical ventilation may decrease pulmonary artery pressure and thus limit the efficacy of change in pulmonary artery resistance in redistributing pulmonary blood flow. On the other hand, pulmonary artery pressure and vascular resistance may both increase during anesthesia. The resulting distribution depends on the pattern of vasoconstriction and transcapillary pressure.[17]

Central Control of Respiration

Ventilation is semiautomatic, in that no apparent conscious control is necessary to maintain the tensions of oxygen and carbon dioxide in arterial blood within relatively narrow limits over a wide range of metabolic rates. This control may be voluntarily interrupted for such activities as phonation or deglutition, or the pattern may be changed for temperature regulation as in the panting dog. In higher vertebrates, carbon dioxide is primarily regulated.[16] Sensors within the brain respond both to tension of carbon dioxide and to the pH changes produced by hydration of carbon dioxide (forming carbonic acid) such that an increase in carbon dioxide in arterial blood is assiciated with more vigorous respiratory movement. With sensors in the carotid body, in bronchi, in lung parenchyma, in muscles, and elsewhere, there are additional integrated reflexes within the central nervous system modulating this fundamental control. With the state of exercise, ventilation increases slightly before the increased load of metabolic carbon dioxide reaches the lung for excretion, presumably via a neural mechanism. The pattern, as well as volume, of respiration is also regulated by reflex by stretch receptors and deflation receptors within the lung (Hering-Breuer reflex), although the relative magnitude of these reflexes varies considerably from animal to animal. The rat and rabbit show rather marked reflexes of this nature, cat and dog show intermediate reflexes, and man and monkey show little or no reflex regulation.

CENTRAL CONTROL OF CARBON DIOXIDE TENSION

The effect of carbon dioxide on ventilation is usually studied by means of the carbon dioxide response curve. Ventilation and alveolar or arterial carbon dioxide are measured simultaneously. Alveolar carbon dioxide is then increased by either rebreathing in a large system without carbon dioxide absorption or by adding carbon dioxide to the inspired gas. The in-

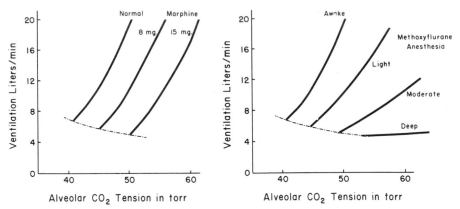

FIG. 14.8. The ventilatory response to carbon dioxide as affected by two different types of respiratory depressants. In the panel on the left, the ventilatory response to carbon dioxide is seen to be a parallel shift of the line to the right; a respiratory stimulant would move the curve to the left, retaining the same slope. With loss of consciousness, such as produced by general anesthesia (methoxyflurane anesthesia is typical), the curve changes slope with a near linear relation between the decrease in slope and the anesthetic depth. In both instances, the curves start at the resting point which is the intersection of the CO_2 excretion hyperbola of Figure 14.6 and the respiratory response indicated on this figure. Since these hyperbolas are quite flat in the range of carbon dioxide tension considered normal, respiratory depression causes a more apparent change in carbon dioxide tension than it does in absolute ventilation.

creased carbon dioxide tension of arterial blood then causes an increase in ventilation. A plot is made of the ventilation as a function of alveolar or arterial P_{CO_2} (Fig. 14.8). These plots are characterstically linear after the first 4 or 5 Torr of increased P_{CO_2} with a slope between 1 and 2 liters/minute/Torr. Two forms of depressed respiration can be identified in such a response. The more common, as produced by narcotics, is evidenced by a curve similar in shape to the control, but shifted to the right so that any given ventilation results from a higher carbon dioxide.[48] A second form of depression of ventilation, produced by general anesthesia, consists of a progressive decrease in the slope of the plot as depth of anesthesia is increased.[19] Of the two forms of depression, the latter is more dangerous because the control mechanism is less effective in maintaining a given P_{CO_2}. A large dose of morphine, for example, may depress the central nervous system and result in an elevated resting carbon dioxide tension of 50 Torr. If, in addition to this depression, there is increased carbon dioxide production from hypermetabolism, or mechanical interference with respiration tending to increase the P_{CO_2}, the brain will respond with increased ventilatory effort, since the slope of the carbon dioxide response is still approximately normal. During deep anesthesia, however, the flatness of the response indicates that an increase in P_{CO_2} evokes little compensatory effort.

HYPOXIC STIMULUS TO RESPIRATION

In addition to the carbon dioxide regulation mechanism, there are chemoreceptors in the carotid and aortic bodies responsive to lack of oxygen. This reflex mechanism is responsible for little of the basic regulatory processes in higher vertebrates breathing room air, but may reflect a considerable portion of the regulatory control in animals exposed to 10 to 12% oxygen, or at higher altitudes.[2, 55] The ventilatory response to hypoxia is less impaired by general anesthesia than the carbon dioxide response and is thought to represent a phylogenetically older control mechanism.

RESPIRATORY CONTROL DURING ANESTHESIA

During general anesthesia, the carbon dioxide response may become nearly a flat line, indicating that the control of respiration is largely by mechanisms other than carbon dioxide stimulation. In this case, interference with respiration such as that produced by large packs or retractors in the abdomen or an abnormal body position will cause an increase in carbon dioxide but no compensatory increase in ventilation. If P_{CO_2} is allowed to increase high enough, above 90 to 100 Torr, there is actually a direct depressant effect of carbon dioxide on the central nervous system. This additional depression can lead to cardiovascular failure and death. Note that the axes for plotting the carbon dioxide response curve are the same as those used for plotting carbon dioxide excretion in Figure 14.6. In the spontaneously breathing animal, carbon dioxide response curves and carbon dioxide excretion curves can be plotted simultaneously as in Figure 14.9 (assuming V_D/V_T remains constant as V_E increases). The intersection of

the two graphs describes the point of P_{CO_2} and ventilation for steady state conditions in a given animal (point A). When the animal is given a respiratory depressant for premedication, the response curve moves to the right and the animal reaches a new steady state (point B), with a slightly decreased ventilation and a slightly increased P_{aCO_2}. When the animal is anesthetized, two events occur: (a) the metabolic production of carbon dioxide is reduced by 10 to 15% as indicated by the dotted hyperbola; and (b) the carbon dioxide response curve is flattened. The insersection of these two curves (point C) describes the steady state condition for a spontaneously breathing, anesthetized animal, with this metabolic production of carbon dioxide and ventilatory responsiveness to carbon dioxide. If ventilation is augmented by assisted or controlled respiration, a new point (D) will be reached, with a lower P_{aCO_2} as a result of the higher ventilation.

When the control of respiration is assumed by the anesthetist, he can alter the alveolar ventilation at will and thus directly alter the P_{aCO_2} of arterial blood, as discussed in the section on ventilation.

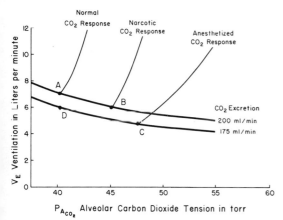

FIG. 14.9. The ventilation-carbon dioxide diagram for premedication with a narcotic followed by general anesthesia. Point A represents the normal ventilation and carbon dioxide tension of man, and point B represents the results of premedication. Since premedicants have little effect on the metabolic rate, both point A and point B lie on the same CO_2 excretion hyperbola. With induction of general anesthesia, the metabolic rate is decreased by 10 to 15%, and the respiratory center responsiveness to carbon dioxide is depressed, resulting in carbon dioxide tension increased to 47 and a decrease of ventilation indicated at point C. If respiration is augmented artificly by increasing the ventilation to 5 liters/minute, the CO_2 tension will fall toward and eventually reach point D

REFERENCES

1. Alexander, S. C., Cohen, P. J., Wollman, H., Smith, T. C., Reivich, M., and Van der Molen, R. A.: Cerebral carbohydrate metabolism during hypocarbia in man: studies during nitrous oxide anesthesia. Anesthesiology, 26: 624, 1965.
2. Arborelius, M., Jr.: Influence of moderate hypoxia in one lung on the distribution of pulmonary circulation and ventilation. Scand. J. Clin. Lab. Invest. 17: 257, 1965.
3. Askrog, V. F., Pender, J. W., Smith, T. C., and Eckenhoff, J. E.: Changes in respiratory dead space during halothane, cyclopropane, and nitrous oxide anesthesia. Anesthesiology, 12: 342, 1964.
4. Bartlett, R. G., Jr., Brubrach, H. F., and Stecht, H.: Demonstration of aventilatory mass flow during ventilation and apnea in man. J. Appl. Physiol. 14: 97, 1959.
5. Bendixen, H. H., Bullwinkle, B., Hedley-Whyte, J., and Laver, M. B.: Atelectasis and shunting during spontaneous ventilation in anesthetized patients. Anesthesiology 25: 297, 1964.
6. Bergman, N. A.: Components of the alveolar-arterial oxygen tension difference in anesthetized man. Anesthesiology 28: 517, 1967.

7. Bergofsky, E. H.: Relative contributions of the ribcage and diaphragm to ventilation in man. J. Appl. Physiol. *19:* 698, 1964.

8. Bernards, J. A., Dejours, P., and Lacaisse, A.: Ventilatory effects in man of breathing successively CO_2 free, CO_2 enriched, and CO_2 free gas mixtures with low, normal, or high oxygen concentration. Resp. Physiol. *1:* 390, 1966.

9. Bohr, C., Hathaba, K. A., and Krogh, A.: Euber, einen in biologischer Beziehung wichtigen Einfluss, den die Kohlensaurespannung des Blunts auf bessen Sauerstoffbindung ubt. Scand. Arch. Physiol. *16:* 402, 1904.

10. Brody, A. W., Stroughton, R. R. Connolly, T. L., Shehan, J. J., Navin, J. J., and Kobald, E. E.: Experimental value of the Reynolds critical flow in the human airway. J. Lab. Clin. Med. *67:* 43, 1966.

11. Campbell, G. S., Houle, D. B., Crisp, N. W., Weil, M. H., and Brown, E. B.: Depressed response to intravenous sympathomimetic agents in humans during acidosis. Dis. Chest *33:* 18, 1958.

12. Cavagna, C. A., Stemmler, E. J., and DuBois, A. B.: Alveolar resistance to atelectasis. J. Appl. Physiol. *22:* 441, 1967.

13. Clements, J. A.: Surface tension in the lung. Sci. Amer., *207:* 120, 1962.

14. Cohen, P. J., Wollman, H., Alexander, S. C., Chase, P. E., and Behar, M. G.: Cerebral carbohydrate metabolism in man during halothane anesthesia: effects of $PaCO_2$ on some aspects of carbohydrate utilization. Anesthesiology *25:* 185, 1964.

15. Colgan, F. J.: Relationship of changing bronchial caliber to respiration in the dog. J. Appl. Physiol. *19:* 803, 1964.

16. Comroe, J. H., Jr.: The Baxter lecture. Central and reflex control of breathing. Anesth. Analg. (Cleveland) *46:* 367, 1967.

17. Cooperman, L., Warden, J., Morris, J., Smith, T. C., and Price, H. L.: Pulmonary hemodynamics during general anesthesia in man. Anesthesiology *30:*629, 1969.

18. Dickson, W. R.: The right heart and the lung with some observations on teleology. Amer. Rev. Resp. Dis. *94:* 691, 1966.

19. Dunbar, B., Ovassapian, A., and Smith, T. C.: The effects of methoxyflurane on ventilation in man. Anesthesiology *28:* 1020, 1967.

20. Eger, E. I., and Severinghaus, J. W.: The rate of rise of PaCO in the apneic anesthetized patient. Anesthesiology *22:* 419, 1961.

21. Egbert, L. D., Laver, M., and Bendixen, H. H.: Intermittent deep breaths and compliance during anesthesia in man. Anesthesiology *24:*57, 1963.

22. Emil, B.: *Clinical Hypothermia.* Chap. 2, pp. 8–108. McGraw-Hill Book Company, New York, 1964.

23. Engstrom, C. G., Hertzark, P., and Norlander, P.: A method for the continuous measurement of oxygen consumption in the presence of soluble gases during controlled ventilation. Acta Anaesth. Scand. *5:* 115, 1961.

24. Finley, T. N., Lenfant, C., Haab, P., Piiper, J., and Rahn, H.: Venous admixture in pulmonary circulation in anesthetized dogs. J. Appl. Physiol. *15:* 418, 1960.

25. Gilfoil, T. M., Youmans, W. B., and Turner, J. K.: Abdominal compression reaction: causes and characteristics. Amer. J. Physiol. *196:* 1160, 1959.

26. Greene, N. M.: *Inhalation Anesthetics and Carbohydrate Metabolism.* The Williams & Wilkins Company, Baltimore, 1963.

27. Hedley-Whyte, W. J., Laver, M. B., and Bendixen, H. H.: Effect of changes in tidal ventilation on physiologic shunting. Amer. J. Physiol. *206:* 891, 1964.

28. Hunt, K. H.: Resistance in respiratory valves and canisters. Anesthesiology *16:* 190, 1955.

29. Jameson, A. E.: Diffusion of gases from alveolus to pre-capillary arteries. Science *139:* 826, 1963.

30. Lloyd, T. C.: Influence of blood pH on hypoxia and pulmonary vasoconstriction. J. Appl. Physiol. *21:* 358, 1966.

31. Lopez-Majano, V., Wagner, H. N., Jr., Twining, R. H., Tow, D. E., and Chernick, V.: Effect of regional hypoxia on the distribution of pulmonary blood flow in man. Circ. Res. *18:* 550, 1966.

32. Mead, J., and Collier, C.: Relation of volume history of lungs to respiratory mechanics in anesthetized dogs. J. Appl. Physiol. *14:* 669, 1959.

33. Nakamura, R., Takashima, T., Sagy, Y., Sasaki, T., and Okubo, T.: A new method of analyzing the distribution of mechanical time constants in the lung. J. Appl. Physiol. *21:* 265, 1966.

34. Ngai, S. H., and Papper, E. M.: *Metabolic Effects of Anesthesia.* Charles C Thomas, Publisher, Springfield, Ill., 1961.

35. Nimbs, R. G., Connor, E. H., and Comroe, J. H., Jr.: The compliance of the human thorax in anesthetized patients. J. Clin. Invest. *34:* 744, 1955.

36. Nisell, O. I., and DuBois, A. B.: Relationship between compliance and FRC of the lungs in cats, and measurement of resistance in breathing. Amer. J. Physiol. *178:* 206, 1954.

37. Nunn, J. F., and Matthews, R. V.: Gaseous exchange during halothane anesthesia: the study of respiratory state. Brit. J. Anaesth. *31:* 330, 1959.

38. Paul, G., Barnauskas, E., and Forsberg, S. A.: Effects of carbon dioxide breathing upon the the circulation of patients with mitral valve disease. Clin. Sci. *26:* 110, 1964.

39. Price, H. L., and Cohen, P. J. (editors): *Effects of Anesthetics on the Circulation.* Charles C Thomas, Publisher, Springfield, Ill., 1964.

40. Price, H. L., Connor, E. H., and Dripps, R. D.:

Some respiratory and circulatory effects of mechanical respirators. J. Appl. Physiol. *6:* 517, 1954.

41. Price, H. L., Linde, H. W., Jones, R. E., Black, G. W., and Price, M. L.: Sympatho-adrenal responses to general anesthesia in man and their relation to hemodynamics. Anesthesiology *20:* 563, 1959.

42. Reeves, J. T., and Leathers, J. E.: Hypoxic pulmonary hypertension of the calf with denervation of the lungs. J. Appl. Physiol. *19:* 976, 1964.

43. Reynolds, R. C., and Haugaard, N.: The effect of variations of pH upon the activation of phosphorylase by epinephrine in perfused contracting heart, liver slices, and skeletal muscle. J. Pharmacol. Exp. Ther. *156:* 417, 1967.

44. Roughton, F. J. W., and Foster, R. E. Relative importance of diffusion and chemical reaction rate in determining the rate of exchange of gases in the human lung with special reference to true diffusing capacity of pulmonary membrane and volume of blood in lung capillaries. J. Appl. Physiol. *11:* 290, 1957.

45. Severinghaus, J. W., and Stupful, M.: Alveolar dead space as an index of distribution of blood flow in pulmonary capillaries. J. Appl. Physiol. *10:* 335, 1957.

46. Severinghaus, J. W., Swenson, E. W., Finley, T. N., Lattagola, M. T., and Williams, J.: Unilateral hypoventilation produced in dogs by occluding one pulmonary artery. J. Appl. Physiol. *16:* 53, 1961.

47. Smith, T. C., and DuBois, A. B.: Effects of scopolamine on the bronchi of man. Anesthesiology 30: 12, 1969.

48. Smith, T. C., Stephen, G. W., Zeiger, L., and Wollman, H.: Effects of premedicant drugs on respiration and gas exchange in man. Anesthesiology *28:* 883, 1967.

49. Staub, N. C.: Interdependence of pulmonary structure and function. Anesthesiology *24:* 831, 1963.

50. Swenson, E. W., Finley, T. N., and Guzman, S. D.: Unilateral hypoventilation in man during temporary occlusion of one pulmonary artery. J. Clin. Invest. *41:* 828, 1962.

51. Theye, R. A., and Tuohy, G. E.: Considerations in the determinations of oxygen uptake and ventilatory performance during methoxyflurane anesthesia in man. Anesth. Analg. (Cleveland) *43:* 306, 1964.

52. West, J. B., Dollary, C. P., and Naimarka, N.: Distribution of blood flow in isolated lung: relation to vascular and alveolar pressures. J. Appl. Physiol. *19:* 713, 1964.

53. Whitteridge, D., and Bülbring, E.: Changes in activity of pulmonary receptors in anesthesia and their influence on respiratory behavior. J. Pharm. *89:* 340, 1944.

54. Wu, N., Miller, W. F., and Luhn, N. R.: Studies of breathing in anesthesia. Anesthesiology *17:* 696, 1956.

55. Winterstein, H.: Chemical control of pulmonary ventilation. I. The physiology of the chemoreceptors. II. Hypoxia and respiratory climitization. III. The reaction theory of respiratory control. New Eng. J. Med. *255:* 216, 272, and 331, 1956.

15
Depth of General Anesthesia

LAWRENCE R. SOMA

Observation of the reaction of the patient to increasing concentrations of an anesthetic agent has been regarded as fundamental for the safe administration of general anesthetics, since safe use involves recognition of various changes before respiratory or cardiac arrest occurs.[7] There is a somewhat predictable sequence of events from the early stages of anesthesia to the stage of complete medullary paralysis. Unfortunately, the sequence will vary somewhat from patient to patient, and not all signs of the depth of anesthesia noted in one will be observed in another. Signs of anesthesia will also be modified by preanesthetic medication, different agents used for the induction of anesthesia, the condition of the patient, and various anesthetic agents. In veterinary anesthesia, variations also occur among species. For example, the signs of diethyl ether anesthesia in the dog and horse may have similar stages but not identical patterns. There are also variations among anesthetic agents; all the changes in the sequence described for diethyl ether anesthesia are not easily recognized during halothane anesthesia. The more rapid the induction of anesthesia, the less obvious is the transition from one plane of anesthesia to another.

The determination of anesthetic depth is important for a number of reasons.[7] (a) The beginner must have some established guidelines to follow in order to develop criteria for safe anesthesia. (b) Patient safety is greater if the depth of anesthesia can be determined with some accuracy. (c) Many reflexes and relaxations of certain muscle groups occur at various levels of anesthesia, and the knowledge of the cessation of function of these protective reflexes is important in anesthetic management. (d) Guidelines in assessing the depth of anesthesia are essential in comparing observations.

The stages of ether anesthesia as described by Guedel and extended by Gillespie are the standard to which all other anesthetics are compared.[11, 12] These signs are based on observation of the patient, changes in the pulse and blood pressure, eye patterns and reflexes, respiratory pattern, chest and abdominal muscles, warmth of the skin, capillary refill, and color. The electroencephalogram has also been used to determine the depth of anesthesia, but this necessitates special skills and equipment. It is a useful tool if used constantly and if the observer becomes expert in its interpretation. The concentration of anesthetic in the arterial blood or the concentration in the inhaled or exhaled gases can be used as a guide to the depth of anesthesia, but this involves laboratory measurements and is not available instantaneously. Monitors have been developed for the measurement of the inhaled or exhaled concentration of an anesthetic agent.

Effects of General Anesthetics

The effects of general anesthetics range from producing a stage of amnesia and analgesia to death. With most of the general anesthetics, a progressive depression of the sensorium and normal physiological mechanisms can be produced by gradually increasing arterial concentrations. Barbiturates, for example, can produce sedation at low doses and deep depression at higher doses. This is also true for the inhalation anesthetics which can be used for analgesia in man at lower inhaled concentrations. Table 15.1 outlines some of the sequential effects of increased arterial concentrations of a general anesthetic. Included are the four basic elements of "the state of anesthesia" as presently accepted: (a) sensory block (afferent input); (b) motor block (afferent output); (c) reduction of reflex activity; and (d) sleep.[23]

Sensory block includes the reduction of the awareness of stimuli arising from the surgical field, and varying degrees of sensory block can be created. Narcotics produce a reduction in the intensity of pain, but do not completely eliminate the awareness of pain. Under light levels of general anesthesia (plane 1) surgical stimulation can produce autonomic response to stimulation with an increase in heart rate and blood pressure, and occasionally slight movement with no conscious expression or remembrance of pain. Deeper planes of anesthesia eliminate both the autonomic and overt response to surgical stimulation. Alterations of the electroencephalogram occur with surgical stimulation. A complete sensory block can be produced by application of a local anesthetic to an afferent nerve.

A motor block which is centrally mediated is created by a state of sleep, unconsciousness, or light levels of anesthesia. Relaxation becomes more profound as anesthesia is deepened, and the peripheral direct motor end plate effects of anesthetics become apparent.[6] In the deep planes of ether anesthesia, an almost flaccid state can be obtained. Complete muscle relaxation is produced by the use of muscle relaxants such as curare and succinylcholine chloride, or regional block is produced by a local anesthetic in the epidural space. Muscle relaxants create a state of apparent anesthesia. It is difficult to judge the depth when relaxants are used in conjunction with general anesthetics, and care must be taken to provide adequate sedation and analgesia. Fortunately, the autonomic nervous system is capable of responding, and such changes as a rise in blood pressure, heart rate, pupillary dilation, salivation, and sweating are subtle indications of pain.[7, 20]

The reduction of reflex activity includes both undesirable and desirable reflexes. Vomiting, laryngospasms, bronchospasms, and salivation are examples of undesirable reflex responses which are eventually blocked by deeper levels of anesthesia. Some reflexes and responses to stimuli are exaggerated during stage 2 anesthesia, increasing the danger of the induction period of anesthesia. The cardiovascular vasomotor reflexes are gradually depressed by increasing depth of anesthesia, thus diminishing the capability to adjust to changes in blood volume, position, and changes in cardiovascular function.

Unconsciousness or sleep is the last criteria of the state of anesthesia; light sleep from which an animal can be easily roused can be produced by tranquilizers, narcotics, and sedative doses of barbiturates. Unarousable sleep is produced by

TABLE 15.1

Effects of general anesthetics

1. Analgesia and amnesia
2. Loss of consciousness and motor coordination
3. Reduction of protective reflexes
4. Blockage of afferent stimuli
5. Muscular relaxation
6. Respiratory and cardiovascular depression
7. Depression of cardiovascular and respiratory reflexes
8. Apnea
9. Cardiac standstill

anesthetic agents. Most of the drugs capable of creating a state of deep sleep will also produce delirium as the patient emerges from or is placed into this state.[23]

The four criteria described can be obtained by the administration of complete anesthetics such as ether, halothane, and methoxyflurane, but can also be produced by a combination of weaker agents. A combination of a narcotic, a thiobarbiturate, nitrous oxide, and a muscle relaxant can produce analgesia, unconsciousness, depressions of reflex activity, and muscle relaxation, without deep planes of an anesthesia.

Stages and Signs of Anesthesia

The stages of anesthesia have been categorized into four specific areas, but the transition from one stage to another is not as clear as the specific stages imply. The stages of anesthesia are more clearly observed with agents that provide gradual increase in the blood concentration, and ether is used for the classic description of the stages and planes of anesthesia. Stage 1 is the subjective stage and stage 2 is the delirium stage. Stage 3 is the "working stage" of anesthesia, within which the anesthetist endeavors to maintain the patient. Because of the importance of stage 3 and because it also has observable levels, it is subdivided into four planes. Here again, and even more so than the defined stages, the transition from one to another is not clear-cut and can be altered by the modifying aspects of previous drugs, condition of the patient, degree of surgical stimulation, and the rapidity in which the arterial concentration increases. The signs of anesthesia during recovery are not necessarily the mirror image of the induction phage, and transition from a deeper plane to a lighter plane may be more rapid.

STAGE 1

Stage 1 of anesthesia is basically subjective in nature and can only be related to man. It has been called the stage of analgesia and consciousness with disorientation.[6, 17] Its boundaries are from the beginning of anesthesia to the loss of consciousness. Although man can respond to verbal commands, he is amnesic. Sensation of pain is not absent and the threshold to pain is not altered, but they will tolerate minor surgical procedures. The subjective signs are warmth, a feeling of suffocation and a dulling of sensations. The body may feel stiff or buoyant with a sense of numbness. All senses and coordinated responses are reduced. Hallucinations and verbalization may ensue. The objective signs are few and are limited to slight increase in respiration and pulse rate; the pupil size is normal (unless modified by atropine or a narcotic) and has a normal reactivity to light.

STAGE 2

In stage 2 there is a loss of consciousness and subsequent excitement (Figs. 15.1 and 15.2). This is the stage of delirium and uninhibited action. The release of control by higher centers will result in uncoordinated movements, struggling, crying, and exaggerated response to painful stimuli and spinal reflexes. This is a most dangerous period because of the hyper-reactivity of the system. The pupils are dilated, but the iris will respond to light. Aternate contractions of the oculomotor muscles will produce a slow rhythmic oscillation of the eyeballs. This seems to vary with the species, being minimal in the dog and well defined in the horse. Laryngeal reflexes are still present, and the oropharyngeal activity is present with chewing and swallowing. Chewing and swallowing is most noticeable in the ruminants, and may even persist into stage 3. Vomiting can occur in the dog and cat especially if the stomach contains food or air. Vomiting during the slow induction of anesthesia can occur in the brachycephalic breeds, despite a 12-hour fast. This may be due to a greater degree of areophagia in these dogs.

Respirations are irregular and breath holding can occur. The transition from stage 1 to stage 2 may be indistinguishable in animals because of the struggling created by the anesthetic mask. The gross manifestation of the excitement pe-

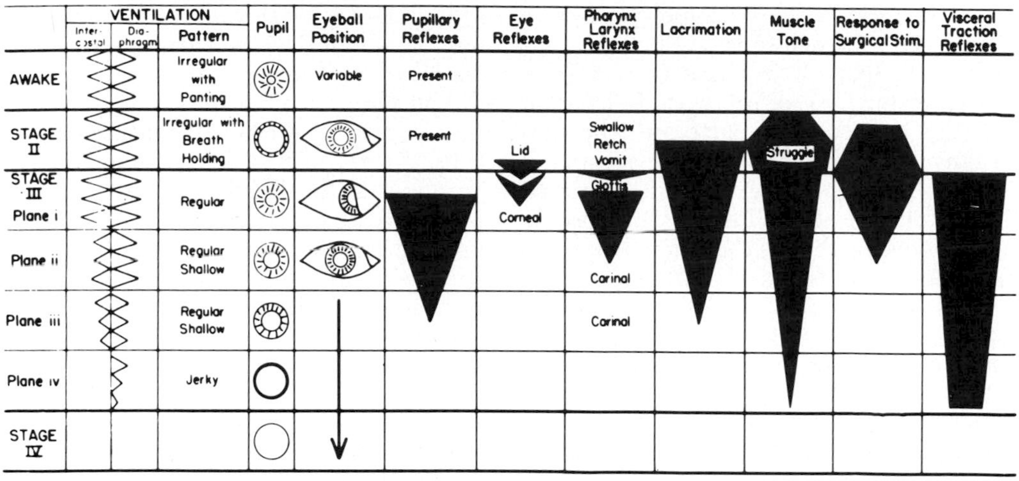

	VENTILATION			Pupil	Eyeball Position	Pupillary Reflexes	Eye Reflexes	Pharynx Larynx Reflexes	Lacrimation	Muscle Tone	Response to Surgical Stim.	Visceral Traction Reflexes
	Inter-costal	Dia-phragm	Pattern									
AWAKE			Irregular with Panting		Variable	Present						
STAGE II			Irregular with Breath Holding			Present	Lid	Swallow Retch Vomit			Struggle	
STAGE III Plane i			Regular				Corneal	Glottis				
Plane ii			Regular Shallow					Carinal				
Plane iii			Regular Shallow					Carinal				
Plane iv			Jerky									
STAGE IV												

FIG. 15.1. The signs and reflex changes of the stages and planes of diethyl ether. These signs are also applicable to methoxyflurane anesthesia. (Modified after Gillespie.[11])

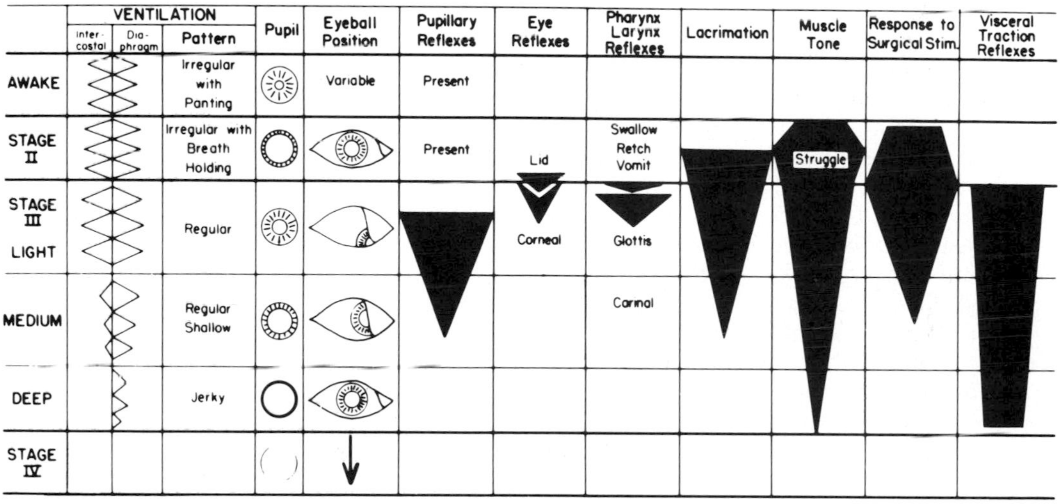

	VENTILATION			Pupil	Eyeball Position	Pupillary Reflexes	Eye Reflexes	Pharynx Larynx Reflexes	Lacrimation	Muscle Tone	Response to Surgical Stim.	Visceral Traction Reflexes
	Inter-costal	Dia-phragm	Pattern									
AWAKE			Irregular with Panting		Variable	Present						
STAGE II			Irregular with Breath Holding			Present	Lid	Swallow Retch Vomit			Struggle	
STAGE III LIGHT			Regular				Corneal	Glottis				
MEDIUM			Regular Shallow					Carinal				
DEEP			Jerky									
STAGE IV												

FIG. 15.2. The signs and reflex changes of the stages and levels of halothane anesthesia. (Modified after Thomas et al.[22])

riod (stage 2) will vary among species. It is more marked in the dog with phonation and struggling, but a lesser degree of excitement is noted in the cat. The induction of anesthesia with an inhalation agent in the horse is comparatively easy, of short duration, and is not accompanied by a great deal of struggling.

The passage through stage 2 is aided by the use of agents with a low partition coefficient or the induction of anesthesia with thiobarbiturates. Inhalation agents can be used more successfully for the induction of anesthesia if the patient is adequately premedicated; under these circumstances the response to the mask placement is minimal and the induction of anesthesia and passage into stage 3 is quickened. The transition period into stage 3 is cessation of struggling, the onset of regular respirations, and constriction of dilated pupils.

STAGE 3

Stage 3 is divided into four planes and is characterized by a progressive depression of respiration, circulation, protective reflexes, and muscle tone.

Plane 1. Plane 1 is characterized by a regular respiratory effort with full use of both the intercostal muscle and the diaphragm; full expansion of the chest and descent of the diaphragm should be noted (Figs. 15.1 and 15.2). Inspiration may be slightly longer than exhalation. The pupils are constricted and still respond to light. The eyeball may oscillate slowly, but usually in the dog and cat they are eccentrically placed at the medial canthus with eversion of the nictitans. Slow oscillations are prominent in the horse at this stage of anesthesia. The lid and palpebral reflexes are still present and in the horse can persist into deeper planes. Pharyngeal and laryngeal reflexes persist, and endotracheal intubation will evoke a response; despite this intubation is still possible in the dog, horse and ruminant. Oral manipulation in the ruminant can evoke a chewing reflex. The cat, as compared to the dog, maintains greater jaw tone in this plane and attempts to place a laryngoscope in the oral cavity can result in spastic closure of the mouth. Salivation persists and can be profuse with ether anesthesia. Muscle tone is still present and painful stimuli can still produce a retraction of limbs and an increase in heart and respiratory rate. Respiratory stridor can occur in the cat in response to surgical stimulation. Tremors of the limbs and an exaggerated extensor reflex may be seen in the cat, but they are transient and will disappear as anesthesia is deepened. Vomiting does not occur unless the animal lightens and passes back into stage 2. Secretion of tears still persists.

Plane 2. The entrance into plane 2 is not easily distinguished with all anesthetic agents. It is defined as the point where the eyeballs become centrally fixed, and this is generally true with ether and methoxyflurane. With halothane, all other signs point to plane 2, but the eyeballs remain eccentrically fixed. Pupil size may not change at this point, especially when narcotics have been used for premedication. Atropine will dilate pupils, also mod-

ifying the response somewhat; in the dog, narcotics will over-ride the mydriasis produced by atropine.

The changes in respiratory pattern are minor except for a general decrease in tidal volume and an increase in rate (Figs. 15.1 and 15.2). Tidal volume changes are primarily due to a reduction in intercostal muscle activity. Here again, variations will occur, the respiratory rate will be increased with diethyl ether, especially in the dog, giving the impression of a continued respiratory drive. With halothane, methoxyflurane, cyclopropane, and barbiturates, respiration is more quiet, and there is an illusion of greater depth of anesthesia. Surgical stimulation usually will produce a respiratory response, especially at the upper portion of this plane. The respiratory drive produced by ether anesthesia is obvious in the dog and minimal in the horse.

Heart rate and blood pressure are well maintained in plane 2, with an increase during ether anesthesia. Halothane, methoxyflurane, and the barbiturates produce a gradual decrease in heart rate and blood pressure. An increase in blood pressure, heart rate, and respiration can occur in response to surgical stimulation in animals under halothane anesthesia.

Oropharyngeal reflexes may not be completely abolished in the cat, and placement of the laryngoscope and intubation may evoke a response. Deep tracheal reflexes still persist and placement of the tube to the carina will evoke a response. Lacrimation and salivation still persist but are diminished, and beginning dryness of the conjunctiva is noted.

Muscle tone lessens, but the degree will vary with species, the anesthetic agent, and from patient to patient. Relaxation of abdominal muscles is easily produced in cats, but deeper planes are necessary in more massive animals.

Plane 3. The respiratory pattern in plane 3 undergoes a noticeable change as intercostal muscle activity decreases further and lags behind diaphragmatic contraction. Obvious intercostal paralysis can be regarded as the beginning of plane 3 and ending with complete paralysis in plane 4. This unequal expansion creates a "rocking boat" type of respiratory movement. Inspirations are shorter, the pause between each is increased, and as a result the depth of ventilation is further reduced. This ventilatory pattern can be detected by observing thoracic and abdominal excursions or by placing the hand on the xyphoid area and palpating the differential expansion. Abdominal muscles are also relaxed.

The eyeball is now centrally fixed with all agents and moderately dilated. Most operative procedures under halothane anesthesia can be performed in the dog and cat with the eyeball eccentrically fixed; its rotation centrally and moderate dilation indicate an unnecessary depth of anesthesia. With methoxyflurane and ether, the eyeballs fix centrally sooner, but at this point with only moderate dilation. Lacrimation, salivation, and oropharyngeal and laryngeal reflexes are abolished, but vagal reflexes due to traction on abdominal or thoracic viscera may persist. The eyes appear dry and muscle relaxation is marked. The depth of anesthesia attained in plane 3 is not necessary for most surgical procedures, with the probable exception of deep abdominal exploration in a large dog or horse.

Plane 4. Intercostal and abdominal muscles are completely paralyzed in plane 4, and ventilation is due completely to diaphragmatic action. This plane begins with complete paralysis of intercostal muscles and ends with apnea. Tidal volume is greatly reduced because of the lack of expansion of the thoracic cavity. This diaphragmatic ventilation produces a "tracheal tug" which is an exaggeration of the passive movement of the trachea and larynx during the inspiratory effort. This posterior movement of the larynx may be such that the mandible may also be moving, which to the novice may be interpreted as lightening of anesthesia. This type of respiratory effort produces excessive abdominal movement which can be annoying during abdominal surgery.

The cornea is dry and dull due to absence of lacrimal secretions. Lid and corneal reflexes are completely absent, as are all other protective reflexes. Pupils are dilated and do not respond to light. Heart rate and pulse pressure are reduced and cardiovascular compensating reflexes are markedly diminished. This is an extremely dangerous level of anesthesia, and no surgical procedure requires this depth. Cessation of ventilatory effort signifies the entrance into stage 4. This apnea should not be confused with that occurring in the lighter planes of anesthesia due to breath holding, manipulation of organs, or reduction of arterial carbon dioxide following a period of hyperventilation.

STAGE 4

Stage 4 is the interval between respiratory arrest and subsequent circulatory collapse. The patient is premortum inasmuch as circulation is failing. The range of this stage depends upon the anesthetic used and oxygenation at the time of respiratory arrest. Cardiac arrest will closely follow respiratory arrest when chloroform, divinyl ether, or ethyl chloride is used. During ether, halothane, or methoxyflurane anesthesia, circulation will be maintained for a short period after apnea if oxygenation has been adequate. Prompt action should be taken to reduce the arterial concentration of anesthetic agent and support cardiovascular function. Intermittent positive pressure ventilation should be initiated, and the breathing bag should be flushed with oxygen and emptied repeatedly. Cardiac filling should be aided by increasing fluid input, and pressor amines should be used when indicated.

Variations

The signs described should be slightly modified for agents which can produce more rapid changes in levels of anesthesia than ether. Because of the respiratory depressant effect of cyclopropane, respiratory arrest occurs long before plane 4. Anesthesia appears deeper than it actually is with halothane and methoxyflurane because of the more quiet type of ventilation. As a consequence, an increase in heart rate, blood pressure, ventilation, and occasional muscular activity will occur upon surgical stimulation. It is generally easier to lighten anesthesia than deepen it, and the induction period should be carried past the point of surgical stimulation. The response to stimuli and the clinical signs should be used together as a guide to an adequate plane of anesthesia. If no response, the delivered concentration can be reduced.

Halothane anesthesia has been divided into three planes because of the difficulty in distinguishing the transition between the various planes as described for ether.[22] The laryngeal and pharyngeal reflexes are abolished earlier with halothane, and even cats can be intubated with less difficulty. The major respiratory change is respiratory depression with a reduction in tidal volume. Changes in ventilatory patterns are not as distinct, and the gradual shift from thoracic to diaphragmatic pattern may not be as perceptible. The pupillary signs upon entrance into the deeper plane of anesthesia are a central fixation, followed by a progressive dilation. Planes 1 and 4 are generally easily recognized with all anesthetic agents; the middle planes as described for diethyl ether are not easy to distinguish because of the more rapid transition.

The pupil and reflex signs of methoxyflurane anesthesia are more compatible with the changes noted with ether because of the slower induction and transition through the planes of anesthesia. All the signs described may not be noted in every clinical case. Preanesthetic medication with a narcotic can exaggerate the respiratory depressant effects of anesthetic agents producing apnea early. Age, conditions of the patient, and the surgical area will also modify the response to anesthesia. Prolonged surgery and hypothermia will exert an influence, and lesser amounts are needed to maintain adequate levels of anesthesia.

Electroencephalogram

The electroencephalogram (EEG) has been used in both clinical and research aspects of general anesthesia as a method to describe the effects of depressants on central nervous system activity. It can be used to determine the depth of anesthesia when other vital signs are difficult to assess, such as during whole body perfusion for cardiopulmonary bypass. It can be used to detect cerebral anoxia and to assess damage in determining immediate effects and, more importantly, to prognosticate recovery. It is important in the teaching of anesthesia and in the clinical evaluation of new drugs, and it is useful in determining and maintaining a steady state of anesthesia in laboratory experiments in which variations in depth of anesthesia are undesirable. The effect of ether on the electroencephalogram was described in 1937[10]; this was followed by a more detailed description in 1950.[5] In this later study, seven patterns were ascribed to ether anesthesia. The continuum discussed related the changes from the induction of anesthesia to complete suppression of central nervous system activity. This has been a guide for the subsequent description of the effect of other anesthetic agents on the EEG.[3, 8]

AWAKE PATTERNS IN THE DOG

Reports vary as to the dominant pattern in the adult awake dog. Low voltage patterns with a frequency of 6 to 8 c/s have been described.[9, 18] This pattern is similar to the awake pattern in man. Other investigators have reported dominant patterns of higher frequencies (30 to 40 c/s) with superimposed moderate voltage lower frequency (4 to 8 c/s).[13, 19] Variation among laboratories in awake patterns can be expected due to different electrode placement and, most important, according to the conditions under which the data was obtained.[15] Dogs paralyzed with muscle relaxants have been used as controls; the question arises whether, in fact, this can be considered a control alert state or an apprehensive state. Frequency patterns under these circumstances have been higher when compared with data from awake nonparalyzed dogs. Paralyzed dogs artificially ventilated can be inadvertently either hyperventilated or hypoventilated.

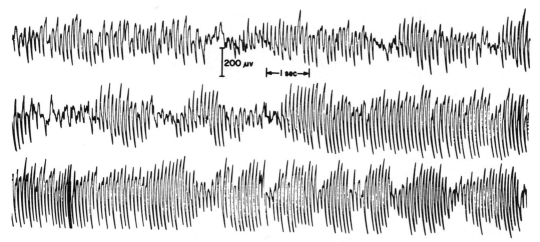

FIG. 15.3. Spindle formation of the rhythmic complex pattern of what can be considered stage 2 of general anesthesia. In this illustration, the dog is emerging from ether anesthesia. *Upper left*, the α-pattern of the lighter plane of anesthesia progressing to stage 2. The dog was paralyzed with succinylcholine chloride, and ventilation was controlled.

Hypoventilation with an increase in arterial carbon dioxide tension will produce a deeper level of anesthesia,[3, 16] and hyperventilation will also alter the EEG, producing a high voltage, low frequency pattern.[16, 21] These patterns described in the EEG's of paralyzed ventilated dogs could be due to changes in arterial carbon dioxide tension or, possibly, atropine which is generally administered to these dogs.

ANESTHESIA PATTERN

Shortly after the induction of anesthesia there is a decrease in amplitude and increase in frequency (20 c/s), which is Courtin's level 1.[3, 4, 8] As the depth of anesthesia is increased, there is a progressive change to a lower frequency, higher voltage pattern (Fig. 15.3). This pattern has a spindle conformation in which the amplitude is lowest at the beginning and end of the grouping. The frequency of the grouping is 8 to 12 c/s at voltage level of 75 to 100 μv. This is Courtin's level 2 or the rhythmic complex. As the arterial concentration is increased, this spindle pattern fades into a dominant lower frequency, high voltage pattern (75 to 200 μv). Superimposed on this slower rhythm is a higher frequency, lower voltage pattern (Fig. 15.4). This superimposed pattern

accounts for the notches in the large delta waves (Table 15.2). As anesthesia is deepened, there is a gradual reduction in the lower superimposed frequency, and the high voltage is the dominant pattern. This is Courtin's level 3 or complex wave form.

The phenomenon of burst suppression occurs as the depth of anesthesia is further increased. This periodic electrical silence is separated by irregular high voltage complexes. The Courtin levels 4 through 7 grade the duration of electrical inactivity: level 4 is less than 3 seconds of electrical silence; level 5 is greater than 3 seconds but less than 10 seconds; level 6 is greater than 10 seconds; and level 7 is complete electrical silence[3, 8] (Fig. 15.4).

Variations from the above descriptions can be expected with different agents, but all anesthetic agents that can produce a state of general anesthesia varying from very light levels to death will follow this continuum. Atropine, tranquilizers, and other depressants even administered in low doses will alter the normal awake pattern[13] and will influence, to some degree, the subsequent pattern produced by a general anesthetic. The EEG reflects the overall state of the central nervous system, and because of this it will also be influenced by changes in cerebral blood flow and body temperature, especially at mod-

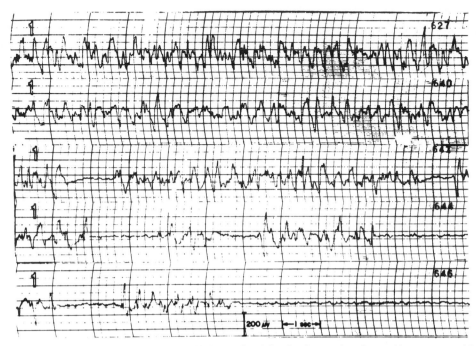

FIG. 15.4. Progressive depression of the EEG of a dog following increasing doses of intravenous thiopental sodium. The EEG progression shown here illustrates the sequence from the complex wave form (*upper left*) to complete electrical silence. With some exceptions, this sequence is noted with most general anesthetics as anesthesia is deepened.

TABLE 15.2

Range of Frequencies

Delta (δ), less than 4 c/s
Theta (θ), from 4 c/s up to but excluding 8 c/s
Alpha (α), from 8 c/s to 13 c/s inclusive
Beta (β), more than 13 c/s

erate and deep hypothermic states. Arterial concentrations of carbon dioxide will affect the EEG directly or through alterations in cerebral blood flow.

Hypoxia causes a recognizable change in the EEG pattern; unfortunately, profound degrees of hypoxia are necessary before obvious pattern changes are noted. It is a catastrophic warning, needing 40 to 30% oxygen saturation levels before a pattern change could be visualized.[2] The EEG can be very useful to prognosticate the recovery from cerebral anoxia.[14] Surgical stimulation will also alter the EEG pattern in the lighter planes of anesthesia; the shift is toward a higher frequency, indicating lighter level of anesthesia.[1]

REFERENCES

1. Backman, L. E., Lofstrom, B., and Widen, L.: Electroencephalography in halothane anesthesia. Acta. Anaesth. Scand. *8:* 115, 1964.
2. Brechner, V. L., Kinnell, J., Bauer, R. O., Bethone, R. W. M., and Dillon, J. B.: Electroencephalographic signs of hypoxia in the anesthetized dog. Anesth. Analg. (Cleveland) *44:* 322, 1965.
3. Brechner, V. L., Walter, R. D., and Dillon, J. B.: *Practical Electroencephalography for the Anesthesiologist.* Charles C Thomas, Publisher, Springfield, Ill., 1962.
4. Burlo, G. M., Sechzer, P., and Rovenstine, E. A.: Electroencephalography with methitural sodium. Anesthesiology, *18:* 140, 1957.
5. Courtin, R. F., Bickford, R. G., and Faulconer, A., Jr.: The classification and significance of electroencephalographic patterns produced by nitrous oxide-ether anesthesia during surgical operations. Proc. Staff Meet. Mayo Clin. *25:* 197, 1950.
6. Drill, V. A.: *Pharmacology in Medicine,* 2nd ed. McGraw-Hill Book Company, New York, 1958.
7. Dripps, R. D., Eckenhoff, J. E., and Vandam, L. D.: *Introduction of Anesthesia,* 3rd ed. W. B. Saunders Company, Philadelphia, 1967.
9. Faulconers, A., Jr., and Bickford, R. G.: *Electroencephalography in Anesthesiology.* Charles C Thomas, Publisher, Springfield, Ill., 1960.

9. Fox, M. W.: Effects of pentobarbital on the EEG of maturing dogs and a review of the literature. Vet. Rec. *76:* 768, 1964.

10. Gibb, F. A., Gibbs, E. L., and Lannox, W. G.: Effect on the electroencephalogram of certain drugs which influence nervous activity. Arch. Industr. Med. *60:* 154, 1937.

11. Gillespie, N.: The signs of anesthesia. Anesth. Analg. (Cleveland) *22:* 275, 1943.

12. Guedel, H. E.: *Inhalation Anesthesia*, 2nd ed. The Macmillan Company, New York, 1937.

13. Herin, R. A., Purinton, P. T., and Fletcher, T. F.: Electroencephalography in the unanesthetized dog. Amer. J. Vet. Res. *29:* 329, 1968.

14. Hockaday, J., Potts, F., Epstein, E., Bonazzi, A., and Schwab, S.: Electroencephalographic changes in acute cerebral anoxia from cardiac or respiratory arrest. Electroenceph. Clin. Neurophysiol. *18:* 575, 1965.

15. Klemm, W. R.: Technical aspects of electroencephalography in animal research. Amer. J. Vet. Res. *26:* 1237, 1965.

16. Marshal, M., Longleg, B. P., and Stanton, W. H.: Electroencephalography in anesthetic practice. Brit. J. Anaesth. *37:* 845, 1965.

17. Mushin, W. M.: The signs of anesthesia. Anaesthesia *3:* 154, 1948.

18. Pampiglione, G.: *Development of Cerebral Function in the Dog*. Butterworth & Co. (Publishers) Ltd., London, 1963.

19. Prynn, R. B., and Redding, R. W.: Electroencephalographic continuum in dogs anesthetized with methoxyflurane and halothane. Amer. J. Vet. Res. *29:* 1913, 1968.

20. Rumble, L., Jr., Cooper, M. N., Bickers, D. S., Schellack, J. K., Waits, E. J., and Hyatt, K.: Observations during apnea in conscious human subjects. Anesthesiology *18:* 419, 1957.

21. Sakai, F., Dakuma, A., Otsuka, Y., and Kumagi, H.: The effect of hypo- and hyperventilation on the electroencephalogram. Naunyn Schmiedeberg Arch. Pharm. Exp. Path. *244:* 145, 1962.

22. Thomas, G. J., Pantalone, A. L., Buchanan, W. K., and Zeedick, J. F.: Summary of stages and signs in anesthesia. Anesth. Analg. (Cleveland) *40:* 42, 1961.

23. Woodbridge, P. H.: Changing concepts concerning depth of anesthesia. Anesthesiology *18:* 536, 1957.

16
Vaporizers for Volatile Anesthetic Agents

LAWRENCE R. SOMA

Volatile anesthetic agents can be vaporized by various means. Ether and chloroform, the first volatile agents used, were inhaled from masks saturated with the liquid. This early method employed the "draw over" principle in which the patient's tidal volume was used in the simple "open drop" technique of anesthetization. This principle is used in the wick-type in-the-circle glass vaporizers, and in emergency portable vaporizers.

The disadvantage of the use of a simple mask saturated with a liquid is its erratic vapor concentration. High concentrations of anesthetic vapor can be attained early in the anesthetic period because of a dry, warm mask and a more rapid rate of evaporation; this could lead to an early overdose. During the later period of anesthesia, cooling of the mask and the accumulation of moisture will reduce the concentration of anesthetic vapor. The erratic delivery, the potential of dangerously elevated concentrations, and the development of drugs of greater potency has stimulated the search for safer methods of vaporization of volatile anesthetic agents.

Techniques have progressed from the simple mask to a slightly more efficient glass vaporizer and finally to the modern calibrated vaporizers. The potency and ease of vaporization of many new agents require that the anesthetic vapor be delivered by calibrated vaporizers. In this manner, known concentrations can be delivered to the anesthesia circuit over a prolonged period of time, thus increasing the relative safety of the anesthestic procedure.

Essential factors in the design of vaporizers are: (a) constant output concentration for a prolonged period of time; (b) concentration maintained over a wide range of gas flows; (c) prevention of changes in liquid temperature or compensation for changes; (d) minimize corrosive effect of volatile anesthetic agents on components of apparatus; (e) the back pressure produced by artificial ventilation should not alter vapor concentration; (f) delineated ON and OFF positions; (g) rugged construction so that movement will not affect calibration; (h) minimal number of moving parts; and (i) the vaporizer should be well marked or the filling funnel "indexed" to prevent filling of the vaporizer with the wrong anesthetic agent.

Basic Principles of Vaporizers

The concentration of a volatile anesthetic agent delivered from a vaporizer depends on several factors[2, 3, 4]: (a) the characteristic vapor pressure of the anesthetic agent and the liquid temperature; (b) the evaporation surface of the vaporizer; (c) the level of the anesthetic agent; and (d) the flow of the carrier gas through the vaporizer.

The saturated vapor pressure varies with the temperature and increases with a rise in temperature (Fig. 16.1). A liquid placed in a closed container is in contact and in equilibrium with the vapor above the liquid so that an equal number of molecules leave the bulk liquid state and an equal number return from the vapor state. The number of molecules which exist in the vapor state (saturated vapor pressure) at a given temperature varies with the physiochemical characteristic of the agent. The concentration above the liquid is far in excess of that needed for the induction of anesthesia, and it is the function of the vaporizer to systematically deliver and dilute this saturated vapor within the proper range.[7]

As the saturated vapor is removed from the vaporization chamber and the process of evaporation takes place, this liquid temperature falls. This will change the pressure of the saturated vapor and less will be available for dilution; therefore, one of the most important functions of a vaporizer is to maintain a constant liquid temperature, despite the cooling process of vaporization, or compensate for the temperature change.

The evaporation surface of a vaporizer can vary with design. In the more simple glass vaporizers, it may be limited only to the gas-liquid interface created by the diameter of the bottle (Fig. 16.2). Under this reduced gas-liquid interface, the output of the vaporizer will be limited. The vaporization surface can be increased without enlarging the vaporizer by placing a series of wicks into the vaporization chamber and therefore increasing enormously the surface for evaporation (Fig. 16.3). A second method used to increase vaporization surface is to place a bubbler in the system (Fig. 16.4).

The level of anesthetic agent reaches a critical level in all vaporizers where it is not sufficient to either saturate the wicks or to cover adequately the bubbling plate. The level of the liquid is more critical in the older bubble through glass vaporizers.

The flow of carrier gas which can be passed through a vaporizer and still deliver a known concentration of vapor is dependent on the design, size, and thermostability of the vaporizer. This will determine the maximum rate of gas flow that can be achieved and still deliver adequate volumes of anesthetic vapor. Because of their inability to compensate for liquid temperature changes, glass vaporizers are more variable in this respect.

Glass Vaporizers

PLENUM-TYPE BUBBLE THROUGH VAPORIZER

Glass vaporizers are generally simple in design and are constructed in such a

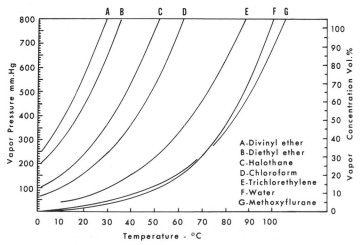

FIG. 16.1. Vapor pressure curves for common volatile anesthetic agents.

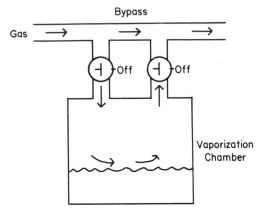

FIG. 16.2. Schematic of a simple glass vaporizer. The vaporization surface (the gas-liquid interface) is limited to the surface of the liquid.

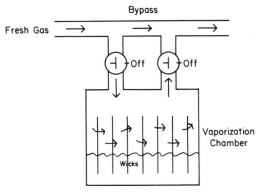

FIG. 16.3. Schematic of a wick-type glass vaporizer. The wick markedly enlarges the surface for vaporization, therefore increasing efficiency. This type is generally used as draw over vaporizer because of the lesser resistance than the bubble type.

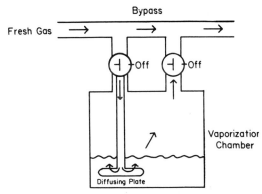

FIG. 16.4. Schematic of a bubble type vaporizer. The liquid-gas interface is increased by the creation of many small bubbles.

manner that a varying amount of carrier gas (oxygen alone or in combination with other compressed gases) can be diverted into the vaporizing chamber. Many glass diversion-type vaporizers have been developed, but their methods of operation are basically similar. When the control valve is closed, the carrier gas bypasses the vaporization chamber, and, as the valve is opened, a greater proportion of the gas flow is diverted into the chamber.[4]

The plenum type differs from the draw over vaporizer in that the fresh gas or carrier gas is delivered from an anesthesia machine and is perfused or forced through the vaporizer; this is the most common type. The anesthetic vapor and carrier gas are then delivered, depending on the system in use, to the patient directly or to the rebreathing system.

In a simple glass jar, evaporation is confined to the surface area of the liquid, which limits the efficiency of the vaporizer. As discussed, methods have been devised to increase the evaporating surface and thereby increase efficiency by the addition of wicks or bubblers. The size of the wick and the depth of the container are varied according to the volatility of the agent. In general, smaller vaporizers can be used for the more highly volatile agents.

A common glass vaporizer is the "bubble through type" which incorporates a stem which can divert oxygen from the manifold into the liquid anesthetic. The carrier gas can be bubbled through the anesthetic agent when high concentrations are desired, or the control lever can be adjusted to surface contact only for lower concentrations. A diffusing plate will disperse the oxygen into many bubbles, providing a larger liquid-gas interface. The finer this dispersion, the greater is the surface area for vaporation. The usual vehicular gas is oxygen, but nitrous oxide or any of the other anesthetic gases can be added to oxygen.

A disadvantage of the glass vaporizer is that the concentration of anesthetic vapor delivered is not constant and will vary with the flow of oxygen, temperature of

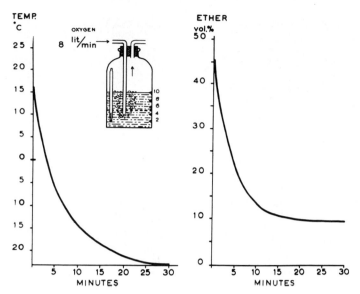

FIG. 16.5. A rapid fall in temperature of the liquid ether occurs during high flows of oxygen (*left*). The drop in delivered concentrations parallels this change in temperature (*right*). (Courtesy of R. R. MacIntosh, W. W. Mushin, and H. B. Epstein: *Physics for the Anesthetist*, 2nd ed. F. A. Davis Co., Philadelphia, 1958.)

the anesthetic liquid, and the amount of liquid anesthetic contained within the vaporizer.[3] When a high gas flow is used, the temperature of the anesthetic liquid will decrease rapidly during vaporization unless an external source of heat is provided. The drop in concentration of vapor parallels the temperature change (Fig. 16.5). The thermal conductivity of glass is poor, and heat is not readily conducted into the liquid. Therefore, the major portion of the heat of vaporization is obtained from the anesthetic liquid. A more constant temperature can be maintained by the addition of an external source of heat or by substituting a metal container for the glass container. If temperature changes can be prevented, a more constant output can be anticipated from any vaporizer.

DRAW OVER VAPORIZERS OR INHALERS

The "draw over" vaporizers differ from the plenum type in the method of propelling the carrier gas through the vaporizer. Instead of bubbling the carrier gas through the vaporizer, the patient draws gas through it during inspiration. The resistance of the plenum vaporizer is too high for use as inhalers. The draw over glass vaporizers have the same deficiencies as the bubble through vaporizers. The gas flows through the inhaler-type vaporizer are intermittent and vary in volume; therefore, calibrations do not hold true under these conditions. A common draw over vaporizer, which can be used for ether or methoxyflurane, is the Ohio Chemical No. 8 (Fig. 16.6).

Precision-Type Vaporizers

The deficiencies of the glass vaporizers are partially eliminated in the precision vaporizers (the thermocompensated vaporizers and the "heat sink" vaporizers). These enable delivery of a controlled concentration of anesthetic vapor for a long period of time, independent of ambient temperature and carrier gas flow.

FLUOTEC VAPORIZERS

The Fluotec vaporizers (Fig. 16.7) are thermocompensating vaporizers which have been designed for halothane only. They contain a mechanism which will respond to the reduction in temperature of the liquid anesthetic as vaporization occurs.[2] As liquid temperature drops, an

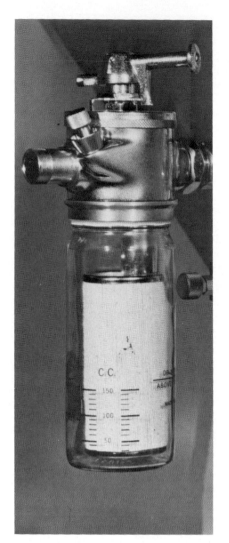

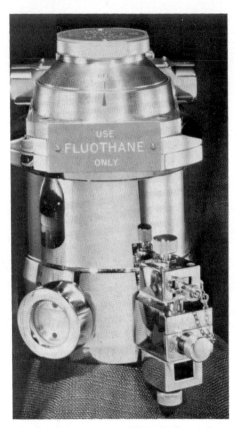

FIG. 16.7. Fluotec Mark III is the latest design of Cyprane series of halothane vaporizers. (Courtesy of Frazer Sweatman Co., Lancaster, N.Y.)

FIG. 16.6. Ohio Chemical No. 8 glass vaporizer. The wick increases the vaporization surface without markedly increasing the resistance to respiration. This is commonly used as a draw over vaporizer, for ether or methoxyflurane.

increased amount of halothane vapor is delivered to the bypass gas flow. Thus, the alterations in vapor concentration which can be produced by changes in temperature during the process of vaporization are minimized. The Fluotec Mark I was the first of this type to become commercially available. The correlation between percent concentration on the dial setting and output concentration is good when oxygen flow rates of 4 liters/minute or greater are used. Below 4 liters/minute, a linear relationship does not exist (Fig. 16.8, *top*), and referral must be made to the flow chart. These high flows are not economical in veterinary anesthesia, and vaporizers designed for accuracy at lower gas flows are advisable.

The Fluotec Mark II, which is similar in construction to the Mark I, is both thermocompensated and flow compensated. This enables the delivery of adequate concentration of halothane at both low and high oxygen flows. Unfortunately, at fresh gas flows of 0.5 liters/minute, there is a marked increase in output at the higher concentration dial settings (Fig. 16.8, *bottom*). Therefore, at the lower gas flows, as with high flows, the output is not linear with the dial settings. The concentration delivered must be determined from the

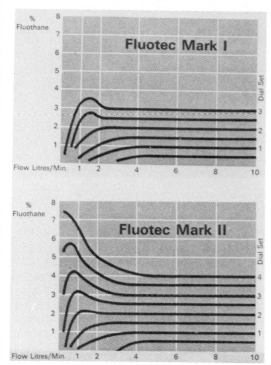

FIG. 16.8. Output performance graphs for the Fluotec Mark I and Mark II. At gas flows of 4 liters/minute, both vaporizers have a linear output. This relationship between the dialed concentration and delivered concentration is not linear at lower gas flow rates. The Mark II will deliver higher concentrations at low gas flow rates. (Courtesy of Frazer Sweatman Co.)

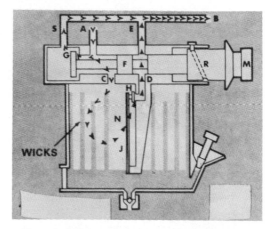

FIG. 16.9. Schematic of the Fluotec Mark I. Carrier gases enter port A. When the dial M-R is pulled forward and rotated clockwise, the block F is removed from port C allowing carrier gases to enter the vaporization chamber N. The passage G is a variable one and according to the concentration dialed, determines how much of the incoming gas flow is diverted through channel C and into the vaporization chamber. The carrier gases pass over a series of wicks and the saturated vapor exits through port H-D. This leaves through channel E and mixes with the bypass gas from S, both emerging through port B. The size of port H is controlled by the bimetallic strip J and varies according to liquid temperature to maintain a constant output concentration of vapor.

chart when carrier gas flows of less than 3 liters are used.

The automatic temperature compensation utilizes the response of a bimetallic strip to adjust the output concentration to changes in liquid temperature (Fig. 16.9). The concentration control knob determines the amount of carrier gas which enters the vaporization chamber and the amount which bypasses the vaporization chamber. The gas entering the vaporization chamber passes over a series of wicks which completely saturates the incoming gas with halothane. The orifice of the outlet of the chamber is controlled by the bimetallic strip which responds to changes in the liquid temperature; as the temperature drops the port opens and allows more vapor to emerge and combine with the bypassed carrier gas. This as-

sures that the output concentration remains reasonably constant.

In the Fluotec Mark III (Fig. 16.7), the output of anesthetic vapor is more independent of the carrier gas flows. As compared to the Mark I and Mark II, the output is linear over a wider range of flows and concentrations. The function of the Mark III differs from the earlier models in that the temperature-sensitive valve regulates the amount of gas which is diverted into the vaporization chamber and not how much saturated vapor is allowed out of the vaporization chamber (Fig. 16.10). The rotation of the concentration dial determines the degree of mixing between the carrier gas flow which enters the vaporization chamber and the bypass flow through the temperature-sensitive valve. The delivered concentration is therefore determined by the resistance to flow created by two contact areas: one is auto-

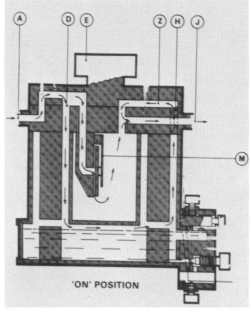

'ON' POSITION

FIG. 16.10. Schematic of the Mark III thermocompensated vaporizer. Metered gas enters channel A and splits into two streams at D. One stream flows into the vaporization chamber and the second stream flows through the temperature-sensitive valve M to outlet J. In this vaporizer, this is the bypass gas flow. As the control knob E is rotated, the size of channel Z is increased, creating a lower resistance to flow through this channel, allowing more carrier gases to enter the vaporization chamber. The temperature-sensitive valve M varies the bypass flow in proportion to liquid temperature. The delivered concentration is determined by the relative resistance to flow created by the channel Z and the temperature-sensitive valve M. (Courtesy of Frazer Sweatman Co.)

matically controlled by alterations in liquid temperature, and the second is manually controlled by selection of an anesthetic concentration.

PENTEC VAPORIZERS

The Pentec vaporizers, Mark I and Mark II, are similar to the Fluotec vaporizers in function, but have been developed for methoxyflurane. The vaporizers are not interchangeable. The Pentec I is the original model, and the maximum concentration delivered at room temperature (20 C) is between 1.3 and 1.7%.[10] At higher

temperatures (25 C), 2.0 to 2.4% methoxyflurane can be delivered. Calibration curves for the Pentec are set for flows of 5 liters/minute and are slightly higher when lower flows are used. The oxygen flow generally used for animals is between 0.5 and 2 liters/minute.

The Pentec II is an advanced model and is somewhat similar to the Fluotec III in design and operation. The main exception is the "safety stop." The thermocompensation calibration portion of the vaporizers is from 0 to 2% methoxyflurane. When the "safety stop" is released and the control lever is set on maximum setting, the thermocompensating portion of the vaporizer is eliminated from the carrier gas flow path, and all of the carrier gas flow is now diverted through the vaporization chamber (channel D, Fig. 16.10). The control setting, when placed in the full ON position becomes a "maximum saturation" vaporizer, and the output concentration is dependent upon room temperature. The concentration of methoxyflurane at 20 C is 3% and at 35 C is 6.6% (Table 16.1). The high concentrations are useful under certain conditions, especially when a rapid induction is desirable in a large patient. It can be very dangerous, especially if the anesthetist is not aware of output at various room temperatures.

FLUOMATIC, PENTOMATIC, AND ETHERMATIC VAPORIZERS

The Fluomatic, Pentomatic, and Ethermatic vaporizers are thermocompensating vaporizers which have been developed for halothane, methoxyflurane, and ether (Fig. 16.11). The problem of maintaining a constant output regardless of temperature has been approached in a unique manner. A silicone cone with a high coefficient of thermal expansion in relation to the valve seat is used instead of a bimetallic strip (Fig. 16.12). As with the Fluotec vaporizers, changes in temperature will automatically alter the diameter of a variable orifice. Resistance change in relation to a fixed orifice will increase or decrease gas flow through the vaporization chamber.

TABLE 16.1

Liquid temperature of methoxyflurane and vapor concentrations

Vaporizer temperature (°C)	20	25	30	35
Vapor pressure: methoxyfluran (torr)	23.0	30.5	39.5	50.5
Concentration (vol %*)	3.0	4.0	5.2	6.6

* The barometric pressure at sea level (760) is assumed in the calculations:

Concentration percent = (vapor pressure/760) × 100

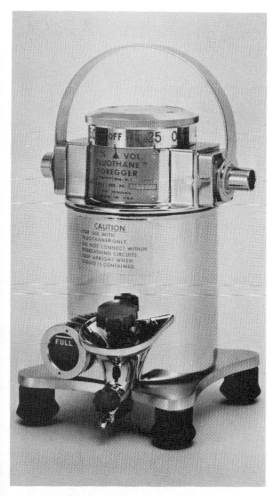

Fig. 16.11. Fluomatic halothane vaporizer. (Courtesy of Foregger Co., Smithtown, N.Y.)

The vaporizer has a spring-loaded vent to prevent a high gas flow (such as full gas flush) from passing through the vaporizer.

The methoxyflurane vaporizer is similar in design to the Fluomatic with the exception of having a double cone, thereby allowing a higher proportional gas flow through the vaporization chamber. This is necessary because of the lower vapor pressure of methoxyflurane.

VAPOR HALOTHANE VAPORIZER

The Vapor vaporizer is not thermocompensating in design (Fig. 16.13). It is based on the principle of a "heat sink." Instead of using the thermocompensating mechanism to adjust to temperature changes, it maintains a constant liquid temperature. It is constructed of copper, a metal of high thermal conductivity. Copper will convey heat from the surrounding air and metal of the anesthesia machine to the liquid anesthetic, supplying the necessary latent heat for the vaporization process. The temperature of the liquid agent will vary with daily changes in room temperature, but will not drop during the vaporization process. This basic concept eliminates the need for the thermocompensating mechanism, which is more susceptible to malfunction. This thermostability allows the delivery of an accurate concentration of halothane over a wide range of carrier gas flows. The output concentration and the dial concentrations are linear over gas flows ranging from 300 ml/minute to 10 liters/minute (Fig. 16.14).

A problem in vaporizer construction results from the difficulty in the design of valves which will split the incoming gas into two proportional flows, regardless of the rate of oxygen flow. This division of the incoming oxygen, regardless of the flow, into two proportional components (one portion bypassing the vaporization chamber and the other entering the chamber) cannot be as easily accomplished in a

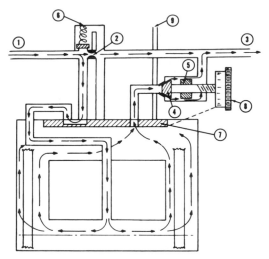

FIG. 16.12. Schematic of the Fluomatic vaporizer (thermocompensated). The gas flow enters inlet *1* and is split into two streams. The bypass stream flows through the fixed resistance *2*, and the other portion flows into the vaporization chamber. As the control dial *8* is rotated, the size of the variable orifice created by the cone *4* will increase or decrease and determine the amount of carrier gas which enters the vaporization chamber. As the dial is rotated toward a higher concentration, the total diameter of the port created by the cone *4* increases, and the relative resistance created by the fixed restriction *2* and the variable restriction *4* favors higher flow into the chamber. The thermocompensation is accomplished by the large coned control needle valve *4* and the valve seat. The silicone needle valve *5* has a high coefficient of thermal expansion and will expand and contract with temperature changes. The isolation valve *7* is moved by way of a linkage to control valve *8*. In the *OFF* position, this valve slides to the right, closing the gas inlet to the chamber and directly venting all gas out through orifice *3*. A relief valve *6* is provided to limit the pressure of the inlet gas in the event that high flows are applied during an oxygen flush. (Courtesy of Foregger Co.)

thermostatic-type system as it can in a heat sink system.

The output concentration in the halothane vapor is controlled both by a fixed and a variable cone (Fig. 16.15). The fixed cone controls the bypass flow and the variable cone controls the amount of saturated carrier gas leaving the vaporization chamber. The resistance changes (pressure drop) across both cones are re-

lated linearly to the volume flow; thus, the splitting of the carrier gas flow is proportional over a wide range. The vapor contains a thermometer, indicating the liquid temperature. To deliver a known

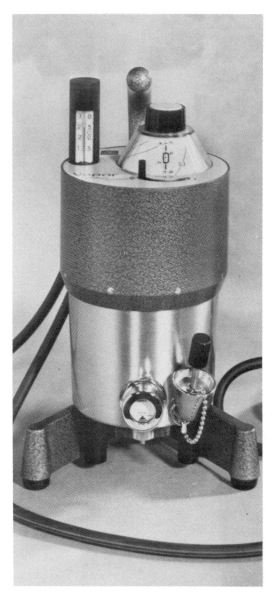

FIG. 16.13. Vapor halothane vaporizer. The vaporizer is operated by switching the side valve to the *ON* position, reading the temperature scale and turning the control knob clockwise, and aligning the percent scale and the vertical temperature scale. (Courtesy of North American Dräger, Telford, Pa.)

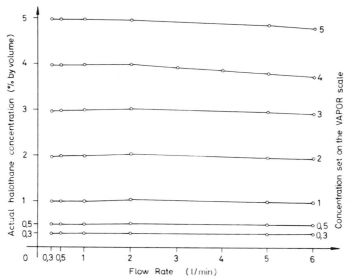

FIG. 16.14. Output curves for the Vapor halothane vaporizer. (Courtesy of North American Dräger.)

concentration of halothane, the concentration curve and the temperature curve are aligned (Fig. 16.13).

The relationship of liquid temperature to the vaporization of a volatile agent can be appreciated by looking at the relationship between the vertical temperature scale and the curved percentage scale (Fig. 16.15). If the ambient temperature is reduced to lower operational limit (16 C), the control knob is rotated clockwise to adjust the 24 C and 2% intersect to the 16 C and 2% intersect position, thereby opening the variable cone (F) to its maximum within the 2% scale reading, and allowing more anesthetic vapor to escape. The Vapor operates at ambient temperatures between 16 C and 28 C, but special models are available for working at ambient temperatures between 18 C and 43 C.

The Vapor is an accurate vaporizer and is very useful as a source of accurate concentration of anesthetic vapor.[6] The lack of a metallic strip or plastic block may assure a longer usage period without vapor concentration alterations.

METHOXYFLURANE VAPOR

The methoxyflurane vapor is similar in design and operation to the halothane vaporizer. The main exception is that channel E (fig. 16.15) is a variable cone instead of a fixed channel. It is linked to the variable cone F, therefore allowing a greater amount of the incoming gas to enter the vaporization chamber. The calibration is from 0 to 2.5% methoxyflurane; when placed in the full dial position, it becomes a "maximum saturation" vaporizer and the output is dependent upon room temperature.

BYPASS VAPORIZERS

The Copper Kettle (Fig. 16.16) and the Verni-Trol are two commonly used vaporizers for the accurate administration of volatile anesthetic agents. As in the Vapor, the bypass vaporizers are constructed of large amounts of copper which maintain constant liquid temperature during vaporization.

In all the systems described previously, the vaporizer splits the carrier gas into proportional parts. This split is basically proportioned by relative resistance between a variable and fixed resistance. The "bypass" vaporizers do not create this dual flow by splitting a single incoming stream of gas, but by delivering two separate flows of gas (Fig. 16.16): one oxygen flow through the vaporizer (for vaporiza-

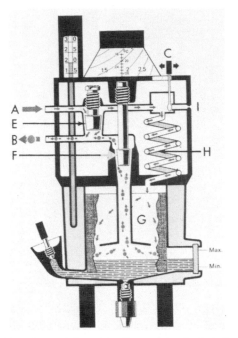

FIG. 16.15. Schematic diagram for the halothane vapor vaporizer. The fresh gas enters the inlet port *A*, and when the lever *C* is closed all the gas is diverted through the fixed channel *E* and out outlet *B*. When the lever *C* is placed in the "ready to use position" some of the inflow gas is diverted into the vaporization chamber *G* through the coiled channel *H*. The amount of gas which passes into the vaporization chamber is determined by the resistance produced between the coned variable channel *F* and the fixed coned channel *E*. As the control knob is rotated clockwise, the variable channel *F* is enlarged, allowing more anesthetic vapor out of the chamber. Both the bypass gas and the saturated carrier gas leave the vaporizer through outlet *B*. Orifice *I* releases any pressure within the vaporizer when the switch is placed in the *OFF* position. (Courtesy of North American Dräger.)

tion) and a second gas flow system which completely bypasses the vaporizer (for metabolic needs).

The oxygen flow through the vaporizer is dispersed through a diffuser which produces a great number of fine bubbles; these provide a large gas-liquid interface, and oxygen flowing through the vaporizer becomes saturated (equilibrated) with anesthetic vapor. A high concentration of anesthetic vapor is delivered to the mixing chamber and mixed with the bypass oxygen and often with other anesthetic gases. This diluted vapor is delivered to the anesthetic circuit. By proper dilution, a specific concentration of anesthetic vapor can be delivered. The metered oxygen flow through the vaporizer is usually labeled for the rapid calculation of the percent of halothane by the thermal percentage system.[1] The amount of anesthetic vapor delivered per milliliter of oxygen carrier gas passed through the vaporizer will vary with the room temperature. As the liquid temperature increases, so will the vapor pressures, producing a greater concentration of anesthetic vapor at any given flow of oxygen. Therefore, at elevated room temperatures, a greater amount of bypass diluting oxygen is needed to produce a given percentage of halothane. A percent of halothane scale, a temperature scale, and thermometer are incorporated in the anesthesia machine for the rapid calculation of halothane concentrations. When the vapor pressure is known, percent of concentration of any volatile anesthetic agent can be calculated by the use of the gas laws or a flow calculator (Fig. 16.17).

The main advantage of a bypass vaporizer is its adaptability to all volatile anesthetic agents. Unfortunately, they are not as simple to use as the other vaporizers and are more difficult to use at low carrier gas flows.

Pumping Effect

When intermittent positive pressure ventilation is used, the concentration of volatile anesthetic agent will increase in many vaporizers. As the pressure pulsation is transmitted from the breathing circuit to the vaporization chamber, a back pressure is created.[5] During the release of pressure to allow exhalation, the contents of the chamber exit not only through the normal exit port, but also through the inlet port to the vaporizer (Fig. 16.18).

The Vapor vaporizers have a built-in back pressure compensator. It is simply

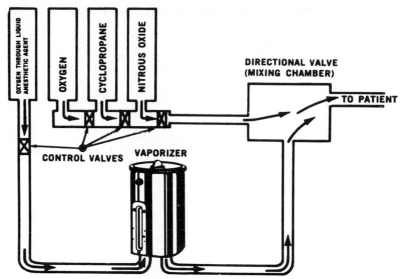

Fig. 16.16. Two sources of gas are used in the Copper Kettle. One is oxygen flow through the vaporizer only, which may be as high as 600 ml/minute. The second source delivers the metabolic source of oxygen and other anesthetic agents. The high concentration of vapor emerging from the vaporizer is diluted in the mixing chamber, thereby delivering (by dilution) a known vapor concentration. (Courtesy of Foregger Co.)

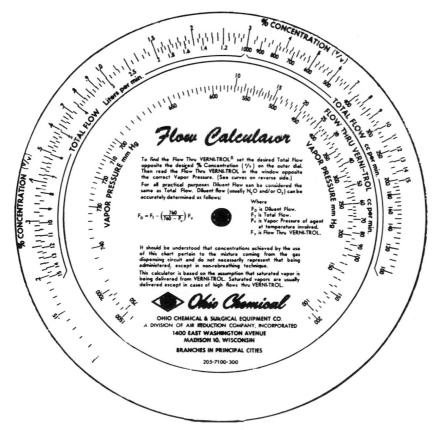

Fig. 16.17. Flow calculator. The flow calculator can be used to calculate the flow through the Verni-Trol or the Copper Kettle to produce a known concentration for any volatile anesthetic agent. The calculator has been set for a 3% concentration of halothane at 1000 ml of total gas flow. The vapor pressure at 20 C is 250 mm Hg, indicating a total flow of 60 ml of oxygen through the Verni-Trol.

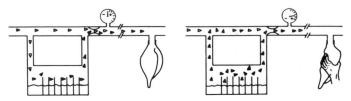

Fig. 16.18. Fresh gas enters the vaporizers and becomes saturated with the vapor of the volatile anesthetic agents; it mixes with the bypass fresh gas as it leaves the vaporizer. When positive pressure is applied downstream to the vaporizer, anesthetic vapor is forced backwards up into the bypass channel by the back pressure created. Under this increased pressure change, the output of the vaporizer is temporarily increased upon release of pressure. (Adopted from Hill and Jackson.[5a])

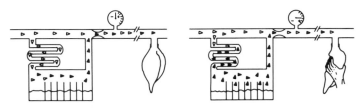

Fig. 16.19. The effect of positive pressure ventilation on the output of a vaporizer can be prevented by heightening the inlet tube to the vaporization chamber. As pressure is applied, the anesthetic vapor now "backs up" into the coiled tube, but does not reach the bypass tube. Under these circumstances there is no surge of anesthetic vapor through the bypass tube. (Adopted from Hill and Lowe.[7])

fitted with a long coiled inlet tube to the vaporizing chamber (tube *H*, Fig. 16.15). The saturated vapor will rise up the long tube during the pressure phase but will not reach the bypass tube (Fig. 16.19).[5a]

The pumping effect increases the concentration in the Fluotec Mark I and Mark II from 0.5 to 1%, the greater increase in concentration at gas flows of 500 ml.[5] Many methods have been devised to reduce this effect. The Fluotec I and Fluotec II can be fitted with a small pressure regulator placed on the outlet to prevent the pressure from being transmitted back into the vaporizer. This effect also occurs in the Copper Kettle and Verni-Trol, and unidirectional valves have been placed distal to the vaporizer to prevent the "pumping effect."[8, 9]

The Fluomatic has two design features to eliminate the "pumping effect." This vaporizer operates at a 6 mm Hg pressure drop between the inlet and outlet. The pressure effect only manifests itself when the back pressure is above 6 torr. The second mechanism is a low gas volume capacity of the chamber which is also used in the Fluotec III.

REFERENCES

1. Abajian, J., Jr.: Thermal Percentage System, Pamphlet VIII. Foregger Company, Smithstown, N.Y., 1965.
2. Brennan, H. J.: A vaporizer for fluothane. Brit. J. Anaesth. 29: 332, 1957.
3. Epstein, H. G.: Principles of inhalers for volatile anesthetics. Brit. Med. Bull. 14: 18, 1958.
4. Faulconer, A.: Anesthetic vaporizers: a physical basis for functional classification. Anesthesiology 18: 372, 1957.
5. Hill, D. W., and Lowe, H. J.: Comparisons of concentrations of halothane in closed and semi-closed circuits during controlled ventilation. Anesthesiology 23: 291, 1962.
5a. Hill, D. W., and Jackson, D. C.: Recent developments in vaporizers. Anaesthesia 19: 191, 1964.
6. Hill, D. W.: Halothane concentrations obtained from a Dräger Vapor vaporizer. Brit. J. Anaesth. 35: 285, 1963.
7. Hill, D. W.: The design and calibration of vaporizers for volatile anesthetic agents. Brit. J. Anaesth. 40: 648, 1968.
8. Keenan, R. L.: Prevention of increased pressure in anesthetic vaporizers with a unidirectional valve. Anesthesiology 24: 732, 1963.
9. Meet, J. E., Valentine, G. W., and Riccio, J. S.: An arrangement to prevent pressure effect in the Verni-Trol vaporizer. Anesthesiology 24: 734, 1963.
10. North, W. C.: Equipment and calibration. In Symposium on Methoxyflurane: an evaluation in 1966. Excerpta Med. (Anesthesiology), April 1966.

17
Systems and Techniques for Inhalation Anesthesia

LAWRENCE R. SOMA

There is a great deal of confusion concerning terminology and basic definitions of the various methods of delivering anesthetic gases or oxygen. Three methods can be used in veterinary anesthesia: (a) semiopen; (b) nonrebreathing; and (c) rebreathing (Table 17.1). The method chosen is usually determined by the equipment available and the size of the animal. The function of the anesthetic system is to provide a means of delivering anesthetic gases and oxygen and adequately removing exhaled carbon dioxide. The carbon dioxide produced by metabolism and exhaled may be eliminated from the delivery system by one of three general ways: (a) dilution; (b) nonrebreathing valves; and (c) chemical absorption.

Removal of carbon dioxide in the awake animal following exhalation is by simple dilution by the surrounding atmosphere (Fig. 17.1). When a face mask is added, the ability of the animal to excrete CO_2 is reduced because of the additional dead space created by the mask (Fig. 17.2). This is an important consideration in the use of a face mask, whether it be for anesthesia or oxygen therapy, especially in small patients. The smallest mask possible must be used to minimize the volume of dead space. Under these circumstances, the patient is exhaling CO_2 into a confined space and not into the infinite environment, and an adequate flow of fresh gas must be provided to avoid rebreathing of exhaled gas. One arrangement, for example, is the placement of the fresh gas flow as near as possible to the patient's nose and the "leak" or outflow downstream from the mask (Fig. 17.3).

The second method used for the removal of exhaled CO_2 is by the use of valves to separate the inhaled gas from the exhaled portion. If the valves are functioning properly, the inspired CO_2 is zero and the delivered concentration of anesthetic vapor and oxygen can be accurately determined. This is a nonrebreathing technique which can be used in small animals.

The third method is the chemical removal of carbon dioxide from the exhaled gas, enabling the reinspiration of the remaining gas which contains oxygen and anesthetic vapor. This is the most common and versatile technique used in anesthesia. It permits economy of the anesthetic agents and oxygen and also permits a better assessment of ventilation by observation of the rebreathing bag. Positive pressure ventilation can be initiated by manually compressing the rebreathing bag.

Semiopen Systems

The semiopen methods can allow the patient's respiratory system to be open to

TABLE 17.1

Delivery systems for inhalation anesthetics

System	Absorption of Carbon Dioxide	Breathing Bag	Rebreathing of Expired Gases	Directional Valves
Semiopen				
Open drop	No	No	Slight	No
Ayre's method	No	No/yes	No	No
Kuhn's system	No	Yes	No	No
Magill system	No	Yes	No	Yes
Nonrebreathing				
Leigh, Fink, Ruben	No	Yes	No	Yes
Timar face mask	No	Yes	No	Yes
Rebreathing closed				
Circle	Yes	Yes	Complete	Yes
To and fro	Yes	Yes	Complete	No
Rebreathing, Semiclosed				
Circle	Yes	Yes	Partial	Yes
To and fro	Yes	Yes	Partial	No

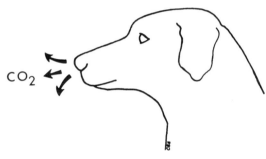

FIG. 17.1. The removal of exhaled carbon dioxide in the animal is by simple dilution.

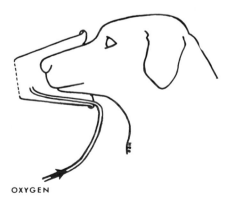

OXYGEN

FIG. 17.2. The addition of a mask adds to the anatomical dead space and decreases effective alveolar ventilation. Rebreathing of exhaled gases can occur unless the mask fits well to facial conformations or high flow of fresh gas is provided to flush out the dead space.

the atmosphere on both inspiration and exhalation. The removal of carbon dioxide is either by simple dilution by room air (open drop method) or by the flow of fresh gas to flush out the exhaled carbon dioxide. Valves are generally not used in this system to produce a unidirectional flow of gas. Three semiopen techniques can be easily used in small animal anesthesia: the open drop method, the Ayre's "T" piece, and the Magill-type systems.

OPEN DROP TECHNIQUE

The "open drop" or "cone method" of delivery is still applicable to the toy canine breeds and to cats and can provide adequate planes of anesthesia with a minimal amount of equipment. The induction of anesthesia in the large dog, however, is difficult because of the restraint, amount of anesthetic agent, and size of the mask which is necessary. The main advantages are that it can be readily applied to the smaller species and that there are no valves to impose a resistance to respiration. Major disadvantages are: (a) it is wasteful and therefore can only be used economically with the older volatile agents; (b) there is considerable variation in anesthetic concentration, and experience is required to provide a constant inspired vapor concentration; (c) there is no

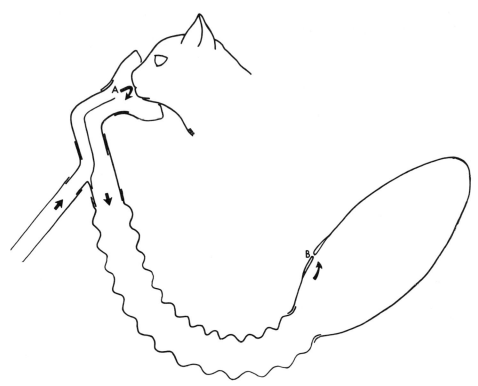

FIG. 17.3. Schematic representation of the Kuhn system, a semiopen method for delivering inhalation anesthetics. The fresh gas enters at A and washes the exhaled gases from the body of the mask and out port B. Positive pressure ventilation can be administered by placing a finger over port B and compressing the breathing bag.

method of supporting ventilation if hypoventilation occurs; and (d) there is some rebreathing of exhaled carbon dioxide and a decrease of oxygen tension because of the increased dead space imposed by the mask.[8]

The equipment consists of a wire mesh mask covered with eight layers of 16-ply surgical gauze (Fig. 17.4). The layers of gauze provide a good surface for vaporization of the volatile anesthetic agent, are a sufficient barrier to prevent facial contamination by the liquid anesthetic, and are thin enough to insure adequate exchange of respiratory gases with room air.

A common fault in this method is the use of a large cone packed at one end with cotton. Cotton or any other dense material will impede the exchange of respiratory gases with room air, and the large cone will create a dead space, further minimizing the ventilatory exchange. The result-

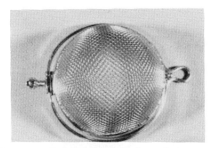

FIG. 17.4. A simple wire mesh mask for open drop anesthesia. This mask is covered by eight layers of 16-ply surgical gauze to provide a surface for the vaporization of a volatile agent.

ing dead space can be a major hazard of the open drop technique. The concentration (partial pressure) of oxygen below the mask when room air is being used will be lower than atmospheric pressure because of its dilution by accumulated water vapor, carbon dioxide, and anesthetic vapor. The proper exchange of gas will depend upon the mask fit, the size of the mask, the thickness of the gauze, and the patient's tidal volume in relationship to the dead space created by the mask. The concentration of carbon dioxide will be markedly increased as the patient's tidal exchange is decreased in the deeper planes of anesthesia. To insure an adequate concentration of oxygen and reduction of the accumulation of carbon dioxide, a flow of oxygen of 200 to 300 ml/minute of oxygen should be maintained below the mask (Fig. 17.2).[8]

The cat or small dog is restrained gently by an assistant or the anesthetist, and the face mask, after application of a few drops of liquid anesthetic, is held close to the face. Initial contact between the face mask and the animal should be avoided. The liquid agent should be dropped on the mask slowly at first in order to accustom the animal to the smell of the vapor. The rate of drip can be increased slowly as sedation occurs and the cat or dog becomes tolerant to the smell of the anesthetic vapor. Cats especially will resist vigorous restraint; therefore, the initial handling should be gentle. The cat should be approached from behind and allowed to back towards the body of the anesthetist as the mask is placed near the face. Struggling will occur when the excitement period (stage 2) is approached, and during

this phase the cat or dog should be held on its side as anesthesia is deepened.

The open drop method is relatively safe and can be used when it is difficult to induce anesthesia by intravenous barbiturates and other techniques are not available. It can be used effectively when a rapid recovery from a short period of anesthesia is desired. Important aspects of the method are as follows. (a) Only eight to nine layers of 16-ply gauze should be used to cover the mask, and tight wads of cotton should not be used. (b) The evaporization surface should be broad enough to insure sufficient area for the vaporization of the liquid agent. (c) The cone or mask should fit closely to the face of the animal, thereby minimizing dead space. (d) The eyes should be protected with a bland ophthalmic ointment. (e) Shortly after the induction of anesthesia, supplemental oxygen should be administered below the mask. (f) The concentration of volatile anesthetic should be increased slowly and discontinued if breath holding occurs. This is to prevent the sudden buildup of high concentrations of anesthetic vapor. (g) The liquid anesthetic should be added evenly over the entire surface of the mask, developing a consistent pattern of application. (h) Cooling of the mask surface will occur with the vaporization and, at this point, the mask should be changed.

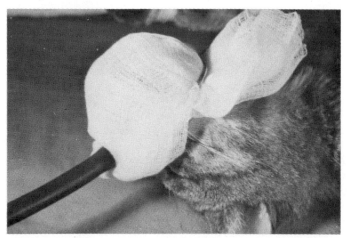

Fig. 17.5. An anesthetic-oxygen mixture is added below an open drop mask through a catheter. (Courtesy of Clifford and Soma.[6])

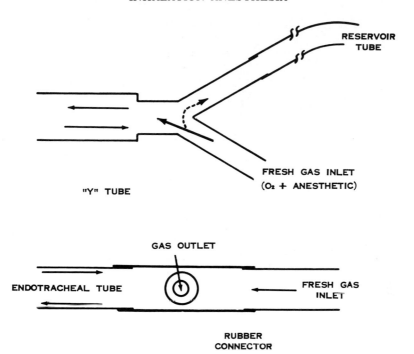

FIG. 17.6. *Top*, schematic representation of a "Y" piece. The reservoir tube prevents dilution of the anesthetic agent and oxygen with room air during inspiration (*bottom*). The "Y" piece has been simplified by the removal of the reservoir arm. Exhaled gases are eliminated through a hole in the rubber connector attached to the endotracheal tube. (Courtesy of Clifford and Soma.[6])

A convenient method of maintaining general anesthesia after the induction of anesthesia is to administer the anesthetic-oxygen mixture below the mask through a catheter (Fig. 17.5). An oxygen source and a vaporizer are necessary.

Diethyl ether is the most commonly used agent in the open drop method. Excessive loss of the anesthetic agent into the room cannot be avoided and large quantities are necessary to maintain general anesthesia. This and the potency of halothane or methoxyflurane preclude their use by the open drop method. A common method is to use more rapid acting agents such as divinyl ether for the induction of anesthesia and diethyl ether for the maintenance of general anesthesia.

Hepatotoxicity can occur when ethylchloride and divinyl ether are used for periods of anesthesia in excess of 20 to 30 minutes. Ideally, these agents should be used only for the induction of anesthesia and short periods of maintenance. Ethyl chloride and divinyl ether are extremely potent agents and can induce anesthesia very rapidly. Respiratory arrest and cardiac arrest can occur simultaneously, if care is not exercised (see Chapter 10).

AYRE'S "T" PIECE SYSTEM

The Ayre technique is a semiopen method of delivering inhalation agents developed originally for pediatric anesthesia and is suitable for cats and the small breeds of dogs.[2, 3, 6] The equipment consists of a simply "Y" or "T" piece connected to an endotracheal tube (Figs. 17.6 and 17.7). One arm of the "Y" piece is attached to a source of oxygen and is the inhalation limb. The second arm acts as an exhalation limb and is connected to a small reservoir (Fig. 17.6). The unidirectional flow of gas is created by a constant flow of gas through one arm of the "Y" piece, and the absence of valves assures a low resistance to respiration. The removal of carbon dioxide and flushing out of the system to prevent rebreathing of exhaled gases is accom-

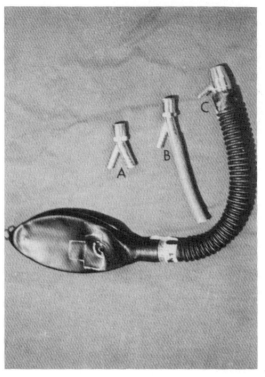

FIG. 17.7. The Foregger "Y" piece (*A* and *B*) and the Kuhn system (*C*) use Ayre's "T" piece principle for the delivery of inhalation agents.

plished by delivering a total flow higher than the patient's respiratory minute volume. The constant flow of oxygen-anesthetic mixture assures the exhalation of respiratory gases through the expiratory limb.

The addition of the reservoir tube is employed in the system to eliminate the dilution of the oxygen-anesthetic mixture with room air during inspiration. The total capacity of the reservoir should be approximately one-third of the animal's tidal volume. The internal diameter of the reservoir should be at least 1 cm; therefore, a piece of tubing 2.5 cm long will contain 2.5 ml of gas. The tidal volume of 2- to 4-kg cats under anesthesia varies between 12 and 25 ml; therefore, the expiratory arm should be between 4 and 8 cm long.

This reservoir can potentially increase the anatomical dead space by providing an area for the accumulation of exhaled carbon dioxide. To prevent rebreathing and assure the proper elimination of carbon dioxide, the size of the reservoir and flow of gas necessary to flush out the system should be considered. The flow of gas into the system should be approximately 2 times the respiratory minute volume.[2, 4] This assures proper flushing of carbon dioxide from the expiratory limb. The respiratory minute volume of cats (2 to 4 kg) under anesthesia is 200 to 1000 ml/minute; this dictates a flow of about 400 to 2000 ml/minute. For most cats, the flows are maintained at 1 to 1.5 liters/minute, and these are increased or decreased slightly depending upon the size of the animal.

A modification involves the addition of a breathing bag which results in a greater capacity in the reservoir tube (Figs. 17.3 and 17.7).[14] This addition adds the capacity of administering positive pressure ventilation. The dilution of inspired gases cannot occur because of the increased capacity of the reservoir, but rebreathing can. To prevent rebreathing, the fresh flow of gas should be at least 2 times the respiratory minute volume. The Kuhn apparatus is an excellent adaptation of this modification and can be used both with a mask or with an endotracheal tube. The fresh gas inlet to the mask is placed close to the patient's nose, and, by this means, removes the exhaled gases (Fig. 17.3).

Ayre's original technique has also been modified by eliminating the reservoir tube (Fig. 17.6, *bottom*).[16] The exhaled gases are eliminated through a hole at the end of the endotracheal tube, which is equal to the internal diameter of the endotracheal tube. With a fresh flow of 2.5 times the respiratory minute volume, approximately 25% of the inspired gas will be room air. This dilution does not prevent the maintence of adequate levels of anesthesia. If the standard "Y" piece is not available, this modification can be easily made. To prevent any dilution of the oxygen-anesthetic agent with room air, 5 times the respiratory minute volume is required in this modification.[16]

The Ayre original method or its modifications are recommended only for animals under 4 to 6 kg. Larger dogs require higher gas flows through the system to provide adequate concentrations of anesthetic agent. The higher flows needed for the larger animals can create an increase in resistance to respiration because of the narrow diameter of the "Y" piece. In small patients, the system is economical because relatively low flows can be used.

THE MAGILL CIRCUIT

The Magill circuit, devised by Sir Ivan Magill, consists of a breathing bag, a length of corrugated tubing, a fresh gas inlet, and a one-way valve adjacent to the patient (Figs. 17.8 and 17.9A). It can be considered a semiopen system[8] and is similar in its application to the Ayre method. As in the Ayre method, fresh gas flows are used to eliminate carbon dioxide; the basic difference is the use of one valve and the direction of flow of the fresh gases.

In the Magill circuit, the fresh gases enter into the distal segment of the system and leave through an exhalation valve at the face piece or endotracheal tube. With this arrangement, the Magill circuit will prevent rebreathing, with a fresh gas flow less than the patient's respiratory minute volume.[15] The efficiency of the system is based on the location of the exhalation valve and less mixing between the exhaled gas and fresh gas. The gas which is initially exhaled is anatomical dead space gas, and is identical in composition with the fresh gas. The remainder of the exhaled gas is alveolar gas, which has been in contact with the gas exchange portions of the lung; the rebreathing of this gas will raise alveolar and arterial carbon dioxide tensions (Fig. 17.9B). Purging of the system begins toward the end of exhalation. At this point in the respiratory cycle, the breathing bag is filling, and the pressure in the system is elevated sufficiently to open the exhalation valve. The fresh gas flow purges the system of alveolar gas. In theory, only the anatomical dead space gas has to be replaced with fresh gas flow to adequately remove exhaled carbon dioxide (Fig. 17.9C). The fresh gas flow necessary to remove the alveolar gas, therefore, must be correlated with the patient's alveolar ventilation and not with respiratory minute volume.[18] Because of this, the fresh gas flows necessary are smaller than measured respiratory minute volumes. There is inherent difficulty in attempting to equate fresh gas flows to body weight because of the variation in ventilation in patients of similar weight when under anesthesia. However, fresh gas flows of between 500 and 600 ml/minute are sufficient to prevent rebreathing in cats between 2 and 4 kg. Understandably, as respiratory rate in-

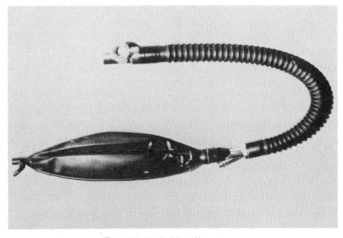

FIG. 17.8. A Magill system.

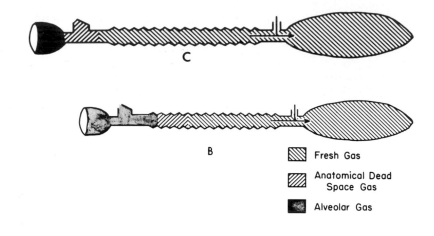

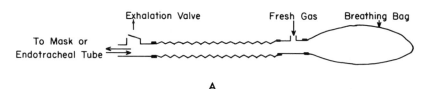

FIG. 17.9. *A*, schematic representation of the Magill system. The fresh gas flow for the removal of CO_2 is opposite in direction to the Ayre system. It enters into the distal portion of the system and leaves through the exhalation valve. *B*, composition of gas in various segments of the Magill circuit during early exhalation. The initial gas exhaled is anatomical dead space gas, which is identical in composition with the fresh gas. The flow of gas at this point is toward the breathing bag; as the breathing bag fills, the exhalation valve opens and the flow of gas is out the valve, purging the system. *C*, the most economical flow would be the replacement of the anatomical dead space gas by the fresh gas flow, thereby purging the alveolar gas from the system. (Adopted in part from Kain and Nunn.[15])

creases, a rise in respiratory minute volume can be anticipated. A greater fresh gas flow may be needed because of the possible increase in alveolar ventilation, but more importantly, the exhalation pause is so short that high fresh gas flows are necessary to flush out the alveolar carbon dioxide prior to inhalation.

The Magill system, like the Ayre system, is well suited for the small patients. As with the Ayre method, it is simple, cheap, and easy to clean. It is not well suited for controlled ventilation, as two hands are necessary, one for compressions of the bag and the second for occluding the exhalation valve. If adequate spontaneous ventilation is anticipated, it is an excellent method for the delivery of anes-

thetic agents. As for other semiopen methods, halothane, methoxyflurane, and nitrous oxide are well suited and similar concentrations are employed.

SEMIOPEN SYSTEM AND MASKS

Masks which conform to the facial structures of cats, small dogs, and laboratory animals can be used with the semiopen systems (Figs. 17.3 and 17.10). For the induction of inhalation anesthesia in smaller animals, this is an excellent method. If the mask conforms somewhat to the facial contours and the gas flows are adequate, the additional respiratory dead space created by the mask can be minimized. In both the semiopen and the nonrebreathing systems, the concentration of the anesthetic agent can be more easily controlled than the rebreathing systems. In these systems, the exhaled gases are expelled into the room and not rebreathed; therefore, the concentration delivered from the vaporizer and the inhaled concentration are the same.

USE OF THE SEMIOPEN SYSTEMS

The mask can be an effective and relatively safe method for the induction and also the maintenance of anesthesia in many small species and in very young animals. Some of the basic principles of the open drop method also apply to the use of the mask. The patient should be restrained as gently as possible and the mask placed near the face. The initial concentration should be low, and then gradually increased as the initial sedating effects are apparent.

A variety of anesthetic agents can be used, particularly halothane, methoxyflurane, and nitrous oxide. Halothane and methoxyflurane can be used alone or in combination with nitrous oxide. Nitrous oxide is odorless and is supplied as a compressed gas (see Chapter 10). It can provide a good base for volatile anesthetic agents, especially when a mask is being used for the induction of anesthesia. The anesthetic agent which induces sedation and anesthesia rapidly (nitrous oxide, halothane, and methoxyflurane, in that

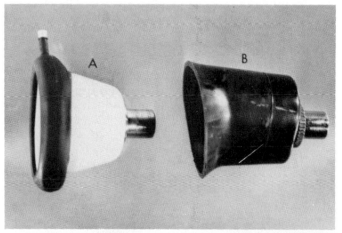

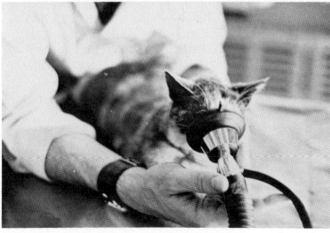

Fig. 17.10. Two types of masks developed especially for cats. *A*, opaque hard plastic mask developed by the Fraser Sweatman Company, Lancaster, N.Y. *B*, hard rubber low dead space mask. (From Mann, P. E. G., and Boretos, J. W.: Laboratory animal care *18:* 657, 1968.)

order) will be the most effective and facilitates the easy induction of anesthesia. Nitrous oxide (75%) and oxygen (25%) is used as the base for the addition of halothane or methoxyflurane. Nitrous oxide-oxygen is started and 0.25% halothane is added and increased by 0.5% increments to 2 to 4%. The rapidity by which the inspired concentration is increased is determined by the animal's reactions to be induction of anesthesia. The maintenance concentration of halothane is approximately 1 to 2.5%, varying with the condition of the patient, preanesthetic medication, and whether nitrous oxide is used. The induction concentrations of methoxyflurane are between 0.5 and 1.5%, and the maintenance is between 0.25 and 0.75%. Anesthesia can be maintained with the mask, or the patient's trachea can be intubated and anesthesia continued with the endotracheal tube. Ultrashort acting barbiturates can be used to speed the induction of anesthesia followed by the inhalation agents.

Nonrebreathing Method

The nonrebreathing method utilizes a set of valves which allows inspiration from a breathing bag (reservoir) and exhalation directly into the atmosphere (Fig. 17.11). If the valves are competent, the only rebreathing which occurs is of the gas contained within the dead space of the valve. The basic design is an inhalation and an exhalation valve incorporated into a metal or plastic tube or mask.[27] These systems have been designed primarily for pediatric anesthesia and therefore can be used for smaller patients in animal anesthesia; several types are available (Fig. 17.12).

There are several primary advantages. (a) The resistance to gas flow is low because of the light weight, and animals with smaller tidal volumes and low inspiratory force can move them easily. (b) The valvular dead space is small and adds little to the anatomical dead space. (c) Compared to the rebreathing system, there is a moment to moment control of the inspired concentration of the anesthetic agent. (d) The nonrebreathing method is economically feasible in the small species, since the respiratory minute volumes are relatively small and only low gas flows are necessary. (e) There is good elimination of carbon dioxide if the valves are competent.

After the induction of anesthesia either with a mask or an ultrashort acting barbiturate and intubation of the trachea, the valve is attached to the endotracheal tube and flow of gas equal to or slightly higher than the animal's respiratory minute volume is added continously to the breathing bag, as judged by watching the bag. If it collapses, the respiratory minute volume of the patient is higher than the delivered gas and should be increased. The fresh gas flow requirements in a 2.5-kg cat or dog are approximately 700 ml. Compared to the semiopen system, the valves prevent the exhaled gases from entering the breathing bag and a flow of gas sufficient to flush out the exhaled gases is not necessary; low gas flows are used.

One of the disadvantages of the nonrebreathing method is the inability of the

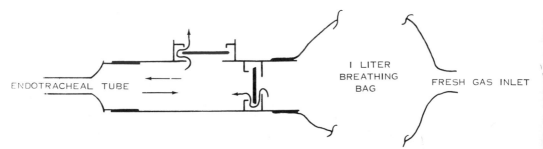

FIG. 17.11. Schematic representation of the Digby-Leigh pediatric nonrebreathing valve and breathing bag. (Courtesy of Clifford and Soma.[6])

system to compensate for a sudden increase in ventilation. If this occurs, the bag will be sucked empty by the increased ventilatory effort of the animal. Maintaining the flow of gas slightly above the actual needs of the patient will prevent this.

The valve resistance is so low that gas from an overfilled bag will leak out through the valve system. A slight positive valve leak is an advantage and will flush out the small dead space between the valves.

Many of these valves are not spring-loaded, and are dependent upon gravity for the closure of the exhalation valve. Periodic inspection of these valves is essential, since they are attached to an endotracheal tube, and mucus can accumulate on the valves, preventing their free movement. Rubber valves will degenerate with time due to the accumulation of moisture and the action of inhalation agents on rubber. It is wise to maintain an extra set of valves for replacement.

The nonrebreathing valves can also be incorporated into a small mask. The feline mask with a breathing bag added can be used to induce and maintain general anesthesia in a cat or small dog without intubation of the trachea (Fig. 17.13).

The basic difference between the semiopen and the nonrebreathing system is the method of preventing the rebreathing of exhaled gases. Both systems are applicable to smaller species of both laboratory and companion animals. Figure 17.14 illustrates the use of the "Y" piece in a lemur. When using the semiopen system, the size of the animal and not the specific

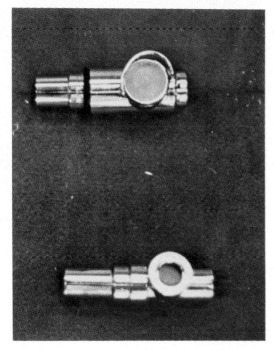

FIG. 17.12. The Digby-Leigh (*bottom*) and the Stephen-Slatter (*top*) nonrebreathing pediatric valves.

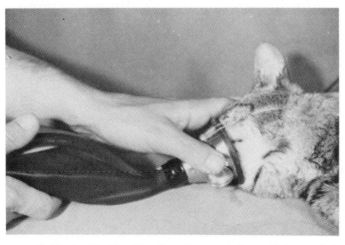

FIG. 17.13. Trimar mask fitted with breathing bag. Oxygen and anesthetic are being supplied through the tail of the bag. Inhalation and exhalation valves are part of the mask. (Courtesy of Clifford and Soma.[6])

species of animal determines the method which is most applicable. The end of the "Y" piece can also be used as a mask when the animal to be anesthetized is very small (Fig. 17.15). Most masks which have been developed for cats can be used for rabbits and large guinea pigs (Fig. 17.16). The anesthetic agents and the concentrations discussed in the previous section are applicable here.

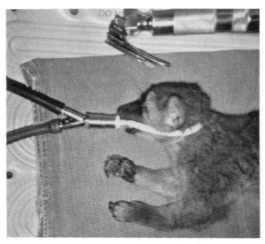

FIG. 17.14. Use of the "Y" piece in a lemur. Anesthesia can be induced with a mask followed by tracheal intubation.

Rebreathing System (Closed and Semiclosed)

In the rebreathing systems, all or part of the animal's exhaled gases are passed back into the system. The differentiation between a completely closed system and the partially closed (semiclosed) is determined primarily by the inflow of fresh gases.

In the semiclosed rebreathing system, part of the animal's exhaled gases is passed back into the system and part escapes into the atmosphere. The amount of exhaled gas which is returned to the system and through the canister for the removal of carbon dioxide is determined for the most part by the inflow of fresh gases. As the fresh gas flow being delivered to the circuit is reduced, the rebreathing system approaches a closed system where more of the exhaled gases, after the removal of carbon dioxide, is inhaled and reused. A closed system has been defined as one with no leaks into which only fresh gas in amounts necessary to supply the animal's metabolic needs is added.[7] In veterinary anesthesia, this can vary a great deal because of the difference in patient size. Two rebreathing systems are used, the circle and the to and fro (Figs.

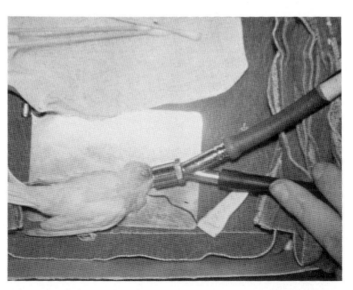

FIG. 17.15. The "Y" piece is being used both as a mask and as an anesthetic delivery system in this small bird.

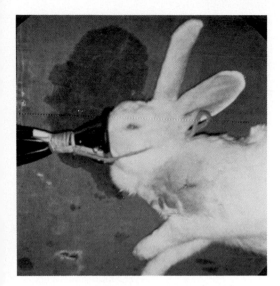

FIG. 17.16. Feline mask is easily applied for the anesthetization of rabbits.

17.17 and 17.20). The circle system is the one most used in both veterinary and human anesthesia, as compared to the to and fro system which has many disadvantages and is not as versatile.

THE CIRCLE SYSTEM

The circle system, regardless of its size or shape, has the following components (Fig. 17.17): (a) a rebreathing or reservoir bag; (b) a canister containing an alkaline earth for the absorption of carbon dioxide; (c) a dome or "Y" piece valves to produce a unidirectional flow of gas; (d) breathing tubes; (e) an inlet for fresh gases; and (f) a "pop off" valve (may be spring-loaded) to allow the escape of excess gases from the circle.

The rebreathing bag, in the absence of high fresh gas flows or a demand valve, is

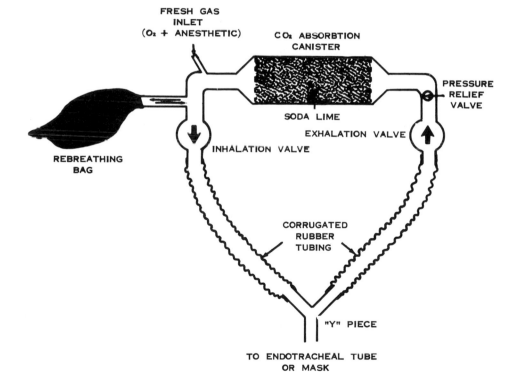

CIRCLE — TYPE REBREATHING SYSTEM

FIG. 17.17. Schematic representation of a rebreathing circle system. (Courtesy of Soma, L. R., and Klide, A. M.: Techniques and equipment for inahalation anesthesia in small animals. J. Amer. Vet. Med. Ass. *152:* 957, 1968.)

a reservoir of gas from which the animal must obtain its tidal volume. The bag is refilled during exhalation by the animal's exhaled volume and by oxygen and other gases from the anesthesia machine. Regardless of oxygen flow into the circuit, the rebreathing bag will provide the animal's respiratory minute volume. A 3-liter bag is generally sufficient for small animal use.

The process of CO_2 absorption is a chemical reaction taking place within the CO_2 absorber.[1] The basic reaction is a combination of CO_2 and water to form carbonic acid, which, in turn, reacts with the hydroxides of alkaline metals. The final product is sodium and/or calcium carbonate, water, and heat. There are two absorbents commercially used; Soda lime (a mixture of barium and calcium hydroxide) and Baralyme. Both absorbents contain a pH-sensitive indicator which will denote the exhaustion of absorbing activity. The absorbents should be checked after active use because the indicator will revert to their original color upon standing. Absorbents with remaining activity will easily crumble when rolled between the fingers; exhausted Soda lime or Baralyme will be hard and brittle, indicating its conversion to the harder carbonates. Improper canister construction or poor

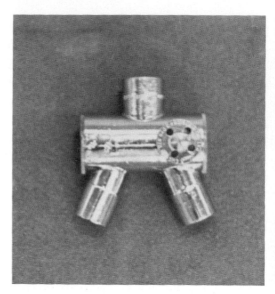

FIG. 17.19. "Y" piece valve for the Bloomquist circle.

packing will decrease the efficiency of carbon dioxide absorption.[10, 11]

A few simple rules should be followed when filling a canister with lime.[21] (a) Soda lime should not be poured through a small orifice as this will cause fragmentation of the granules. (b) The canister should be tapped gently after lime has been added. This aids in filling the canister completely and removes any alkaline dust. (c) Reseal supply stocks of absorbent to prevent drying, because the moisture content is important in the absorption reaction. (d) Do not fill the canister with an excessively dusty absorbent.

Valves are an essential part of the circle system, and most of the resistance in the system is created by them. Two valves are incorporated in the system to create a unidirectional flow of gas. There are generally two types: dome valves, which are placed on the circle (Fig. 17.18), and "Y" piece valves (Fig. 17.19), which are incorporated into the endotracheal tube connector. The dome valves are generally preferable to the "Y" piece valves, as they are easier to maintain, easily visualized, and any malfunction can be quickly noted. Dome valves are made of plastic or

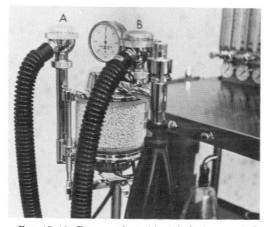

FIG. 17.18. Dome valves (A, inhalation, and B, exhalation) on a circle system suitable for veterinary anesthesia.

mica, making them less subject to the corrosive action of anesthetics.

The body of the "Y" valve is made of plastic or metal, and the flaps usually are of rubber. The disadvantages of "Y" piece valves are numerous, and they are not recommended unless well maintained and periodically inspected. When made of rubber, they are more subject to the corrosive action of anesthetics. Because of their proximity to the endotracheal tube, rubber or plastic valves will become caked with mucus, making them sticky. Their position and construction does not allow easy inspection of valves and valve seats, and some, if not positioned properly, may not completely close or open due to gravitational forces.

The sticky valves increase the resistance to respiration and the work of breathing, and incompetence valves allow the inhalation of exhaled gases. The circle system will not complete the function of removing carbon dioxide if one valve is missing or remains in the open position. High concentrations or carbon dioxide can develop.

The diameter of corrugated breathing tubes on circle systems is either 1.9 cm (equipment designed for adult usage) or 1.3 cm (pediatric size). Both sizes are used in equipment designed or adapted for veterinary use.

The fresh gas inlet on the circle system is generally placed directly on the canister or on the inhalation side. The "pop off" valve, depending upon the circle design, is generally located on the exhalation portion of the circle canister or the "Y" piece. Because they are spring-loaded, some of the "pop-off" valves may impose a resistance to exhalation in very small animals. Valves are available which will "pop off" at pressures of less than 1 cm of water. The tail of the rebreathing bag can be used in place of a "pop off" valve by partially clamping it with a butterfly clamp.

TO AND FRO SYSTEM

In the to and fro technique, the gases pass back and forth through the carbon dioxide absorber instead of in a circular pattern. No valves are necessary, and it is the most efficient method for the absorption of carbon dioxide, since the gases pass through the canister twice (Fig. 17.20). The main advantages are the small resistance offered to respiration because of the absence of valves and the ease of cleaning. Disadvantages of the system preclude its value for routine use. The accumulation of heat is greater in this system because the canister is directly attached to the endotracheal tube and the warm gases from the canister are inhaled directly. This is a potential hazard in animals which depend upon the respiratory system for the dissipation of heat. The inhalation of alkaline dust is always a possibility, and channeling of gases through the canister is more likely because of its horizontal position.

To minimize dead space, the canister must be attached directly to the endotracheal tube with no intermediate attachments. The canister dead space increases with time because of the exhaustion of the activity of the absorbent at the end close to the patient. This portion of the absorbent, when exhausted, is no longer absorbing carbon dioxide and is additive to the anatomical dead space. This disadvantage

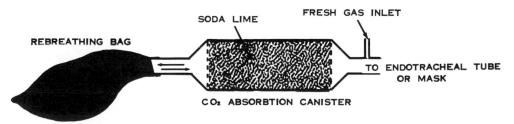

FIG. 17.20. Schematic representation of the to and fro rebreathing system.

can be minimized by turning the canister at intervals or choosing a canister which more easily nearly matches the animal's tidal volume. This requires a series of canisters for various size animals.

The Position of the Vaporizer in Relation to the Circle

There are two locations for the placement of the vaporizer in relation to the circle: outside the circle (VOC) and in the circle (VIC) (Fig. 17.21). In the outside the circle position, the oxygen is passed through the vaporizer and the oxygen anesthetic mixture is delivered to the circle. In the in the circle position, the vaporizer is placed within the circle and the animal's tidal volume is utilized to vaporize the volatile anesthetic. There are differences in the concentrations attained within the circle when each of the two methods of vaporization is employed.

From a practical standpoint, the out of the circle technique is a more versatile

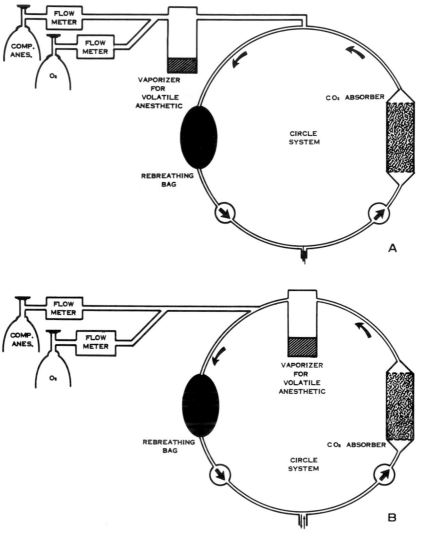

Fig. 17.21. Schematic representation of anesthetic system with the vaporizer out of the circle (VOC) and vaporizer inside the circle (VIC). (Courtesy of Soma, L. R., and Klide, A. M.: Techniques and equipment for inhalation anesthesia in small animals. J. Amer. Vet. Med. Ass. *152:* 957, 1968.)

TABLE 17.2

Comparison of vaporizer outside (VOC) and inside (VIC) the breathing circuit

Ventilation	
VOC	VIC
Changes in ventilation will not affect the output of the vaporizer.	An increase in ventilation due to light anesthesia will automatically increase the inspired concentration.
An increase in ventilation will reduce inspired concentration because of an increased uptake of anesthetic agent by the animal and a constant output of the vaporizer.	Sudden changes in ventilation can produce dangerously high inspired concentrations.
Assisted or controlled ventilation can be used with a greater degree of safety.	Assisted or controlled ventilation at any given setting will greatly increase inspired concentrations.
Fresh Gas Flow	
For any setting, the lower the fresh gas flow, the lower will be the inspired concentration in relation to the concentration being delivered from the vaporizer. The lower the fresh gas flow, the greater the economy.	For any setting, the lower the fresh gas flow, the higher the inspired concentration.
	The lower the fresh gas flow, the greater the economy.
Economy does not introduce the risk of high concentrations.	Economy is at the expense of potentially high inspired concentrations.
Vaporizer	
High efficiency vaporizers are essential.	Low efficiency vaporizers can be used.
Known concentrations can be delivered to the breathing circuit, and an estimate of the inspired concentration can be made with no difficulty.	Calibrated vaporizers are meaningless because ventilation affects the inspired concentration to a marked degree.

system, as vaporizers and circles can be interchanged and a rebreathing system can be easily converted to a nonrebreathing or a semiopen system by simply detaching the delivery hose from the circle. Another advantage is that water vapor from the animal's water-saturated breath cannot condense in the vaporizer and no contamination of the vaporizer from pulmonary disease will occur. There are four factors which determine the concentration of the volatile anesthetic in the rebreathing system: (a) the animal's ventilation; (b) fresh gas flow into the system; (c) vaporizer in use; and (d) anesthetic uptake by the animal. Assuming a constant removal of anesthetic agent regardless of the type of system used, the final three factors will be discussed in relationship to VOC and VIC (Table 17.2).[17, 20]

Vaporizers inside the Circle

VENTILATION

When the vaporizer is placed within the circle, the animal's ventilation controls the vaporization of the anesthetic agent and a draw over type of vaporizer is used (see Chapter 16). As ventilation increases, the flow of gas through the vaporizer increases, and the concentration of anesthetic rises. Doubling the ventilation will double the inspired concentration of anesthetic.[17, 20] This can become serious if breathing is vigorous, and high inspiratory levels of anesthesia are created. Serious cardiac and respiratory depression can occur rapidly. A more common danger is when the animal is artificially ventilated. Manual compression of the rebreathing bag is, in effect, creating a higher gas flow through the vaporizer, producing a higher inspired concentration. Back pressurization of the vaporizer is also a factor (see Chapter 16). Unless the control setting is markedly reduced, extremely high levels of anesthetic vapor will be produced. This is illustrated in Figure 17.22: as the respiratory minute volume of the patient increases, there is a major increase in the inspired concentration of halothane. The fresh gas flows into the circuit, and the tap settings remain the same.[17]

The opposite effect can occur (an inadequate concentration of anesthetic agent) if a very small animal with a low tidal volume is placed on the system. The ventilation may be so small that the flow of gas through the vaporizer may be insufficient to vaporize adequate quantities of anesthetic agent. This is more likely to occur with anesthetic agents such as methoxyflurane which has a low vapor pressure.

The vaporization of an anesthetic agent being dependent upon the ventilation of the patient, in theory, may seem desirable. This concept is referred to as autoregulation, and implies that as ventilation

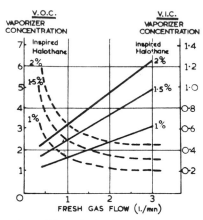

FIG. 17.23. The relationship of the inspired concentration of a volatile agent and fresh gas flow in both the VIC and the VOC. (Courtesy of Mushin and Galloon.[20])

increases due to a lighter level of anesthesia, the increase in ventilation and the subsequent increase in inspired concentration will result in deepening of anesthesia. The risk inherent in this system is the danger of a sudden vigorous respiratory effort or controlled ventilation.

FRESH GAS FLOW

With the vaporizer placed inside the circuit, the inspired concentration of anesthetic increases as the oxygen entering the system is reduced (Fig. 17.23). When the fresh gas flow is increased, the inspired concentrations decrease. This is understandable, because the greater the fresh gas flow in relation to the metabolic needs of the animal, the greater is the amount of exhaled gas which will be discharged through the "pop off" at each breath. As the system approaches a closed system, the inspired concentration will increase at any vaporizer setting. Regardless of the fresh gas flow, the inspired concentration will progressively increase because of the repassage of exhaled gases containing anesthetic vapor through the vaporizer and the decreased anesthetic uptake by the body. When the concentration is to be reduced, the vaporizer is turned off and the fresh gas flow is increased as an aid in a more rapid removal of the anesthetic agent from the system.

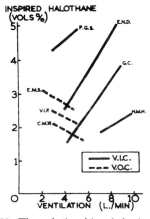

FIG. 17.22. The relationship of the inspired concentration of a volatile agent and ventilation in both the VIC and VOC. (Courtesy of Mushin and Galloon.[20])

VAPORIZERS

Not all vaporizers are satisfactory for the VIC system. High efficiency vaporizers such as the Vapor or Fluotec are only designed as plenum vaporizers (see Chapter 16). The lower resistance "draw over" vaporizers are generally used, but still should be used with caution. For example, a vaporizer with maximum delivered concentration of 1.5% halothane (Goldman vaporizer) when placed in a VIC position can deliver an inspired concentration of 7.5% halothane.[20] Under these circumstances, a low efficiency vaporizer still delivers a too potent concentration for safe use. Potent, easily vaporized agents such as halothane should not be used in conjunction with in the circuit vaporizers. Agents such as diethyl ether and methoxyflurane have been used with greater safety in this system. Methoxyflurane, despite its high potency, can be used with some safety because of its low vapor pressure; unfortunately, when controlled ventilation is used, dangerous concentrations can be delivered. Diethyl ether has been used for many years in the VIC system. Its lower potency adds a margin of safety despite high volatility.

The trend is toward the use of calibrated vaporizers which can deliver a known concentration of a volatile agent over a prolonged period. The VIC defeats this concept in that changes in ventilation and the changes in the exhaled concentration will make the calibrations on the vaporizer useless or at best only a gross approximation.

Vaporizers outside the Circle

VENTILATION

With the vaporizer outside the circle, changes in ventilation will not affect the concentration delivered from vaporizer. The gas flow through the vaporizer in this case is determined by the anesthetist, not by the patient's ventilation. When ventilation increases, the inspired concentration will actually decrease (Figs. 17.22 and 17.24). As ventilation increases, there is an increase in alveolar ventilation with a subsequent increase in the uptake of the anesthetic by the pulmonary blood and a decrease in the concentration in the circle system. In contrast to the VIC, the output of the vaporizer remains the same in the VOC. As ventilation increases, the in-

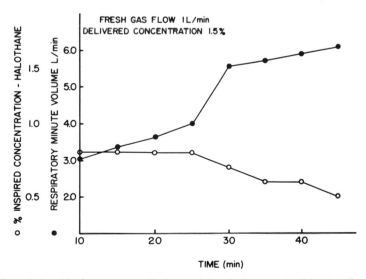

FIG. 17.24. The relationship between ventilation and inspired concentration at a fixed delivered anesthetic concentration and fresh gas flow in a 17-kg dog. As ventilation increases, a drop in inspired concentration occurs. Because of the low fresh gas flow in this large dog, the inspired concentration is considerably lower than the delivered concentration.

spired concentration will decrease as the anesthetic uptake increases.

Despite the increase in the arterial concentration of the anesthetic agent, the overall effect of increased ventilation on the level of anesthesia in the VOC is less in magnitude than a comparable change in the VIC.[17] This means that assisted or controlled ventilation can be utilized with a greater degree of safety, and there is less fear of a marked increase in inspired concentration. Because the patient's ventilation plays no part in the vaporization of the anesthetic agent, a more accurate estimate of the inspired concentration can be made.

FRESH GAS FLOW

In VOC the inspired concentration during the induction and maintenance of anesthesia may approach the concentration being delivered from the vaporizer but is not higher. The change in inspired concentration in the VOC is directly opposite to the VIC: the higher the fresh gas flow from the vaporizer, the more rapidly the inspired concentration approaches the concentration being delivered from the vaporizer (Fig. 17.23).

This can be more easily understood if the following is considered. The exhaled concentration, because of continuous extraction of the anesthetic agent by body tissues, is lower than the inspired concentration; therefore, the gas contained within the circle at each exhalation is being diluted by a gas containing a lesser amount of anesthetic vapor. The maintenance of an inspired concentration equal to the delivered concentration is dependent upon the rapidity by which this dilution is replaced by the incoming gas. This can be easily equated if grams of vapor or milliliters of liquid agent are considered instead of volume percent. At a concentration of 1% and a fresh gas flow of 2 liters/minute, the equivalent in anesthetic vapor of 5 ml of halothane per hour will be delivered to the anesthesia circuit (Fig. 17.25). When the flow is reduced to 1 liter/minute, a concentration of 2% halothane is necessary to deliver an equal amount of halothane. Therefore, the inspired concentration necessary to maintain an adequate plane of anesthesia can be provided by a higher volume percent at a lower gas flow, or a lower percentage at a higher rate of gas flow.

As the fresh gas flow is increased in the VOC, there is a greater turnover of gas

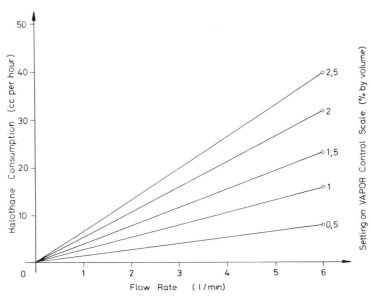

FIG. 17.25. The amount of consumption in milliliters of liquid halothane at various fresh gas flows through the Vapor vaporizer at various concentration settings. (Courtesy of North American Dräger, Telford, Pa.)

within the circle, and the inspired concentration more rapidly approaches the concentration being delivered from the vaporizer. This is one reason for increasing the fresh gas flows during the initial anesthetic period, which is an aid in a more rapid induction of anesthesia.

VAPORIZERS

High efficiency, precision vaporizers are recommended for the VOC circuit (see Chapter 16). Vaporizers for volatile agents have been developed which will deliver known concentrations for prolonged periods of time. Vaporizers which will deliver 4 to 5% halothane and 2 to 2.5% methoxyflurane are advised for the VOC system, which enables the maintenance of an adequate inspired concentration, even at low fresh gas flows.

Fresh Gas Flows in the Rebreathing System

The rebreathing system can be used as a closed (minimal oxygen flows) or semiclosed system (high oxygen flows). In the completely closed system, only the patient's minimum metabolic needs of oxygen and anesthetic are being delivered, and all exhaled gas minus the removed carbon dioxide is rebreathed. As the fresh gas flow containing oxygen or oxygen and other gaseous agents delivered to the anesthetic machine-lung system exceeds the needs of the patient, the system is no longer completely closed, but is semiclosed. Under these conditions, not all of the oxygen-anesthetic mixture is being "taken up" by the patient and the excess is being discharged or "popped off" into the room by the "pop off" valve. The term semiclosed only indicates that the fresh gas flow is greater than the needs of the patient, and, when describing the system, the flows being used and the size of the patient should be indicated.[9]

The volume of fresh gas delivered to the patient per minute through the rebreathing system has many functions. (a) It supplies the oxygen requirements of the patient resulting from metabolic needs and leakage through poor connections. (b) It

is used to deliver induction and maintenance concentrations of anesthetic agents. (c) It will wash out nitrogen or other gas from the lung and breathing circuit.[8]

FRESH GAS FLOW AND OXYGEN
REQUIREMENTS

The amount of rebreathing is determined by the relationship of the fresh gas flow delivered to the anesthetic machine-patient system and by the patient's ventilation and oxygen consumption. If the fresh gas flow equals the patient's respiratory minute volume, little or no rebreathing will occur, and the system almost functions as a nonrebreathing system. This is important in veterinary patients because of the great variation in size. For example, the respiratory minute volume of a 5-kg dog under anesthesia would approximate 600 ml, with a fresh gas flow of 600 ml/minute, little or no rebreathing would occur. On the other hand, the respiratory minute volume of a 50-kg dog would approach 5 liters, and with similar fresh gas flows (600 ml/minute) almost complete rebreathing of exhaled gases occurs. In both cases, adequate amounts of oxygen are being delivered; in one case, in great excess of metabolic needs and in the other, minimal amounts. The approximate oxygen needs must be considered in establishing flows necessary for various size patients.

The oxygen consumption of the smaller dog approximates 50 ml/minute, and with a fresh gas flow of 600 ml/minute 550 ml of the fresh gas being discharged into the room. In this small dog, the oxygen consumption is only 10% of the fresh gas flows. On the other hand, the oxygen consumption of the larger dog is in the range of 550 ml, and over 90% of the delivered oxygen is used for the animal's metabolic needs; rebreathing is maximal and the oxygen flows being delivered barely match the patient's metabolic requirements.

The minimal amount of fresh gas flow containing oxygen which can be delivered to the rebreathing system is determined primarily by the metabolic needs of the patient and loss through the leakage in the system. When nitrous oxide is used in conjunction with volatile anesthetic agents, the flows of oxygen in proportion to nitrous oxide must be such that the metabolic requirements of the animal are met. In the examples cited, both fresh gas flows of oxygen are in excess of the metabolic requirements of the patient, and both are satisfactory. The exact oxygen consumption of the patient is generally not known and cannot be easily calculated, and from a clinical use point of view, such information is not necessary. However, it does point out the fact that the flows of gas delivered to the rebreathing system should be chosen with some appreciation of the range of the oxygen requirements of the veterinary patients.

The economic aspects of the system would dictate that lower flows would be the most advantageous, but two other functions of the fresh gas flow, delivery of adequate volumes of anesthetic vapor and

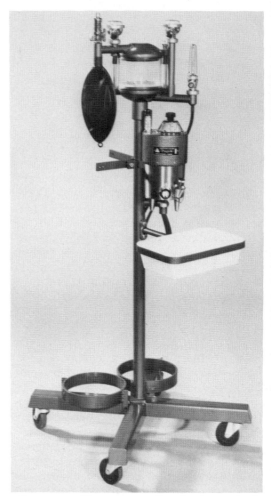

FIG. 17.27. Narcovet small animal anesthesia machine. (Courtesy of North American Dräger.)

denitrogenation also must be considered especially during the induction phases of anesthesia. These two aspects of fresh gas flow mandate higher initial fresh gas flows for the induction of anesthesia which can be followed by lower flows for the maintenance of anesthesia.

DELIVERY OF ADEQUATE CONCENTRATIONS OF VAPOR

In the use of the semiopen and the nonrebreathing system, a change in the delivered concentration of the agent from the vaporizer or flowmeter will alter the inspired concentration within a few breaths. As discussed in previous sections, the in-

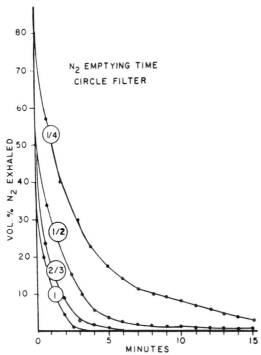

FIG. 17.26. Curve showing denitrogenation from a healthy volunteer breathing oxygen from a circle system. The series of curves show denitrogenation at the volunteer's minute volume (1) and ¼, ½, and ⅔ of minute volume. (Courtesy of Miles, et al.[19])

spired concentrations and delivery concentrations are similar. In the rebreathing system, because of the internal volume of the system, changes in the concentration of anesthetic agents delivered from the vaporizer or flowmeter will not immediately be reflected in a change in the inspired concentration. The relationship of the inspired concentration to the delivered concentration will be dependent upon the volume of the circle and the patient's ventilation, the fresh gas flow into the system, and the placement of the vaporizer in relationship to the circle (VIC or VOC). These factors have been discussed in the sections entitled "Vaporizers inside the Circle" and "Vaporizers outside

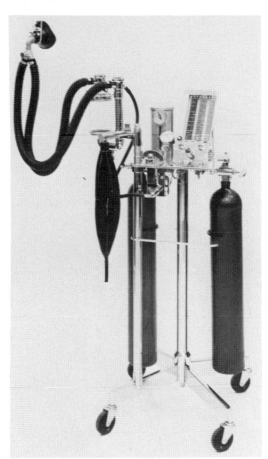

FIG. 17.29. Foregger Compact "50." (Courtesy of Foregger Company, Smithtown, N.Y.)

the Circle," but are worthy of a brief repetition.

When the vaporizer is placed outside of the circle, the higher the fresh gas flow and the higher the patient's ventilation, the more rapid will be the turnover or equilibration time in the rebreathing circuit. Under these circumstances, the inspired concentration will more rapidly approach the concentration being delivered to the system. Again equating this to our previous examples, the delivered concentration necessary to maintain an inspired concentration of 1.25% in the 5-kg dog may be only slightly higher, whereas in the larger dog (with the lower gas flows), a delivered concentration of 2.5 to 3% may be necessary to maintain an adequate inspired concentration. This is well

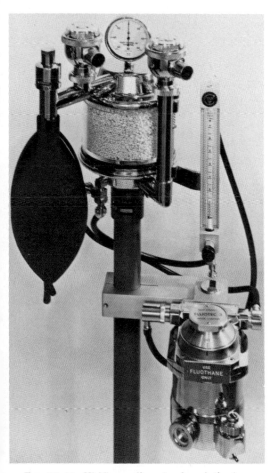

FIG. 17.28. VMS small animal anesthesia machine. (Courtesy of Fraser Sweatman, Lancaster, N.Y.)

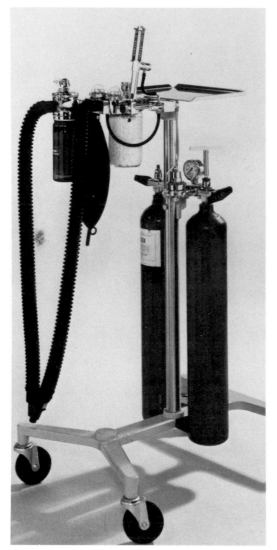

Fig. 17.30. Pitman Moore model 960 small animal machine. This model contains an in the circuit vaporizer for ether or methoxyflurane. (Courtesy of Pitman Moore Company, Fort Washington, Pa.)

demonstrated in equine anesthesia. Following the induction of anesthesia, a semiclosed system with low flows is used with fresh gas flow of oxygen of 2 to 2.5 liters/minute, which is about equal to the horses's metabolic needs. The vaporizer concentration of halothane necessary to maintain general anesthesia is between 2.5 and 3%; the measured inspired con-

centration approaches 1.0 within the first hour.

The relationship of fresh gas flow and inspired concentration is reversed when the vaporizer is placed within the circle. The higher the fresh gas flow, the lower is the inspired concentration. In the VIC system, alterations in ventilation have a greater effect on the inspired concentration than the VOC.

DENITROGENATION

Denitrogenation is the process of eliminating nitrogen from the lung and body tissues by breathing a gas not containing nitrogen. In the semiopen and nonrebreathing systems, denitrogenation is rapid because of exhalation of the patient's respiratory volume into the room. Under these circumstances, the phase of lung denitrogenation occurs within 2 to 3 minutes.[13] Denitrogenation of slowly perfused tissue such as bone, fat, hollow organs, and tendonous tissue is much slower, but for all practical purposes only the lung, blood, and highly perfused tissues are considered. In the rebreathing systems, denitrogenation is accomplished by initial high gas flows or by periodic flushing of the system during the induction of anesthesia. The removal of nitrogen from the rebreathing system is of concern when weak anesthetic agents such as nitrous oxide are used in a semiclosed system. The system must be denitrogenated to minimize the dilution of oxygen with the anesthetic agent and nitrogen.

When using more potent anesthetic agents such as halothane or methoxyflurane in oxygen, the accumulation of nitrogen is of concern only when very low flow or completely closed rebreathing techniques are used. High fresh gas flows during the induction of anesthesia will minimize this problem. Fresh gas flows to the rebreathing system equal to the patient's respiratory minute volume will reduce the nitrogen concentration to almost zero within 2 to 3 minutes (Fig. 17.26).[7, 13, 19] Denitrogenation is more of a problem in large animal anesthesia where, for economy, metabolic flows are used for the maintenance of anesthesia. With fresh gas flows of 1.5 to 2.5 liters/minute, which equal the metabolic needs of a 500-kg horse, the nitrogen concentration ranges between 23 and 57% after 2 hours of anesthesia.[29] The concentration of oxygen can be appreciably increased by flushing the system five or six times during the first 15 minutes of anesthesia.

The Use of Nitrous Oxide

Nitrous oxide is delivered to the patient by any of the techniques described above. Nitrous oxide is not a potent anesthetic, and adequate anesthesia can only be attained with adjunctive drugs or when supplemented with the other agents.

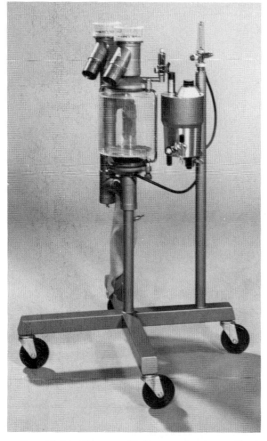

FIG. 17.31. Narcovet-E large animal anesthesia machine. (Courtesy of North American Dräger.)

Many drugs, including barbiturates and narcotic analgesics, have been used to supplement nitrous oxide. This combination, and muscle relaxants, can be used in veterinary anesthesia and is a useful technique under certain circumstances.

In veterinary anesthesia, nitrous oxide is commonly used as an adjunct to halothane or methoxyflurane. Because of its low solubility in blood and body tissues, the induction of anesthesia is rapid; but, because of its low potency, stage 3 of general anesthesia cannot be attained (see Chapter 10). When combined with volatile anesthetic agents, it can facilitate the induction of anesthesia by its analgesic effects and the production of unconsciousness. In unpremedicated healthy animals, when used alone, the depth of anesthesia is not sufficient for intubation of the trachea or even minor surgical procedure. Nitrous oxide in combination with halothane or methoxyflurane is considered supplemental to the volatile anesthetic agent and is not necessarily more desirous than either agent used alone. It does, however, reduce the concentration of the other anesthetic when using a mask and provides a more rapid recovery from anesthesia, especially when combined with very soluble agents.

For effective anesthesia, the nitrous oxide must replace the nitrogen in the alveoli and blood and should be administered in concentrations in excess of 50% in oxygen. For maximal efficiency in the use of nitrous oxide, especially during the induction of anesthesia, 80% in oxygen has been administered. This concentration is not recommended beyond the induction period of anesthesia. The inspiration of 20% oxygen during anesthesia is not an adequate concentration to assure proper oxygenation. Increased physiological shunting, changes in ventilatory patterns (see Chapter 14), and increased anatomical dead space contribute to hypoxemia during anesthesia and surgery.[5, 23, 28] This implies that higher concentrations in oxygen should be delivered with nitrous oxide. It is strongly recommended that the inspired oxygen concentration in the anesthetic mixture contain not less than 30 to 33% oxygen.[22, 23, 24] The delivery of adequate concentrations of oxygen to the inspired line can be easily determined in the semiopen and in the nonrebreathing systems. With the use of the rebreathing systems for nitrous oxide-halothane-oxygen

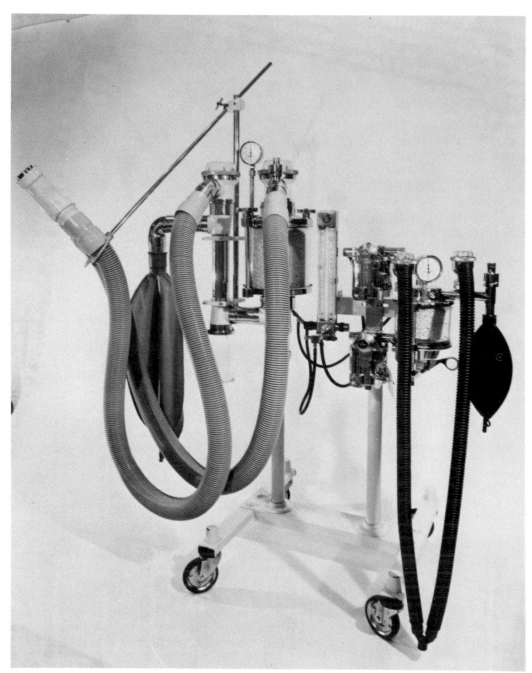

FIG. 17.32. VMS large animal anesthesia machine. (Courtesy of Fraser Sweatman.)

anesthesia, for example, high flows should be used to assure adequate inspired concentrations of oxygen.

There is difficulty in establishing guidelines in animals for both a safe and economical concentration of nitrous oxide and oxygen. The lower the flows, the more unpredictable is the inspired concentration in relation to total gas flow.[25] The lack of a relationship is due to variations between patients in ventilation, oxygen comsumption, and uptake of the anesthetic agent. It is suggested that in order to maintain an adequate inspired oxygen concentration, the estimated oxygen consumption of the patient should be exceeded by at least 4 to 5 times. The oxygen consumption of a dog under anesthesia ranges from 6 to 8 ml/kg/minute.[26, 30] Using this estimate of metabolic needs, the oxygen flow for a 15-kg dog should be 500 ml/minute of oxygen, with nitrous oxide added to produce a calculated delivered concentration of 30% oxygen. The above calculations are based on average values for oxygen consumption, which may vary from patient to patient and should be used only as guidelines. If an oxygen analyzer is not available for measurement of inspired concentrations, the error should be on the side of higher gas flows.

The elimination of nitrous oxide is at the reverse of the uptake rate, and none is detected in the blood stream after 10 minutes. The rate of removal, because of its low solubility in blood and body tissues, is extremely rapid during the first 2 to 3 minutes.[13] Because of this, a complication called diffusion hypoxia during the early elimination phase may occur.[12] A large volume of nitrous oxide pours into the alveoli, and when the patient begins to breathe room air, only a small amount of nitrogen is absorbed into the blood stream. The effect of alveolar dilution of oxygen by nitrous oxide and nitrogen can cause hypoxemia. The period of danger is within the first 5 minutes of elimination.

The complication can be prevented by the use of high flows of oxygen in the circle system during the early elimination phase of nitrous oxide. Following 2 to 3 minutes of high flow oxygen, the patient can be switched to room air without danger.

Anesthesia Machines for Veterinary Use

Compact anesthesia machines for veterinary use are available commercially (Figs. 17.27, 17.28, 17.29, and 17.30). The Narcovet (Fig. 17.27), VMS (Fig. 17.28), and the C Compact "50" (Fig. 17.29) are very versatile in that other vaporizers and flowmeters can be easily added or are contained in the original model. In this manner, the veterinarian can obtain a basic machine with the possibilities of expansion at a later date. These machines have diameters and fittings which are identical with the standards established by the Sectional Committee of Standards of the American Society of Anesthesiologists.

REFERENCES

1. Adriani, J.: *The Chemistry and Physics of Anesthesia*, 2nd ed. Charles C Thomas, Publisher, Springfield, Ill., 1962.
2. Ayre, P.: Endotracheal anaesthesia with the T tube. Brit. J. Anaesth. *28:* 520, 1956.
3. Ayre, P.: Anesthesia for intracranial operations. Lancet *1:* 561, 1937.
4. Baratta, A., Brandslater, B., Muallem, M., and Seraphim, C.: Rebreathing in a double T-piece system. Brit. J. Anaesth. *4:* 47, 1969.
5. Campbell, E. J. M., Nunn, J. F., and Peckett, B. W.: Comparison of artificial ventilation and spontaneous respiration with particular reference to ventilation-blood flow relationships. Brit. J. Anaesth. *30:* 166, 1958.
6. Clifford, D. H., and Soma, L. R.: *Feline Medicine and Surgery*, 1st ed., chap. 22. American Veterinary Publications, Inc., Santa Barbara, Calif., 1964.
7. Collins, V. J.: *Principles of Anesthesiology*. Lea & Febiger, Philadelphia, 1966.
8. Dripps, R. D., Echenhoff, J. E., and Vandam, L. D.: *Introduction to Anesthesia*, 2nd ed. W. B. Saunders Company, Philadelphia, 1961.
9. Editorial: Anesthesiology *25:* 3, 1964.
10. Elam, J. O.: Channeling and overpacking in carbon dioxide absorbents. Anesthesiology *19:* 403, 1958.
11. Elam, J. O.: The design of circle absorbers. Anesthesiology *19:* 99, 1958.
12. Fink, B. R.: Diffusion anoxia. Anesthesiology *16:* 511, 1955.

13. Fruman, M. J., Salanitre, E., and Rackow, H.: Excretion of nitrous oxide in anesthetized man. J. Appl. Physiol. *16:* 720, 1961.

14. Harrison, G. A.: Ayre's T-piece: a review of its modifications. Brit. J. Anaesth. *36:* 118, 1964.

15. Kain, L. M., and Nunn, J. F.: Fresh gas economics of the magill circuit. Anesthesiology *29:* 964, 1968.

16. Lewis, A., and Spoerle, W. E.: A modification of Ayre's technique. Canad. Anaesth. Soc. J. *8:* 501, 1961.

17. Mapelson, W. W.: The concentration of anesthetics in closed circuits with special reference to halothane. I. Theoretical study. Brit. J. Anaesth. *32:* 298, 1960.

18. Mapelson, W. W.: The elimination of rebreathing in various semi-closed anesthetic systems. Brit. J. Anaesth. *26:* 323, 1954.

19. Miles, G. G., Martin, N. T., and Adriani, J.: Factors Influencing the elimination of nitrogen using semi-closed inhalers. Anesthesiology *17:* 213, 1956.

20. Mushin, W. W., and Galloon, S.: The concentrations of anesthetics in closed circuits with special reference to halothane. III. Clinical aspects. Brit. J. Anaesth. *32:* 324, 1960.

21. Neff, W. B.: Annotation on the handling of carbon dioxide absorbing substances. Anesthesiology *3:* 688, 1942.

22. Nunn, J. F.: Factors influencing the arterial oxygen tension during halothane anesthesia with spontaneous respirations. Brit. J. Anaesth. *36:* 327, 1964.

23. Sara, C.: The oxygen content of anesthetic mixtures, Med. J. Aust. *2:* 581, 1961.

24. Slater, E. M., Nilsson, S. E., Leake, D. L., Parry, W. L., Laver, M. B., Hedley-Whyte, J., and Bendixen, H. H.: Arterial oxygen tension measurements during nitrous oxide-oxygen anesthesia. Anesthesiology *26:* 642, 1965.

25. Smith, T. C.: Nitrous oxide and low flow circle systems. Anesthesiology *27:* 266, 1966.

26. Soma, L. R., and Kenny, R.: Respiratory cardiovascular metabolic and electroencephalographic effects of Doxapram hydrochloride in the dog. Amer. J. Vet. Res. *28:* 191, 1967.

27. Sykes, M. K.: Non-rebreathing valves. Brit. J. Anaesth. *31:* 450, 1959.

28. Taylor, S. H., Scott, D. B., and Donald, K. W.: Respiratory effects of general anesthesia. Lancet *1:* 841, 1964.

29. Tevik, A., Sharpe, J., Nelson, A. W., Berkely, W. E., and Lumb, W. V.: Effect of nitrogen in a closed circle system with low oxygen flows for equine anesthesia. J. Amer. Vet. Med. Ass. *154:* 166, 1969.

30. Theye, R. A., and Messick, J. M.: Measurements of oxygen consumption of spirometry during halothane anesthesia. Anesthesiology *29:* 361, 1968.

18
Intubation of the Trachea

LAWRENCE R. SOMA

Intubation of the trachea affords many advantages during general anesthesia. Anatomical dead space is reduced, the patency of the airway is more readily assured, and secretions from the oral cavity and stomach contents can be prevented from entering the tracheobronchial tree. Secretions can be easily removed from the tracheobronchial tree by passage of a suction catheter through the tube. Inhalation anesthetics are more easily delivered, and artificial ventilation can be applied without danger of inflating the stomach. This problem is greater in the brachycephalic breeds and ruminants where intermittent positive pressure ventilation is difficult with a mask. Various head positions can also be assumed with less chance of airway obstruction.

Equipment

ENDOTRACHEAL TUBES

Tubes are categorized on the basis of their consistency, use, and also by designation of the designer. Tubes classified on the basis of consistency are (a) soft; (b) semirigid; and (c) metal.[7] The soft and semirigid tubes are used for endotracheal intubation, and the metal tubes are generally used for bronchoscopy. The tubes commonly used for tracheal intubation are of soft consistency and are made of rubber or plastic (Table 18.1; Fig. 18.1). The soft tubes will kink when the radius is reduced to a critical point as determined by the wall thickness and consistency (Figs. 18.2 and 18.3). This varies with the age of the tube. The semirigid tubes are composed of stainless steel coiled wire covered with latex rubber. Spiral tubes will not collapse or kink when bent at various angles and are preferred for oral surgery or when extreme head positions are necessary. Tubes are also designated by their original designer; the two most commonly used are the Magill and the Murphy (Fig. 18.4; Table 18.1). The basic difference between the two is an eye on the Murphy tube which is placed opposite to the bevel. This is intended to prevent complete obstruction if the bevel of the tube rotates against the wall of the trachea.

Endobronchial intubation of either the right or left bronchus is possible with specially designed tubes. The tube is provided with a bronchial and tracheal cuff enabling the complete separation of the right and left bronchus (Fig. 18.5).

The choice between rubber tubes and plastic tubes generally is one of personal preference. Natural rubber tubes are more porous than vinyl plastic tubes and may absorb secretions and also germicides used for sterilization, with possible irritation of the tracheal structures.[20] Rubber tubes are more difficult to clean than the less porous plastic tubes. Plastic tubes will stiffen with age, and their consistency will alter with changes in temperature, being stiff at room temperature and softening at body temperature. The possibility of trauma to the larynx is greater when intubating with a stiffer plastic tube, but less damage due to prolonged intubation can be expected of a tube which can soften and mold to the tracheal comformation.

Size Designation. The size of an endotracheal tube can be designated by one of

TABLE 18.1

Commonly used endotracheal tubes

Composition	Designer or Name
Rubber (soft)	Magill, Murphy, or Cole
Natural or Neoprene	(infant)
Plastic (soft)	Magill, Murphy,
Vinyl, clear	Lonnecken
Opaque white	(infant)
Semitransparent	Cole (infant)
Latex (soft)	Sanders
Continuous spiral of nylon embedded in latex	
Latex (semirigid)	L.A. woven catheter
Continuous spiral of stainless steel embedded in latex	(anode)
Rubber (semirigid)	Carlens (left bronchus)
Double lumen endo-	White (right bronchus)
bronchial tubes	Bonica (right bronchus)
with carinal hook	

five systems which is very confusing when various types of tubes are purchased. Obviously a single system is necessary for optimum reference purposes (Tables 18.2 and 18.3). The five systems used are: (a) the French catheter gauge; (b) the Magill number, which is an arbitrary scale) (c) the Daval scale, which also is an arbitrary scale; (d) the external diameter in millimeters, and (e) the internal diameter in millimeters. The internal diameter in millimeters has been designated as the American Standard by the American Society of Anesthesiologists (Table 18.3), with an

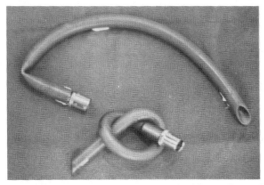

Fɪɢ. 18.2. Comparison of a soft rubber tube and an anode tube for resistance toward kinking. The anode tube should be used when unusual head positions will reduce the radius of the tube.

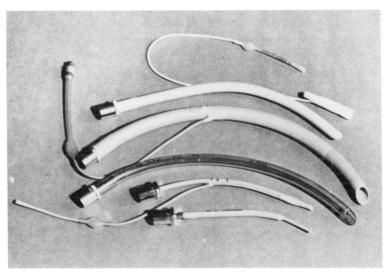

Fɪɢ. 18.1. Commonly used endotracheal tubes. *Top to bottom,* replaceable cuff, opaque plastic, streamlined cuffed rubber tube, clear plastic tube, cuffed rubber tube, and Cole pediatric tube.

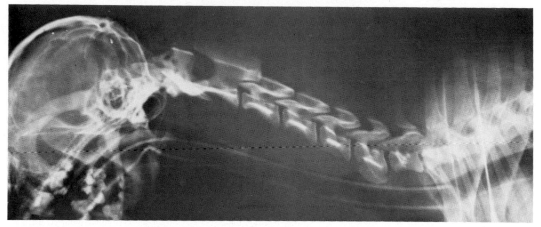

FIG. 18.3. Two possible complications of endotracheal intubation: Kinking of the endotracheal tube due to excessive flexion of the head and possible endobronchial intubation by too caudal placement of tube.

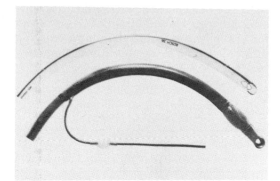

FIG. 18.4. Murphy tube which features an eye opposite to the bevel. Clear plastic and rubber.

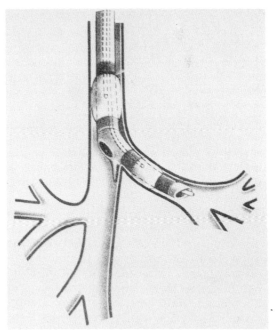

FIG. 18.5. Endobronchial tube, enabling the complete separation of both bronchi. (Courtesy of Rusch Company, New York, N.Y.)

accepted tolerance of 0.2 mm. The internal diameter is marked on the outside of the tube. The British Standard also utilizes the internal diameter as the official size designation.

With the exception of very large breeds of dogs and larger farm animals, tubes used for veterinary anesthesia are identical with those used for humans. Larger tubes are needed for the giant breeds of dogs and for large farm animals. The Association of Veterinary Anesthetists of Great Britain and Ireland has established essential requirements for veterinary endotracheal tubes in farm animals (Table 18.4), which include size range, size designation, materials, and basic definitions. Table 18.5 lists the size recommendations for dogs and cats.

Inflatable Cuffs. The inflatable cuff, which can be placed on plain tubes or tubes with built-in cuffs, permits the maintenance of a completely sealed system. When inflated, the cuff reduces the possibility of passage of foreign matter from the oral cavity into the trachea. When replaceable cuffs are used, they

TABLE 18.2

Magill, French, internal diameter endotracheal tube comparison scale and guide to replaceable cuff sizes

Magill Scale	French Scale	Internal Diameter Scale	Cuff Size
		mm	
00	13	4.0	
0	16	5.0	
	18		5 mm (3/16 inch)
1	20	5.0	
2	22	6.0	
3	24	7.0	6.5 mm (¼ inch)
4	26	8.0	
5	28	8.0	
6	28	9.0	
7	30	9.00	8.0 mm (5/16 inch)
8	32	10.00	
9	34	11.00	
10	36	12.00	9.5 mm (3/8 inch)
	38		
	40		
	42		11.0 mm (7/16 inch)
	44		
	46		12.5 mm (½ inch)
	48		

should be placed at least ½ inch from the end of the tube to prevent overlapping of the cuff over the end of the tube when inflated.

Inflation of the cuff should be done carefully, with an amount of air just necessary to occlude the space between the outer wall of the tube and the inner wall of the trachea. The adequacy of inflation can be tested by listening for the escape of air around the tube either during spontaneous respiration or, preferably, by compressing the breathing bag. A small pilot balloon is usually a part of the cuff to indicate the state of inflation.

Care of Endotracheal Tubes. Mechanical scrubbing of an endotracheal tube with soapy water is one of the most important aspects of tube care. The external surface should be cleansed thoroughly with a soft brush, and the inside should be cleaned with a test tube brush, rinsed, and allowed to dry to be stored in clean dry containers. Sterilization of tubes and storage in sterile packages is practiced by some and deemed unnecessary by others.

Tubes can be sterilized by various means: boiling, steam autoclave, liquid chemical, and ethylene oxide. Unfortunately, deterioration of rubber and plastic compounds is accelerated by the various means of sterilization.[4] All rubber products are susceptible to damage by heat and chemical sterilization; the clear plastic tubes are least affected.[4] The specific effect of various means of sterilization varies with the composition of the tube, and if tubes are to be sterilized, the recommendations of the manufacturer should be considered.

The most practical approach to tube care is as follows: (a) proper cleansing of both the internal and external surface; (b) soaking in a chemical sterilizing solution for 20 minutes (benzalkonium chloride, hexachlorophene) if contamination is a

TABLE 18.3

*Endotracheal tube internal diameters and lengths**

Internal Diameter (Tolerance ± 0.20)	Minimum Tube Length
mm	cm
2.5	12.0
3.0	14.0
3.5	16.0
4.0	18.0
4.5	20.0
5.0	22.0
5.5	24.0
6.0	26.0
6.5	28.0
7.0	30.0
7.5	31.0
8.0	32.0
8.5	33.0
9.0	34.0
9.5	35.0
10.0	36.0

* Internal diameters and tolerances established by the American Standards Association and the American Society of Anesthesiologists. Under this system all tube sizes are indicated by internal diameter in millimeters.

TABLE 18.4

*Sizes of veterinary endotracheal tubes for farm animals**

Internal Diameter	External Diameter	Length	Length of Cuff	Distance of Cuff from End	Size of Animal
mm	mm	cm	cm	cm	
35	43	100	20	5	Large thoroughbred and large draught horses.
30	38	100	20	5	Thoroughbreds and hunters. Bulls and some large cows.
25	31	80	15	5	Large and medium ponies, most cows. Yearling thoroughbreds and hunters.
20	26	80	15	4	Medium and small ponies. Young foals. Yearling cattle.
18	22.5	60	10	4	Large rams and boars. Pony foals and 6-month calves.
16	19.5	60	10	3	Adult sheep and pigs. 3-month calves.
14	17	50	8	3	Yearling sheep and pigs (of pork to bacon size). Young calves.
12	15	40	8	3	Younger sheep and pigs. Newborn calves.

* Recommendations of the Association of Veterinary Anesthetists of Great Britain and Ireland.

TABLE 18.5

*Guide for a selection of veterinary endotracheal tubes**

	Body Weight	Magill Size	Internal Diameter
	lb		mm
Cats	2.5	00	4.0
	4.5	0	5.0
	9.0	1	5.0
Dogs	5	2	6.0
	10	4-5	8.0
	15	6-7	9.0
	20	8	10.0
	25	9-10	11.0-12.0
	30	9-10	11.0-12.0
	35	10-11	12.0
	40	11-12	
	45	11-12	

* Modified from Le Roux.[17]

LARYNGOSCOPES

Laryngoscopes to aid in the intubation of small animals are to be recommended over the use of the finger to depress the epiglottis or the use of forceps to grasp the epiglottis or tongue. Laryngoscopes are available with straight or curved blades. The blades are detachable, and various sizes can be used interchangeably on a battery-containing handle (Figs. 18.6 and 18.7). The choice of a straight blade or a curved blade in animals is generally one of personal preference. The curved blades can be used more effectively and are advantageous in small dogs, cats, and the brachycephalic breeds.

Techniques of Endotracheal Intubation

Methods of intubation vary with the species, but generally three methods are employed: (a) direct vision with a laryngoscope which is the method of choice in dogs, cats, and the smaller farm animals; (b) blind intubation through the oral cavity which is the method used in the horse; and (c) tactile intubation with insertion of the tube by touch which can be used in the dog and cat, but is the common method in the larger ruminants. Nasal intubation, a method employed in man, is not advised in veterinary patients, because the ventral meatus of the nasal cavity is too small in proportion to the trachea, and a large enough tube cannot be passed.

concern; (c) rinsing well in clear water; and (d) storage in dry, clean containers.

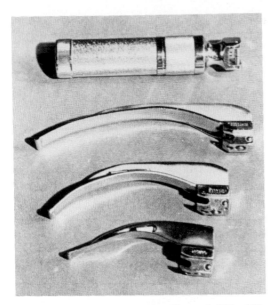

FIG. 18.6. Laryngoscope handle and 158-, 130-, and 108-mm MacIntosh curved laryngoscope blades. A small 87-mm blade is also available.

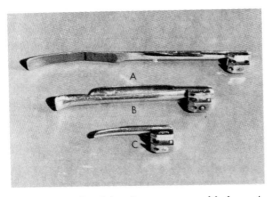

FIG. 18.7. Straight laryngoscope blades, A, standard straight blade modified by the addition of an extension for intubation of small ruminants; B, Wis-Foregger straight blade; C, a 75-mm Millar premature infant straight blade.

DIRECT VISION

Direct vision of the larynx is the commonly employed method of orotracheal intubation in small animals. The anesthesia must be deep enough to provide adequate muscle relaxation and suppression of orotracheal reflexes. Complete muscle paralysis to produce apnea is not necessary for routine intubation of most veteri-

nary patients. The apneic technique is the method of choice for the intubation of man. It necessitates greater speed because of the possibility of hypoxia if intubation is delayed. When the apneic technique is used, preoxygenation by use of the mask will delay a decline in oxygen saturation to a dangerous level.[16]

Positioning and Laryngoscopy. The proper angulation and positioning of the head facilitates intubation of the trachea. In the standing dog, for example, an angle is formed between straight lines drawn parallel to the oral cavity and one drawn through the trachea. This orotracheal axis (Fig. 18.8) prevents ease of intubation unless reduced by head positioning and depression of the epiglottis (Fig. 18.9). The position for intubation in the dog can be either lateral recumbancy or supine. Large dogs with long and flexible necks can remain in lateral recumbancy with the head twisted to a more supine position (Fig. 18.10). Cats and small dogs can be easily rolled into the supine position (Fig. 18.11).

The laryngoscope is grasped in the left hand (right-handed person) while the thumb of the right hand is used to depress the mandible and open the mouth. The blade is inserted slightly to the right of the midline of the tongue to push it to the left of the oral cavity. In very large dogs, because of the size of the tongue, it may have to be held between the small and ring finger of the left hand to prevent it from sliding over the laryngoscope blade.

When using a curved blade, the tip is placed at the base of the tongue at the glossoepiglottic fold (Fig. 18.12). The laryngoscope is lifted upward, and the blade is rotated slightly backward, the base of the blade being the rotational fulcrum. In this manner the entire mandible is lifted upward. The suspension and the slight rotation of the base of the tongue at the glossoepiglottic fold will lift the epiglottis, exposing the glottis and related structures (Figs. 18.13, 18.14, and 18.15). The use of the curved blade is advantageous for exposure of the glottis (Fig. 18.14). The base

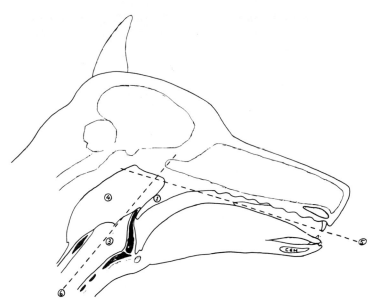

FIG. 18.8. Structures and angulation of the orotracheal axis in the dog. *1*, soft palate; *2*, epiglottis, *3*, glottis; *4*, nasopharyngeal cavity; *5*, oral axis; *6*, tracheal axis.

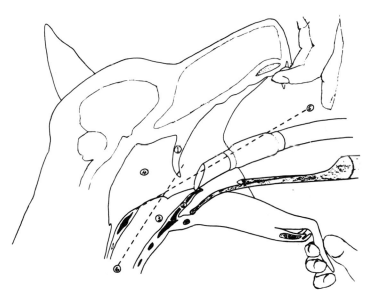

FIG. 18.9. Structures and angulation of the ortracheal axis for intubation of the trachea in the dog.

of the laryngoscope handle, because of the curvature of the blade, does not impede direct vision.

A straight blade can be used in a manner described for the curved blade, but because of the lack of a curve, the rotation of the laryngoscope is not as effective in lifting the epiglottis upward. The straight blade is generally placed on the tip of the epiglottis and pressed toward the base of the tongue. When the laryngoscope blade is used in this manner, the blade can partially block the view of the glottis, obscuring its true diameter. An inexperienced

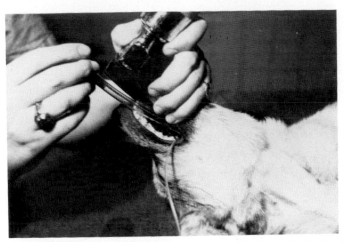

FIG. 18.10. Positioning of the dog for tracheal intubation. The dog can also be intubated in the lateral position. An assistant can aid intubation by opening the mouth.

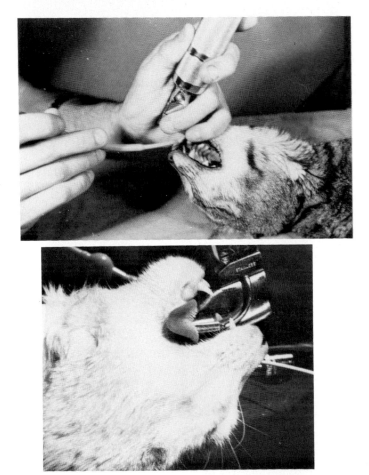

FIG. 18.11. Positioning of the cat for tracheal intubation. *Top*, view from the right side; *bottom*, view from the left side. (Courtesy of Clifford, D. H., and Soma, L. R.: *Feline Medicine and Surgery*, 1st ed. American Veterinary Publications, Inc., Santa Barbara, Calif., 1964.)

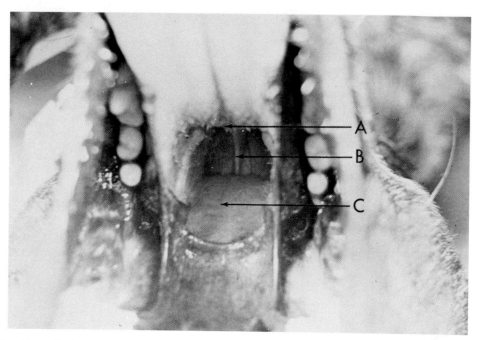

FIG. 18.12. Oral cavity of the dog. The laryngoscope blade is placed at the glossoepilgottic fold (A), lifting the epiglottis (B), for exposure of the glottis. The soft palate (C) usually is in position below the epiglottis. The dog is in a supine position.

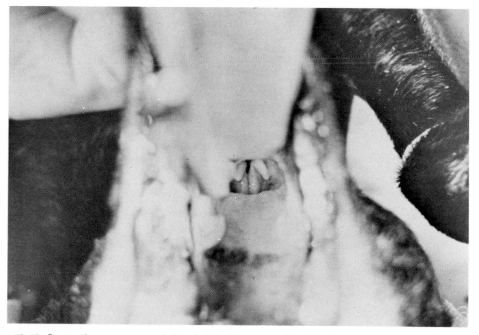

FIG. 18.13. Incomplete exposure of the glottis. The jaw is lifted further upward, and the laryngoscope rotated to expose the glottis and surrounding structures.

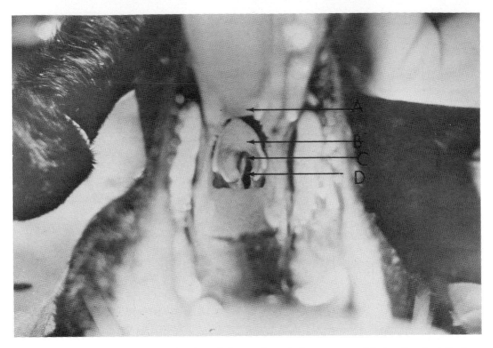

FIG. 18.14. Larynx exposed for intubation of the trachea. *A*, laryngoscope blade placed at the base of the tongue; *B*, epiglottis, *C*, vocal fold; *D*, glottis.

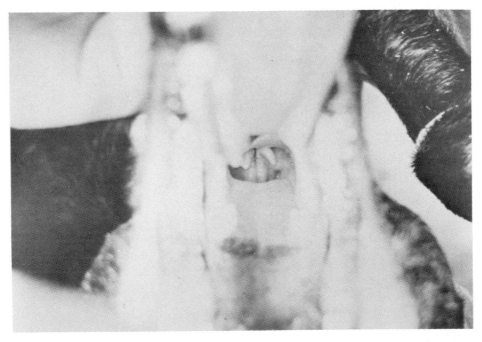

FIG. 18.15. Partial closure of the arytenoid cartilages in a lightly anesthetized dog.

clinician, under these circumstances, will generally intubate with a smaller tube.

The soft palate of the dog is located below the epiglottis and may interfere during tracheal intubation. This is a problem particularly in the brachycephalic breeds, and the palate may have to be depressed with the endotracheal tube during intubation (Fig. 18.12). The soft palate may be touching the glottis in some brachycephalics.

Placing the Tube. Upon exposure of the glottis, a clean tube is inserted. The tube should be held with the thumb and first finger and supported with the middle finger (held like a pen) and passed preferably during inspiration, when the degree of abduction of the vocal cords is greatest.[7] The tube is inserted with a slight rotary motion and is not pushed directly through the vocal folds.

Occasionally, intubation is attempted in animals under very light planes of anesthesia. Laryngeal tone is still present, and partial closure of the glottis can occur if attempts are made to force the tube through the closed larynx. At this point, the level of anesthesia should be deepened, or the patient paralyzed with succinylcholine chloride, ventilated with oxygen, and intubation attempted once more.

Occasionally it may be necessary to intubate a patient under light anesthesia because of an emergency situation. The tip of the bevel should be placed in the laryngeal opening and during the next inspiration the tube rotated and gently pushed into the trachea. Adequate lubrication of the tube will facilitate passage under these circumstances. An undersized tube can be placed temporarily until adequate levels of anesthesia are achieved, and it can then be replaced with a larger tube.

Intubation of the Cat. The mechanical aspects of intubation of the cat do not vary greatly from the dog (Fig. 18.11). The cat can be easily placed in the supine position and a small curved laryngoscope blade placed in the mouth. The tongue is proportionately smaller in this species

than in the dog; therefore, it can be pushed aside with the blade by placing the blade to the right of midline of the tongue. As in the dog, the tip of the curved blade is placed at the base of the tongue, and the laryngoscope is lifted upward and forward.

The anatomy of the larynx of the cat, and of the feline family in general, differs somewhat from that of the dog. It is "dome-like" in shape with thinner arytenoid borders[21] (Figs. 18.16 and 18.17). The soft palate is shorter and therefore the trailing edge is not located under the epiglottis when the mouth is opened for placement of the laryngoscope blade. Commonly, under moderate levels of anesthesia, passive movement of the arytenoid structures with respiration will be noted. This should not be confused with spastic closure of the glottis.

Cats, nonetheless, are more difficult to intubate because of a greater tendency toward laryngospasms and a persistence of jaw tone during the lighter planes of anesthesia. Intubation during barbiturate anesthesia necessitates deeper planes in order to avoid spasms. Barbiturates, due to their increase in parasympathetic tone, tend to predispose the larynx to spasms, but halothane produces good jaw relaxation and reduces laryngeal reflexes in the lighter planes, thus facilitating tracheal intubation.[1, 23] For ease of intubation under light planes of anesthesia, succinyl-

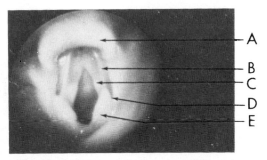

FIG. 18.16. Larynx of the cat. *A*, curled epiglottis; *B*, vestibular fold; *C*, vocal fold; *D*, aryepiglottic fold; *E*, arytenoid cartilage. (Courtesy of Dr. J. O'Brien, University of Pennsylvania, School of Veterinary Medicine.)

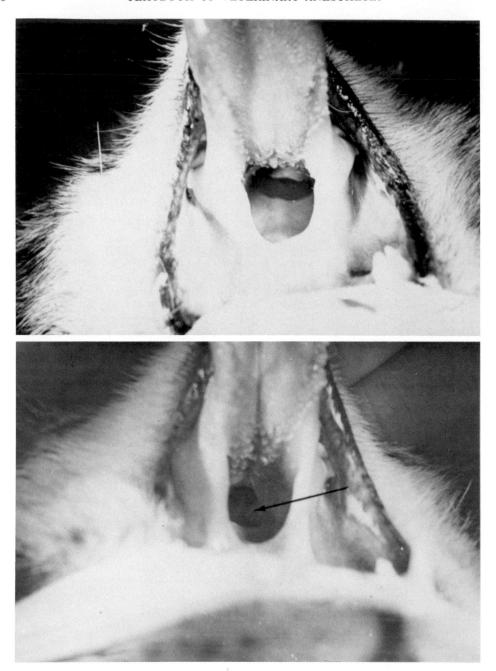

FIG. 18.17. Positioning for intubation in the cat. As compared to the dog the epiglottis of the cat is small-er, the soft palate is shorter, and the larynx has a dome-like structure. (Courtesy of Clifford, D. H., and Soma, L. R.: *Feline Medicine and Surgery*, 1st ed. American Veterinary Publications, Inc., Santa Barbara, Calif., 1964.)

choline chloride can be used to abolish or prevent laryngospasms and provide complete muscle relaxation. Spraying the larynx with a local anesthetic will reduce laryngeal sensitivity and decrease the occurrence of laryngospasms. After induction of anesthesia with a mask, the larynx can be sprayed with a local anesthetic and then anesthesia continued until a plane of anesthesia is obtained which is adequate for intubation.

Other Species. Tracheal intubation by direct vision is the method of choice in a variety of animals. The subhuman primates are approached in a manner similar to that of the dog and cat. Laryngospasms in the subhuman primates are of more concern than the dog, and intubation should be performed under moderate levels of anesthesia or the larynx sprayed with a local anesthetic prior to intubation.

The smaller ruminants and the pig can also be intubated by direct vision; the laryngoscope blade should be at least 250 mm long. This length can be achieved by adding an extension to a standard blade (Fig. 18.7), or by the use of the Rowan laryngoscope which has been developed for farm animals (see Chapter 27). In sheep or goats, a curved tube with a wire stylet to maintain the curvature will facilitate intubation. The herbivores have a large tongue, and the larynx is far back in the oral cavity; in most instances only the dorsal aspect of the laryngeal inlet is viewed. The sheep retains some of its laryngeal and swallowing reflexes at a depth of anesthesia that produces apnea. Under these circumstances intubation may be difficult. Succinylcholine chloride in doses of 40 to 60 mg can be used to produce muscle paralysis to aid intubation in the sheep. Intubation must be rapid because of the inability to ventilate ruminants with a mask. Some laryngeal tone has been noted to persist even when complete paralysis of other muscle systems has been accomplished with succinylcholine.

BLIND INTUBATION

Tracheal intubation of the horse is accomplished by blind intubation. The long oral cavity coupled with bulky cheeks and the minimal posterior extension of the commissures of the lips makes it impossible to open the mouth sufficiently for direct vision of the larynx. The orotracheal axis can be easily aligned in the horse by simply extending the head (Fig. 18.18).

The mouth is opened and a bite block is placed between the teeth. The tongue is held in the forward position as the tube is passed. The tongue should not be pulled forward, but just immobilized as the tube is passed toward the larynx. Damage to the hyoid bones can occur if excessive tension is placed on the tongue.[24] To prevent laceration of its walls by the sharp molar teeth, the tube should be passed on the midline. A slight curve to the tube is beneficial in aiding passage along the tongue to its base and into the larynx. Occasionally, the tube will bypass the larynx and slip into the esophagus; the tube should be partially withdrawn and redirected into the larynx. When the tip of the tube is in the region of the larynx, the larynx can be grasped externally, and passage of the tube into the larynx is easily detected. The tube should be passed into the larynx during inspiration (see Chapter 26).

Blind intubation has been performed in small ruminants. When using this technique, spontaneous ventilation aids in tracking the tube into the larynx.

TACTILE INTUBATION

Intubation of the trachea by palpation is easily accomplished in the large ruminants. A bovine speculum or a bite block is used to open the mouth, and the arm is passed into the oral cavity, a maneuver which can stimulate the chewing reflex. The arm should be maintained in the midline to prevent injury by the large molars. The epiglottis is depressed by the index and middle finger and the tube passed through into the larynx. A small stomach tube can also be passed by palpation, followed by threading the endotracheal tube over the stomach tube into the larynx (see Chapter 27).

Palpation has also been used for the

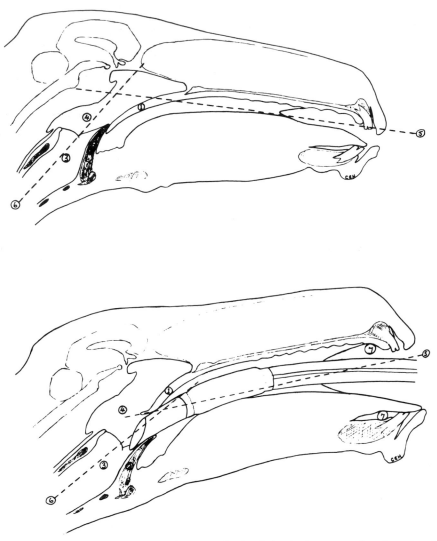

Fɪɢ. 18.18. Structures and angulation of the orotracheal axis in the horse. *1*, soft palate; *2*, epiglottis; *3*, glottis; *4*, nasopharyngeal cavity; *5*, oral axis; *6*, tracheal axis.

intubation of dogs and cats but this technique is not recommended.

Complications of Tracheal Intubation

The complications of tracheal intubation are markedly reduced as skill in the method and the ability to recognize abnormal reactions to the tube increase. The advantages afforded by intubation far outweigh the potential complications. Mishaps can be categorized into: (a) trauma; (b) misplacement of tube; (c) res-

piratory effects; and (d) cardiovascular effects.

TRAUMA

Damage to the mucous membrane of the oral cavity, larynx, and trachea can occur. This is most likely to result from repeated attempts to intubate. Damage to teeth can occur easily in man[3, 18] but is uncommon in animals because of the greater width of the oral cavity. Lips and tongue can be traumatized by pinching them between the laryngoscope and the teeth-or by tying them between the tube and the teeth when securing the tube in the oral cavity. Marked edema of the tip of the tongue has occurred by pinching it between the incisor teeth and the tube, especially when the tube is secured by gauze to the mandible. Abrasions or lacerations of the mucous membrane of the upper respiratory tract can occur by the pushing of a dry tube into the larynx, especially if relaxation is incomplete.

The incidence of sore throat following tracheal intubation in man varies a great deal[10], an effect which cannot be easily determined in veterinary patients. Laryngitis and tracheitis have been noted in some cases. Following endotracheal anesthesia, excessive swallowing and a persistent dry cough have also been observed.

Pressure on the larynx and trachea by the placement of an oversized tube for a short period of time has produced histological changes in a series of experimental monkeys.[30] Ulcers and edema occurred over the cricoid cartilages, and polymorphonuclear infiltration was seen in the 24- to 48-hour specimens. Steroids in a single dose after the intubation period decreased the number of inflammatory cells. Varying degrees of damage, including inflammatory cell infiltration, ciliary destruction, hyperemia, exudation, and erosion were noted when dogs were sacrificed following a 3-hour period of tracheal intubation.[13]

Temporary damage to the larynx and trachea does occur, but these effects do not negate the advantages of the technique. Gentleness and intubation at adequate levels of anesthesia will minimize trauma. The respiratory tract changes in length during the respiratory cycle; therefore, the endotracheal tube should be loosely tied to the jaw to allow free movement up and down with the trachea. This movement is exaggerated during intermittent positive pressure ventilation.

Prolonged orotracheal intubation in veterinary patients is not a common practice, because of the measures necessary to prevent destruction of the tube. The endotracheal tube can be maintained in place safely only when the animal is paralyzed, under anesthesia, or comatose. Prolonged intubation in man varies considerably and may be from 3 days to 3 weeks. Complications occurring during the period of intubation include occlusion by secretions or edema, hemorrhage, ulceration of the mucous membrane, and swelling of the cords. Complications following the intubation include hoarseness, persistant airway obstruction, a subglottic web, stenosis, and granuloma or papilloma of the vocal cords.[2, 8, 9, 19, 28, 29]

If prolonged intubation is contemplated, a sterile tube should be passed under maximal relaxation. If positive pressure ventilation is not indicated, a tube one size smaller than necessary should be inserted to minimize pressure on the larynx. When inflation of the cuff is essential, it should be deflated every 2 to 3 hours for a short period of time. It is essential that the tube be cleaned of secretions by the instillation of 0.5 to 1 ml of sterile saline and suctioned out with a sterile catheter. Adequate fluid balance must be maintained to prevent thickening of tracheobronchial secretions. Atropine is contraindicated because it produces secretions which are thicker and more viscous, rendering them more difficult to remove. The tracheostomy tube is more commonly used for prolonged treatment of upper airway obstruction in animals, and the general care is similar to that of the endotracheal tube.

MISPLACEMENT OF THE TUBE

Misplacement during intubation or displacement during anesthesia can result in a partial or complete respiratory obstruction. Endotracheal tubes are used to assure a patent airway; their insertion into the esophagus defeats this purpose. Lack of familiarity with the orotracheal structures, a hurried intubation, light anesthesia, or an oversized tube are the common causes of an esophageal placement. As the tip of the tube is placed into the glottis, vision of the inlet and surrounding structures is lost. If the tube is oversized or the larynx poorly relaxed, the tube can slip over the larynx into the esophagus.

An endotracheal tube can be inserted too far into the trachea and into the right bronchus, producing left lung collapse. After intubation, the chest should be checked for equal expansion or auscultated for equal breath sounds on both sides. Displacement also can occur due to movement of the animal or weight of the anesthesia connections dislodging a poorly secured tube. Inflation of the cuff which is only partially in the larynx can push the tube out of the glottis.

RESPIRATORY EFFECTS

The process of intubation in the lightly anesthetized dog or cat can produce transient increase in respiration or coughing (bucking) on the tube. This is an attempt to expel the tube—a response of the trachea to a foreign body. Apnea can occur shortly after intubation due to reflex inhibition of respiration under very light planes of anesthesia. Placement of the tip of the tube to the area of the carina can stimulate respiration because of the persistence of the tracheal reflex. The respiratory pattern will be irregular in nature.

Sensitivity of the larynx and its response to external stimuli varies from species to species.[26, 27] Unfortunately, detailed information on many species is not available. The larynx of the cat is very reactive, and spastic closure is common. On the other hand, the horse can tolerate a high concentration of diethyl ether or other stimuli with no signs of laryngeal or tracheopulmonary sensitivity. Complete closure of the larynx, where no egress and ingress of air occurs, is impossible in most animals except some arboreal species and man.[21] Man, the gibbon, the chimpanzee, and the gorilla are capable of preventing the escape of air by closure of the ventricular bands, a function dogs, cats, and most domestic species do not have. The arboreal species can fix the volume of the chest by preventing the escape of air, an aid in pulling themselves directly upward.

Animals that climb, grasp, hug, or strike (e.g., cat, bear) do have more developed inlet valvular closure, either by a vaulted type of larynx, as seen in the cat, or a secondary inlet valve produced by a thyroartenoid fold.[21] It has been noted clinically that some animals with a more highly developed inlet valve (man, cat, subhuman primates) are more prone to laryngospasms during tracheal intubation.

During light planes of anesthesia, spasms can occur even with the tube in place. Spasms of the larynx against the tube can produce damage to the cords.[7] Bronchospasms can occur under light planes of anesthesia but generally are not readily apparent in animals.

Respiratory obstruction, partial or complete, can occur during endotracheal anesthesia due to a mechanical obstruction. The cuff can be overinflated, compressing the lumen of the tube, or, if the cuff is placed too close to the beveled portion of the tube, a bubble can ride over the bevel producing an obstruction. Excessive flexion of the neck can kink a rubber or plastic tube (Fig. 18.2 and 18.3), or the tube can kink in or out of the oral cavity due to the weight of the equipment connections or extreme positions of the head. Veterinary patients have bitten down on tubes, creating an obstruction, or chewed a tube in half, with the distal half sliding into the trachea. Foreign matter can accumulate in the tube due to improper cleaning, bleeding, or excessive mucous secretions.

Respiratory obstruction may be detected by an increase in respiratory effort without a noticeable increase in movement of the breathing bag. This increase in resistance produced by a partial obstruction can be missed by a casual observer. If anesthesia is deep, apnea may occur because of the lack of muscle power to overcome the increased resistance.

CARDIOVASCULAR EFFECTS

The cardiovascular effects of manipulation of the larynx and intubation vary among species. There is minimal information in this area in all animals except man. The general effect in man is an increase in blood pressure and heart rate during manipulation of the epiglottis and intubation.[6, 22] Electrocardiographic changes in the form of bigeminal rhythms, ectopic ventricular contractions, and sinus tachycardia have been reported in man.[18, 22] These electrocardiographic changes have also been noted in the dog and cat, a response which may be caused by an increase in sympathetic activity or reflex excitation of the vagus nerve. Arrhythmias under anesthesia and during intubation may be caused by an imbalance between the parasympathetic and sympathetic system, in many instances created by the predominant effect of drugs. For example, narcotics and barbiturates are vagotonic. This effect, coupled with the release of catecholamines during the induction of anesthesia or intubation, can produce arrhythmias.

The cardiovascular changes in the dog are opposite to those of man; the common effect in the dog is bradycardia and hypotension.[15] The vagotonic effects of narcotics, barbiturates, and halothane, for example, may exaggerate these effects.[5, 14, 25] In the dog, the vagolytic effects of atropine will minimize the effects of intubation and should be used. Atropine will not prevent laryngospasms, but its reduction of secretions may prevent inadvertent stimulation by these secretions.

The cardiovascular effects in the cat are more similar to those in man, where an increase in blood pressure and heart rate can be expected. Cardiac arrest during intubation has been reported in man[18] and has occurred in dogs. Hypoxia, hypercarbia, severe cardiovascular disease, hypovolemia, and a combination of compromising conditions can predispose the patient to extreme cardiovascular changes during intubation.

Extubation

The effects of intubation can be mimicked during extubation (removal of tube), but unless hypoxia or hypercarbia occur, the effects are only transient.[11, 12] Of a greater concern can be obstruction or aspiration following extubation. Obstruction due to spasms is more likely in the cat, and following extubation the mask should be replaced and the patient allowed to breathe oxygen until the patency of the airway is assured. A stridor may be noted for a brief period following extubation. Obstruction due to an elongated soft palate and relaxation of maxilla allowing the tongue and epiglottis to fall backward and partially occlude the glottis is a real danger in the brachycephalic breeds. Extubation should be accomplished under light planes of anesthesia when the laryngeal reflexes and oral tone are present. Even under these circumstances obstruction can still occur, and the tongue should be pulled forward and head extended. The patient should be carefully observed until the animal is sternal and the airway patent.

Regurgitation occasionally occurs in dogs and cats during the recovery period, and the tube should remain in place until the swallowing and laryngeal reflexes have returned. Regurgitation and excessive salivation can be a continuous problem in the ruminants, and the tube should remain in place as long as possible. Placing sand bags under the neck will elevate the esophagus and minimize regurgitation in ruminants and will also foster drainage of secretions from the oral cavity.

REFERENCES

1. Abajian, J., Jr., Brazell, E. H., Dente, G. A., and Mills, E. L.: Experience with halothane (Fluothane) in more than 5000 cases. J. A. M. A. 171: 535, 1959.
2. Allen, T. H., and Steven, I. M.: Prolonged endotracheal intubation in infants and children. Brit. J. Anaesth. 37: 566, 1965.
3. Bamforth, B. J.: Complications during endotracheal anesthesia. Anesth. Analg. (Cleveland) 42: 727, 1963.
4. Bosomworth, P. B., and Hamelberg, W.: Effects of sterilization technics on safety and durability of endotracheal tubes and cuffs. Anesth. Analg. (Cleveland) 44: 576, 1965.
5. Burn, J. H., Epstein, H. G., Feigan, G. A., Paton, W. D. M., Burns, T. H. S., Mushin, W. W., Organe, G. S. W., and Robertson, J. D.: Fluothane: a report to the Medical Re-

search Council by the Committee on Nonexplosive Anesthetic Agents. Brit. Med. J. 2: 479,
1957.

6. Burstein, C. L., LoPinto, F. J., and Newman,
W.: Electrocardiographic studies during endotracheal intubation; effects during usual routine technics. Anesthesiology 11: 224, 1950.

7. Collins, V. J.: Principles of Anesthesiology. Lea
& Febiger, Philadelphia, 1966.

8. Fearon, B., MacDonald, R. E., Smith, C., and
Mitchell, D.: Airway problems following prolonged endotracheal intubation. Ann. Otol. 75:
975, 1966.

9. Harrison, G. A., and Tonkin, J. P.: Some serious laryngeal complications of prolonged endotracheal intubation. Med. J. Aust. 1: 605,
1967.

10. Hartsell, E. J., and Stephen C. R.: Incidence
of sore throat following endotracheal intubation. Canad. Anaesth. Soc. J. 11: 307, 1964.

11. Hutchinson, B. R.: Changes in pulse rate and
blood pressure after extubation. Brit. J. Anaesth. 36: 661, 1964.

12. Hutchinson, B. R.: Electrocardiographic
changes in children following extubation. Med.
J. Aust. 1: 151, 1967.

13. Incze, F., Csernohorszky, V., Karacsonyi, S.,
and Adam-Molnar, M.: Bacteriological and
morphological aspects of endotracheal anesthesia. Acta Chir Acd. Sci. Hung. 2: 365, 1961.

14. Johnstone, M.: Pethidine and general anesthesia. Brit. Med. J. 2: 943, 1951.

15. King, B. D., Harris, L. C., Jr., Greifenstein, F.
E., Elder, J. D., Jr., and Dripps, R. D.: Reflex circulatory responses to direct laryngoscopy and tracheal intubation performed during general anesthesia. Anesthesiology 12: 556,
1961.

16. Lachman, R. J., Long, J. H., and Krumper-
man, L. W.: Changes in blood gases associated with various methods of induction of
endotracheal anesthesia. Anesthesiology 16:
29, 1955.

17. Le Roux, P. H.: A graph expressing body weight

in relation to the size of an endotracheal catheter for dogs and cats. J. South African Vet.
Med. Ass. 34: 231, 1963.

18. Lewis, R. N., and Swerdlow, M.: Hazards of
endotracheal anesthesia. Brit. J. Anaesth. 36:
504, 1964.

19. Markham, W. G., Blackwood, M. J. A., and
Conn, A. W.: Prolonged Nasotracheal intuba-
tion in infants and children. Canad. Anaesth.
Soc. J. 14: 11, 1967.

20. McDonald, W. L. J., Welch, H. J., and Keet,
J. E.: Antisepsis of endotracheal tubes and
face masks. Anesthesiology 21: 103, 1960.

21. Negus, V.: Biology of Respiration. E. S. Livingstone, Ltd., Edinburgh, 1965.

22. Orr, D., and Jones, I.: Anesthesia for laryngoscopy. Anaesthesia 23: 194, 1968.

23. Pittinger, C. B.: Halothane—its usefulness in
otolaryngologic procedures. Western J. Surg.
Obstet. Gynec. 69: 189, 1961.

24. Raker, E. W.: Clinico—pathologic conference,
University of Pennsylvania, School of Veterinary Medicine. J. Amer. Vet. Med. Ass. 144:
895, 1964.

25. Redgate, J. D., and Gellhorn, E.: The tonic effect of the posterior hypothalamus on blood
pressure and pulse rate disclosed by the action
of intra-hypothalamically injected drugs.
Arch. Int. Pharmacodyn. 105: 193, 1956.

26. Rex, M. A. E.: Stimulation of laryngospasms in
the cat by volatile anesthetics. Brit. J. Anaesth. 38:569, 1966.

27. Rex, M. A. E.: The laryngeal reflex. New Zeal.
Vet. J. 15: 222, 1967.

28. Striker, T. W., Stoal, S., and Downes, J. J.:
Prolonged nasotracheal intubation in infants
and children. Arch. Otolaryng. (Chicago) 85:
210, 1967.

29. Tonkin, J. P., and Harrison, G. M.: The effects
on the larynx of prolonged endotracheal intubation. Med. J. Aust. 2: 581, 1966.

30. Way, W. L., and Sooy, F. A.: Histologic changes
produced by endotracheal intubation. Ann.
Otol. 74: 799, 1965.

19
Intravenous Techniques

ALAN M. KLIDE

A most important aspect of venipuncture in animals is proper control. This may range from firm but gentle physical restraint to aggressive management. Sites for venipuncture in many of the domestic species and related wild species are similar, but the latter often require special cages or chemical restraint.

Sites of Venipunctures

CEPHALIC VEIN

The cephalic vein is used commonly for intravenous injection in most species except the very large (horse and cow). It is located on the dorsomedial aspect of the forearm.[4, 10, 12] This site provides an area on which a needle can be well stabilized for prolonged use and where perivascular infiltration is quickly seen. To restrain the animal for cephalic venipuncture, the assistant stands on the side of the animal opposite the vein to be punctured; e.g., if the needle is going in the right cephalic vein, the assistant stands on the left side (Fig. 19.1). The assistant's left arm is placed around the animal's neck and in this manner the head is held against the assistant's chest. With his right hand, the assistant grasps the animal's right elbow, which should nestle in the palm of the hand, preventing the animal from pulling his leg away from the needle. The thumb is passed over the proximal end of the radius, and the hand is rotated so as to pull the cephalic vein slightly lateral. This oc-

cludes the vein, straightens it, and makes it more accessible and visible (Figs. 19.1, 19.2, and 19.3a).

Sometimes the owner has to aid in the restraint of the pet. When this is the case, the vein can be occluded with a tourniquet, or the individual doing the venipuncture can occlude it with one hand and insert the needle with the other. One disadvantage of the latter method is inability to fix the vein with the free hand and prevent it from rolling away from the advancing needle. When working alone, the animal can be tied with a short leash and the vein occluded as above.

The cephalic vein may be used nearer the site of origin. It is located medially emerging from the palmar surface of the paw around the attachment of the first digit. This is sometimes useful in chondrodystrophic dogs (e.g., dachshunds); however, it is more difficult to stabilize a needle in this area. The accessory cephalic vein on the dorsal aspect of the carpus and metacarpus in the dog and subhuman primate is occasionally useful. For prolonged infusion into the cephalic vein, the paw should be stabilized by taping a tongue depressor or other suitably sized support to the ventral surface of the paw and forearm.

JUGULAR VEIN

The jugular veins are the largest diameter superficial veins available.[4, 10, 12] In large animals (horse and cow), this vein

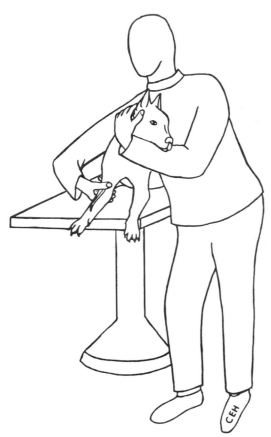

FIG. 19.1. Assistant restraining dog and occluding right cephalic vein.

lies in the jugular furrow which is located on the ventrolateral surface of the neck.[12] Its ventral border is the sterno-cephalicus muscle, and its dorsal border is the brachiocephalicus. In small animals the jugular vein is in the same approximate position as above; however, it is more mobile and its position varies with the position of the head and neck.[4, 10] In some small birds, the left jugular vein may be more prominent than the right.[1]

These veins are suitable for taking blood samples or giving intravenous injections; however, there are some disadvantages to using them. Movement of the head and neck can easily dislodge the needle and perivascular infiltration may not be obvious at the time of injection. For prolonged infusions in this site, it is useful to use a plastic catheter as described below. These catheters are also

useful in the horse or cow which is going to be anesthetized. If the catheters are placed before the animal is brought to the anesthesia and surgical area, venipuncture is avoided in an apprehensive animal.

Horses are restrained with a halter and lead shank; a twitch may occasionally have to be used. The site for injection is the middle third of the neck. The vein is occluded with the thumb proximal to the site of puncture. In most cases the vein is visualized as it fills. When tapped with a finger, fluid waves can be seen and felt with the occluding finger. Initially the needle should be almost perpendicular to the skin, inserted into the vein, and then threaded further down or up the vein.

Cattle may be held by a lead shank and halter, with or without a nose lead. Pulling the head away from the side on which the venipuncture is to be performed usually aids in visualization of the vein. The puncture is done as in the horse; however, the skin is more difficult to penetrate.

To perform a jugular puncture in small animals, they are placed on their sternum

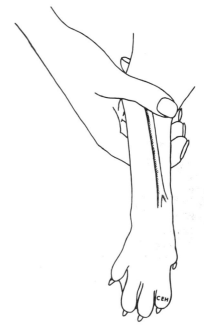

FIG. 19.2. Close-up view of the right cephalic vein, the most common vein for venipuncture.

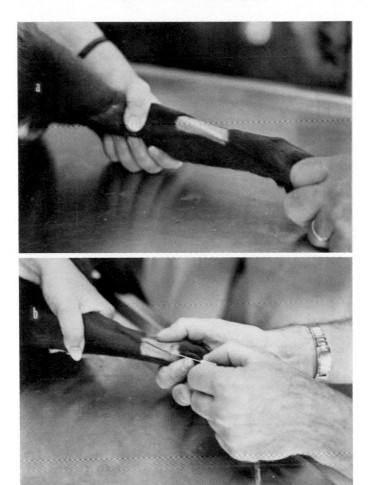

Fig. 19.3. *a*, left cephalic vein being occluded; *b*, occlusion and left-handed venipuncture of the dorsal branch of the left lateral saphenous vein of a dog.

on a table. The neck and forelegs should be positioned over the edge of the table. The forelimbs are pulled down and the head and neck dorsoflexed and the vein occluded at the thoracic inlet (Fig. 19.4). It may be necessary to rotate the head from side to side to make the vein more obvious, and in very fat animals the vein may be difficult to visualize or palpate.

SAPHENOUS VEIN

The saphenous veins located on the hind limb are useful in small animals. There is some difference in the naming of the vessels in the dog, cat, and primate,

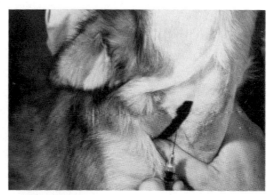

Fig. 19.4. Venipuncture of the right jugular vein of a dog. The head is extended upward and the forelegs pulled over the edge of the table.

but the vessels are in similar positions.[3, 4, 9, 10]

In the dog and cat, a vein arises at the anterior lateral surface of the hock and progresses upward toward the posterior surface of the stifle (Fig. 19.3). This is the dorsal branch of the lateral saphenous vein in the dog[10] and the dorsal branch of the small saphenous vein in the cat.[4] The dorsal branch of the medial saphenous arises at the anterior medial surface of the hock in the dog and cat and extends dorsally toward the femoral triangle.[4, 10] The dorsal branch of the medial saphenous vein joins the medial saphenous at the stifle, both ultimately joining the femoral vein.[10] In the cat, this sequence of vessels is the dorsal branch of the great saphenous vein, the great saphenous vein, and the femoral vein.[4] In the primate the great saphenous vein extends along the medial surface of the leg. The small saphenous vein is on the posterolateral aspect of the lower leg, emptying into the popliteal vein at the posterior aspect of the stifle.[3, 9]

Dogs and cats can be placed on their side, with the assistant standing at the animal's back and holding both hind legs in one hand and both forelegs in the other, and with the forearm, the neck is held against the table (Fig. 19.5). Small primates can be restrained for a venipuncture by holding both arms behind their backs or by utilizing a restraining cross.

EAR VEINS

These are most useful in the rabbit and pig and occasionally have been used for intravenous infusions in dachshunds. The marginal ear veins are located on the margins of the convex (outside) surface of the ears. These can be occluded at the base of the ear by finger pressure or a tourniquet. In the smaller animals, it is generally difficult to aspirate blood; however, it is very easy to see if injected material is within the vein or perivascular.

ANTERIOR VENA CAVA

The anterior vena cava of the pig has been used for the collection of large volumes of blood. The needle is inserted into a notch found somewhat cranial to and on a line connecting the manubrium with the base of the ear.[13] Small pigs are placed on their back with the front and hind legs extended.

Venipuncture

The area for venipuncture should be prepared, when possible, by clipping the hair and cleansing the skin. Clipping allows for better observation and cleaning of the site. Swabbing with isopropyl or ethyl alcohol removes loose hair and dirt and aids in better visualization of the vein. There is some question whether alcohol is efficacious in the disinfection of the site.[2, 5, 11]

There are several procedures which may be used to distend the vein and make it more obvious. The most common is the use of a tourniquet. This tourniquet may be an assistant's hand, the operator's hand, a length of latex rubber tubing, or a commercial unit such as the Nye tourniquet. The latter is useful in that it can be released by the operator with one hand.

Other procedures such as tapping or rubbing the site, squeezing the limb distal

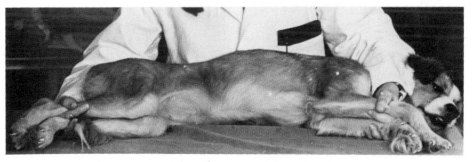

FIG. 19.5. Dog being restrained on its side by an assistant.

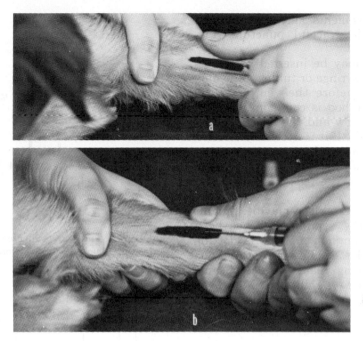

FIG. 19.6. Vein stabilization. *a*, use of the thumb to prevent movement of the vein; *b*, downward skin tension with the thumb and forefinger prevents the vein from moving away from the advancing needle (left-handed puncture).

to the venipuncture, making the limb dependent, warming, or moistening the site will increase appreciably the visualization of the vessel. Whether the vein is apparent or not the site should be palpated with the fingers. Palpation provides information on the tension of the vessel wall and the diameter. Sometimes the vein is not visually apparent and palpation may be the only method for finding it.

Once the vessel has been located, it should be fixed in position as securely as possible. One way is to tense the skin around the vessel; *e.g.*, for cephalic vein puncture the palm of the free hand is placed on the ventral (ulnar) surface of the forearm to pull the skin down. Another method is to place the thumb of the free hand against the side of the vessel to prevent the rolling of the vessel (Fig. 19.6).

VENIPUNCTURE

The vein can be approached from above or from the side with the bevel of the needle up or down. The simplest method is from above with the bevel up. The needle

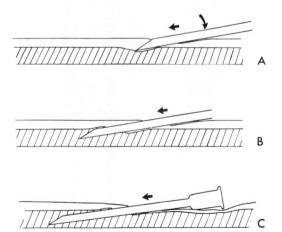

FIG. 19.7. Schematic representation of a venipuncture. *A*, needle through the skin with shaft of needle close to the skin; *B*, needle advanced into vein followed by (*C*) threading into vein.

is held in one hand and the vein fixed with the other. The two main structures to be penetrated are the skin and the vein wall. This may be done in one or two motions; *i.e.*, the needle placed through the skin and then in a separate movement the needle inserted through the vein wall, or these two movements may be combined into one single graceful puncture (Fig. 19.7).

The needle may be inserted before attaching it to a syringe or tubing, or it may be connected before the venipuncture. The former method is commonly used in the horse and cow and the latter method is small animals. If it is necessary to use a large syringe, one with an eccentric tip or a venotube connected between the syringe and needle is suggested (Figs. 19.8 and 19.9).

The aspiration of blood may be difficult even though the venipuncture has been successful. A common problem is clotting of blood in the needle. If repeated attempts are being made with the same needle, it should be flushed after each attempt to insure its patency. In a small vessel or one with a low flow, the negative

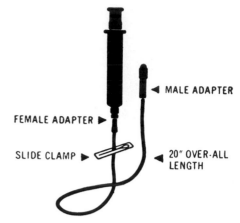

FIG. 19.9. Venotube connected to a syringe. (Courtesy of Abbott Company, North Chicago, Ill.)

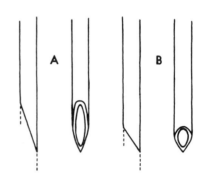

FIG. 19.10. Hypodermic needles. A, regular bevel; B, short bevel.

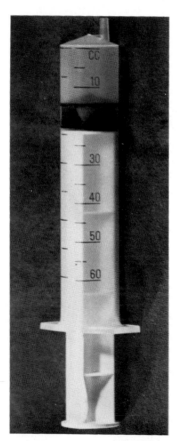

FIG. 19.8. Large syringe with eccentric tip.

pressure produced by aspiration may collapse the vein and pull the wall of the vein against the bevel of the needle. Sometimes blood is withdrawn but the needle is not in a vein. This can occur with multiple attempts which have produced a hematoma. During the subsequent attempts, the hemotoma may be the source of blood obtained instead of the vein.

Inadvertent intra-arterial puncture has occurred during attempted jugular vein punctures in the horse,[8] but can also occur in any species. The expected signs of arterial puncture are pulsatile flow, high pressure, and bright red color. If a small gauge needle is used, the only sign may be bright red color. When this is noted, no injection should be made, the needle should be withdrawn, and pressure applied at the site to minimize the possibility of a hematoma.

For the placement of a large gauge needle in a fractious animal, it may be useful to inject a small amount of a local anesthetic around the vein with a smaller needle. Care must be taken to prevent intravenous or intra-arterial injection of the local anesthetic.

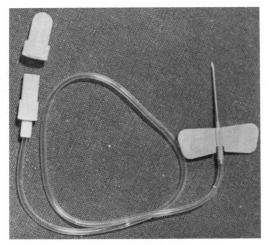

FIG. 19.11. Butterfly Infusion Set.

EQUIPMENT

The most commonly used hypodermic needles are those with regular beveled points. These may be more difficult to thread up the vessel and can penetrate both walls easily. Needles with short bevels are easier to thread and maintain in the vessel without penetration (Fig. 19.10). Thin wall needles provide a larger than normal bore without an increase in external diameter. A system which can be useful, especially in difficult venipunctures, is the Butterfly Infusion Set or the Scalp Vein Set (Fig. 19.11). These needles are equipped with plastic wings, which are a useful aid in the venipuncture and for fixing the needle to the leg. When the needle enters the vein the blood flows out into the clear plastic tube and confirms proper placement.

For prolonged infusions it is best to insert a plastic catheter in the vessel. There are many different types available; however, they can be classified in two major groups. One has the catheter around the outside of the placement needle and the other has the catheter inside the place-

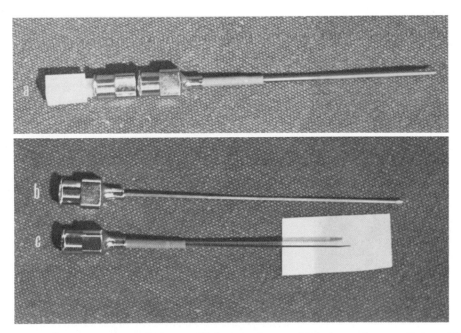

FIG. 19.12. Jelco I.V. Catheter Placement Unit. a, unit assembled; b, needle; c, catheter with radiopaque line.

ment needle (Figs. 19.12 and 19.13). An example of the first group is the Jelco I.V. Catheter Placement Unit which is placed in the following manner (Fig. 19.12). The site may or may not be infiltrated with a small amount of local anesthetic. The needle is inserted a small distance into the vein. The needle is then held still and the catheter advanced off the needle and down the vein. The needle is removed, the intravenous set connected, and the catheter taped in position.

The second type of catheter has a needle which is short in relation to the length of the catheter and through which the catheter is passed. An example of this type is the Venocath (Fig. 19.13). When placing either type, great care should be taken not to pull the catheter back through or onto the needle when in the vein; this procedure can cut the catheter, and a piece of it is then free in the circulatory system. Some catheters have a radiopaque line so that they can be located. In the first type the catheter is slightly larger than the needle, whereas in the second type the catheter is much smaller than the venipuncture needle.

The Venopak is an example of a system of tubing for dispensing fluids. The pack contains a screw cap with an air vent and drip chamber connected to a long length of plastic tubing. On the end of the tubing is a short gum rubber sleeve and a fitting for connecting to a needle (Fig. 19.14). The gum rubber sleeve can be used for additional injection; however, if a large needle is used or repeated punctures made, the sleeve may leak. Other units are available with a short side arm containing an injection port, which is advantageous when many injections have to be given (Fig. 19.14). Drugs may be added to the fluid in the bottle by injecting directly into the air vent after removing the air filter. With the regular Venopak system, the delivery rate is approximately 15 drops/ml. When giving intravenous fluids to small animals, a piece of tape should be placed on the bottle to show the starting level; this is useful for keeping track of the volume administered. For a more accurate method of delivery of small volumes, the Venopak Microdrip is recommended (Fig. 19.14). This system delivers smaller drops, the rate being approximately 60 drops/ml. The

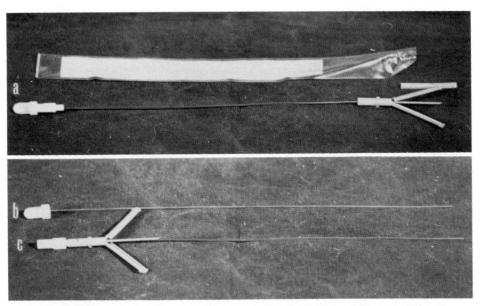

Fig. 19.13. Venocath. *a*, the protective sheath has been removed; the needle is in position for venipuncture; *b*, stylet removed; *c*, catheter has been advanced through needle.

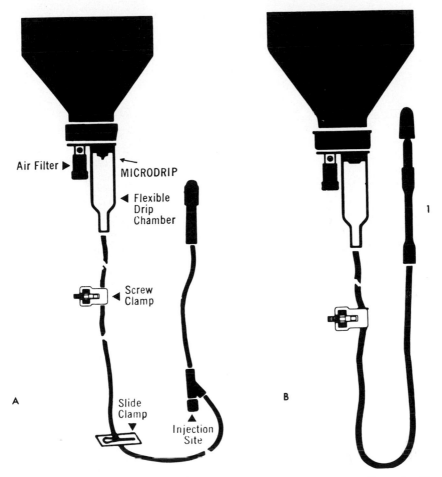

Air Filter ▶ ◀ MICRODRIP

◀ Flexible Drip Chamber

◀ Screw Clamp

A

Slide Clamp ▼ ▲ Injection Site

B

FIG. 19.14. Fluid dispensing systems. *A*, Microdrip with side arm injection port; *B*, regular Venopak with gum rubber sleeve (*1*). (Courtesy of Abbott Company.)

most accurate method for delivering small volumes is a system such as the Precision Volume Soluset-100. This unit prevents giving a greater volume of fluid than desired. Several bottles of one type of solution or compatible solutions can be connected by secondary delivery tubing. These are caps with an air inlet, filter, and a plastic tube. In such a series the last bottle connected will be the first to empty (Fig. 19.15).

Blood is dispensed from bottles with a blood administration set (Fig. 19.16). If the blood has to be administered rapidly, there are several methods for increasing the volume being delivered per unit of

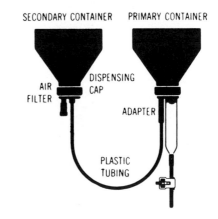

SECONDARY CONTAINER   PRIMARY CONTAINER

AIR FILTER   DISPENSING CAP

ADAPTER

PLASTIC TUBING

FIG. 19.15. Secondary Venopak connecting two fluid containers. (Courtesy of Abbott Company.)

time. Since flow is directly proportional to hydrostatic pressure, raising the height of the bottle will increase flow. The pressure in the bottle can also be increased by the injection of air into the air inlet of the bottle. This will markedly increase the flow; however, the system has to be watched very carefully since the compressed air will run into the vein after the fluid has left the bottle if it is not discon-

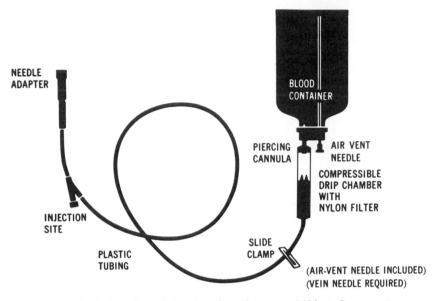

Fig. 19.16. Blood Administration Set. (Courtesy of Abbott Company.)

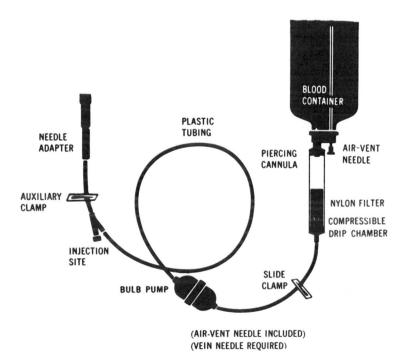

Fig. 19.17. Blood Pump Administration Set. (Courtesy of Abbott Company.)

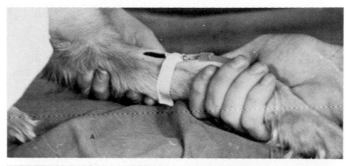

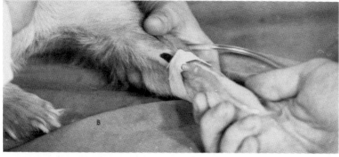

FIG. 19.18. Taping needle in place. *A*, narrow strip of tape was placed between the limb and needle with adhesive side against the needle. The ends of the tape are then crossed over the needle and attached to the limb. *B*, a loop has been put in the tubing and tape passed over the needle, tubing, and around the limb for a secure placement.

nected or the pressure relieved. The Blood Pump Administration Set can also be used to increase blood flow (Fig. 19.17). This unit has included in the delivery tube a bulb pump. The system is used in the normal manner; however, when flow has to be increased, the bulb pump is manually squeezed.

When deciding on the diameter of needle for fluid infusion, one which is as large as practical should be used, especially in a situation where large quantities of fluid may be needed. Since flow is directly proportional to the 4th power of the diameter, a doubling of the lumen size of a needle will increase flow 16 times.[6]

NEEDLE FIXATION

To fix the needle to the leg, a strip of tape is placed over the needle and around the limb. If an infusion set has been attached to the needle, a small loop should be made in the distal delivery tubing and fixed with tape. This loop will prevent the needle from being pulled out should any tension be placed on the delivery tubing.

A more secure method for fixing a needle is to use a strip of narrow tape placed between the needle and the skin with the sticky side toward the needle. The tape is then crossed over the needle and around the leg and back over the needle, a loop made in the tubing, and another tape placed around the needle and tube (Fig. 19.18).

ANESTHETIC DISPENSING CAPS

Caps are available for use on bulk volume containers of ultrashort acting barbiturates such as thiopental and thiamylal. These allow removal of the drug with syringes without repeated insertions of a needle.

Collecting Arterial Samples

When arterial blood is needed for measurement of blood gases and pH, it should be collected in heparinized glass syringes. The heparin (1000 units/ml) is drawn into the syringe and then expelled. The amount remaining in the syringe dead space is enough to prevent the blood from clotting. After collecting the sample, the syringe is held vertically to expel the small amount of air from the syringe and needle. The needle is then inserted into a rubber stopper, and the syringe is placed in ice water.

The most common site of collection in the dog is the femoral artery. This can be done in the unsedated dog only if the dog is very cooperative. A small amount of local anesthetic should be infiltrated to avoid movement with the needle placement and to try to minimize local arterial spasm. Generally a 22-gauge needle is used. When the needle is in the artery, the syringe begins to fill without aspirating because of the arterial pressure. After the sample is collected, strong finger pressure should be applied to the site of puncture to prevent a hematoma.

In the anesthetized horse, arterial blood is most easily obtained from the great metatarsal artery. Samples may be obtained in the standing awake horse by carotid artery puncture.[7]

REFERENCES

1. Amand, W. B.: Personal communication.
2. Berggren, R. B., Batterton, T. D., McArdle, G., and Erb, W. H.: Clostridial myositis after parenteral injections. J. A. M. A. *188:* 1044, 1964.
3. Bessinger, O. M., Jr., Browning, F. M., and Schroeder, C. R.: *An Atlas and Dissection Manual: Rhesus Monkey Anatomy.* Anatomy Laboratory, Tallahassee, Fla., 1966.
4. Crouch, J. E.: *Text-Atlas of Cat Anatomy.* Lea & Febiger, Philadelphia, 1969.
5. Dann, T. C.: Routine skin preparation before injection: an unnecessary procedure. Lancet *2:* 96, 1969.
6. Dripps, R. D., Eckenhoff, J. E., and Vandam, L. D.: *Introduction to Anesthesia,* 34th ed., chap. 26. W. B. Saunders Company, Philadelphia, 1967.
7. Gabel, A. A., Hamlin, R., and Smith, C. R.: Effects of promazine and chloral hydrate on the cardiovascular system of the horse. Amer. J. Vet. Res. *25:* 1151, 1964.
8. Gabel, A. A., and Koestner, A.: The effects of Intracarotid artery injection of drugs in domestic animals. J. Amer. Vet. Med. Ass. *142:* 1397, 1963.
9. Gardner, E., Gray, D. S., and O'Rahilly, R.: *Anatomy,* 2nd ed. W. B. Saunders Company, Philadelphia, 1963.
10. Miller, M. E., Christensen, G. C., and Evans, H. E.: *Anatomy of the Dog.* W. B. Saunders Company, Philadelphia, 1964.
11. Price, P. B.: The meaning of bacteriostasis, bactericidal effect, and rate of disinfection. Ann. N.Y. Acad. Sci. *53:* 76, 1950.
12. Sisson, S., and Grossman, J. D.: *The Anatomy of the Domestic Animals,* 4th ed. revised. W. B. Saunders Company, Philadelphia, 1953.
13. Westhues, M., and Fritsch, R.: *Animal Anesthesia: General,* p. 219. J. B. Lippincott Company, Philadelphia, 1965.

20
Preanesthetic Evaluation

DONALD CLIFFORD

The preanesthetic examination and evaluation of the patient are extremely important since the choice and dose of the preanesthetic drug and the selection of anesthetic agent and technique of administration are influenced by them.[18] Some veterinarians use only one, or at the most, two anesthetic techniques and may argue that individual preanesthetic evaluation is not necessary. Such individuals may be denying their patients a shorter or safer anesthesia. In experimental procedures, it is frequently necessary to adhere to a standardized anesthetic technique, but this does not preclude the investigator from making a careful preanesthetic examination.

Most conditions which affect the animal will also influence the anesthetic and postanesthetic period. Fright, vitamin deficiencies, the administration of drugs, and previous activities of the animal may drastically influence the anesthetic period, but are often not considered. Some of the important factors which influence the preanesthetic evaluation of the animal and subsequent anesthesia are discussed below.

Physical Status or "Risk"

The term "risk" is commonly used to describe the animal's potential for surviving anesthesia and surgery. This expression refers not only to the condition of the animal, but includes the competence of the anesthetist and the surgeon. The risk is greater when the surgeon and/or anesthetist have limited experience, despite the physical status or condition of the animal. The term "poor risk patient" is often used after a surgical or anesthetic death to excuse errors of omission, poor management, faulty judgment, or poor technique.

Classification of the physical status reflects an attempt to define the condition of the animal, and thereby alert the clinician, anesthetist, surgeon, or investigator to problems which may occur during anesthesia and surgery.[24] It also is used as a means of correlating and evaluating anesthetic problems and methods with the status of the animal.

The following is, in part, the classification adopted by the American Society of Anesthesiologists and applied in the preoperative evaluation of animals.[16]

Class 1. Animals with no organic disease or in whom the disease is localized and causes no systemic disturbance. Animals submitted for elective surgery or "normal" animals used in research would fit this category.

Class 2. Animals with slight to moderate systemic disturbances which may or may not be associated with the surgical complaint, and interfere only moderately with the normal activities and general physiological equilibrium. Some of these conditions are not associated with signs that can be detected by the clinician on routine physical examination. Slightly dehydrated or obese animals and those with simple fractures are examples.

Class 3. Animals with slight to moderate systemic disturbances that may or may not be associated with the surgical complaint, and may interfere with the patient's normal activities. Animals with compensated nephritis or valvular insufficiency are examples.

Class 4. Animals with extreme systemic disturbances which may or may not be associated with the surgical complaint, interfere seriously with the patient's normal activities, and have become a threat to life. Animals in this category are not able to compensate for the condition, and, frequently, surgery is required to save the animal's life. Rupture of the urinary bladder and strangulated hernias exemplify this category.

Class 5. Animals in a moribund condition.

The assignment of a rating will vary with the clinician or investigator but the classification of physical status serves as a reference point for subsequent observations.

Many animals such as the dog, cat, rabbit, and horse, sheep, and cow lend themselves to an individual physical examination. A detailed case history is frequently available to guide the clinician or investigator in making this physical examination. Body temperature, pulse, and respiration should be taken initially, followed by an examination of each system. For clinical patients, a hematological profile (hemoglobin, hematocrit or red blood cell count, white blood count) should be obtained prior to anesthesia and surgery. In older animals, urinalysis and blood urea nitrogen and a cardiac examination should be included.

An inspection rather than an examination is usually made with wild or zoological animals and small rodents; however, this compromise is not without danger. The inspection will be infinitely more valuable when supplemented by the observations of keepers or animal attendants. Good keepers and attendants can provide a great deal of information about the consumption of food, general activity, and behavior.

Presence of Disease

Disease may have a limited or wide effect on systems of the body, and hence upon anesthesia.[2, 19, 46] Those diseases which influence the respiratory, cardiovascular, and central nervous systems are most likely to exaggerate the effects of anesthetic agents. Shock, loss of blood, leucocytosis, anorexia, dehydration, anemia, obesity, malnutrition, uremia, diabetes, and most debilitating conditions will influence the anesthetic and postanesthetic period. Generally speaking, the patient is less able to compensate for alterations in body functions produced by anesthesia and surgery. Cardiovascular, respiratory, renal, and acid-base changes are amplified. This is not to say that anesthesia is contraindicated in these conditions, but greater care is necessary. Specific anesthetic agents and techniques are indicated in certain diseases (see Chapter 22).

Many species of animals have latent infectious diseases which can render anesthesia extremely hazardous, and in the event of investigation of the anesthetic agent itself, they might lead the investigator to a false conclusion. Three examples of such disease are distemper in dogs, chronic respiratory infection in rats, and pasteurellosis or snuffles in rabbits.

Size, Species, and Genetic Background

Large animals have a slower basal metabolic rate and generally require less anesthetic agent on the basis of their weight or body mass than smaller animals. For example, when the intravenous dose of pentobarbital for the mouse (60 mg/kg), the rat (40 mg/kg), and the dog (30 to 33 mg/kg) are compared, one might quickly conclude that the difference may be due to species rather than a size. This is partially true, but in the canine species, a large dog generally requires less anesthetic than smaller animals of the same sex and age.

There are species and subspecies differences. Some strains of mice or breeds of dogs require more or less anesthetic than others.[12] Respiratory distress observed in the brachycephalic breeds of dogs is usually due to poor airway and not to susceptability to anesthetics and can be prevented by endotracheal intubation. Cats, which require about the same amount of pentobarbital as dogs, need approximately twice as long to recover from anesthesia.[16] Large *Felidae* (lions and tigers) metabolize barbiturates much more slowly than the domestic cat.[17] Racing greyhounds have a longer recovery period and a greater incidence of excitement after the use of thiobarbiturates.[15]

Individual variation in the metabolism and elimination of drugs in a homologous population of animals can be large.[44] In controlled anesthetic experiments where precise measurements are being made, the genetic background can be controlled by selection and randomization of the population.

Age

Age is an important consideration, although it is not a completely independent variable and can be correlated with basal metabolic rate, nutritional status, activity, and function of various systems. The metabolic rate is less in the newborn and old animal than in the young adult.[36, 46] The sensitivity to many drugs is greater at these periods and lower doses must be administered.

Young dogs, 3 to 12 months of age, recover from barbiturate anesthesia more rapidly than older animals.[23] There also is a greater survival rate in dogs 3 to 12 months of age when serial injections are administered every 15 minutes. In rats, the lethal dose and anesthetic dose of pentobarbital is less on a weight basis in old rats (over 12 months) than in young animals (less than 9 months).[8, 9]

Sex

The sex of the animal has an influence on the dose of intravenous anesthetic agents in small laboratory animals. Female animals usually are more sensitive to anesthetic agents than males.[20, 35, 48] Although there is a rise in the basal metabolic rate during pregnancy, there does not appear to be a corresponding rise in dose of barbiturates required to produce anesthesia. Unspayed female rats are less sensitive to pentobarbital than spayed females.[7] Uncastrated males are less susceptible to bar-

biturate anesthesia, and castrated males are as susceptible as females. The effect of testosterone on hepatic detoxification may be responsible for this.[7]

Not all authors have observed differences between sexes in laboratory animals,[34, 38] and in clinical anesthesia these differences are difficult to distinguish.[25] When these differences occur, they modify but do not replace changes resulting from such factors as temperament, preanesthetic medication, and presence of disease.

Nutritional State, Intake of Food, and Fluid Balance

Malnutrition can be considered as a chronic disease, and metabolism of drugs is impaired during this state. Dogs and cats are carnivores and must be fed a diet which is relatively high in protein in order to bear the stress of anesthesia and surgery. Malnourished dogs remain anesthetized longer with barbiturates than those which are well fed.[23]

Some animals have exceptional dietary requirements for certain food ingredients. The guinea pig requires more vitamin C than other rodents, and guinea pigs which were fed diets deficient in this vitamin were more profoundly depressed and recovered more slowly from ether, chloroform, and divinyl ether anesthesia.[3] A similar relationship exists between avitaminosis C and barbiturate anesthesia in guinea pigs.[31] In dogs, volatile agents were found to increase the plasma ascorbic acid levels. Deficiencies in other nutrients as well as excessive deposits of fat reduce the anesthetic requirements.[3, 11, 46]

Digestible food in the alimentary canal increases the metabolic rate, but carnivores do not attain the maximum nutritional value until 12 to 18 hours after ingestion. Thus, a recent meal does not benefit the animal. Conversely, if an animal has eaten during the preceding 6 hours, vomiting is more common, and abdominal surgery is more difficult. Nonruminant animals should be fed a nutritious, low residue meal on the afternoon prior to anesthesia, and water should not be withheld until the day of surgery. Dehydration has been shown to increase sleeping time in mice.[4]

Handling and Environmental Factors

These usually are less important considerations in the preanesthetic evaluation, but in special instances they can greatly influence general anesthesia. Unfamiliar surroundings are apt to excite or produce fear in animals. When an animal is handled roughly or brought into a strange environment, it may become unmanageable and require larger doses of preanesthetic medication for sedation and greater amounts of anesthetics for induction of anesthesia. If barbiturates are used, the resulting plane of anesthesia may be deeper than is desired. Epinephrine released in an excited animal may sensitize the heart to certain volatile agents (chloroform, cyclopropane, trichlorethylene, halothane, and ethyl chloride) and result in cardiac irregularities.[32] Cardiac arrhythmias during the induction of anesthesia with barbiturates are not uncommon in an extremely excitable animal. This can be a potentially dangerous situation leading to cardiac arrest. Some complications can be prevented by adequate premedication and gentle handling.

Hypothermia will usually prolong the recovery from preanesthetic medication and barbiturate anesthesia.[13, 14, 29] Hypothermia will also delay the recovery from inhalation anesthesia if ventilation is depressed. Animals that are anesthetized with oxybarbiturates are very susceptible to environmental temperatures because of the slow detoxification of those agents.[40, 45] In large dogs, hyperthermia can pose a problem during summer unless air conditioning is provided.

There are daily as well as seasonal changes in animals and their response to drugs.[21, 22, 43] Digestion, fatigue, activity, metabolic rate, and urinary excretion are reasons for these differences. Many of these variables are undefined in anesthetic experiments and may explain differences which are not otherwise apparent.

Stress

Changes in the animal's condition or environment can be considered as forms of stress. Crowding, transportation, changes in lighting, and the introduction of new animals are common stresses which render animals more susceptible to disease and weight loss. The condition known as "shipping fever" is a prime example of this form of stress. Unfortunately, this disturbance to a normal physiological equilibrium is difficult to definitively define and measure physiologically. However, it can alter the animal's response to drugs, and this ill-defined alteration in body homeostasis should be taken into consideration during the preanesthetic handling and hospitalization. Pain is a form of physical and "emotional" stress and will increase basal metabolic rate. It will also increase the amount of drugs needed to produce sedation and analgesia. Endocrine function has received some study as it relates to anesthesia but further investigation is needed.[5, 33, 49]

Previous Medication

Tranquilizers, narcotics, anticonvulsants, and barbiturates are drugs which will potentiate the effect of preanesthetic medication and also influence general anesthesia. The duration of administration, the amount, and the depressant effect on the animal should always be taken into consideration.

Sulfonamides potentiate barbiturate, ether, and chloroform anesthesia.[1, 6, 46] The effect of 2½ days of oral administration of sulfanilamide on the duration of pentobarbital anesthesia was more pronounced than a single intravenous injection of this drug.[6] Other antibiotics, neomycin, kanamycin, streptomycin, and polymixin-B-sulfate may potentiate the neuromuscular block of muscle relaxants.[47] Disulfiran, metabolic inhibitors, antihistamines, atropine-like substances, glucose, megimide, and other drugs have been reviewed concerning their effect on anesthesia.[19, 27]

Intimately associated with previous

medication is tolerance, a condition which may be defined as a decrease in response to a drug because of prior administration of the same or similar drug. Animals quickly acquire a tolerance to narcotics and barbiturates; thus, larger doses are necessary to produce the same effect. Repeated injections of a short acting barbiturate may result in an increase in the dose necessary to produce anesthesia and/or a decrease in the duration of anesthesia.[10, 26, 28, 37] In drugs that have a long duration of action, the agent may not be completely detoxified at the time of the second injection so that a decrease rather than an increase in anesthetic dose, will be required.[39] The anesthetic drug, species, and the time interval between injections are factors to be considered when determining the response to previous administration of drugs.[41] In cats and dogs, tolerance to pentobarbital is not observed if 10 days or more are allowed to elapse between injections,[42] while in dogs acquired tolerance disappears in less than 2 weeks.[37, 39] Cross-tolerance between depressants does occur.[30, 42] Development of tolerance to barbiturates in animals does not appear to be accompanied by a concomitant decrease in the lethal dose.

REFERENCES

1. Adriani, J.: Effects of anesthetic drugs upon rats treated with sulfanilamide. J. Lab. Clin. Med. 24: 1066, 1939.
2. Adriani, J.: Anesthesia for patients with uncommon and unusual diseases. Anesth. Analg. (Cleveland) 37: 1, 1958.
3. Beyer, K. H., Stutzman, J. W., and Hafford, B.: The relation of Vitamin C to anesthesia. Surg. Gynec. Obstet. 79: 49, 1944.
4. Borzelleca, J. F., and Manthei, R. W.: Factors influencing pentobarbital sodium sleeping time in mice. Arch. Int. Pharmacodyn. 111: 296, 1957.
5. Bunker, J. P.: Neuroendocrine and other effects on carbohydrate metabolism during anesthesia. Anesthesiology 24: 515, 1963.
6. Butler, T. C., Dickison, H. L., Govier, W. M., Greer, C. M., and Lamson, P. D.: The effect of sulfanilamide and some of its derivatives on the reaction of mice to anesthetics. J. Pharmacol. Exp. Ther. 72: 298, 1941.
7. Cameron, G. R.: Some recent work on barbiturates. Proc. Roy. Soc. Med. 32: 309, 1938.
8. Carmichael, E. B.: The average lethal dose of Nembutal (pentobarbital) for young and old rats. J. Pharmacol. Exp. Therm 60: 101, 1937.
9. Carmichael, E. B.: Nembutal anesthesia. III. The median lethal dose of Nembutal (pentobarbital sodium) for young and old rats. J. Pharmacol. Exp. Ther. 62: 284, 1938.
10. Carmichael, E. B.: Observations on effect of repeated administration of Nembutal in guinea pigs. Proc. Soc. Exp. Biol. Med. 30: 1329, 1932.
11. Caster, W. O., and Ahn, P.: Electrocardiographic notching in rats deficient in essential fatty acids. Science 139: 1213, 1963.
12. Clark, A. J., and Raventos, J.: Dynamic variation in response to barbiturates. Quart. J. Exp. Physiol. 30: 187, 1940.
13. Clifford, D. H.: Effect of preanesthetic medication on barbiturate anesthesia, hypothermia, traumatic shock and lethal dose of pentobarbital in feline species. Ph.D. thesis. University of Minnesota, Minneapolis, 1959.
14. Clifford, D. H.: Effect of preanesthetic medication with promazine and promethazine on anesthesia with pentobarbital and subsequent hypothermia in the cat. J. Amer. Vet. Med. Ass. 137: 251, 1960.
15. Clifford, D. H., and Jha, S. K.: A comparison between oxymorphone (Numorphan®) and morphine sulfate prior to pentobarbital anesthesia in the dog. Anesth. Analg. (Cleveland) 40: 645, 1961.
16. Clifford, D. H., and Soma, L. R.: Anesthesiology. Feline Medicine and Surgery, 1st ed., p. 392. American Veterinary Publications, Inc., Santa Barbara, Calif., 1964.
17. Clifford, D. H., Stowe, C. M., and Good, A. L.: Pentobarbital anesthesia in lions with special reference to preanesthetic medication. J. Amer. Vet. Med. Ass. 139: 111, 1961.
18. Collins, V. J.: Principles and Practice of Anesthesiology. Lea & Febiger, Philadelphia, 1952.
19. Cooney, A. H., and Burns, J. J.: Factors influencing drug metabolism. In Advances in Pharmacology, vol. 1. Academic Press, New York, 1962.
20. Crevier, M., D'Iorio, A., and Robillard, E.: Influence of the sexual glands on detoxication of pentobarbital by the liver. Rev. Canad. Biol. 9: 336, 1950.
21. Davis, W. M.: Day-night periodicity in pentobarbital response of mice and the influence of socio-psychological conditions. Experientia 18: 235, 1962.
22. De Beer, E. J., Hjort, A. M., and Fassett, D. W.: Analysis of relationships between environmental changes and duration of anesthesia in albino mice. J. Pharmacol. Exp. Ther. 66: 241, 1939.
23. De Boer, B.: Factors affecting pentothal anesthesia in dogs. Anesthesiology 8: 375, 1947.
24. Dripps, R. D., Eckenhoff, J. E., and Vandam,

L. D.: *Introduction to Anesthesia*, 2nd ed. W. B. Saunders Company, Philadelphia, 1961.

25. Dundee, J. W.: Influence of body weight, sex and age on dosage of thiopentone. Brit. J. Anaesth. *26:* 164, 1954.

26. Dundee, J. W.: Acquired tolerance to intravenous thiobarbiturates in animals. Brit. J. Anaesth. *27:* 165, 1955.

27. Elliot, H. W.: Influence of previous therapy on anesthesia. Clin. Pharmacol. Ther. *3:* 41, 1962.

28. Ettinger, G. H.: Duration of anesthesia produced in dog by repeated administration of Dial and Nembutal. J. Pharmacol. Exp. Ther. *63:* 82, 1938.

29. Fuhrman, F. A.: Effect of body temperature on drug action. Physiol. Rev. *26:* 247, 1946.

30. Green, M. W., and Koppanyi, T.: Studies on barbiturates. XXVII. Tolerance and cross tolerance to barbiturates. Anesthesiology *5:* 329, 1944.

31. Green, M. W., and Musulin, R. R.: Studies on barbiturates: effect of vitamin C level on barbiturate depression in guinea pigs. J. Amer. Pharm. Ass. *30:* 613, 1941.

32. Hall, L. W.: Anesthetic accidents and emergencies. Vet. Rec. *70:* 888, 1958.

33. Hayes, M. A., and Goldenberg, I. S.: Renal effects of anesthesia and operation mediated by endocrines. Anesthesiology *24:* 487, 1963.

34. Holck, H. G. O., Kanan, M. A., Mills, L. M., and Smith, E. L.: Studies upon the sex-difference in rats in tolerance to certain barbiturates and to nicotine. J. Pharmacol. Exp. Ther. *60:* 323, 1937.

35. Holck, H. G. O., Mathieson, D. R., Smith, E. L., and Fink, L. D.: Effects of testosterone acetate and propionate and of estradiol dipropionate upon resistance of rate to Evipal sodium, Nostal, Pernoston and pentobarbital sodium. J. Amer. Pharm. Ass. *31:* 116, 1942.

36. Homburger, E., Etsten, B., and Himwich, H.E.: Some factors affecting susceptibility of rats to various barbiturates: effect of age and sex. J. Lab. Clin. Med. *32:* 540, 1947.

37. Hubbard, T. F., and Goldbaum, L. R.: The mechanism of tolerance to thiopental sodium in mice. J. Pharmacol. Exp. Ther. *97:* 488, 1949.

38. Kennedy, W. P.: Sodium salt of C-C-cyclohexenylmethyl-N-methyl barbituric acid (Evipal) anaesthesia in laboratory animals. J. Pharmacol. Exp. Ther. *50:* 347, 1934.

39. Kinsey, V. E.: The use of sodium pentobarbital for repeated anesthesia in rabbit. J. Amer. Pharm. Ass. *29:* 292, 1940.

40. Krog, J.: Notes on rectal temperature variations in dogs during Nembutal anaesthesia. Acta Physiol. Scand. *45:* 308, 1959.

41. Masuda, M., Budde, R. N., and Dille, J. M.: Investigation of acquired tolerance to certain short-acting barbiturates. J. Amer. Pharm. Ass. *27:* 830, 1938.

42. Maynert, E. W., and Klingman, G. I.: Acute tolerance to intravenous anesthetics in dogs. J. Pharmacol. Exp. Ther. *128:* 192, 1960.

43. Mirsky, J. H., and Giarman, N. J.: Studies on potentiation of thiopental. J. Pharmacol. Exp. Ther. *114:* 240, 1955.

44. Papper, E. M., and Kitz, R. J.: *Uptake and Distribution of Anesthetic Agents.* McGraw-Hill Book Company, New York, 1963.

45. Raventos, J.: Influence of room temperature on action of barbiturates. J. Pharmacol. Exp. Ther. *64:* 355, 1938.

46. Richards, R. K., and Taylor, J. D.: Some factors influencing distribution, metabolism and action of barbiturates. A review. Anesthesiology *17:* 414, 1956.

47. Sabawala, T. B., and Dillon, J. B.: The action of some antibiotics on the human intercostal nerve-muscle complex. Anesthesiology *20:* 659, 1959.

48. Streicher, E., and Garbus, J.: Effect of age and sex on duration of hexobarbital anesthesia in rats. J. Geront. *10:* 441, 1955.

49. Van Brunt, E. E., and Ganong, W. F.: The effects of preanesthetic medication anesthesia and hypothermia on the endocrine response to injury. Anesthesiology *24:* 500, 1963.

21
Intravenous Anesthetic Agents

LAWRENCE R. SOMA

The intravenous anesthetics in their broadest coverage would include a multitude of drugs, ranging from barbiturates, which are the most commonly used, to many nonbarbiturates. The nonbarbiturates represent a wide number of nonrelated chemical compounds many of which are primarily used for basal narcosis; like the barbiturates, many are classified as hypnotic-sedative, e.g., glutethimide, chloral hydrate, and hydroxydione. On the other hand, drugs such as narcotics, tranquilizers, local anesthetics, and alcohol, which generally are not considered intravenous agents, have been used in this manner in moderate amounts, and many times in combination to produce a state of deep sedation almost bordering on general anesthesia. Unconsciousness is not produced with these latter compounds, and arousal is possible. The unconscious state can be quickly created by the superimposition of small amounts of a barbiturate or an inhalation agent. The cyclohexamines, although discussed as preanesthetic agents (see Chapter 13), have been used both intramuscularly and intravenously to create levels of sedation bordering on general anesthesia.

The veterinary clinician generally associates barbiturates with intravenous anesthesia; from a pragmatic aspect this is true, but in the modern usage of drugs, many agents are used intravenously alone or in combination to establish varying degrees of central nervous system depression. Unfortunately, many clinicians approach and compare many new compounds which can be injected intravenously as substitutes for the barbiturates, despite dissimilar actions, in the hopes that the disadvantages of intravenous barbiturates can be eliminated and the advantages preserved.

Barbiturates

The barbiturates are a widely used and very versatile group of agents. They are classified as hypnotic-sedatives based on their primary use for the production of sedation as prenaesthetic drugs. In veterinary anesthesia, they are used primarily for the induction or the maintenance of general anesthesia. The central nervous system actions of barbiturates are diverse and progressive, ranging from sedation, which implies mild depression, to hypnosis, which indicates a stronger degree of depression leading to sleep. The sedation and hypnosis produced by barbiturates can be considered gradations of the stage of general anesthesia, inasmuch as higher doses will produce excitement (stage 2) followed by general anesthesia (stage 3). An important distinction in comparing the actions of the sedative-hypnotic drugs with the actions of narcotics and tranquilizers is that increasing doses of barbiturates will produce anesthesia.

The parent compound was derived by Adolf van Bayer in 1867, and, since then, thousands of "barbituric acid" compounds have been developed (Fig. 21.1). One of the first sedative compounds, diethyl barbituric acid, was discovered by Fischer and von Mering in 1903. This compound, Veronal (barbital), was one of the first to be used clinically. The barbiturates for comparison can be classified in two ways: one, according to the basic chemical substitutions of the barbituric acid molecule and the other, according to the duration of action.

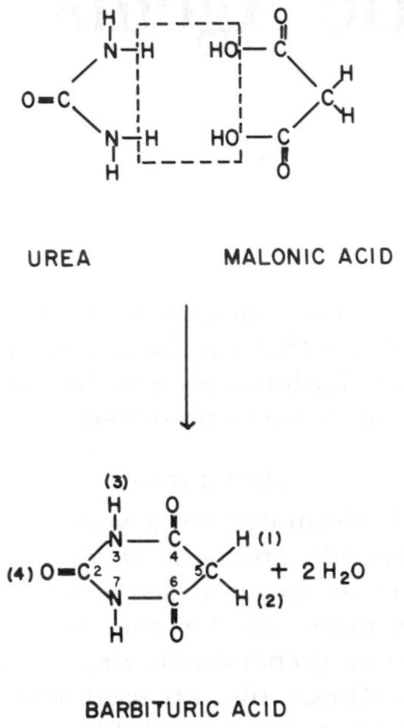

FIG. 21.1. Barbituric acid molecule with the major locations for substitution of radicals indicated.

Chemically, three basic groups are used clinically: (a) oxybarbiturates, which include pentobarbital, phenobarbital, barbital, and secobarbital; (b) methylated oxybarbiturates, which include hexobarbital and methohexital; and (c) thiobarbiturates, which include thiopental, thiamylal, and thialbarbital. The parent compound barbituric acid is a combination of malonic acid and urea and has no sedative properties (Fig. 21.1). The barbiturates have many structural functional relationships which are dependent upon substitution at positions *1, 2, 3,* and *4* on Figure 21.1. For the creation of sedative compounds, the hydrogens 1 and 2 at carbon position 5 must be substituted. Sodium barbital, the original barbiturate, was produced by the substitution of diethyl radicals at this position (Fig. 21.2). Lengthening the side chain beyond the two carbons, but not longer than five, shortens the onset of action and diminishes the duration of action. For example, the short side chained (diethyl) oxybarbiturate sodium barbital has a longer period of action than the longer chained (ethyl methylbutyl) oxybarbiturate sodium pentobarbital, which is a short acting drug in compar-

OXYBARBITURATES

	R-1	R-2	R-3	R-4
BARBITAL	$-CH_2-CH_3$	$-CH_2-CH_3$	$-H$	$-O-$
PHENOBARBITAL	$-CH_2-CH_3$	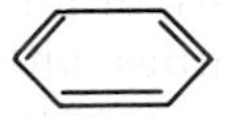 ⬡	$-H$	$-O-$
PENTOBARBITAL	$-CH_2-CH_3$	$-CH-CH_2-CH_2-CH_3$ $\quad CH_3$	$-H$	$-O-$
SECOBARBITAL	$-CH_2-CH=CH_2$	$-CH-CH_2-CH_2-CH_3$ $\quad CH_3$	$-H$	$-O-$
METHOHEXITAL	$-CH_2-CH=CH_2$	$-CH-C=C-CH_2-CH_3$ $\quad CH_3$	$-CH_3$	$-O-$

FIG. 21.2. Structural formulas for commonly used oxybarbiturates.

THIOBARBITURATES

	R-1	R-2	R-3	R-4
THIOPENTAL	$-CH_2-CH_3$	$-\underset{\underset{CH_3}{\mid}}{C}H-CH_2-CH_2-CH_3$	$-H$	$-S-$
THIAMYLAL	$-CH_2-CH=CH_2$	$-\underset{\underset{CH_3}{\mid}}{C}H-CH_2-CH_2-CH_3$	$-H$	$-S-$
THIALBARBITAL	$-CH_2-CH=CH_2$	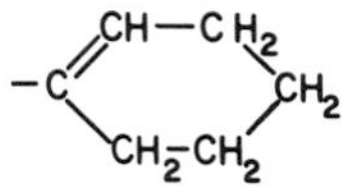 (cyclohexenyl ring)	$-H$	$-S-$

FIG. 21.3. Structural formulas for commonly used thiobarbiturates.

TABLE 21.1
*Classification of barbiturates according
to duration of action*

Type	Name
Long acting	Phenobarbital, barbital, butabarbital
Short or intermediate acting	Pentobarbital, secobarbital, hexobarbital
Ultrashort acting	Thiopental, thiamylal, methohexital

ison. The oxybarbiturate sodium methohexital is an ultrashort acting drug by virtue of the longer chained methyl pentynyl group (Fig. 21.2). As the side chains at carbon number 5 are increased beyond five carbons in length, the hypnotic properties are reduced and convulsive properties appear. Different radicals may enhance one property; for example, the addition of a phenyl group at R_1 or R_2 (5-carbon position) as in sodium phenobarbital renders greater anticonvulsant properties than the diethyl radicals in the same position. The replacement of the oxygen molecule with the sulfur molecule was a major alteration of the barbituric acid (Fig. 21.3). This markedly increases its lipid solubility, en-

hancing transfer across biological membranes. Because of this, the thiobarbiturates have actions which are ultrarapid in onset and ultrashort in duration. The longer carbon side chain oxybarbiturate compounds, like the thiobarbiturates, have a more rapid onset and shorter duration of action. However, unlike the sulfur substitutes, the longer carbon side chained oxybarbiturate, e.g., methohexital, has a more rapid rate of metabolic degradation and is not as dependent on redistribution into non-nervous tissue for its ultrashort actions (see Chapter 11).

Barbiturates are also commonly classified according to their duration of action (Table 21.1). The ultrashort acting barbiturates are used principally for the induction of anesthesia and maintenance with an inhalation agent or for short periods of a light plane of barbiturate anesthesia. The short to intermediate acting drugs are used in small animals for 2 to 3 hours of general anesthesia. The prolonged and stormy recovery period, particularly in the horse, makes the short acting drugs unsuitable for use in this species. These compounds are used as hypnotic-sedatives in man and can be used for this purpose in the horse when combined with tranquilizers (see Chapter 13). The longer acting compounds are also used for the treatment of convulsive disorders in veterinary medicine. The duration of actions of these drugs is subject to marked fluctuation in each individual and species of animal. Sleeping time as high as 48 hours has been reported following the use of short acting barbiturates (*e.g.*, sodium pentobarbital) in wild and domestic cats, a duration of actions more similar to phenobarbital.

Determination of the Depth of Barbiturate Anesthesia

As with the inhalation agents, it is difficult to define as specific depth of anesthesia in an individual at a given moment in the time course of a barbiturate anesthetic. All that can be presented are some guidelines. The effects of barbiturates on the central nervous system, as with the inhalation agents, are progressive in nature. At low doses there is a loss of discrimination, cloudiness of vision, and impairment of speech and cerebellar function. This can be followed by sleep. Sleep induced by oxybarbiturates overtly resembles physiological sleep, but more definitive sleep studies utilizing electroencephalographic activity and rapid eye movements as criteria for judgment have shown this to be false.[26] Rapid eye movement time is diminished with barbiturate-induced sleep, which is made up on subsequent nights.[38] Barbiturate-induced sleep is not as refreshing as one might anticipate; although the hypnotic effects may last for 2 to 3 hours, a performance decrement may still persist for 10 to 22 hours.[26] Granted, low doses are not used in veterinary medicine and definitive performance testing in animals is not routinely used in other than laboratory situations, but alterations in performance of highly trained animals can be anticipated following low doses of drugs or conceivably after many hours following the usual therapeutic doses.

Although the observations of veterinary anesthesia are limited to the more objective effects of stages 2 and 3, some observations can be made which relate to the subjective changes described in man during stage 1. These changes are notable when the rapid acting thiobarbiturates are administered slowly intravenously. Following the initial injection of low doses in the dog, drowsiness and a quieting effect are produced; some head weaving occurs, indicating possible dizziness. Licking and swallowing are common, possibly due to a slight feeling of nausea or the bitter taste of the barbiturate, which has been noted in man. These effects are transitory, and, as the intravenous administration continues, some manifestation of stage 2 (excitement stage) can be observed. As with other anesthetic agents, this stage is manifested by a loss of consciousness, excitement, and hyperexcitability (see Chapter 15). This hyperexcitability is due to the loss of the inhibitory function of the reticular activating system following lower doses of anesthetic agents. The excitatory phase is very mild or nonexistent when thiobarbiturates are used for the induction of anesthesia. When occurring, the excitement is transitory and limited to dilation of the pupils, slight increase in muscle tone, and slight movement. Whining and thrashing about are uncommon. The transition into stage 3 is noted by muscle relaxation, constriction of pupils, and transformation from an irregular to a regular respiratory pattern. The slow intravenous injection of an oxybarbiturate such as pentobarbital, because of the slower transfer across the blood-brain barrier, produces considerable excitement which includes vocalization, paddling of the legs, urination, defecation, and involuntary uncoordinated movement. The passage through stage 2 with pentobarbital is slow unless a high arterial concentration of the barbiturate is attained rapidly.

Stage 3 of barbiturate anesthesia can be divided into three planes, and, admittedly, their distinct separation is difficult. As with inhalation drugs, the planes are separated by presence or usually absence of reflex signs. The neurological signs used are the wink, corneal, swallowing, and patellar reflexes.[37] These are assessed along with response to painful stimuli, spontaneous movements, ventilation (rate and depth), heart rate, pulse pressure, and pupil size.

In the lighter plane of anesthesia (plane 1) the animal is hypoactive to painful stimuli but will withdraw the leg if the toe webbing is pinched. The corneal reflex, a contraction of the orbicularis muscle induced by touching the cornea and the inner canthus of the eye, respectively, is still present. The cornea at this time is covered by the prolapsed nictitans membrane. The patellar reflex, an extension of the hind leg in response to tapping of the quadriceps tendon, is still present. Jaw muscle tension still persists and reflex closure of the larynx will occur with attempts at endotracheal intubation. The tracheal reflex persists, and a coughing or breath holding will occur following introduction of the tracheal tube. Respiratory rate is reduced, but tidal volume is adequate. The responses indicated will, of course, be modified by the condition of the animal and preanesthetic drugs.

Plane 2, or moderate surgical, is distin-

TABLE 21.2
Physiological values in dogs in deep surgical anesthesia with sodium pentobarbital (38.1 mg/kg)*

Sign	Value
Respiratory rate (breaths/min)	5.3 ± 0.37
Exhaled minute volume (ml/kg/min)	98.4 ± 9.15
Arterial pH	7.25 ± 0.019
Arterial carbon dioxide tension (Torr)	53.0 ± 2.13
Arterial oxygen tension (Torr)	71.1 ± 5.29
Standard bicarbonate (mEq/liter)	20.2 ± 0.45
Heart rate (beats/min)	141.5 ± 1.99
Systolic pressure (Torr)	150 ± 3.61
Oxygen consumption (ml/kg/min)	6.8

*Mean dose of the drug administered with no preanesthetic medication. Data are the mean values for 14 dogs $\pm$ 1 S.E. of the mean.

TABLE 21.3
Determinants of effective arterial levels of barbiturates

1. Injected dose
2. Ionized versus unionized form
3. Amount of plasma binding
4. Rate of redistribution
5. Rate of biotransformation
6. Renal excretion of drug

guished by the absence of all of the aforementioned reflexes with the possible exception of the patellar. The pupils are constricted as in plane 1.

Plane 3, or deep surgical, is distinguished from the previous plane by marked ventilatory depression with a reduced respiratory rate and tidal volume. Respiratory acidosis is marked, and when breathing room air, arterial oxygen tensions are low (Table 21.2). The electroencephalographic pattern is depressed as has been described in Chapter 15. Stage 4 of general anesthesia is universal in its signs, irrespective of the drug used.

Determinants of an Effective Plasma Level

The effective plasma level of a barbiturate is the fraction of the drug which is capable of transferring across the blood-brain barrier. There are many factors which modify and finally determine this effective concentration (Table 21.3). The considerations listed in Table 21.3 are physiochemical and do not take into consideration the hemodynamic forces which influence blood flow to the brain and other organs and therefore the delivery rate of the agent per unit of time. The hemodynamic forces will partially affect the induction time, the rate of redistribution and equilibration into non-nervous tissues and finally the rate of renal excretion or hepatic metabolism.

DOSE

The most obvious and initially controllable factors which determine the initial plasma level are the dose, the route of administration, and, if given intravenously, the speed of injection, Regardless of the route of administration once given, retrieval is impossible and the effect and the time course of the recovery are dependent upon hemodynamic and physiochemical factors, most of which are beyond the control of the clinician. The remaining determinants of an effective plasma level are obviously difficult to assess, but in the routine use of these drugs as anesthetics an awareness of their contribution is important.

IONIZATION

Barbiturates are weak acids, and for both weak acids and bases the ionized and nonionized portions have different lipid solubilities.[39] The ionized group, because of their strong interaction with water dipoles,

penetrate poorly or not at all into lipoidal cell membranes.[25, 36] For drugs which are partially ionized at body pH, the nonionized form is the diffusable component; therefore, the rate of entry into cells is strongly dependent upon pH. The arterial pH will determine the equilibrium between the two plasma forms and the fraction of the plasma concentration available for entry into cells. A simple expression of the two forms is as follows:

$$B\ Na \rightleftarrows B^- + Na^+$$

A decrease in pH (increase in hydrogen ion concentration) will shift the equilibrium to the left, increasing the concentration of the nonionized drug and therefore the movement out of plasma into extravascular compartments, including the central

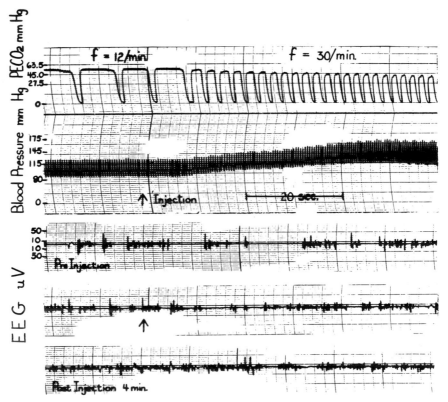

FIG. 21.4. The electroencephalogram (*EEG*), systemic blood pressure, and end expired carbon dioxide (*PECO₂*) of a dog under deep pentobarbital anesthesia. The hypoventilation is demonstrated by the elevated expired CO₂ and the depth of anesthesia by the burst suppression pattern of the electroencephalogram. The injection of a respiratory stimulant produced a transient improvement in ventilation, reducing carbon dioxide tensions and increasing arterial pH. There is an improvement in the electroencephalogram indicating a lightening of anesthesia. The change in the pattern is not related to any direct effect of the stimulant.

TABLE 21.4
*Physical properties of three barbiturates**

Drug	pK_a	Fraction Nonionized at pH 7.4	Fraction Bound to Plasma Protein at pH 7.4	Partition Coefficient of Nonionized Form n-Heptane/Water
Thiopental	7.6	0.613	0.75	3.3
Pentobarbital	8.1	0.834	0.40	0.05
Barbital	7.5	0.557	0.02	0.002

* Data from Goldstein *et al.*[25]

nervous system. For example, a change in pH from 7.36 to 6.89 pH units, which represents an increase in hydrogen ions from 43.6 to 129 μmEq, causes a decline in the plasma concentration of thiopental from 33.4 to 20.8 mg/liter; following a pH return to 7.33, the plasma level increased to 29.0 mg/liter.[14] An increase in hydrogen ion concentration will occur with the hypoventilation which is common during deep barbiturate anesthesia. This shift to the nonionized fraction produced by an increase in hydrogen ion concentration occurs with all barbiturates, including the long acting phenobarbital and the short acting pentobarbital (Fig. 21.4). The pK_a's of the barbiturates are similar but not identical; therefore, the nonionized fraction of each drug will vary at a given pH (Table 21.4). As compared to the other commonly used barbiturates, pentobarbital has the highest degree of nonionized portion at pH 7.4.

Alterations in pH and its effect on transfer into nervous tissue is an important consideration during barbiturate anesthesia, and as with all anesthetics, the tendency is toward hypoventilation and respiratory acidosis. Fortunately, the hypoventilation can be corrected by assisted or controlled ventilation.

PLASMA BINDING

Plasma proteins bind a large number of organic and inorganic molecules, the principal protein being albumin.[14, 21, 22, 23, 25] As would be expected because of their high lipid solubility, the thiobarbiturates have a higher degree of plasma binding (Table 21.4). Of the more commonly used drugs, thiopental is highly bound, being in the order of 65%, with pentobarbital, 40%, phenobarbital, 20%, and barbital, 5% bound at a given pH.[21, 22, 23] The degree of binding to plasma protein is pH-dependent, and reaches maximum binding at a pH of between 7.6 and 8. As with the relationship between pH and the ionized and the nonionized fraction of the barbiturate, an increase in hydrogen ions (acidemia) decreases the amount of drug bound to albumin, therefore increasing the fraction of drug capable of crossing biological membranes. The change in binding power produced by pH changes over the physiological pH range (6.8 to 7.6) is not great and varies with the drug, the alteration being greater with the highly bound thiopental and minimal with barbital.

Common to all biological reactions, the percent of binding is reduced with increasing concentrations of barbiturates, although the total amount bound is greater.[14, 21] The stronger bound thiopental, due to its greater affinity, is capable of displacing the weaker bound molecules on the albumin molecule. Included in this effect are highly bound nondepressant compounds which can influence the depth and duration of a barbiturate anesthetic (see "Variations in Response to Barbiturates"). When attempting to correlate the plasma concentration of a barbiturate with the physiological effects, the physiological active concentration must be used; because of this, the plasma binding and arterial pH should be determined.

REDISTRIBUTION

The shorter duration of the ultrashort thiobarbiturates and methylated oxybarbiturate as compared to other barbiturates is the result of a more rapid fall in plasma levels and therefore brain concentration. Thiobarbiturates as compared to the methylated oxybarbiturates are rapidly redistributed into non-nervous tissue.[41, 42, 43] The rapid redistribution is initially into highly perfused visceral tissues (see Chapter 11). There is a simultaneous uptake by lean body tissues which is slower but meaningful in the time course of this initial injection. The maximal uptake by the lean body tissues coincides with a lightening of anesthesia in 10 to 15 minutes (Fig. 21.5). The rapid redistribution into non-nervous tissues other than fat accounts for the ultrashort actions of these drugs. The thiobarbiturates are very soluble in fatty tissues, but because of the slow perfusion of adipose tissue, the initial contribution to the reduction in plasma level is not great. The uptake by fatty deposits does become significant in a longer time period, and the amount of fatty tissue can influence the final recovery.

The characteristic steep decline in plasma concentrations occurs within the first 10 minutes and is followed by a slower decline as redistribution continues into tissues with reduced perfusion. Maximal distribution into fatty tissues occurs within 4 hours in the dog, with final stabilization (equilibration) of the fat/plasma ratio in about 6 hours.[46] The fat concentrations of thiopental in the dog at the 24- and 36-hour periods are 22 and 5%, respectively. Because of the extreme affinity for fat, the plasma levels of the thiobarbiturates are so low that no clinical signs are detectable. The only clinical implications at the 24-hour period would be the administration of subsequent anesthesia and a delayed final recovery because of partially saturated fatty tissues. In the same study, peak fat concentrations in man were measured within 2 ½ hours; it must be noted that the dose used in the dog was 2 ½ times greater than in man on a milligram per kilogram basis.[46] When this distribution is complete, the final decline in the plasma concentration is dependent primarily on metabolic degradation.

The oxybarbiturate methohexital attributes its short action to rapid detoxification. Because of this, there is less residual depressant effect, and greater performance capability should be expected following recovery when this drug is used for the induction of anesthesia.

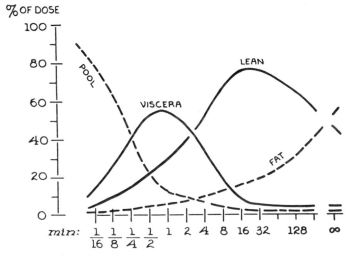

Fig. 21.5. Distribution of thiopental sodium in tissues at various times after intravenous injection. (Courtesy of Price *et al.*[43])

BIOTRANSFORMATION AND RENAL EXCRETION

The anesthetic and sedative effects of the short acting barbiturates are terminated largely by biotransformation in hepatic tissue and to a limited degree by other tissues.[26, 34, 35] The sole area of detoxification of the oxybarbiturates is in the liver, whereas the thiobarbiturates undergo some change in kidney and brain tissue. The metabolic by-products are eliminated primarily in the urine. These drugs are detoxified by four routes: (a) oxidation of radicals at carbon 5, which is the most important route; (b) dealkylation of the alkyl group; (c) desulfuration of the thiobarbiturates; and (d) destruction of the barbituraic acid ring, which is of minor importance.[26] The longer acting barbiturate phenobarbital undergoes some metabolism, but is primarily excreted by the kidneys unchanged.[11, 53] The diethyl analogue barbital is not metabolized and is excreted unchanged in the urine.

A major urinary metabolite of thiopental in the dog is the alcoholic derivative of pentobarbital. Pentobarbital has been isolated from rat liver microsomal preparations and from the blood of dogs administered thiopental, indicating the desulfuration of the thiobarbiturates and oxidation to the oxybarbiturate. The pentobarbital pharmacologically does not contribute significantly to thiopental anesthesia at the time when the level of anesthesia is most profound.[19] Whether this process might contribute to postoperative central nervous depression has not been determined.

Despite the ultrashort action of the thiobarbiturates, their ultimate removal is through biodegradation and excretion of the by-products. The rate of metabolism into nonsedative by-products will vary with age, species, and, in some species, sex. Within a species of animals, marked variation will occur, depending upon the individual's physcial condition. The rate of detoxification of pentobarbital in the dog is 15% of the total dose per hour, that of thiopental, 5%/hour. The rates in man are 4% for pentobarbital and 15%/hour for thiopental.[9, 46] The extremes of this variation are exemplified by many members of the family Felidae, which can have prolonged recovery from pentobarbital anesthesia, and the adult reminants in which duration of anesthesia is short. In the sheep, pentobarbital is cleared from the plasma at the rate of 49%/hour, and thiopental at the rate of 17%/hour. This is following tissue equilibrium.[44] The short duration of action pentobarbital in sheep is due to a more rapid metabolism by this species.

The binding of the barbiturates to tissue, especially hepatic, is indicative of the degree and rate of metabolism. For example, the variations in drug-protein interaction for in vitro rat tissue parallels some differences in drug metabolism. The binding of pentobarbital and phenobarbital is greater than the nonmetabolized barbital. As would be expected, adult binding power is greater than newborn.[49] Sexual differences in the duration of pentobarbital anesthesia could not be explained on this basis.

Administration and Dosage

SHORT ACTING BARBITURATES

The most commonly used short acting barbiturate is sodium pentobarbital, and the safest method of administration is intravenously. Oral, intraperitoneal, intrapleural, intramuscular, and even subcutaneous routes have been used but are less reliable, more apt to produce tissue damage, and are not recommended. The risk from the administration of a fixed dose which other routes necessitate should be obvious and is exceptionally dangerous when ill or aged animals are encountered. All animals to be subjected to venipuncture should be handled quietly and with a minimum of physical restraint (see Chapter 19), and in many instances preanesthetic drugs may be necessary to allow safe handling. Sodium pentobarbital for veterinary use is usually supplied as a 6 to 6.5% solution (60 to 65 mg/ml). When being administered to cats and other smaller animals, it is advisable to dilute the solution with an equal amount of saline or water for injection.

The recommended method of anesthetizing a healthy dog or cat with pentobarbital is to inject rapidly one-third to one-half of the calculated dose (25 to 30 mg/kg or approximately 60 mg/5 lb). The rapid initial injection of a relatively large amount is important when using the short and intermediate acting drugs. This rapid injection of at least one-third of the dose produces a high plasma level, and the excitement period (stage 2) of general anesthesia is rapidly passed, thereby avoiding massive excitement. If, following this initial injection, there are some indications that the animal is about to enter stage 2, a small additional amount should be given promptly before the needle is dislodged. When stage 3 has been established, the remaining amount of drug necessary to produce a surgical plane of anesthesia should be administered slowly to effect, while testing the animal's reflexes (see previous section). The time period to produce general anesthesia is markedly slower than with the ultrashort acting drugs, and the injection time should be at least 5 minutes in duration. This allows sufficient time for the anesthetic to cross the blood-brain barrier and equilibration of the plasma-brain concentration. A too rapid injection of a large amount can cause apnea which will be prolonged because of the slow decline of the plasma level of pentobarbital. Alternately, too slow an administration of the initial dose will lead to excitement, which subsequently will necessitate an increased amount of barbiturates to produce adequate planes of anesthesia. This will increase the sleeping time and delay full recovery.

The total amount of pentobarbital required to produce surgical planes of anesthesia will vary according to the animal's age, nutritional state, weight, preanesthetic medication, and many other factors.[3] Because of this, the recommended doses should only be used as a rough guideline for an approximation of the final total dose. There is marked variation in the dose range and preanesthetic medication will consistently reduce the amount but does not reduce the scatter (Fig. 21.6).

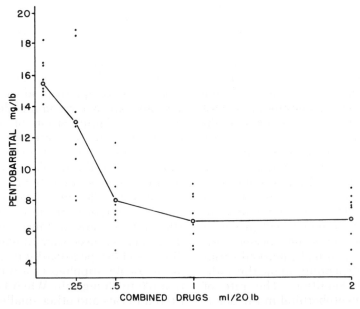

FIG. 21.6. The effect of Innovar-Vet on the anesthetic dose of pentobarbital sodium. The horizontal axis represents Innovar-Vet at ¼ to 2 times the dose of 1 ml/20 lb of body weight (1 ml/9 kg). There is a marked variation in the control doses of the barbiturates. The dose level is reduced, with a greater variation, after premedication. The maximal potentiation occurs at 1 ml/20 lb. At the higher dose levels of this combination of drugs, an exaggeration of spinal reflexes was noted.

The suggested dose range is from 30 to 40 mg/kg. This range should be scaled down by about one-third when preanesthetic medication has been administered; here again, this is approximate depending on the drug, amount, and sedative effect on the animal.

ULTRASHORT ACTING BARBITURATES

The use of the thiobarbiturates, thiopental and thiamylal in small animal practice has closely paralleled that of the oxybarbiturate pentobarbital. The use of the ultrashort drugs is also common in large animal practice, especially in the equine for the induction of anesthesia. Methohexital, although not a thiobarbiturate, can be included in this group because of its ultrashort actions.

As with the oxybarbiturates, the preferred route of administration is intravenously. Although other routes have been used, these methods injure surrounding tissues. The perivascular injection of a 6% solution of pentobarbital or a 5% solution of a thiobarbiturate can cause necrosis and eventual sloughing of tissue, whereas a 2.5% solution of a thiobarbiturate is less likely to produce tissue damage unless large amounts are inadvertently injected subcutaneously. With the exception of the large domestic animals where a 10% solution is used primarily for the convenience of containment of the total dose in one syringe, the more dilute solutions are suggested for safety and to facilitate more accurate administration, especially in smaller animals. Rectal thiopental has been used in cats for examination and minor surgery,[7] but its use in this manner is presently outmoded.

In contrast to pentobarbital, the thiobarbiturates can be given more slowly and to effect. The transfer from plasma to brain is very rapid, and the effect of an injection can be noted within one circulation time of 10 to 15 seconds. Because there is no delay in the transfer of drug from perfusing blood into brain, the maximum effect from the intravenous injection of a quantity (bolus) of the drug is attained quickly and with no lag period (Fig. 21.7). Subsequent

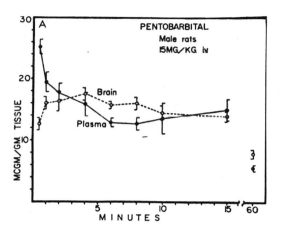

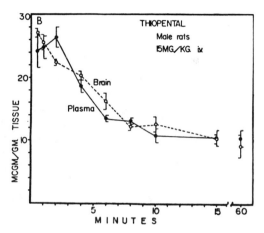

FIG. 21.7. Brain and plasma levels of thiopental sodium and pentobarbital sodium after intravenous injection in rats. For thiopental, the maximal brain concentration is achieved quickly, followed by a decline to a plateau at 6 to 8 minutes. The brain levels of pentobarbital are initially low and do not attain equilibrium with plasma for 4 minutes. (Courtesy of Goldstein, A., and Aronow, L.: The duration of action of thiopental and pentobarbital. J. Pharmacol. Exp. Ther. *128:* 1, 1960.)

doses can be given at short intervals to attain the desired depth of anesthesia slowly and carefully. With careful observation this "foreleg to central nervous system time" can be used to somewhat assess the animal's circulation time and judge the subsequent effects of additional anesthesia. Again, using the skills of simple observation, differences can be noted in circulation when comparing the healthy animal with those, for example, in shock or with cardiovascular disease.

The capability of injecting thiobarbiturates slowly with minimal expectation of excitement is an important asset, especially when anesthetizing ill and debilitated animals. The drug can be administered to effect slowly. In handling excitable or overly nervous animals, very low doses can be given initially in an attempt to quiet the animals; once a more serene state has been established, the induction of anesthesia can be continued. It must be pointed out that the induction of anesthesia in an extremely excitable dog is dangerous because of the tendency to induce anesthesia rapidly. Under these circumstances where maximal physical restraint is needed, the induction of anesthesia should be abandoned until sedation can be produced with additional narcotics or tranquilizers.

It should be remembered that thiobarbiturates are more potent than the oxybarbiturates; this combined with a more rapid effect can lead to respiratory arrest quickly and early in the induction period if given rapidly. As compared to the short acting drugs, the respiratory arrest with the ul-trashort acting drugs is shorter in duration and can be easily managed by controlling ventilation for a period of time (see Chapters 22 and 36). The amount of thiopental and thiamylal necessary to produce surgical planes of anesthesia is approximately 18 to 26 mg/kg. As with the oxybarbiturates, considerable variation can occur which is not minimized by the addition of pre-anesthetic medication (Fig. 21.8).

The ultrashort acting barbiturates, and the thiobarbiturates in particular, are commonly used to induce anesthesia prior to maintenance with the inhalation anesthetics. The amount necessary under these circumstances of use is considerably less than required for surgical intervention; all that is necessary is adequate depth to produce sufficient muscle relaxation for tracheal intubation. A dose guide for this purpose is approximately 10 mg/kg with a very marked dose range (Fig. 21.9). The number of dogs in Figure 21.9 represents unselected clinical cases, which understandably range from critically ill dogs where no premedication is indicated to health patients. The histogram simply illustrates the variation in the induction

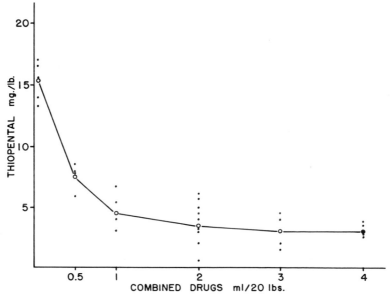

FIG. 21.8. The effect of Innovar-Vet on the anesthetic dose of thiopental sodium. The Innovar-Vet was administered in doses of ½ to 4 times the dose of 1 ml/20 lb of body weight (1 ml/9 kg). As with pentobarbital, maximal potentiation occurs at 1 ml/20 lb.

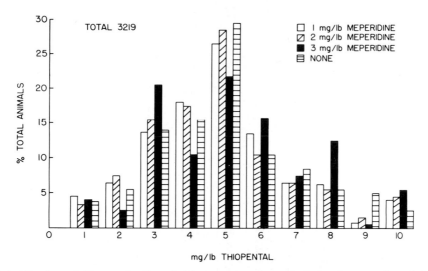

FIG. 21.9. The dose of thiopental sodium for the induction of anesthesia in a large number of clinical cases. The dose range of meperidine (Demerol) varied from 0 to 3 mg/lb (6.6 mg/kg). The clinical cases were unselected and included critically ill dogs, where no narcotic premedication is indicated, and healthy dogs. The histogram simply illustrates the variation in the induction dose of a thiobarbiturate. The physical status of the animal, its disposition, the time period between the administration of the drug and induction of anesthesia, and many other variables will influence the amount of barbiturate used for the induction of anesthesia regardless of the amount of premedication.

dose of thiopental. The physical status of the dog, its disposition, the time period between the administration of the preanesthetic drug and the induction of anesthesia, and many other variables will influence the induction dose of a barbiturate, regardless of the amount of preanesthetic medication.

Thiamylal is approximately 1.5 times as potent as thiopental; unfortunately, the criteria for establishing a definite relationship are difficult to control, and opinions vary as to the actual figure.[14] If both drugs are administered slowly to effect, it is difficult to distinguish between the two. Figure 21.10 shows a histogram of the dose of thiopental and thiamylal against the frequency of use. The impression is that thiamylal is somewhat more potent by the fact that over one-half of the cases received from 1 to 3 mg/lb of thiamylal, whereas one-half of the cases of thiopental received from 1 to 4 mg/lb. As can be seen by the scatter, the mean dose indicated has very little meaning. The amount administered was not for surgical planes of anesthesia, but for the intubation of the trachea.

Thialbarbital (33 to 36 mg/kg) and methitural (45 mg/kg) are less potent than thiopental or thiamylal, and higher doses are necessary to produce surgical planes of anesthesia.[8] Methohexital is more potent than thiopental or thiamylal, the median effective dose being 5.8 mg/kg.[4, 15]

Variations in Response to Barbiturates

In the administration of general anesthesia, whether intravenous or inhalation, there is no dose which is suitable for all animals within a species, and the smallest amount compatible with surgical requirements should be used. When administering inhalation anesthetics the requirements can be adjusted to the animal's needs on an almost moment to moment basis. The inhalation agents are in physical solution with blood and body tissues, undergo little chemical degradation and only minimal excretion by body excretory organs other than the lung and because of this these agents can be removed rapidly by increasing ventilation. There are many pathological and physio-

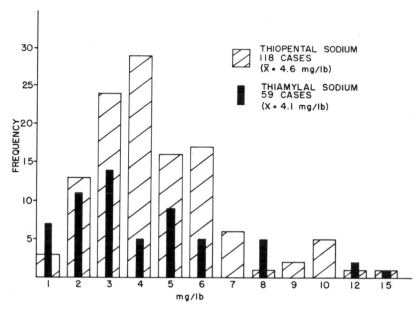

FIG. 21.10. The scatter in the induction dose of both thiamylal sodium and thiopental sodium. The mean dose for each drug has very little meaning. These dogs were premedicated with Innovar-Vet, 1 ml/40 lb of body weight.

logical conditions which will alter the response and recovery of animals when subjected to inhalation anesthesia, but these are primarily confined for all practical purposes to alterations in the cardiopulmonary system. These within certain limits can be manipulated to effect a more rapid change in the level of anesthesia and the dose increased or decreased following assessment of effect on these two systems.

The physio-chemical relationship of a parentally administered drug is more complex, and such factors discussed in preceding sections such as plasma binding, pH, metabolic degradation, and redistribution are potential factors which can intensify their actions or prolong recovery.[33, 34] Unfortunately, these many factors may be somewhat beyond the control of the clinician.

BODY WEIGHT

Understandably, the most common relationship attempted is the body weight to dose relation, and doses are usually expressed in this manner. Unfortunately, the administration of a fixed dose on a body weight basis produces marked variation in response, and many animals would be barely anesthetized and many grossly overdosed (Figs. 21.6, 21.8, 21.9, and 21.10). In assigning a fixed dose, the size of the liver, heart, and kidneys and the blood volume are assumed to be in proportion to the animal's body weight, but body fat and muscular stature are not easily proportioned in a body-weight and organ-size relationship. Particularly with the very fat-soluble thiobarbiturates, the amount of body fat is an important consideration in the final recovery from anesthesia. Because of the more delayed redistribution in fatty tissues, body fat does not contribute as much to the immediate recovery but does have a greater influence on the longer term complete recovery from the drug. This becomes more obvious at the extremes of the spectrum, when comparing an extremely thin cat, for example, with an obese one. Here, because of final redistribution of the drug into body fat, the attainment of the righting reflex and full recovery from anesthesia should be expected sooner in the obese animal. This would be especially so following multiple doses. Ataxia has been observed up to 24 hours following thiobarbiturate anesthesia in extremely thin cats; in these animals both lean body tissue (muscle) and fatty tissues are reduced and the final reduction of the plasma level is more dependent upon metabolic degradation than redistribution in muscle and fat. In rats, a 5% decrease in body fat resulted in a 100% increase in recovery time with a fixed dose of thiopental.[29] Body fat is a lesser consideration in mitigating final recovery when using the oxybarbiturates due to their limited lipid solubility, but should influence the final dose administered.

The racing greyhound can have a prolonged recovery from thiopental anesthesia, especially following larger single or intermittent doses. This is attributed to general lack of fatty tissues in this breed.[50] If low doses are used and the administration is confined to the induction of anesthesia with maintenance with inhalation agents, recovery problems are minimized. The ultrashort acting oxybarbiturate methohexital has been suggested as an alternative.[18] The average period from the induction to breast recumbency for methohexital (9 mg/kg) was 25 minutes as compared to 2 hours for thiopental (22 mg/kg). When administering barbiturates, the muscular stature, the proportion of fatty tissue, and activity should be considered in relation to body weight. Larger amounts on proportional weight basis are necessary for the induction of anesthesia in larger muscled active animals.

AGE AND SEX

In most domestic animals, both large and small, no statistics are available demonstrating a sex or specific age relationship to doses of barbiturates. The exceptions to this again lie at the extremes, the very young and the very old. It is well appreciated that the very young do not have mature enzyme systems, and detoxification may be delayed. Younger rats have decreased hepatic binding power for barbiturates.[49] Young calves (10 to 84 days) have a prolonged sleeping time when administered thiobarbiturates and may remain ataxic for 18 to 24 hours,[31] whereby adults detoxify barbiturates very rapidly.

There has been no clinical documentation in domestic animals on variations attributable to sexual differences. Alterations in sleeping time have been reported in rodents following castration. Female rats slept longer with pentobarbital anesthesia than comparable males, and the sleeping time of males was increased by castration. Castration had no effect on females, and the administration of estrogens to males prolonged their recovery time.[10]

REDUCED BLOOD VOLUME

Pathological or physiological conditions which reduce blood or plasma volume, e.g., hemorrhage, peritonitis, shock, or other conditions which have altered the relationship of the vascular bed to vascular volume, have in effect reduced the central pool of blood into which a drug is being injected. The mortality in shocked animals can be extremely high if the physiological changes accompanying this condition are not understood (see Chapter 37).

The peripheral vasoconstriction which occurs during the initial shock period physiologically attempts to maintain perfusion of vascular beds which are immediately essential to the maintenance of life, producing a redistribution of blood from the peripheral organs to more centrally located ones. In essence, the intravenous anesthetic or the inhalation anesthetic is being delivered into a more restricted central pool, with a greater percentage of the remaining blood volume being delivered to the more critical organs, e.g., heart, lung, brain, etc. During the induction of anesthesia the actions are intensified.

In animals in shock and other low perfusion situations, liver perfusion is reduced, interfering with detoxification of barbiturates, thus further prolonging final recovery from the anesthetic agent. Understandably, the restriction of blood volume is not the only condition which renders anesthesia of these patients dangerous. Low oxygen tension, acidosis, changes in body temperature, and poor perfusion all contribute to anesthetic difficulties. Animals can be anesthetized if necessary, but extreme care must be exercised. Attempts must be made to increase fluid volumes before and during the induction of anesthesia by the infusion of balanced salt solutions, and, when hemorrhage has been a contributing factor, whole blood.

FAILURE OF DETOXIFICATION

For the short and ultrashort acting drugs, the final removal of the drug is dependent upon liver detoxification and excretion of metabolic products. Liver damage, whether acute or from chronic disease, has to be considerable due to the reserve capacity of this organ. Understandably, hepatic dysfunction would have a greater impact on the short acting barbiturates, e.g., pentobarbital, than on the ultrashort acting thiobarbiturates used only for induction of anesthesia.

There are many experiences of prolonged recovery from pentobarbital anesthesia in apparently healthy dogs and cats which, certainly, from clinical examination, would not indicate hepatic problems. The major contributor to a decreased rate of detoxification by hepatic tissue is hypothermia, which creates general reduction and impairment of body function (see Chapter 38)

Moderate degrees of hypothermia are common during routine anesthesia and surgery, especially in air-conditioned operating rooms, during prolonged surgery on the smaller patients. Open body cavities and cold fluids add to this cooling effect. Many of the prolonged recoveries might be directly attributable to hypothermia. Acidosis, reduction in oxygen tension and hypotension, other complications of general anesthesia, and the recovery period also contribute to reduced hepatic function.

UREMIA

The production of experimental uremia in dogs increases considerably the duration of thiopental narcosis. This increase in the final recovery time was markedly out of proportion to the duration of surgical anesthesia.[16] In uremia, whether clinical or exprimentally produced, electrolyte imbalances also occur which might contribute to the prolonged sleeping time. In nephrectomized rabbits, plasma binding was reduced, increasing the duration of anesthesia.[51]

Clinical implications are obvious for animals with renal disorders but are also important especially when anesthetizing the elderly dog with the potential of interstitial nephritis. Because of the possibility of a prolonged period of narcosis, barbiturates should be used sparingly and only for the induction of anesthesia. The possible mechanisms of reduced plasma binding and general electrolyte imbalance have been mentioned. Another mechanism may be related to the barbiturate molecule itself, which has urea as a component. Endogenous urea may be preferentially handled.

ANEMIA

Prolonged recovery from barbiturate anesthesia occurs in anemic patients when comparing a hemoglobin of 8 to 9 g % to patients with concentrations of 12 to 13 g %.[14] Similar studies are not available in veterinary medicine, but occasional observations of prolonged recovery have been made (author) which should at least serve as a warning of a similar existing problem, but certainly not a confirmation. Anemia in veterinary patients, whether due to acute hemorrhage or chronic disease, should not be taken lightly as a potential source of problems. Unfortunately, many clinicians bypass the determination of hemoglobin or hematocrit as a routine analysis prior to anesthesia and surgery with the basic excuses of time, expense, and the surgery being only a routine procedure. This laboratory test and the physical examination should be mandatory prior to anesthesia, with few exceptions.

The effects of chronic anemia may not be readily apparent, especially in the sedentary pet animal. The oxygen-carrying and buffering capacity of blood is decreased by virtue of the reduced hemoglobin content. The cynosis of oxygen deprivation is caused by the continued circulation of desaturated hemoglobin and the potential hypoxemia of hypoventilation when breathing room air is less apparent with a reduced hemoglobin concentration. Cyanosis is an unreliable index of the degree of oxygenation in normal dogs and totally useless under conditions of reduced hemoglobin concentration. The cardiopulmonary system is more sensitive to barbiturates inasmuch as adequate oxygenation to vital organs in anemic patients is maintained by increasing cardiac output (see Chapter 36). The increased flow can partially compensate for the decrease in oxygen-carrying and buffering capacity. This reserve capability is diminished during anesthesia, reducing oxygenation and creating a situation in which organs are more susceptible to the depressant effects of anesthetic agents.

CARDIOVASCULAR DISEASE

The effects of barbiturates on patients with cardiovascular disorders are basically similar to the overall effects of other general anesthetics, and similar precautions must be observed (see Chapter 21). Barbiturates depress the myocardium directly, and the reduction in cardiac output and blood pressure is generally related to the dose and speed of injection. The rapid injection of barbiturates produces a fall in blood pressure which slowly returns to control levels. The diseased myocardium is more sensitive to the depressant effects, and the cardiovascular reserve capabilities are reduced. The reduction in cardiac output, blood pressure, and peripheral vasodilation which occur are compensated for by the nondiseased system, but the diseased system may undergo profound changes with only small amounts of barbiturate. As discussed in the preceeding section, the foreleg to brain circulation time is reduced in these patients, and the induction of sleep with the thiobarbiturates and other barbiturates is delayed. This should be appreciated and the induction of anesthesia not rushed. Secondary to the effects on the cardiovascular system are the effects on ventilation. The resulting hypercarbia and hypoxemia, if ventilation is not immediately assisted, can further compromise cardiovascular function.

Not all patients with cardiovascular disease should be placed in the highest physical status grouping, but some basic principles should be followed. (a) The anesthesia must be induced in a quiet animal. (b) The rate of administration of the thiobarbiturate should be slow and a dilute solution used. (c) When possible, an intravenous drip should be running slowly, and the barbiturate injected into the drip. (d) The periods of delay in the induction should be frequent to allow the maximum time period for the drug to take effect and observations made. (e) The patient should be intubated as soon as possible, and ventilation controlled or assisted. (f) Emergency drugs should be readily available. (g) The electrocardiogram should be monitored when possible.

GLUCOSE EFFECT

When glucose is administered during the emergence from pentobarbital anesthesia, the dog will relapse into a clinically observable deeper plane of anesthesia. This can be repeated on successive occasions during the awaking period. This phenomenon does not seem to occur during the deeper surgical planes of anesthesia. Objective monitoring of the electroencephalogram, blood pressure, heart rate, and ventilation did not indicate an increased depth of pentobarbital anesthesia.[28] It appears that the administration of glucose is not contraindicated during the surgical planes of pentobarbital anesthesia.

POTENTIATING COMPOUNDS

A host of substances and drugs will potentiate and prolong the depressant effects of barbiturates, especially the short acting ones. Among these are the many other sedatives and hypnotics, narcotics, tranquilizers, inhalation anesthetics, antihistamines, and alcohol. The additive or potentiating effects of these compounds are understandable, inasmuch as they all have depressant properties. The mechanism of actions of other compounds which in themselves do not produce central nervous system depression is more obscure. These other compounds can exert an effect through alterations in pH or protein binding which will modify the relationship between the diffusable and nondiffusable component. For example, sodium acetrizoate (Urokon), a contrast media, has been shown to potentiate pentobarbital anesthesia by competitive protein binding. The dye is more highly bound, displacing the bound barbiturate from the albumin, increasing the diffusable component.[32]

Other possible mechanisms would be altered cellular permeability, renal excretory patterns, or blockage of metabolic enzyme systems.[32] Metabolic breakdown is the final means of terminating pentobarbital anesthesia, and interference with its biodegradation is not uncommon. The rate of barbiturate metabolism is dependent upon species, age, nutrition, and previous exposure to drugs. Other drugs can also interfere with this metabolic transformation. Therapeutic doses of chloramphenical, for example, significantly prolong the duration of pentobarbital anesthesia.[1] The prolongation is through inhibiting the action of the microsomal enzymes that inactivate pentobarbital by hydroxylation.[1]

The interaction of various drugs in the determination of the intensity of action and final recovery from injectable anesthetics is intriguing and certainly important clinically. The feeding of large amounts of corn oil in rats reduces the thiopental sleeping time by 30%.[54] The initial assumption of the mode of action is the trapping of the barbiturate in the chylomicrons within the blood stream. These chylomicrons do contain large amounts of neutral fat, but because of an envelope of protein and phospholipids, the globules of fat do not exhibit the actions of neutral fat, and little trapping of the barbiturate occurs.[54] The thiobarbiturate enters the intestine and is trapped by the unabsorbed corn oil. The fatty material within the intestine is the primary depositing area instead of the normal fatty deposits. Heparin will reverse the corn oil effect, but

through a totally different mechanism. Heparin does play a role in the plasma clearance of chylomicrons and lipoproteins.[27] This involves the disruption of neutral fat into unesterified fatty acids, which will compete for binding sites on albumin, making it less available for thiopental.[54]

The above illustrations are used to exemplify complexities of interaction of drugs and their effect on each other. The clinician is very much attuned to the synergistic or additive effect of many of the depressant drugs on each other, but most often has little appreciation of the potential effects of unrelated compounds on recovery and metabolic breakdown.

POLYVINYL COLLARS AND INSECTICIDES

Polyvinyl collars impregnated with the anticholinesterase dichlorvos (phosphoric acid, 2,2-dichlorovinyl dimethyl ester) are being used for the control of fleas and other ectoparasites. Published comments have suggested that clinical interaction may occur with barbiturate anesthesia, potentiating and prolonging anesthesia.[47, 48] As has been described, barbiturate anesthesia may be altered by many factors, and the incrimination of one factor in a clinical situation may be extremely difficult. In a control study using 96 dogs in three age groups exposed to dichlorvos flea collars for 28 days, all dogs exposed and anesthetized with pentobarbital recovered normal function as rapidly as the control dogs.[56] The exposure produces no significant effect on any of the measured clinical laboratory parameters other than the reduction of erythrocyte and plasma cholinesterase levels. In a comparable study with thiamylal sodium anesthesia, a tendency toward a greater degree of respiratory depression was noted in dogs following exposure to the flea collars impregnated with dichlorvos. In this study the dogs were their own controls. Oxygen tensions under general anesthesia were further decreased, and carbon dioxide tensions were elevated more after the exposure to the flea collar. Although this tendency was noted, the difference was not significant.[45] All studies to date have been on experimental animals, and no information is available in clinical patients. The clinical data would be extremely difficult to evaluate because of the variation in the exposure of the dog or cat to the collar. The data available indicate that there is a tendency toward a greater degree of ventilatory depression; if the clinician is forewarned and greater care exercised during the induction of anesthesia, the potential danger should be minimal.

RESISTANCE OR TOLERANCE

The terms resistance, tolerance, addiction, or dependency are interrelated in that they imply an adaptation of the central nervous system to the presence of a drug.[26] The most commonly referred to terms are addiction or dependency, indicating a long-term adaptation, complicated with the need for a drug for the maintenance of normal daily existence. The criteria for addiction or dependency are the absolute need for a drug and withdrawal signs when denied. Resistance or tolerance can be divided into "drug disposition tolerance" or "pharmacodynamic tolerance."[26] Drug disposition tolerance is resistance developed through the activation of drug-metabolizing enzymes by the previous exposure of the animal to a similar drug. This tolerance is manifested by a more rapid recovery from the effects of the barbiturate. Pharmacodynamic tolerance involves the development of resistance to the effects of the drug, necessitating a greater amount to produce comparable effects.

Acute tolerance develops during a single administration of a drug, notably the thiobarbiturates. It had been observed that the duration of sleeping times was similar in two groups of patients receiving high (15.1 mg/kg) and lower (4.6 mg/kg) doses of thiopental.[17] It was concluded that the peak concentration attained in the brain during the induction or maintenance of anesthesia determined the blood level at which the patient will awaken.[17] The higher the peak level of thiopental, the higher is the plasma level at awakening. This tolerance occurs during the time course of the anesthetic. The mechanism of action is unknown. In studies where repetitive anesthetics are to be administered, a waiting period of at least 10 to 14 days should be allowed to assure regression of acute or chronically acquired tolerance.

Pharmacological Actions

VENTILATION

Barbiturates are respiratory depressants, and ventilation is reduced as anesthesia is deepened by a reduction of respiratory rate and tidal volume. As with other depressants of the central nervous system, the barbiturates decrease the response to increasing concentrations of carbon dioxide, the consequence of which is a respiratory acidosis with moderate and deep planes of anesthesia (Table 21.2). Under deep barbiturate anesthesia, the control of respiration is shifted from the centrally located respiratory centers to the more peripherally located chemoreceptors located at the bifurcation of the carotid artery.[13] Because of the depression of the respiratory centers, the stimulus for respiration is the reduction in oxygen tension. The impulses originate primarily from the peripheral chemoreceptors. The administration of oxygen will further depress ventilation by virtue of removal of the anoxic drive, and the accumulation of carbon dioxide can further depress the respiratory centers. It is advisable under moderate to deep planes of anesthesia that ventilation be controlled to maintain adequate oxygenation and the removal of carbon dioxide.

HEMODYNAMICS

The reports of the hemodynamic changes produced by barbiturates (pentobarbital) are conflicting.[2] This is expected because of the variation in experimental model, dose, and preanesthetic medication. Studies in precannulated dogs, which enabled the comparison of the anesthetized state to the awake control period, indicated some basic agreement.[2, 20, 40] There was an initial fall in mean blood pressure followed by a rise to control or above within 30 to 60 minutes. The changes in mean pressure can be deceiving. A significant drop in systolic pressure and a rise in diastolic pressure can balance out, with no significant change in mean pressure.[6, 40] Cardiac output increased within the first 30-minute period, followed by a gradual 25% decrease to below control levels during the remaining 2½- to 4-hour study period. Heart rate increased and remained elevated throughout. Contractile force and stroke volume were significantly reduced from control levels. Peripheral resistance was elevated in all studies. The reduction in packed cell volume, hemoglobin, and leukocyte count due to the splenic vasodilation was confirmed in these studies.[2, 20, 40] The reduction in leukocytes also occurred in splenectomized dogs[20, 52] and appears to result from pooling of leukocytes in the pulmonary bed.[20]

The thiobarbiturates have different actions on the vascular smooth muscle. Thiamylal produces vasoconstriction decreasing spleen, kidney, and leg volume. Similarly, thiamylal produced vasoconstriction of the pulmonary bed, with no change during pentobarbital anesthesia.[24]

Renal function during moderate levels of pentobarbital anesthesia remains unchanged, with no significant alteration from the awake state of glomerular filtration rate, renal blood flow, and tubular reabsorption of water.[5] Sodium pentobarbital in this study produced no antidiuretic effect.[6] Unfortunately, as with many attempts to determine the effects of general anesthesia on renal function, reports are conflicting.

Nonbarbiturate Intravenous Drugs

Most of the nonbarbiturate intravenous drugs are generally not used to any great extent and have not endured the test of time.

PROPANIDID

Chemically, the drug is a 3-methoxy-4-(N-diethyl-carmindomethoxy)phenyl acetic acid-n-propyl ester.[12] The major advantage of this drug is its rapid metabolism and freedom from postanesthetic sedation. The duration of anesthesia is about 5 minutes

with good recovery within 10 to 12 minutes. The does of propanidid is 7 to 11 mg/kg, the drug having one-fifth the potency of methohexital.[30] It has had extensive trials in man but has gained little continuous use.[55] Its major disadvantages are its thick consistency, tendency toward the production of phlebitis, and high incidence of larnygospasms. It has not been used in the United States.

OTHER DRUGS

Chloral hydrate, paraldehyde, tribromethanol, and gluthethimide have been described elsewhere (see Chapters 13, 23, and 24). These agents are used only sparingly, with the exception of chloral hydrate, which is used somewhat in large animal anesthesia. The cyclohexylamines have greater promise as drugs which will remain in the clinical armamentarium. Their current use has been described in Chapter 13.

Solutions of Barbiturates

Barbituric acid compounds are not soluble in aqueous solutions, but the sodium salts are readily soluble, forming alkaline solutions (pH 10 to 11). These solutions can absorb carbon dioxide from the air, reducing the alkalinity which can result in some precipitation. The thiobarbiturates are obtained in powdered form, ready for the addition of known amounts of saline or water for injection. Pentobarbital is commercially available in solutions of 5, 6, or 6.5%, depending upon the manufacturer. Most of the short and long acting drugs are available in oral and rectal forms.

REFERENCES

1. Adams, H. R., and Dixit, B. M.: Prolongation of pentobarbital anesthesia by chloramphanicol in dogs and cats. J. Amer. Vet. Med. Ass. *156:* 902, 1970.
2. Barlow, G., and Knott, D. H.: Hemodynamic alterations after 30 minutes of pentobarbital sodium anesthesia in dogs. Amer. J. Physiol. *207:* 764, 1964.
3. Bazett, H. C., and Erb, W. H.: Standardization of dosage of sodium ethyl (1-methyl-butyl) barbiturate (Nembutal) for anesthesia in cats and dogs. J. Pharmacol. Exp. Ther. *49:* 352, 1933.

4. Bellville, J. W., Fennel, P. J., Murphy, T., and Howland, W. S.: The relative potencies of methohexital and thiopental. J. Pharmacol. Exp. Ther. *129:* 108, 1960.

5. Blake, W. D.: Some effects of pentobarbital anesthesia on renal hemodynamics, water and electrolyte excretion in the dog. Amer. J. Physiol. *191:* 393, 1957.

6. Blatteis, C. M., and Horvath, S. M.: Renal and cardiovascular effects of anesthetic doses of pentobarbital sodium. Amer. J. Physiol. *192:* 353, 1958.

7. Branker, W. M.: The sedation of cats. Advances Small Anim. Prac. *4:* 9, 1962.

8. Brodey, R. S., and Martin, J. E.: Preliminary studies on some effects of a new thiobarbiturate in the dog. Amer. J. Vet. Res. *18:* 158, 1957.

9. Brodie, B. B., Burns, J. J., Mark, L. E., Lief, P. A., Bernstein, E., and Papper, E. M.: The fate of pentobarbital in man and dog and a method for its estimation in biological material. J. Pharmacol. Exp. Ther. *109:* 26, 1953.

10. Buchel, L.: Influence des glandes sexuelles sur la sensibilité des rats blancs a quelques hypnotixues. Anesth. Analg. (Paris) *11:* 229, 1954.

11. Butler, T. C., Mahaffee, C., and Waddell, W. J.: Phenobarbital: studies of elimination, accumulation, tolerance, and dosage schedules. J. Pharmacol. Exp. Ther. *111:* 425, 1954.

12. Collins, V. J.: *Principles of Anesthesiology.* Lea & Febiger, Philadelphia, 1966.

13. Comroe, J. H.: *Physiology of Respiration.* Year Book Medical Publishers, Inc., Chicago, 1966.

14. Dundee, J. W.: *Thiopentone and Other Thiobarbiturates.* E. S. Livingstone, Ltd., London, 1956.

15. Dundee, J. W.: Alterations in response to somatic pain associated with anaesthesia. XVI. Methohexitone. Brit. J. Anaesth. *36:* 798, 1964.

16. Dundee, J. W., and Annis, D.: Barbiturate narcosis in uraemia. Brit. J. Anaesth. *29:* 114, 1955.

17. Dundee, J. W., Price, H. L., and Dripps, R. D.: Acute tolerance to thiopentone in man. Brit. J. Anaesth. *28:* 344, 1956.

18. Fabry, A.: Methohexital sodium anesthesia in greyhounds. Vet. Rec. *75:* 1049, 1963.

19. Furano, E. S., and Greene, N. M.: Metabolic breakdown of thiopental in man determined by gas chromatographic analysis of serum barbiturate levels. Anesthesiology *24:* 796, 1963.

20. Gilmore, J. P.: Pentobarbital sodium in the dog. Amer. J. Physiol. *209:* 404, 1965.

21. Goldbaum, L. R., and Smith, P. K.: The binding of barbiturates by human and bovine serum albumin. Fed. Proc. *7:* 222, 1948.

22. Goldbaum, L. R., and Smith, P. K.: Binding of barbiturates by rabbit tissue homogenates. Fed. Proc. *9:* 275, 1950.

23. Goldbaum, L. R., and Smith, P. K.: The interaction of barbiturates with serum albumin and its possible relation to their disposition and pharmacological actions. J. Pharmacol. Exp. Ther. *111:* 197, 1954.

24. Goldberg, S. J., Linde, L. M., Gaal, P. G., Momma, K., Takahashi, M., and Sarna, G.: Effects of barbiturates on pulmonary and systemic haemodynamics. Cardiovasc. Res. *2:* 136, 1968.

25. Goldstein, A., Aronaw, L., and Kalman, S. M.: Principles of drug action. In *The Basis of Pharmacology.* Harper & Row, Publishers, New York, 1969.

26. Goodman, L. S., and Gilman, A. (editors): *The Pharmacological Basis of Therapeutics,* 4th ed. The Macmillan Company, New York, 1970.

27. Gordon, R. S., Jr., and Cherbes, A.: Mechanism of action of lipoprotein lipase. J. Clin. Invest. *35:* 206, 1956.

28. Hamlin, R. L., Redding, R. W., Rieger, R. C., and Prynn, R. B.: Insignificance of the "Glucose Effect" in dogs anesthetized with pentobarbital. J. Amer. Vet. Med. Ass. *149:* 238, 1965.

29. Hermann, G., and Wood, H. C.: Influence of body fat on duration of thiopental anesthesia. Proc. Soc. Exp. Biol. Med. *80:* 318, 1952.

30. Howells, T. H., Harnitt, E., Keller, G. A., and Rosenoer, V. M.: Propanidid and methohexitone: their comparative potency and narcotic action. Brit. J. Anaesth. *39:* 31, 1967.

31. Jennings, S.: The use of β-β-methyl-ethyl glutarimide for terminating barbiturate anesthesia in calves. Vet. Rec. *70:* 594, 1958.

32. Lazzer, E. C., Elizand-Martel, G., and Granke, R. C.: Potentiation of pentobarbital anesthesia by competitive protein binding. Anesthesiology *24:* 665, 1963.

33. Mark, L. C.: Factors modulating barbiturate action. Far East J. Anesth. *4:* 1, 1963.

34. Mark, L. C.: Metabolism of barbiturates in man. Clin. Pharmacol. Ther. *4:* 504, 1963.

35. Mark, L. C., Brand, L., Kamuyssi, S., Britton, R. C., Perel, J. M., Landrau, M. A., and Dayton, P. G.: Thiopental metabolism by human liver in vivo and in vitro. Nature (London) *206:* 1117, 1965.

36. Mayer, S., Maickel, R. P., and Brodie, B. B.: Kinetics of penetration of drugs and other foreign compounds into cerebrospinal fluid and brain. J. Pharmacol. Exp. Ther. *127:* 205, 1959.

37. Maynert, E. W.: The usefulness of clinical signs for the comparison of intravenous anesthetics in dogs. J. Pharmacol Exp. Ther. *128:* 182, 1960.

38. Oswald, I., Berger, R. J., Jaramillo, R. A., Keddie, K. M. G., Olley, R. C., and Plunkett, G. B.: Melancholia and barbiturates: a controlled EEG, body and eye movement study of sleep. Brit. J. Psychiat. *109:* 66, 1963.

39. Papper, E. M., and Kitz, R. J. (editors): *Uptake and Distribution of Anesthetic Agents.* McGraw-Hill Book Company, New York, 1963.

40. Priano, L. L., Traber, D. L., and Wilson, R. D.: Barbiturate anesthesia: an abnormal physio-

logic situation. J. Pharmacol. Exp. Ther. *165:* 126, 1969.

41. Price, H. L.: A dynamic concept of the distribution of thiopental in the human body. Anesthesiology *21:* 40, 1960.

42. Price, H. L., Dundee, J. W., and Conner, E. H.: Rates of uptake and release of thiopental by human brain; relation to kinetics of thiopental anesthesia. Anesthesiology *18:* 171, 1957.

43. Price, H. L., Kovnat, P. J., Safer, J. N., Conner, E. H., and Price, M. L.: Uptake of thiopental by body tissues and its relation to duration of narcosis. Clin. Pharmacol. Ther. *1:* 16, 1960.

44. Rae, J. H.: The fate of pentobarbitone and thiopentone in the sheep. Res. Vet. Sci. *3:* 399, 1962.

45. Ritter, C., Synder, G., Hughes, R., and Weaver, L.: Dichlorvos-containing dog collars and thiamylal anesthesia. Amer. J. Vet. Res. *31:* 2025, 1970.

46. Shideman, F. E., Gould, T. C., Winters, W. D., Peterson, R. C., and Kilner, W. K.: The distribution and in vivo rate of metabolism of thiopental. J. Pharmacol. Exp. Ther. *107:* 368, 1953.

47. Small, E.: Toxicity of flea collars. Mod. Vet. Pract. *49:* 20, 1968.

48. Smith, H. M. S.: Safety of chemically impregnated devices questioned. J. A. M. A. *153:* 1264, 1968.

49. Soyka, L. F.: Determinants of in vitro binding of barbiturates by rat hepatic subcellular fractions. Proc. Soc. Exp. Biol. Med. *128:* 322, 1968.

50. Stevenson, D. E.: Advances in the pharmacology of thiopentone sodium. Vet. Rec. *70:* 103, 1958.

51. Taylor, J. D., Richards, R. K., Davin, J. C., and Asher, J.: Plasma binding of thiopental in the nephrectomized rabbit. J. Pharmacol. Exp. Ther. *112:* 40, 1954.

52. Usenik, E. A., and Cronkite, E. P.: Effects of barbiturate anesthetics on leukocytes in normal and splenectomized dogs. Anesth. Analg. (Cleveland) *44:* 167, 1965.

53. Waddel, W. J., and Butler, T. C.: The distribution and excretion of phenobarbital. J. Clin. Invest. *36:* 1217, 1957.

54. Winters, W. D., Conrad, A., Lenartz, H. F., and Blaskovics, J. B.: Influence of corn oil, heparin and albumin on thiopental action in rats. Anesthesiology *23:* 27, 1962.

55. Wynands, J. E., and Fox, G. S.: A clinical comparison of propanidid and thiopentone as induction agents to general anesthesia. Canad. Anaesth. Soc. J. *13:* 505, 1966.

56. Young, R., Jr., Johnson, L. G., and Brown, L. J.: The effects of pentobarbital sodium on the sleeping time of dogs wearing placebo or dichlorvos-containing flea collars. Veterinary Medicine Department, Shell Development Company, Modesto, Calif., 1970.

22
Anesthetic Management

LAWRENCE R. SOMA

The management of patients with various disease processes or functional disorders can be both a surgical and anesthetic challenge, particularly in the critically ill. The following chapter discusses the management, in a broad sense, of some commonly encountered conditions. The initial section on thoracic anesthesia is applicable in the management of animals with cardiopulmonary or respiratory deficiencies produced by trauma or disease. Anesthetic management suggested in many of the sections is generally applicable in the critically ill.

Specific areas were selected which include anesthesia for thoracic surgery, cesarean section, cardiac disease, obesity, diabetes mellitus, vomiting, and aspiration pneumonitis.

Anesthesia for Thoracic Surgery and Cardiopulmonary Dysfunction

The anesthetic requirements for animals undergoing thoracic surgery basically do not vary greatly from methods and techniques employed for other surgical needs. What does set it apart is the need for controlled ventilation, the possible greater flow of secretions from the diseased lungs, and the possibility of concurrent cardiopulmonary disease. Generally, these patients are in higher physical status categories, and greater preanesthetic and postanesthetic care is needed. Diaphragmatic hernias and other conditions which encroach upon the pleural cavity or lungs, thereby reducing lung capacity, are common needs for thoracic surgery. Partial displacement of the lungs or actual lung collapse will reduce the patient's ventilatory reserve which is further compromised by anesthesia and positional changes. Anesthesia for cardiovascular surgery usually presents both cardiovascular and pulmonary complications.

The awake animal with cardiopulmonary disease, under most circumstances, can adequately eliminate CO_2 by increasing ventilation. This is also true for animals with medical or surgical problems with some encroachment on lung capacity. Unfortunately, cardiopulmonary disease with its reduced cardiac and pulmonary capabilities can seriously impair the patient's capability of maintaining adequate oxygenation, especially when placed under stress. Hypoxemia can occur when the patient is breathing room air and can be a serious problem following thoracic surgery.[8] Oxygenation usually can be maintained during anesthesia when high concentrations of oxygen are used in the gas mixture, but they may be lower than expected despite vigorous efforts to maintain an adequate oxygen tension.

Reduced arterial oxygenation following thoracic surgery occurs in man and stems from the disruption of ventilation and perfusion, the reduction of ventilatory capabilities by pain and a static position, and the lingering depressant effects of anesthetic agents.[8] All contribute to poor cardiopulmonary function. Unfortunately, definitive published clinical studies in veterinary patients are not available, but similar problems exist following thoracic surgery.

PREMEDICATION

The premedication of patients for thoracotomy and of those with respiratory problems related to cardiopulmonary disease depends more upon the condition of the animal than the specific condition or operative procedure. The management is based primarily on the degree of dysfunction and not necessarily the specific disease. An important consideration is the degree of respiratory insufficiency (see Chapter 36). In the face of a respiratory insufficiency, handling of the patient and the administration of depressants must be judicious. Many animals with encroachment on the pulmonary system (e.g., diaphragmatic hernia) can maintain near normal blood-gas tensions by utilizing their pulmonary reserve, maintaining a sitting position, fixing the chest at its maximum position, and increasing the rate of ventilation. The administration of depressants will compromise the animal's ability to compensate for alterations in pulmonary function. All premedication will depress ventilatory effort, and positional changes from sitting to lying may in themselves produce severe hypoventilation. Under these circumstances only atropine for premedication is indicated.

Heavy preanesthetic medication may be necessary to facilitate handling of unmanageable animals. These patients with respiratory problems should be carefully watched and anesthetized as soon as they are tractable. Animals with a respiratory problem, traumatic or nontraumatic, but adequately compensating, can be given small doses of synthetic narcotic derivatives for premedication. Morphine, with its high incidence of emesis following its use, is not recommended. Emesis can be particularly dangerous in an animal with a diaphragmatic hernia. Meperidine, 2.5 to 5 mg/kg, or another comparable synthetic derivative is suggested. Tranquilizers or barbiturates can also be used for preanesthetic sedation, but narcotics are perferred because of their reversibility. It cannot be overly emphasized that the administration of depressants to animals with respiratory insufficiency can create a state of respiratory failure, and these animals should be watched carefully.

GENERAL ANESTHESIA

The choice of a general anesthetic for animals with respiratory disease or for thoracic surgery is secondary to its proper administration. The basis of the proper management of diseased animals is careful handling and providing adequate ventilation and oxygenation during the induction and the maintenance of anesthesia. The immediate threat to life is hypoxia, especially during the induction of anesthesia and prior to tracheal intubation. The utmost must be done to minimize struggling which can increase oxygen needs beyond the animal's capability of proper reoxygenation of venous blood. Clipping of hair, particularly in cats, may have to be deferred until general anesthesia has been established. If the veterinary patient will tolerate a face mask, oxygen should be given 2 to 3 minutes prior to and during the induction of anesthesia. This is not always possible in the conscious animal but should be done if feasible.

Thiobarbiturates are advised for the induction of general anesthesia followed by inhalation agents for maintenance. In extremely ill animals, only sleep doses of thiobarbiturates should be administered slowly until the animal becomes unconscious. The trachea should be intubated quickly and ventilation controlled. If relaxation of the jaw is not sufficient or laryngeal reflexes are not obtunded, the oxygen mask should be applied and anesthesia deepened further with the thiobarbiturate.

Succinylcholine chloride can be used in combination with low doses of thiobarbiturates, thus producing muscle paralysis at very light levels of anesthesia. This facilitates tracheal intubation and ventilatory control. This technique is especially applicable in critically ill animals. With this method, complete muscle relaxation is produced without having to attain deep planes of general anesthesia. It is also recommended for cats in poor condition because of the greater difficulty in intubating this species without deeper planes of anesthesia.

An important consideration in anesthetic management of most patients with cardiopulmonary dysfunction, whether traumatic or spontaneous, is the rapid control of ventilation. All drugs administered depress the patient's ventilatory capabilities, and spontaneous ventilation will be inadequate for proper oxygenation, removal of carbon dioxide, and a smooth transition to the inhalation anesthetic.

In the anesthetic management of animals for thoracic surgery with cardiopulmonary problems, as with other patients with a higher physical status rating, inhalation agents with low solubilities are advised. Cyclopropane and halothane as compared to methoxyflurane and diethyl ether allow a more rapid induction, greater controllability during anesthesia,

and a more rapid recovery. The rapid recovery from anesthesia aids in the return to a more normal physiological state. There is always great danger in stating various concentrations or doses of anesthetic agents, both for maintenance and induction of anesthesia. The inherent variation from one animal to another and the disease state make strict recommendations impossible. Suffice it to say that concentrations anywhere from 0.25 to 2% halothane and 0.25 to 1% methoxyflurane may be necessary for thoracic anesthesia. It is advised to reduce the concentration of delivered anesthetic agent when intermittent positive pressure ventilation is started. The increase in alveolar ventilation and the slight increase in partial pressure of the inhalation agent created by intermittent positive pressure ventilation will produce a higher arterial concentration (Fig. 22.1).

INTERMITTENT POSITIVE PRESSURE
VENTILATION

Intermittent positive pressure ventilation (IPPV) for maintaining adequate oxygenation and removal of carbon diox-

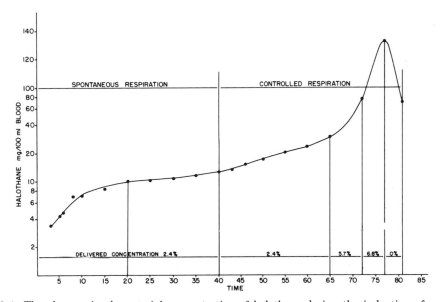

FIG. 22.1. The changes in the arterial concentration of halothane during the induction of anesthesia. There is a subsequent increase in the arterial level when intermittent positive pressure ventilation is initiated at the same delivered concentration and fresh gas flow. The increase in arterial levels are extremely rapid during controlled ventilation upon increase of the delivered concentration.

ide in the open chested animal was demonstrated by Vesalius in 1555.[43] However, it has only been in recent times that IPPV has been adapted as the method of choice during thoracic surgery. Experiments in the ability of this technique to sustain life in an open chested animal were reported by Robert Hook in 1667. Physiologists at the turn of the century used this technique to maintain proper ventilation in experimental animals.[43] The gap between experimenter and practitioner during this period was very obvious. IPPV for thoracotomy was not fully publicized and universally accepted until the late 1930's. It was indeed a misfortune that a technique which had been experimentally used in the 16th century was not used to solve the ventilation problem during thoracic surgery until less effective methods had been utilized.[17, 26]

The need for IPPV is not limited only to thoracic surgery, but during general anesthesia in general, and is a procedure which should be initiated whenever respiratory insufficiency is anticipated or suspected. The effectiveness of assisted or controlled respiration by the use of IPPV is well established, and it should be initiated before the ensuing anoxia and accumulation of carbon dioxide further depress the cardiopulmonary and central nervous systems.

PHYSIOLOGICAL ASPECTS OF IPPV

Intrapulmonary and Intrapleural Pressure. During spontaneous respiration, gas flows into the alveoli are created by the difference between alveolar and ambient pressure. The negative pressure is created by the caudal movement of the diaphragm, the outward expansion of the rib cage, and the subsequent expansion of the lungs. In normal respiration, the pressure difference during the inspiratory phase between the lips and alveoli is approximately -3 to -5 torr (Fig. 22.2). The difference disappears at the end of in-

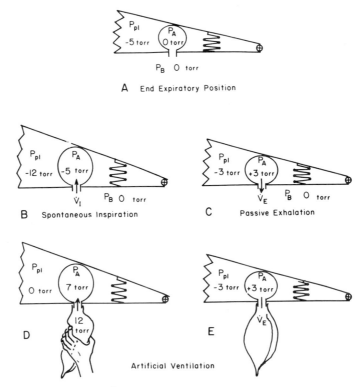

FIG. 22.2. The changes in alveolar pressure (P_A) and intrapulmonary pressure (P_{pl}) during the various phases of spontaneous and artificial ventilation. (Courtesy of Theodore Smith. See also Chapter 14.)

spiration, and alveolar pressure finally becomes positive during expiration. During quiet respiration, these pressure differences are small in magnitude, since it is only necessary to overcome the resistance to flow imposed by the conducting system. Constriction of these conducting tubes, the attachment of anesthetic equipment with high resistance, or improper intubation of the trachea can increase this resistance. Intrapleural or transpulmonary pressures also change during spontaneous respiration; the transpulmonary pressure normally varies between −3 and −12 torr during passive expiration and active inspiration.

These pressure changes which induce the flow of gases also influence the flow of blood from the great veins into the right atrium. The negative transpulmonary pressure produced by inspiration augments the flow of blood back to the heart; this is the respiratory pump mechanism. In the "closed chest dog," application of intermittent positive pressure ventilation reverses the pulmonary pressure during the inspiratory phase. At the expansive inspiratory phase of controlled ventilation, the normally negative transpulmonary pressure is now positive, so that a pressure change of between 7 and 12 torr is now transmitted to the soft tissue within the thoracic cavity (Fig. 22.3). The pressure alterations can be considerably more if the airway pressure necessary to inflate the lungs is high. The alveolar, transpulmonary, and airway pressures approach normal only when full exhalation is allowed. The circulatory changes are exaggerated when the pressures are excessive and improperly applied.

Harmful Effects. Despite the effectiveness and safety of controlled respiration, the method creates considerable alteration of normal physiology. The potential harmful effects are: (a) air embolism; (b) mediastinal emphysema; and (c) circulatory depression.[64] The first two occur only when abnormally high pressures are used. Pressures of 100 to 110 torr will produce fatal air embolism in the intact dog, and pressures of 70 to 100 torr can produce mediastinal emphysema in the tho-

ractomized dog. These pressures are far in excess of the pressure needed for proper expansion of the normal chest and lung and are not usually obtained during properly applied IPPV. Circulatory depression is the most common sequel of pressure ventilation and can occur during its routine application.

Circulatory Changes. During the positive inspiratory portion of controlled ventilation, the increase in intrapulmonary pressure is transmitted to the soft structures within the thoracic cavity, vena cava, atria, right ventricle, and pulmonary veins (Fig. 22.3). The changes in pressure are not uniform throughout the thorax but tend to be higher in the region of the base of the heart.[25] The cardiac compression created interferes with cardiac filling by elevating right atrial pressure. The increased right atrial pressure, together with compression of caval veins and elimination of the respiratory pump mechanism, hinders venous return and cardiac filling. This, in turn, is reflected by a rise in peripheral venous pressure which parallels the transpulmonary pressure changes.[19, 47] The systemic venous pressure increases during the positive inspiratory period and returns toward normal during the exhalation period.

The reduced cardiac filling imposed upon the heart during the now positive inspiratory phase is manifested by a drop in both cardiac output and arterial blood pressure.[51] The changes in arterial pressure and cardiac output are proportional to the duration of the increased airway pressure and not necessarily to the peak pressures attained.[10, 15] The duration of application of positive pressure or the area below the pressure curve is a more important aspect of the pressure cycle in producing circulatory embarrassment (Fig. 22.4)[16]

Normally the reduced pressure gradient between the right side of the heart and the peripheral venous system will be reestablished by a compensating vasoconstriction, which tends to reduce the peripheral pooling of blood and to enhance venous return.[50, 67] The restoration of venous return is essential if cardiac output

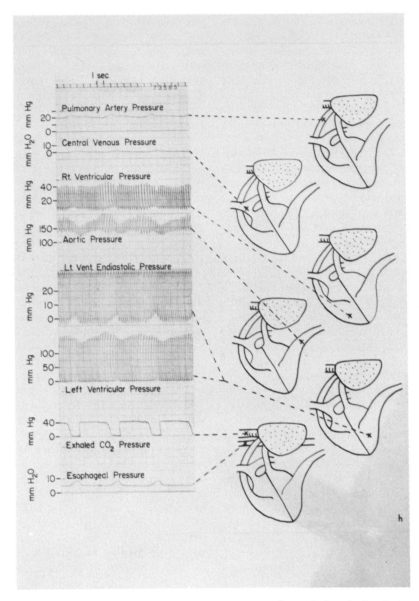

FIG. 22.3. The changes in pressure of the vascular system are shown during the inspiratory and expiratory phases of controlled ventilation. As esophageal pressures rise, the changes in pressure throughout the cardiopulmonary system can be compared. The rise in left ventricular end diastolic pressure emphasizes the effect on the left side of heart despite the greater wall thickness as compared to the right side.

is to be maintained as near normal as possible. This is dependent upon the ability of the circulatory system to adjust to the imposed pressures by the vasomotor reflex mechanisms.[4]

The vascular status of the animal will determine its ability to tolerate the cardi-ovascular alteration imposed on the system during the pressure cycle. Animals with low blood volume due to dehydration, chronic disease, anemia, and acute hemorrhage are less able to tolerate IPPV. Deeper planes of anesthesia depress the cardiovascular reflex mechanisms and render the animal less tolerant to increased intrapulmonary pressures.[7, 10, 52] Epidural anesthesia and drugs which block the sympathetic nervous system (e.g., tranquilizers) also deter reflex compensation. Such physiologically embarrassed animals will experience an even greater depression of circulation due to the inability of the circulatory system to compensate for the increase in airway pressure.

Pulmonary Blood Flow. As with the other soft structures within the thorax, the pulmonary capillaries will be compressed as the pressures within the alveoli are increased above atmospheric. Subsequent to the pressure increase, there is blockage of the venoatrial system and a reduction of venous inflow to the lungs.[1] During the positive inspiratory phase, pulmonary pressure and resistance are increased, with a reduction in pulmonary blood flow.[23, 33, 55] This reduction in right ventricular output is transmitted to the left side of the heart and results in reduc-

tion of left ventricular output and decrease in arterial blood pressure (Fig. 22.3). The increase in resistance to pulmonary blood flow adds an extra burden on the right ventricle and can be significant in patients on the verge of decompensation.

Open Thorax Versus Closed Thorax. In the dog with closed thorax, the aforementioned changes which occur during the positive phase are due to the elimination of the thoracic pump mechanism, cardiac compression, and an increase in pulmonary resistance. In the dog with an open thorax, the importance of the three ways in which controlled ventilation interferes with circulation should be reconsidered. In the open as compared with the closed thorax, cardiac compression is minimized because of the nearly free expansion of the lungs and only becomes important when forces are applied by excessive lung packing or heart manipulation. It would seem logical that opening the chest in the dog would remove the effect of compression of the pulmonary capillaries between the gas under pressure and the chest wall, and higher pressures of longer duration could be applied without further adverse effects to the circulation. Thoracotomy in the dog has been shown to produce a further depression of cardiac output. This change in circulatory status exceeds the alterations expected by the application of intermittent positive pressure ventilation.[9, 25]

The further reduction in cardiac output was ascribed primarily to an even greater reduction in venous return. This is through the complete elimination of negative pressure on the great veins and their further collapse. Assisting venous return by means of a pump in the experimental dog resulted in an increase of cardiac output.[9] Thoracotomy produced a decrease in pulmonary arterial pressure and no further increase in pulmonary resistance. The immediate inference is that the greater reduction in cardiac outputs upon opening the thorax is primarily due to a further reduction in venous return despite the decrease in pulmonary resistance.

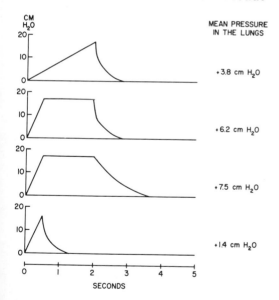

Fig. 22.4. Diagram illustrating the mean pressure in the lungs during IPPV. In each case, the pressure cycle lasts 5 seconds with a tidal volume of 800 ml. The major difference is the ventilatory pattern which includes the shape of the inspiratory and expiratory parts and the inspiratory/expiratory ratio. (Courtesy of Mushin et al.[44])

METHOD OF INTERMITTENT POSITIVE PRESSURE VENTILATION

The immediate undesirable manifestations of the alteration of physiological mechanisms produced by controlled ventilation are its effects on cardiovascular function. Normally the resultant changes can be sustained and are a small price to pay for adequate ventilation. Generally, in a healthy patient, properly applied IPPV is well tolerated; unfortunately, if improperly applied and combined with deeper planes of anesthesia, it can markedly depress cardiovascular function, especially in the debilitated patient.

During controlled ventilation it is necessary to insure uniform alveolar ventilation and thus provide adequate arterial oxygenation and carbon dioxide elimination without producing severe circulatory depression. The pressure cycle must be considered in four major parts: (a) peak pressure; (b) mean pressure; (c) shape of inspiratory and expiratory parts; and (d) inspiratory/expiratory ratio.

In the normal dog and larger species peak airway pressures between 15 and 20 torr are sufficient to overcome the resistance to lung expansion.[28] In a smaller animal (e.g., cats) slightly higher peak pressures may be necessary because of lower lung compliance. The guideline to adequate ventilation is not determined by the measurement of the peak pressure but by the visual bilateral expansion of the chest wall or lungs, or by measurement of exhaled tidal volume (Fig. 22.5). The ideal guideline is either arterial or end expired CO_2 levels, a measurement which is not routine during general anesthesia.

A prolonged pressure phase, whether it be during the inspiratory or expiratory portion, is the component which causes the greatest change in circulation. Therefore, the components of the respiratory cycle must be coordinated in a manner that will minimize the duration of positive pressure but will still insure an adequate tidal volume. Circulatory embarrassment is caused by the maintenance of an elevated mean airway pressure and not by the peak pressure attained.[34] The mean

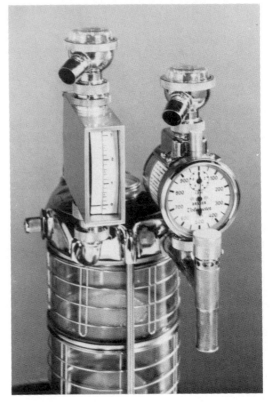

FIG. 22.5. Ventimeter attached to the exhalation line of an anesthesia circuit. This can be used as a guide for determination of respiratory minute volume. (Courtesy of North American Dräger, Telford, Pa.)

pressure is related to the area below the pressure curve (Figs. 22.4 and 22.6).[43] To provide for adequate cardiac compensation, the duration of inspiration should be short in comparison to the exhalation period. In this manner the mean pressure on the lung is reduced. This inhalation period should be composed of an increasing pressure curve rising to a short plateau lasting for about 1 second. This is to insure adequate lung expansion without prolonging the period of positive pressure.[16, 28] Marked prolongation of the plateau or holding the tidal volume at the peak pressure will not increase the tidal exchange but will elevate the mean airway pressure. Once the inspiratory volume has been attained, expiration must be unhindered in order to allow the increased pressures to return to ambient as quickly as possible. The above stresses avoiding prolonged inspiratory periods of increased airway pressure and emphasizes the importance of its release once the volume exchange has been attained.

The rapid return to normal airway pressure, and therefore normal alveolar and intrapleural pressures, will aid in the reestablishment of venous return prior to the next cycle. The inspiratory phase should occupy less than one-half of the total cycle and should not last longer than 1 second.[28] The exhalation phase should be a minimum of 1.5 times as long. A 1:2 inspiratory/expiratory ratio is suggested as one which can be easily achieved either by manual or mechanical means and one which will provide an adequate period for cardiac compensation. A respiratory rate of 20/minute will enable the maintenance of this ratio.

The essentials of manual (Fig. 22.7) or automatic ventilation are relatively simple. The peak pressures, the flow rate (the time during which the peak pressure is attained), and the duration of inspiration

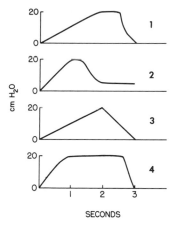

FIG. 22.6. Examples of improper pressure cycles. *1*, the inspiratory portion is too long in proportion to the exhalation phase. Under certain circumstances, this ventilatory pattern may have to be used, especially in a crushed chest or other low compliance situations. *2*, the inspiratory phase is correctly applied but positive pressure is being sustained during the expiration. *3*, the inspiratory and expiratory phases are being sustained. *4*, the state of lung inflation is being maintained for a prolonged time period.

to exhalation should only be of such magnitude and duration to allow adequate expansion of the lungs. The pressures and times suggested are only guidelines, which are adequate in most cases. There are conditions under which higher peak pressures or slower flow rates may have to be used to attain an adequate tidal volume. For example, pneumothorax, hemothorax, or a diaphragmatic hernia will decrease lung compliance (stiffer lung); under these conditions higher peak pressures may be necessary for adequate ventilation.

ASSISTED OR CONTROLLED VENTILATION

In the anesthetized, paralyzed, or sedated patient, ventilation can be assisted or controlled, either manually or mechanically. With assisted ventilation, the patient initiates the ventilatory effort and determines the rate of ventilation. The primary object of assisted ventilation is to augment tidal volume and in this manner to assure adequate alveolar ventilation. In small animal anesthesia, this may be difficult because of the usual rapid ventilatory rate. With respiratory rates of 30 to 40 breaths/minute it may be difficult to assist respiration both by manual and mechanical means. Assisted ventilation by manual means is accomplished by synchronizing the anesthetist's manual effort with the patient's pattern and augmenting slightly the tidal volume. Most mechanical ventilators can be triggered by the animal's inspiratory effort and in this manner assist ventilation. With high respiratory rates, this is difficult to accomplish, and ventilation can be more easily completely controlled.

Controlled ventilation is complete management of both rate and tidal volume. This is invariably the simpler of the two methods, and the technique is commonly used during anesthesia. The anesthetist can gain control of the animal's respiratory patterns by initially assisting respirations.[24] The anesthetist synchronizes his ventilatory pattern with that of the animal and increases tidal volume and improves alveolar ventilation. The anesthetist's own pattern of ventilation is slowly

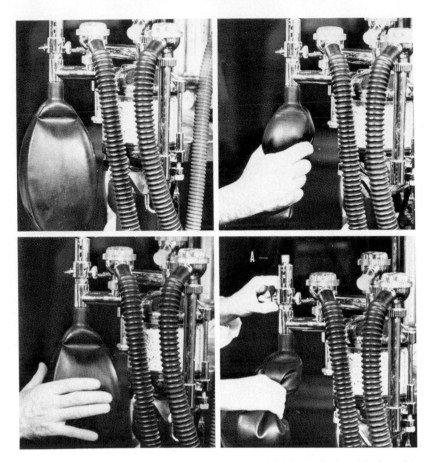

Fig. 22.7. Manual compression of the rebreathing bag for artificial ventilation. The breathing bag should be approximately one-half to three-quarters full (*upper left*) and attempts should be made to maintain the end exhaled volume constant. The bag is grasped, making sure that both the palm of the hand and fingers are in contact with the rebreathing bag, allowing maximal surface for contact. Contact with the bag should continue during the exhalation phase without maintaining positive pressure on the system. The end exhaled volume is maintained constant by adjusting both the fresh gas flow and the "pop off" valve (*A*). If the bag continues to increase, the valve should be opened further to allow a greater amount of gas to escape during the positive pressure phase of the cycle. The breathing bag should not be allowed to be maintained in an overfilled state during the exhalation phase. When the bag overinflates, the volume should be readjusted by opening the pop off valve and dumping the system.

imposed, and by this means the patient is moderately hyperventilated. This method is easily accomplished when halothane, methoxyflurane, cyclopropane, or the barbiturates are used for general anesthesia. The lack of respiratory drive with these agents enables the anesthetist to easily hyperventilate and lower the arterial carbon dioxide tension of most of the smaller veterinary patients and thus control ventilation. This is more difficult with diethyl ether because of the greater respiratory drive as compared to the other anesthetics but can be accomplished at deeper planes of anesthesia.

There may be some difficulty in initially controlling respiration in some patients. A combination of a light plane of anesthesia and surgical stimulation can produce a situation whereby the patient has excessive respiratory effort which is difficult to control. The control of respiration necessitates the removal of reflex stimulation of the respiratory center.[24, 32]

The situation can be remedied by additional intravenous thiobarbiturates, increasing the concentration of the inhalation agent, or the use of muscle relaxants. The additional barbiturate or inhalation agent will centrally raise the threshold of the respiratory center to both carbon dioxide and reflex stimuli. The greater depth of anesthesia also reduces reflex response peripherally, thus allowing easier control of respiration. Muscle relaxants permit ventilatory control without deepening anesthesia by eliminating the respiratory muscles' capabilities of responding to afferent nerve impulses. Narcotics and other premedication also raise the threshold of the respiratory center to carbon dioxide and afferent stimuli, allowing ease of ventilatory control.

The sudden increase in the concentration of an anesthetic agent can be dangerous at this time, and in the diseased animal the use of succinylcholine chloride has its advantages (see Chapter 12). The administration of 0.05 to 0.1 mg/kg will completely paralyze a dog for 10 to 15 minutes, thus allowing a gradual increase in the depth of anesthesia. Usually after the first dose of succinylcholine chloride, unless very light levels of anesthesia are used, subsequent doses are not necessary.

GUIDELINES FOR ADEQUATE VENTILATION

The elimination of carbon dioxide by the patient is the best determinant of adequate alveolar ventilation. It, unfortunately, is best determined by the measurement of arterial pH and carbon dioxide or end expired CO_2, all of which necessitate specialized equipment. The tidal volume necessary to maintain the arterial pH and P_{CO_2} at near normal levels will depend upon many factors, some of which are obvious and others which are not. Obvious determinants are body size and metabolic rate. Metabolic rate can vary according to species and alterations in body temperature produced by fever and increased muscular work. Shivering, restlessness, convulsions, and an increase in room temperature will also affect body temperature. Alterations in respiratory dead space, whether it be anatomical or alveolar, are the less obvious variables which will affect the choice of both rate and tidal volume. These can be measured in animals under anesthesia or those which are sedated, but are certainly not done routinely.

The Radford Nomagram can be used as a guide to determine the initial tidal volume and respiratory rate; unfortunately, these figures are based on average values for CO_2 production which vary considerably (Fig. 22.8). Values for adequate ventilation of various species have not been established in veterinary anesthesia, and despite the inherent criticism, some guidelines would be helpful. In determining the volume to be delivered, the compressibility of gases and the flexibility of the rubber and plastic components result in a volume loss. The compressibility of gases is a function of Boyle's law, and variations in atmospheric pressure and airway pressure will negate the possibility of applying a fixed value. Stiff corrugated tubing should be used to minimize the loss due to tube expansion. Both of these variables belie the use of a nomagram for other than a beginning guide to establish a tidal volume. Other means must be used to determine if an adequate volume is being delivered. Measurement of CO_2 tensions, measurements of volume, or at least observation of chest wall expansion should be used.

Respiratory dead space is increased during IPPV. This adds emphasis to the need for larger tidal volumes when artificial ventilation is initiated than those measured during spontaneous ventilation. There is also an increase in the alveolar arterial oxygen tension difference and venous admixture during anesthesia and controlled ventilation.[63] The venous admixture is reduced when larger tidals are used for ventilation. The inspired mixture should be no less than 30% oxygen when nitrous oxide-oxygen anesthesia is used.[63]

MECHANICAL VENTILATORS

The use of mechanical ventilators in veterinary practice is generally increasing,

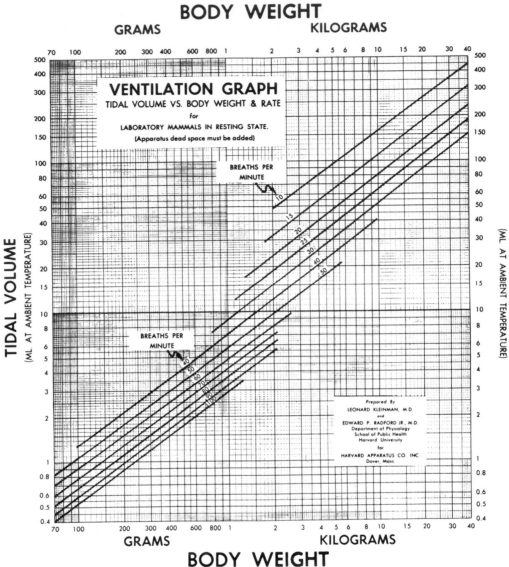

FIG. 22.8. Radford Nomagram. This graph can provide initial guidelines for choosing tidal volume and respiratory frequency in relation to body weight. Any apparatus dead space, expansion of anesthesia tubing, and compression of gases must be added to the tidal volume. (Courtesy of Theodore Smith. See also Chapter 14.)

especially with the greater use of inhalation anesthesia. Unfortunately, they are costly, and many practitioners are reluctant to invest in equipment they poorly understand and that has not been well developed for veterinary use.

There is also confusion in distinguishing equipment which can be used for inhalation anesthesia with a rebreathing system and equipment which has no rebreathing capability; for example, the Burns valve and the AVR ventilator have been used in veterinary medicine but cannot be easily adapted to inhalation equipment.

Mode of Action. To expand the lungs, airway pressure must be raised by some energy source. This source may be from a tank of compressed gas or an electric blower, both of which can be used to actuate a bag, piston, or bellows. Mechanical ventilators are difficult to classify into a specific type because some have a dual mode of operation or characteristics which are similar. The most meaningful description as it applies to their use is to classify them according to method used to end the inspiratory phase.

PRESSURE-LIMITED VENTILATORS. Pressure-limited or pressure-cycled ventilators will continue to inflate the patient's lung until a preset pressure has been attained; once reached, inspiration stops and exhalation starts (Fig. 22.9). They can be further

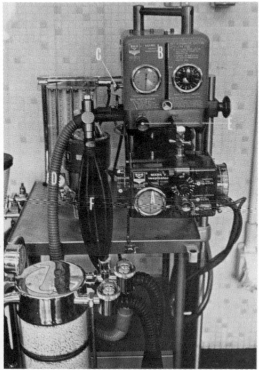

FIG. 22.9. Pressure-limited, flow-generated Bird ventilator (A). The ventilator has volume-limited capabilities when combined with the assistor-controller (B), and the mechanical stop (C) is used to limit the exertion of the bellows. Nonexpandable tubing (D) is used to connect the bellows to the circle. The bellows in the assistor-controller has replaced the breathing bag. The system can be returned from the bellows to manual ventilation by switching (E) the system to the breathing bag (F).

classified into flow- or pressure-generated ventilators. The flow pattern of the pressure-generated system is determined by the flow characteristics of the patient's tracheobronchial tree and lungs. Therefore, any alterations in compliance and resistance within the lung, endotracheal tube, or anesthesia equipment will alter inspiratory flow patterns and subsequent tidal volume. Because of the considerable alteration in lung characteristics, more frequent checks of the patient's tidal volume and adjustment may be necessary. This is especially true during thoracic surgery with opening and closing of the chest and traction and packing of the lungs.

With the flow-generated ventilators, the inspiratory flow pattern is established by the ventilator and not the mechanical aspects of the tracheobronchial tree and lungs. As opposed to the pressure-generated ventilator, the flow-generated type can maintain a flow against a wide range of back pressures.[22]

With the pressure-limited systems, the tidal volume delivered at any one cycle is dependent upon the resistance in the conduction system and lungs at a fixed cut-off pressure; as the resistance within the pulmonary system or the anesthesia equipment increases, the inspiratory period will become shorter and the tidal volume smaller; under these circumstances, a higher pressure has to be preset. Among the pressure-limited types, the flow-generated ventilators are preferred.

VOLUME-LIMITED VENTILATORS. The inspiratory phase of a volume-limited or volume-controlled ventilator ends when a preset volume or time has been attained. The ventilators allow the maintenance of a constant tidal volume and minute volume despite alterations in pulmonary resistance and compliance. Volume-limited ventilators (Fig. 22.10) and time-cycled ventilators (Fig. 22.11) necessitate less observation and resetting to maintain a constant tidal volume. Because of the preset volume, the ventilators cannot compensate for suddenly developed leaks within the system. Most volume-limited

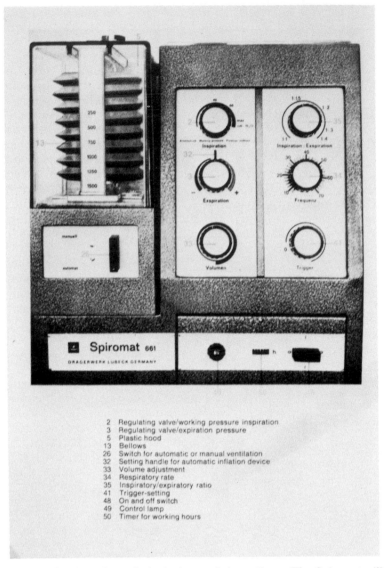

2   Regulating valve/working pressure inspiration
3   Regulating valve/expiration pressure
5   Plastic hood
13 Bellows
26 Switch for automatic or manual ventilation
32 Setting handle for automatic inflation device
33 Volume adjustment
34 Respiratory rate
35 Inspiratory/expiratory ratio
41 Trigger-setting
48 On and off switch
49 Control lamp
50 Timer for working hours

FIG. 22..10. An example of a volume-limited, time-cycled ventilator. The Spiromat will deliver a tidal volume irrespective of changes in resistance and lung compliance. The inspiratory/expiratory ratio and the inspiratory flow rate can be varied independently. This allows the selection of the time period in which the tidal volume will be delivered, the rate of delivery, and the exhalation time irrespective of alterations in lung mechanics.

ventilators also have incorporated in them a safety valve which will prevent the attainment of high pressures. Many pressure-limited ventilators can have volume-limited characteristics by the addition of a bellows with a volume-stop mechanism. When used in this manner, the cut-off pressure is set higher than necessary in order to compensate for any changes in resistance. Most ventilators, whether they are of the volume- or pressure-limited type, allow the adjustment of inspiratory flow rate and pressures developed within the system (Fig. 22.12).

The inspiratory/expiratory ratio is determined in some ventilators by the simultaneous adjustment of the inspiratory time and the respiratory frequency. Generally, volume-limited ventilators have a preset ratio or a multiple choice of ratios. If necessary, the exhalation of the patient can be aided by means of negative pressure or retarded by slowing the exhaust system. An extensive account of automatic ventilators, their function, and construction can be found in the text *Automatic Ventilation of the Lungs.*[44]

Equipment for the ventilation of large animals is not readily obtainable. Most of the equipment in use has been constructed by the individual anesthetist. (Figs. 22.13 and 22.14).

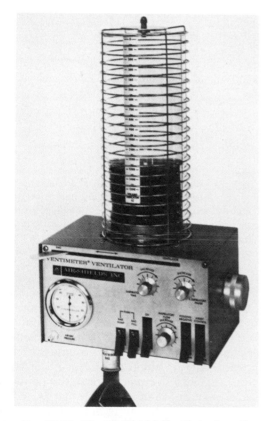

FIG. 22.11. The Air-Shield Ventilator is a time-cycled ventilator with fixed volume capabilities. The tidal volume is established by a combination of inspiratory flow rate and inspiratory time. Because the ventilator is a flow-generated and not a pressure-generated system, flow will continue until a pretimed inspiratory period has ended. This reduces its sensitivity to changes within pulmonary system.

RE-ESTABLISHMENT OF SPONTANEOUS VENTILATION

Controlled breathing during anesthesia usually results in hyperventilation and a respiratory alkalosis, especially in the smaller species. Spontaneous ventilation is resumed in a nonparalyzed veterinary patient, in many instances, following a considerable delay. The conditions which contribute to prolonged apnea are: persistent deep plane of anesthesia, preanesthetic medication, hypocarbia, hypothermia, and lack of external stimuli. Prolonged periods of controlled ventilation and surgical exposure of the abdominal and thoracic cavity can lead to hypothermia in the small dog or cat unless precautions are taken (Fig. 22.15). This reduction in metabolism contributes both to the ease in which hypocarbia is produced and the slow re-establishment of normal CO_2 levels when IPPV is terminated. Under these conditions, prolonged hyperventilation in a cool room will contribute to the delay in the re-establishment of spontaneous ventilation.

Carbon dioxide has a major stimulatory effect on the respiratory system primarily through the respiratory centers in the central nervous system. The degree of wakefulness will determine the sensitivity of the respiratory center to carbon dioxide.

Deep barbiturate or inhalation anesthesia, for example, will increase the threshold of the respiratory centers to CO_2, necessitating a higher arterial blood level to initiate spontaneous respiration. With this in mind, it is possible with inhalation agents to lighten anesthesia during the terminal portions of the surgical period, thereby reducing the depressant effects on the respiratory center. The rate of rise of CO_2 is the same, irrespective of the type of anesthesia, and is related to the metabolic rate. With the many variables, most important of which is the depth of anesthesia and body temperature, it is impossible to predict the duration of apnea following artificial ventilation. Reducing ventilation to allow the accumulation of CO_2 is a most important aspect of initi-

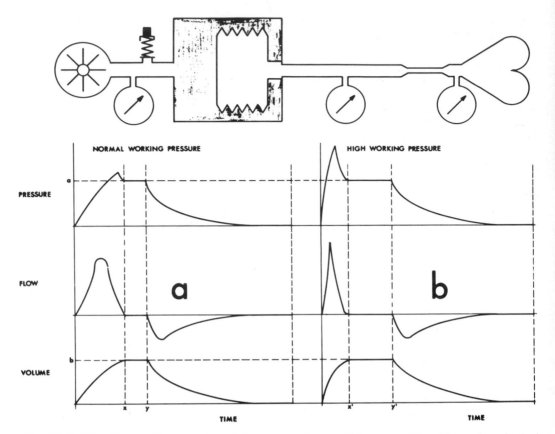

FIG. 22.12. The diagram illustrates two of the many patterns which are possible with a volume-limited time-cycled ventilator. In both cases, the inspiratory/expiratory ratios and the tidal volumes are identical. In *b*, the inspiratory flow rate and pressure are higher, thereby attaining the volume peak in a shorter time period. With a preset volume and ratio, changes in compliance and resistance will not alter tidal volume. The advantage of this system is the capability of allowing equalization of pressures throughout the tracheobronchial tree prior to exhalation. The final mean airway pressures are the same. (Courtesy of North American Dräger.)

ation of spontaneous ventilation. Arterial oxygen tension levels should be maintained by reduced but periodic inflation of the lungs and maintaining the patient attached to the anesthesia equipment. Periods of apnea for a minute or more can be tolerated in most animals especially when attached to an oxygen source. Some external stimulation may be an aid in the establishment of spontaneous respiration, which can be movement of a limb, endotracheal tube, or the placement of the final skin sutures.

The re-establishment of negative pressure within the thoracic cavity can be done by an underwater seal or gentle suction on a chest tube. Irrespective of the method, a chest tube must be placed prior to complete sealing of the chest cavity. The tube is best placed 2 to 3 ribs caudal to the incision. This will provide for removal of air or blood after closure of the chest wall and during the recovery period. Simple expansion of the lungs just prior to complete chest closure is not sufficient in itself to assure complete removal of trapped air. Suction should be applied during expansion of the lungs and at intervals during the recovery period. The tube should remain in place as long as air or blood is removed from the chest cavity. This may mean as long as 24 to 48 hours.

When continuous drainage is necessary due to injury to the lung, a simple one-way valve can be created by an underwater trap. A bottle containing 2.5 cm of water is placed at least 70 to 80 cm below the animal and the drain tube extended into the water. The water acts as a one-way valve; the water moves up the tube a short distance during inhalation and during exhalation as air is expelled from the chest cavity. The extension of the chest tube below the patient is necessary to prevent the aspiration fluid from going into the chest during the negative inspiratory phase.

Anesthesia for Cesarean Section

Cesarean section in small or large animal surgery is usually an emergency procedure due to either maternal or fetal dystocia. Occasionally, in small animal prac-tice, they are planned through knowledge of previous maternal dystocia and known breeding dates, but these are the exceptions.

The unpredictable aspect of delivery and the general tendency for the owner to delay in seeking veterinary aid can create a situation in which the condition of the mother may not be optimal and the condition of the fetuses or fetus unknown. A dead fetus may be emphysematous if the bitch has been in labor for 24 hours or more. The uterus may be devitalized with the potential of uterine rupture and maternal peritonitis. Under these conditions, the prime concern is the mother and an ovariohysterectomy with preoperative and postoperative considerations similar to a toxic pyometra should be considered.

Uterine inertia is a common maternal indication for cesarean section and fre-

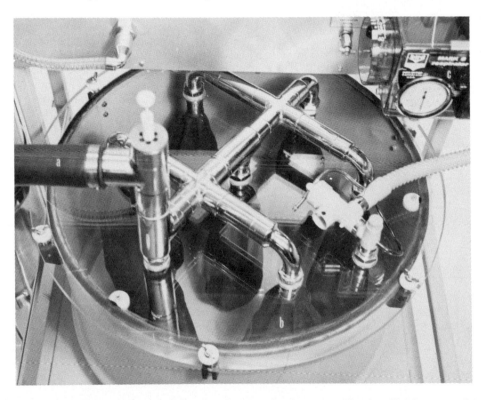

FIG. 22.13. An equine ventilator utilizing the "bag in a box" concept. The six 5-liter bags are ultimately connected to the horse by a common hose (a). The hermetically sealed box (b) is pressurized by a Bird ventilator (c). The equipment contains an anesthesia circuit, flowmeter, and vaporizer for halothane. (Courtesy of the Dupaco Company, Arcadia, Calif.)

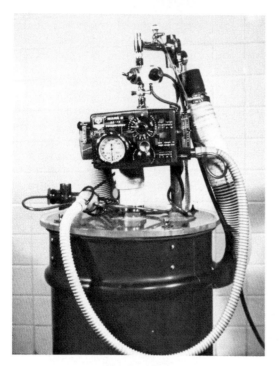

FIG. 22.14. A home-made equine ventilator, utilizing a steel drum and a 30-liter bag sealed within. The Bird Mark 9 is the power source. To expedite evacuation of the box during exhalation, two exhalation valves are placed in series. This ventilator is attached to the anesthesia circuit and, in effect, replaces the rebreathing bag. The ventilator can be used to assist or control ventilation.

quently occurs in the older obese animal. The attending veterinarian has to consider both the potential hazards of an anesthetic in the older obese patient and the effects of drugs and uterine manipulation on the fetus.

PLACENTAL TRANSFER OF DRUGS

Drugs and other foreign substances diffuse across the placenta according to their lipid solubility, molecular size, state of dissociation, concentration gradient, and the characteristics of the placental membrane.[41, 48] The concept of the lipid barrier which has been suggested for the blood-brain barrier also may apply to the placenta,[41] and the rate of entry can be equated to the fat solubility of the nonionized molecule. Common examples are the rapid transfer of thiobarbiturates and inhalation anesthetics which are known for their lipid solubility. Conversely, the muscle relaxants such as *d*-tubocurarine chloride and succinylcholine chloride have low fat solubility and therefore poor penetration. These two drugs also have large molecules with a high degree of dissociation, further reducing their penetrability through biological membranes. This is only speculative information, because like the blood-brain barrier, there is no formal

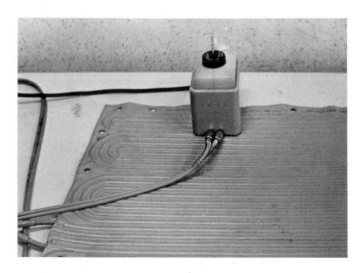

FIG. 22.15. Hot water blanket and circulator.

concept of the relationship of the placental membrane and foreign substances.[41]

The size of the molecule and the charge will also determine its rate of passage across biological membranes. Drugs which have molecular weights of less than 600 pass easily across the placenta as compared to compounds with weights above 1000.[42] Muscle relaxants, for example, have large highly dissociated molecules, as compared to thiobarbiturates which have relatively small primarily undissociated molecules. The undissociated, uncharged molecule is the form which easily crosses biological membranes. Eventually, most molecules will diffuse across the placenta to some extent regardless of size or charge, but in the clinical anesthetic time period they are of no significance.

Regardless of size, charge, and solubility characteristics, the concentration achieved in the fetus is related to the amount administered to the mother.[42] A concentration gradient must exist for the transfer. Conversely, the recovery phase in the fetus is partially dependent upon the rate of removal from the maternal blood. How important the relative binding of drugs in the maternal and fetal plasma is in the uptake and elimination of drugs has not been determined for drugs used in anesthesia.

There are species differences in the placental-fetal membrane relating to the number of membranes separating the fetal and maternal blood and also to the type of placentation. What effect this has on the rates of drug transfer is unknown. From a pragmatic point of view, anesthetic drugs and other depressants administered to the mother will be found in the fetus regardless of type of maternal-fetal membrane.

Inhalation Anesthetics. All inhalation anesthetics, because of their low molecular weight, lipid solubility, and undissociated form readily transfer across the placenta. Umbilical samples obtained shortly following birth in humans indicate an inconsistent relationship between the maternal and fetal blood. A 50 to 60% difference has been reported for nitrous oxide and a 48 to 71% difference in maternal-fetal methoxyflurane concentrations.[61] The great variability in the data is understandable due to the variation in the duration of anesthesia, the progression of delivery, and sampling after birth.

The relationship between the maternal and fetal concentration would be an aid in the evaluation of fetal depression during cesarean section. The ratio of the maternal/fetal arterial concentrations of halothane is constant when measured in a chronically prepared maternal-fetal preparation (Fig. 22.16). During the induction of anesthesia, the maternal-fetal relationship was a constant 30%, followed by a reduction to 20%, difference during steady state anesthesia. As expected, the change in maternal arterial concentration is more rapid than the fetal as the delivered concentration is reduced from an induction concentration of 2.5% to 1% and finally to recovery (Fig. 22.16).

Barbiturates. The ultrashort acting thiobarbiturates are commonly used for the induction of anesthesia for cesarean section in both man and animals. Correlations between amounts administered to the mother and maternal-fetal differences at cesarean section are available from studies in humans.[37] Transfer of thiobarbiturates is extremely rapid and fetal samples were measurable within 45 sec-

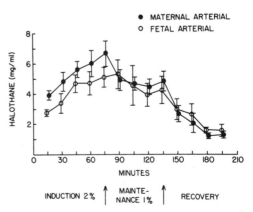

FIG. 22.16. Maternal and fetal arterial concentrations of halothane during the induction, maintenance, and recovery from anesthesia.

onds following maternal injection. Equilibration between the maternal and fetal circulation occurred within 3 to 4 minutes. As expected, the reduction in fetal levels paralleled the reduction in maternal concentration (Figs. 22.17 and 22.18). Maternal doses lower than 8 mg/kg did not produce detectable fetal depression following delivery, and in this series of studies in man, the combination of thiobarbiturate-succinylcholine-oxygen sequence of anesthesia seemed safe for elective cesarean section.[37] After delivery of the baby, an inhalation agent was started for the maintenance of anesthesia for the completion of surgery. This method is difficult in veterinary surgical obstretrics because of the need for more than one dose of the thiobarbiturate and trained personnel for the use of succinylcholine chloride and artificial ventilation.

The absolute transfer of data from man to animals is fraught with the possibility of species differences as is the reverse transfer. Nevertheless, the assumption can be made that the transfer to the fetus, the maternal-fetal gradient, and degradation are similar. An exception is that the initial dose of the thiobarbiturate would be higher in the maternal dog. The fetal concentration is low at the 10-minute period following an initial injection of 4 mg/kg (Fig. 22.17).

As would be expected, the peak concentration and maternal-fetal equilibration of sodium pentobarbital occurred much later in fetal puppies, with a much slower decline (Fig. 22.19).[11] This certainly confirms both veterinary observations and clinical data in man[5] that even sleep doses of the short acting oxybarbiturates (e.g., sodium pentobarbital) produced a marked and prolonged depression in the newborn. As opposed to the thiobarbiturates, the peak concentration in the fetuses occurs within 10 minutes, the approximate time period for surgical delivery.

Narcotics. Narcotics are commonly used for preanesthetic sedation in dogs and for analgesia in women during labor, and their transmission across the placenta is well established. Meperidine reaches the fetal circulation within 90 seconds after intravenous administration to the mother, and equilibrium between maternal and fetal blood is achieved in approximately 6 minutes.[60] The ratio of fetal cord and maternal blood levels ranged from 0.7 to 1.3, indicating an equal to higher blood level in the fetus at delivery.[6, 12, 21] The higher concentration in fetal blood may be explained on the basis of greater concen-

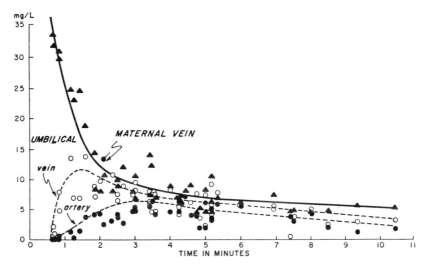

FIG. 22.17. The maternal and fetal concentration of thiamylal sodium following the single injection of 4 mg/kg. Samples were obtained during cesarean section prior to clamping of the cord. (Courtesy of Kosaka, Y. et al.[37])

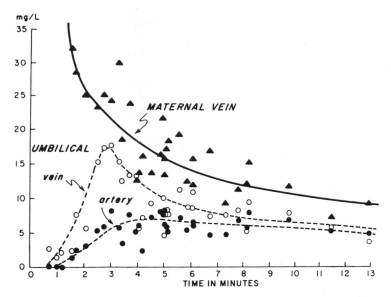

FIG. 22.18. The maternal and fetal concentrations of thiamylal sodium following the single injection of 8 mg/kg. (Courtesy of Kosaka *et al.*[37])

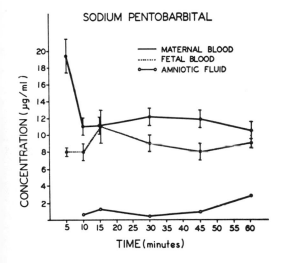

FIG. 22.19. The changes in concentration of pentobarbital in the maternal and fetal blood and amniotic fluid following the intravenous administration of 30 mg/kg to the pregnant dog. (Courtesy of Carrier *et al.*[11])

trations of a basic drug in a more acid media. The pH of the fetus and the newborn is lower than the maternal pH; because of this the transferred un-ionized drug would be in greater concentrations in the more acid medium.[6] Alterations in pH have similar effect on the dissociation of barbiturates, but despite this a maternal-fetal gradient is maintained. Quantitative measurement of narcotics is difficult, and the higher fetal concentrations may be a function of measurement error, especially at the point of equilibrium when maternal-fetal concentrations may be very similar.

Unfortunately, the assessment of the specific effects of the narcotics on the viability of pups in the immediate postnatal period is difficult. Clinical impressions indicate that moderate maternal doses will not produce serious depression in the neonatal pup. Studies in women during delivery indicate that babies born to mothers not given analgesics tend to be less depressed as determined by Apgar scoring.[21]

Tranquilizers. The investigation of the placental passage of phenothiazine tranquilizers has been hindered by the difficulty in the measurement of these compounds in biological material.[18] The drug has been identified in newborn cord blood 2 minutes after intravenous administration to the mother and equilibration reached within 4 to 5 minutes.

Skeletal Muscle Relaxants. The muscle relaxants have large molecules with a quaternary ammonium group. As a result, they are highly ionized in the pH range of blood and also possess low lipid solubility. Their transfer is minimal, and when clinical doses are used, significant amounts are not detectable in fetal blood.[42]

Local Anesthetics. Numerous reports have indicated that local anesthetics administered to the mother by any route cross the placental barrier.[58, 66] High fetal levels of local anesthetics have been associated with fetal depression, arrhythmias, and methemoglobinemia.[66] The rate of absorption from various sites into the maternal blood is related to the vascularity of the area injected and the addition of epinephrine to the anesthetic solution. Local anesthetics are absorbed rapidly from all areas used in obstetrics, which include epidural, intrathecal, caudal, or paralumbar. The umbilical venous lidocaine concentrations found at birth were approximately 52% of the maternal arterial concentration.[59] Lidocaine appears in the umbilical venous blood of the fetus within 2 to 3 minutes following intravenous injections.[58] The maternal/fetal ratio

became stable within 6 minutes and was maintained relatively constantly during the period of decline (Fig. 22.20).

ANESTHETIC TECHNIQUES

Regional analgesia is generally accepted as the form of anesthesia which is least depressant to the fetus. Local anesthetics absorbed from the site of local infiltration or from the epidural space crossing the placenta rarely achieve high levels in the fetus. This is especially true if limited to single injections,[59] which would be the method for cesarean section in veterinary patients.

The potential complications are primarily maternal, an extensive cranial block creating ventilatory difficulties or hypotension. The threat to the fetus is anoxia attributable to reduced uterine blood flow or maternal hypoventilation. Excluding maternal complications, excessive fetal depression ascribed to epidural analgesia is rare. For details on the epidural technique, the reader is referred to Chapter 32.

A concern during regional analgesia is

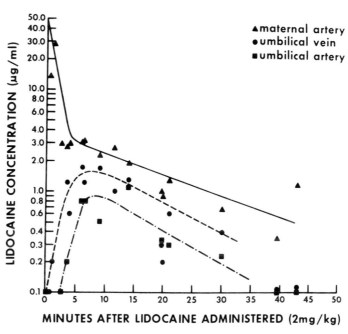

FIG. 22.20. The maternal and fetal concentrations of lidocaine following the single intravenous injection of 2 mg/kg of the drug to the mother. (Courtesy of Shnider and Way.[58])

need for sedation of the mother. Many animals, for cesarean section, will tolerate the supine position following the block without additional sedation. If sedation is necessary for the placement of the epidural block or to comfortably maintain the supine position, a narcotic is suggested. Narcotics can be reversed in both the mother and newborn if excessive cardiovascular or ventilatory depression occurs.

The neonatal respiratory depression can be prevented by the intravenous administration of a narcotic antagonist to the mother 3 to 4 minutes prior to the presentation of the pup or given to the neonate following delivery if respiratory depression is present. Narcotic depression in the newborn is treated by the injection into the umbilical vein of $^1/_{10}$ of the adult dose of a narcotic antagonist.

Inhalation anesthetic agents such as halothane, methoxyflurane, or diethyl ether are secondary choices to epidural analgesia because of the fetal depression occurring following prolonged anesthesia. When inhalation anesthetics have to be used because of circumstances which disallow epidural analgesia, the control of the depth of anesthesia and surgical speed are important. The lightest level of anesthesia comparable with surgical intervention should be administered, and, if possible, the bulk of surgical preparation should be done prior to the induction of anesthesia.

The ultrashort acting barbiturates can be safe for cesarean section if excessively high amounts are not used. Studies in man indicate a dose level of less than 8 mg/kg will not produce marked depression in the newborn.[37] This dose level may not be completely transferrable to the dog because of the higher requirements, but is certainly useful as a guide for the administration of thiobarbiturates. This dose, in most dogs, would not be sufficient for surgical planes of anesthesia, and, as in man, would require supplementation by other depressants or anesthetic agents.

Thiobarbiturates can be used for the induction of anesthesia followed by nitrous oxide and succinylcholine chloride for the maintenance of anesthesia until the pups are delivered. This anesthetic technique may be difficult for the practitioner with untrained personnel, and under this constraint, very light levels of a volatile anesthetic such as halothane could be used to supplement the nitrous oxide. It must be emphasized that only induction doses of the thiobarbiturates should be used, the trachea intubated, and the inhalation agent administered at low concentrations. When general anesthesia must be used, the anesthetic period should be used as efficiently as possible to avoid continuous exposure of the fetus to the anesthetic agent.

Oxybarbiturates (e.g., pentobarbital sodium) or intermittent doses of thiobarbiturates sufficient for the maintenance of general anesthesia are contraindicated if viable pups are to be delivered.

Anesthesia and Cardiac Disease

An often stated cliché in the preparative management of patients for cardiac surgery or heart disease is that the patient has severe heart disease and should receive 100% oxygen, cardiac output should be maintained, and hypotension should not be allowed to occur. Only a cursory knowledge of pharmacological action of depressants and general anesthetic agents indicates to the clinician that this is an impossible request.[36] All anesthetic agents depress respiratory and cardiovascular function and diminish the functional reserve of the patient. The anesthetic and surgical management should be approached with these facts in mind. The remedy is proper preparation and a carefully administered anesthetic—an often stated fact, but nonetheless true.

HEART DISEASE AND PHYSICAL STATUS

The most common acquired heart diseases in the dog are chronic valvular and myocardial disease with a higher prevalence ratio in the older animal. Many of these animals have to be subjected to anesthesia and surgery and a not infrequent question is whether or not they will survive. Unfortunately, many times the danger involved is equated to the difficulty of the surgical procedure as implied in the definition of major or minor surgery. There is no such thing as minor or a "little anesthesia," especially in the patient with advanced cardiovascular disease.[54] No anesthetics which produce unconsciousness or eliminate sensation from a major portion of the body can be considered minor, irrespective of the surgical intervention. Anesthesia in a patient with cardiac disease, even for a short procedure such as cleaning teeth, involves the realization on the part of the clinician of a greater susceptibility of the patient to the respiratory and cardiovascular effects of general anesthesia.[49, 50]

EVALUATION OF THE PATIENT

It is not within the scope of this section to discuss the specific examination of the patient for the diagnosis of cardiovascular disease. There are a multitude of tests which can be used to determine not only the specific disease, but also the degree of debilitation produced by the disorder. These, of course, range from the determination of blood volume and cardiac catheterization to examination of ventilatory capabilities. Usually these are beyond the scope of most veterinary clinics with the exception of research institutes. An evaluation can be completed by most clinicians by use of available techniques: palpation, auscultation, radiographic examination, electrocardiography, and examination of the animal's exercise tolerance.

As essential as auscultation, palpation, and a general overall physical examination, is the radiographic examination of the canine thorax. This permits the determination of the changes in the cardiac silhouette and the state of the great vessels and lungs. Common changes are caudal (left-sided) or cranial (right-sided) cardiac enlargement, secondary to mitral insufficiency. The radiographic existence of cardiac enlargement does not contraindicate general anesthesia, but it does become more meaningful if there are clinical signs of cardiac or pulmonary insufficiency. It serves as a warning of potential problems during anesthesia and surgery.

Electrocardiography is of value in establishing a diagnosis and also determining the potential hazards of added stress of anesthesia and surgery on the myocardial conduction system. Exercise tolerance is an important aspect of the determination of the patient's cardiovascular reserve, and it entails the evaluation of the patient's response to mild exercise. Animals with cardiovascular disease who tolerate running up and down the stairs with no signs of distress should be able to sustain general anesthesia well. Patients with clinical indications of subacute failure usually show signs of cardiopulmonary insufficiency when stressed. Marked increase in ventilation, coughing, discoloration of the mucous membrane, and a marked increase in pulse rate are indications of a poor reserve capacity.

The decision to proceed with anesthesia and surgery has to be based on the severity of the cardiovascular problem coupled with the need for surgery. It has been our experience that animals with mild heart disease, including grade II to III murmurs and moderate enlargement of the cardiac silhouette can tolerate general anesthesia and most operative procedures when care is taken. Animals with beginning signs of congestive heart failure present a greater problem and may have to be digitalized prior to surgery. The basic concept of preanesthetic evaluation of the patient is an attempt to establish the impact of the cardiac disease on the patient's cardiopulmonary reserve. General anesthesia and surgical trauma do have a major effect on the cardiopulmonary system, and patients who are barely sustaining cardiovascular function in the awake state need considerable support prior to and during the anesthetic and postanesthetic period.

PREMEDICATION

There are no hard and fast rules for premedication or the administration of other drugs to cardiac patients or in animals to undergo cardiac surgery. A generalized rule for all older or ill patients is to avoid oversedation with all agents and especially tranquilizers. Tranquilizers are sympatholytic as are most general anesthetics, and the combination can cause a greater degree of cardiovascular depression. Meperidine (4 to 6 mg/kg) or other synthetic narcotic derivations which do not produce vomiting in dogs are suggested for sedation. Narcotics can also produce hypotension, especially upon movement, and the dose of narcotic should be selected with care. The main criteria should be adequate sedation for proper management of the patient prior to the induction of anesthesia. Under certain conditions of advanced disease, sedative preparations should be avoided, especially if animals can be managed without them.

Atropine sulfate is an effective anticholinergic drug for patients with or without heart disease, and vagal inhibition is more effective with atropine than with scopolamine. The effect on heart rate should be considered, especially if digitalis therapy has been initiated. Under these circumstances, a marked increase in heart rate can result in a still greater reduction in ventricular output and a further compromise of the animal.

Preoperative digitalization should be approached in a conservative manner. If the early signs of congestive heart failure are present and surgery is indicated, the patient should be digitalized over a period of several days, sodium intake should be reduced, diuretics should be administered, and the patient operated on when stabilization has occurred. The borderline patients are the most difficult to appraise. These patients, at the time of examination, do not require digitalization for the maintenance of normal function but do have a reduced cardiac reserve, and with the progression of the disease state might necessitate cardioglycosides in the future.

The use of digitalis has been advocated in borderline patients to protect them from the deleterious effects of anesthesia and surgery. Cardioglycosides have an inotropic effect and can strengthen cardiac contractions in the failing heart. This inotropic effect does require an increase in oxygen consumption and production of energy-rich intermediates.[14, 30]

Hemodynamic studies in man have demonstrated that the drug has no detectable effect on cardiac output in the nonfailing heart. This and the failure to present clinical proof to substantiate the theoretical prophylactic advantage has led some to seriously question this practice.[57] Until clinical data become available indicating the prophylactic efficacy of digitalis in the borderline or nonfailing heart, preanesthetic digitalization is not recommended.

GENERAL ANESTHESIA

The induction of anesthesia should be only attempted in a quiet animal requiring minimal physical restraint. The induction of anesthesia in a struggling, muzzled patient is always dangerous and should be avoided, and this is especially true in patients with cardiovascular diseases. If sedation is not adequate, the induction of anesthesia should be delayed. The amount of preanesthetic sedation necessary may have to be determined by the manageability of the patient and, on occasion, only atropine is administered.

A mask induction is generally not recommended, because of the struggling which can occur from both the placement of the mask and the excitement stage of anesthesia. The use of moderate doses of thiobarbiturates to effect it is advised. The rapid acting barbiturates can be administered slowly to the desired level of anesthesia for intubation of the trachea or placement of a mask for the induction of inhalation anesthesia.

Anesthesia should be maintained with light levels of inhalation anesthesia, using controlled ventilation.[65] The importance of the maintenance of adequate oxygenation and removal of carbon dioxide cannot be overemphasized, especially in patients with cardiac disease. The hypertrophied heart has reduced perfusion, and the reduction of oxygen tension and elevation of carbon dioxide tension is especially hazardous. Patients with existing electrical abnormalities generally are more sensitive to the electrocardiographic effects of anesthetic agents, hypercarbia, and reduced oxygen tension. One of the more important aspects of the anesthetic management of the cardiac patient is the maintenance of a normal arterial carbon dioxide and oxygen tension, and adequate ventilation should be established from the onset of anesthesia. Techniques described in previous sections for the induction of anesthesia in animals with respiratory insufficiency are applicable here.

Obesity and Anesthesia

The problem of excess body weight has been recognized as a public health problem in human medicine. Considerable information has been accumulated on the reduction in life expectancy of the extremely overweight individual. In man, medically speaking, a 20% increase in body weight is considered pathological.[56] Unfortunately, data in veterinary patients are not available, and little consideration has been given in both veterinary medicine and surgery to the obese animal. It is recognized in veterinary surgery that obesity does interfere with wound healing, and most surgeons have the clinical impression that surgery on the obese animal presents more difficulty. This impression carries over to general anesthesia. Unfortunately, no specific data are available to confirm or add substance to this impression, especially in the field of anesthesia. Therefore the explanations for some of the problems encountered in the obese veterinary patient have to be partially based on clinical observations in animals and a few studies in man.

RESPIRATION AND CIRCULATION

Studies in the obese man have shown an increase in total respiratory compliance, especially during recumbancy, which indicates greater pressure requirements per volume of air moved. The 1/3 increase in the mechanical work of breathing was primarily due to the increased elastic work of the chest.[27, 45] Respiratory effort is less efficient because of weakness of the respiratory musculature and general interference of movement of both the diaphragm and the chest wall.[35] This increased cost of breathing can lead to hypoxia and hypercarbia under circumstances of stress.

In the extremely obese man, total lung capacity is reduced due to a decrease in vital capacity, but residual volume may be normal. Both the inspiratory capacity and the respiratory reserve volume are reduced.[38] In the obese man, no abnormalities have been found in the physical properties of the lung. The diminished capacity is primarily due to the change in properties of the chest wall, muscle weakness, the increased elastic recoil of the thoracic wall, and alterations in the natural movement of the diaphragm and the chest wall.[38] There is no direct evidence at the present that some of the ventilatory problems noted in man can be extrapolated to the veterinary patient.

An increase in plasma volume and total red cell mass is correlated with the increase in body weight.[13, 40] Cardiac output rises with increasing amounts of excess weight with considerable variation. There can be an increased demand upon the heart with increasing weight; unfortunately, the effects in the veterinary patient are unknown.

TECHNICAL PROBLEMS

Specific differences in the response to general anesthesia in the obese animal and the normal animal cannot be documented at the present time with specific data, but general impressions can be noted. The induction of anesthesia with an inhalation agent will be generally longer and with more excitement in the obese animal. The problem is a function of reduced ventilatory capabilities, thus prolonging the induction of anesthesia. A reduced ventilatory exchange decreases the amount and the speed at which the inhalation agent can reach the pulmonary circulation and ultimately the systemic circulation.

In the obese dog, the surgical plane of anesthesia is more difficult to maintain. It is a combination of the poorer ventilatory status of the patient and the continuous uptake of anesthetic agent by body fat. The margin between adequate surgical levels of the anesthetic and inadequate levels is generally narrow in the obese animal with spontaneous ventilation. Hypoventilation and relatively deep planes of anesthesia may be noted prior to surgical stimulation. Stimulation can produce bucking on the endotracheal tube, increased muscle tension, and an irregular and forced ventilatory effort. Controlled ventilation may have to be used to maintain adequate levels of anesthesia and prevent hypoventilation.

Occasionally, difficulty may be encountered in controlling ventilation in a lightly anesthetized obese dog. Compression of the breathing bag and inflation of the lung stimulates exhalation. In effect, the patient is counteracting the efforts to expand the lungs. This seems to be a more common occurrence in the lightly anesthetized obese dog. A possible explanation is a greater response of the Hering-Breuer deflation reflex.

Generally, inhalation agents have a greater effect on tidal volume and respiratory rate in the obese patient. The rate is more rapid, and tidal volume is very shallow. Under these circumstances of a diminished alveolar ventilation, the delivered concentration of an anesthetic agent may have to be higher to maintain anesthesia. This gives the impression that higher concentrations of anesthetic agents are necessary. In most cases, the increase in delivered amount is necessary to maintain an adequate alveolar concentration because of the decreased alveolar ventilation. Controlled ventilation is strongly recommended.

The recovery phase may be longer, especially if a very soluble anesthetic agent has been used. The uptake by fat and subsequent slow release coupled with a generally poorer ventilatory effort both contribute to a longer recovery period. The postanesthetic complications of hypoventilation, obstruction, and atelectasis are also considered a more serious problem.[29]

The use of ultrashort acting barbiturates for the induction of anesthesia may also be a problem in the obese animal. Venipuncture may be more difficult because of fatty tissue and generally poorer veins. The respiratory depressant effects are also more manifest in the obese patient.

REGIONAL ANALGESIA

The choice of epidural analgesia may not necessarily eliminate the additional complications of anesthesia in the obese animal. Bony landmarks are difficult to palpate and longer epidural needles may be necessary. The level of analgesia can be higher in the obese because of the difficulty in the establishment of the animal's real weight and a greater amount of fat in the epidural space. The reduction in size of the epidural space decreases the amount of drug necessary for an adequate block (see Chapter 32).

Anesthesia for the Diabetic Patient

The management of older veterinary patients with diabetes has become more of a routine in veterinary medicine. Their management includes diet control and the administration of insulin. Animals which are stable generally present few problems related to their diabetes during the anesthetic and postanesthetic period if certain precautions are taken.

The patient is placed off food for at least 6 hours prior to the induction of anesthesia, and the daily injection of insulin is omitted. The rationale for this is that the insulin requirements of the patient during the operative and postoperative period cannot be determined.

The daily doses of insulin are determined during the stabilization period by periodic checks of both urine and blood glucose. This dose is established by the animal's daily activity, which for most house pets is predictable.

The insulin requirements generally will fall during the operative and immediate postoperative period, and it is better to have a moderate degree of hyperglycemia. Under these circumstances, the hyperglycemia would not be associated with metabolic acidosis, ketosis, and dehydration. Hypoglycemic shock cannot be diagnosed under anesthesia and is only distinguished by blood glucose determination. Small amounts of glucose in water can be administered during the anesthetic and postanesthetic periods.

One of the most important aspects of the anesthetic period is rapid recovery from anesthesia and the re-establishment of the animal's feeding routine. Only then are the daily doses of insulin re-established. The problems of postoperative anorexia can be managed by the intravenous administration of glucose and half-doses of insulin. If control becomes difficult during this period, glucose and ketone analysis are necessary.

Vomiting and Aspiration during Anesthesia

Vomiting can be a sudden occurrence during the induction of general anesthesia but is not necessarily limited to this period. Vomiting during the recovery from anesthesia is not as common in animals as it is in man but does occasionally occur. It is more likely in the brachycephalic breeds and in cats after cyclopropane anesthesia.

VOMITING AND REGURGITATION

Vomiting is an active process which includes the co-ordination of abdominal, thoracic, and diaphragmatic muscles. Fortunately, vomiting during the induction of anesthesia is at such a time period that semiconsciousness still persists, and protective oropharyngeal reflexes may still be present, although obtunded.

The mechanism for vomiting during the induction stages of anesthesia is an apparent increased sensitivity of the emetic center to stimuli. Thus, the presence of a full stomach, whether food, fluid, or air, would be more likely to provoke vomiting during this state than the awake state. This hypersensitivity is consistent with the stage of hyperexcitability that exists during stages 1 and 2 of anesthesia. During this phase the emetic center will respond to weak stimuli.

Regurgitation is not a highly integrated process and is passive in nature. It is not as dramatic as vomition, but it is insidiously more common and can occur in simple stomach animals even following proper fasting. When dye is introduced into the stomach, small amounts can be found in pharynx and trachea following anesthesia and surgery.[2] The gastroesophageal junction is not an active sphincter, and its closure is a valvular mechanism consisting of flaps of gastric mucosa. Passive regurgitation involves the opening of this junction.[31] The resistance to caudal flow is small, but it can sustain high reverse pressure differences.[20] The angle at which the esophagus enters the stomach is important in maintaining this valvular function. Normally the angle between the stomach and the esophagus is an acute one, and under these circumstances, the valvular mechanism can withstand reverse pressures up to 28 cm of water. Reducing the angle to 90° diminishes the leaking pressure to 3 cm of water.[39] Traction on the stomach flattens the mucosal fold, reducing the competence of the valve,[46] and gradual distention of the stomach will also produce a similar effect, with leakage.[53] Airway obstruction can also create valvular incompetence, with actual opening of the valve when quiet breathing is converted to an obstructive type.[46, 62] It is apparent that regurgitation in the simple stomach species is most likely to occur during obstructive breathing, gastric traction, gastric distention, and external gastric pressure commonly produced by abdominal packs.

Regurgitation is extremely common in ruminants because of the impossibility of completely reducing gastric contents. Endotracheal intubation or positioning of the head is mandatory to avoid aspiration of ruminal contents.

PREVENTION OF VOMITING

Gastric emptying time in dogs can vary from 1½ to 6 hours. Conditions exist which can delay gastric emptying and may precede the presentation of an animal in need of anesthesia for emergency surgery. Excitement, as with pain and fear, can delay gastric emptying and can be a common situation when patients are admitted for routine elective surgery. It is not uncommon for owners to feed animals prior to hospital admittance. Accidental trauma with or without hypotension or blood loss and sedative drugs will delay gastric emptying.

When the history indicates feeding as long as 4 to 6 hours prior to trauma, the patient should be anesthetized with the assumption that it may have a full stomach, even with a delay between presentation and surgery. Displacement or torsion of stomach, abdominal masses, and impending parturition will completely prevent or delay gastric emptying.

The management of a full stomach necessitates rapid induction of anesthesia and tracheal intubation. Suction apparatus for the removal of vomitus should be available; this includes a bite block to prevent closure of the mouth during light anesthesia.

MANAGEMENT FOLLOWING VOMITION

The most important aspect of management of sudden vomition during the induction of anesthesia is the establishment of a clear airway. The head should be lowered and the animal placed in a lateral position when possible. The pharyngeal cavity should be suctioned and solid food cleared with a gauze sponge. The patient should be intubated as soon as possible and the small suction catheter passed into the trachea and bronchi for the removal of any aspirated material. Oxygen should be administered between suctioning of the trachea.

The possibility of developing aspiration pneumonitis can be predicted by both the pH of the solution and the volume inspired. Pneumonitis can be expected when the liquid material has a pH of less than 2.5. Semisolid, partially digested foods produced a pneumonitis regardless of the pH.[2, 3] Aspiration pneumonitis was easily produced by the introduction of hydrochloric acid solutions into the lungs of anesthetized rabbits.[2] The attempt at preventing this experimentally produced pneumonitis by introducing diluent solutions such as normal saline, sodium bicarbonate, sodium hydroxide, sodium lactate, and calcium gluconate had no beneficial effects. In most cases, the condition was worsened because of the greater spread of the acid solution.[2]

SIGNS AND MANAGEMENT OF ASPIRATION PNEUMONITIS

Aspiration pneumonitis has a triad of signs: persistent cyanosis, tachypnea, and tachycardia. These signs may not appear for 3 to 4 hours after aspiration. Other signs are rhonchi or rales in the chest, wheezing, and an increase in body temperature. Radiographic examination may disclose diffuse pneumonia or consolidation, particularly of the right apical lobe.

The management is primarily symptomatic treatment of oxygen hunger and the inflammatory condition. Steroids alone or in combination with antibiotics alleviate the severity of experimentally produced pneumonitis. Steroids can ameliorate the overwhelming inflammatory reaction, and these combined with antibiotic and oxygen therapy are the basis for symptomatic treatment.

REFERENCES

1. Ankeney, J. L., Hubay, C. A., Hackett, P. R., and Hingson, R. A.: The effect of positive and negative pressure respiration on unilateral pulmonary blood flow in the open chest. Surg. Gynec. Obstet. 98: 600, 1954.
2. Bannister, W. K., and Sattilaro, A. J.: Vomiting and aspiration during anesthesia. Anesthesiology 23: 251, 1962.
3. Bannister, W. K., Sattilaro, A. J., and Otis, R. D.: Therapeutic aspects of respiration pneumonitis in experimental animals. Anesthesiology 22: 440, 1961.
4. Barach, A. L., Eckman, M., Ginsburg, E., Rumsey, C. C., Jr., Korr, I., Eckman, I., and Besson, G.: Studies on positive pressure respiration. I. General aspects and types of pressure breathing. II. Effects on respiration and circulation at sea level. J. Aviation Res. 17: 290, 1946.
5. Batt, B.: Are large doses of intravenous barbiturates justified for use as premedication in labor. Amer. J. Obstet. Gynec. 102: 591, 1968.
6. Beckett, A., and Taylor, J. F.: Blood concentrations of pethidine and pentazocine in mother and infant at time of birth. J. Pharm. Pharmacol. 19: 505, 1967.
7. Beecher, H. K., Bennett, H. S., and Bassett, D. L.: Circulatory effects of increased pres-

sure in the airway. Anesthesiology *4:* 612, 1943.

8. Bendixen, H. H., Egbert, L. D., Hedley-Whyte, J., Laver, M. B., and Pontoppidan, H.: *Respiratory Care.* The C. V. Mosby Company, St. Louis, 1965.

9. Caldini, P., Ho, C., and Zingg, W.: Effect of thoracotomy on cardiac output and pulmonary hemodynamics in dogs. J. Thorac. Cardiovasc. Surg. *44:* 104, 1962.

10. Carr, D. T., and Essex, H. E.: Effects of positive pressure respiration on circulatory and respiratory systems. Amer. Heart J. *31:* 53, 1946.

11. Carrier, G., Hume, A. S., Douglas, B. H., and Wiser, W. L.: Disposition of barbiturates in maternal blood, fetal blood, and amniotic fluid. Amer. J. Obstet. Gynec. *105:* 1069, 1969.

12. Cipgar, V., Burns, J. J., Brodie, B. B., and Papper, E. M.: The transmission of meperidine across the human placenta. Amer. J. Obstet. Gynec. *64:* 1368, 1952.

13. Cole, V. W.: The circulation in extreme obesity. Heart Bull. *10:* 108, 1960.

14. Coleman, H. N.: Role of acetylstrophanthidin in augmenting myocardial oxygen consumption. Circ. Res. *21:* 487, 1967.

15. Coryllos, P. H.: Mechanical resuscitation in advanced forms of asphyxia: A clinical and experimental study in the advanced forms of resuscitation. Surg. Gynec. Obstet. *66:* 698, 1938.

16. Cournand, A., Motley, H. L., Werko, L., and Richards, D. W.: Physiological studies of the effects of intermittent positive pressure breathing on cardiac output in man. Amer. J. Physiol. *152:* 162, 1948.

17. Crafoard, C.: Pulmonary ventilation and anesthesia in major chest surgery. J. Thorac. Cardiovasc. Surg. *9:* 237, 1940.

18. Crawford, J., and Rudofsky, S.: Placental transmission and neonatal metabolism of promazine. Brit. J. Anaesth. *37:* 303, 1965.

19. Dern, R. J., and Fenn, W. O.: The effect of varying pulmonary pressure on the arterial pressure in man and anesthetized cats. J. Clin. Invest. *26:* 460, 1947.

20. Dornhurst, A. C., Harrison, K., and Pierce, J. W.: Observations on normal oesophagus and cardia. Lancet *1:* 695, 1954.

21. Duncan, L. B., Ginsburg, J., and Morris, N. F.: Comparison of pentazocine and pethidine in normal labor. Amer. J. Obstet. Gynec. *105:* 197, 1969.

22. Edwards, W. L., and Sappenfield, R. S.: Pressure-cycled ventilators and flow-rate control. Anesth. Analg. (Cleveland) *47:* 77, 1968.

23. Edwards, W. S.: The effects of lung inflation and epinephrine on pulmonary vascular resistance. Amer. J. Physiol. *167:* 756, 1951.

24. Evans, F. T., and Cray, C.: *General Anesthesia,* vol. 2. Butterworth & Co. (Publishers) Ltd., London, 1959.

25. Finlayson, J. K., Luria, M. N., and Yu, P. N.: Some circulatory effects of thoracotomy and intermittent positive pressure respiration in dogs. Circ. Res. *9:* 862, 1961.

26. Frenchner, P.: Bronchial and tracheal catheterization and its clinical application. Acta Otolaryng. (Stockholm) (suppl.) *20:* 100, 1934.

27. Gilbert, R., Sipple, J. H., and Auchincloss, J. H.: Respiratory control and work of breathing in obese subjects. J. Appl. Physiol. *16:* 21, 1961.

28. Gordon, A. S., Frye, C. W., and Langston, H. T.: J. Thorac. Cardiovasc. Surg. *32:* 431, 1956.

29. Gould, A. B.: Effect of obesity on respiratory complications following general anesthesia. Anesth. Analg. (Cleveland) *41:* 448, 1962.

30. Gousios, A. G., Felts, J. M., and Havel, R. J.: Effects of ouabain on force of contraction, oxygen consumption, and metabolism of free fatty acids in the perfused rabbit heart. Circ. Res. *22:* 445, 1967.

31. Greenan, J.: The cardio-oesphageal junction. Brit. J. Anaesth. *33:* 432, 1961.

32. Guedel, A. E., and Treweek, D. N.: Ether apneas. Anesth. Analg. (Cleveland) *13:* 263, 1934.

33. Hubay, C. A., Brecher, G. A., and Clement, F. L.: Etiological factors affecting pulmonary arterial flow with controlled respiration. Surgery *38:* 215, 1955.

34. Hunter, A. R.: The duration of inspiration during artificial ventilation of the lungs. Anaesthesia *17:* 3, 1962.

35. Kautmen, B. J., Ferguson, M. H., and Cherniak, R. H.: Hypoventilation in obesity. J. Clin. Invest. *38:* 500, 1959.

36. Keown, K. K.: *Anesthesia for Surgery of the Heart,* 2nd ed. Charles C Thomas, Publisher, Springfield, Ill., 1963.

37. Kosaka, Y., Takahashi, T., and Mark, L. C.: Intravenous thiobarbiturate anesthesia for caesarean section. Anesthesiology *31:* 489, 1969.

38. Lambert, I. E.: Obesity and anesthesia. In *Clinical Anesthesia: Common and Uncommon Problems in Anesthesiology,* Series 3. F. A. Davis Company, Philadelphia, 1968.

39. Marchand, P.: The gastro-oesophageal "sphincter" and mechanism of regurgitation. Brit. J. Surg. *42:* 504, 1955.

40. Miller, W. F., and Bashour, F. A.: Cardiopulmonary changes in obesity. Clin. Anesth. *3:* 187, 1963.

41. Moya, F., and Smith, B. E.: Uptake, distribution and placental transport of drugs and anesthetics. Anesthesiology *29:* 465, 1965.

42. Moya, F., and Thorndike, V.: Passage of drugs across the placenta. Amer. J. Obstet. Gynec. *84:* 1778, 1962.

43. Mushin, W. W.: History of thoracic anesthesia. In *Thoracic Anesthesia,* chap. 10. F. A. Davis Company, Philadelphia, 1963.

44. Mushin, W. W., Rendell-Baker, L., Thompson, P. W., and Mapleson, W. W.: *Automatic Ventilation of the Lungs.* F. A. Davis Company, Philadelphia, 1969.

45. Naimark, A., and Cherniack, R. M.: Compliance of the respiratory system and its components in health and obesity. J. Appl. Physiol. *15:* 377, 1960.

46. O'Mullane, E. J.: Vomiting and regurgitation during anesthesia. Lancet *1:* 1209, 1954.

47. Otis, A. B., Rahn, H., and Fenn, W. O.: Venous pressure changes associated with positive intrapulmonary pressure: their relationship to the distensibility of the lung. Amer. J. Physiol. *146:* 307, 1946.

48. Page, E. W.: Transfer of materials across the human placenta. Amer. J. Obstet. Gynec. *74:* 505, 1957.

49. Papper, E. M.: Selection and management of anesthesia in those suffering from disease and disorders of the heart. Canad. Anesth. Soc. J. *12:* 245, 1965.

50. Pierce, A. K.: Assisted respiration. Ann. Rev. Med. *20:* 431, 1969.

51. Pollack, L., McDonald, K. E., Kjartansson, K. B., Delin, N. A., and Schenk, W. G., Jr.: Influence of hyperventilation on cardiac output and renal blood flow. Surgery *55:* 299, 1964.

52. Price, H. F., King, B. D., Elder, J. D., Libien, B. H., and Dripps, R. D.: Circulatory effects of raised airway pressure during cyclopropane anesthesia in man. J. Clin. Invest. *30:* 1243, 1951.

53. Robson, J. G., and Welt, P.: Regurgitation in anesthesia: report on some exploratory work with animals. Canad. Anesth. Soc. J. *6:* 4, 1959.

54. Rodmen, T.: The effect of anesthesia and surgery on pulmonary and cardiac function. Amer. J. Cardiol. *12:* 444, 1963.

55. Rowe, G. G., Castillo, C. A., and Crumpton, C. W.: Effects of hyperventilation on systemic and coronary hemodynamics. Amer. Heart J. *63:* 67, 1962.

56. Schwartz, H.: Problems of obesity in anesthesia. New York J. Med. *55:* 3277, 1955.

57. Selzer, A., Kelly, J. J., Gerbode, F., Kerth, W. J., Osborn, J. J., and Popper, R. W.: Case against routine use of digitalis in patients undergoing cardiac surgery. J. A. M. A. *195:* 549, 1966.

58. Shnider, S. M., and Way, E. L.: The kinetics of transfer of lidocaine (Xylocaine) across the human placenta. Anesthesiology *29:* 944, 1968.

59. Shnider, S. M., and Way, E. L.: Plasma levels of lidocaine (Xylocaine) in mother and newborn following obstetrical conduction anesthesia. Anesthesiology *29:* 951, 1968.

60. Shnider, S. M., Way, E. L., and Lord, M. J.: Rate of appearance and disappearance of meperidine in fetal blood after administration of narcotic to the mother. Anesthesiology *27:* 227, 1966.

61. Siker, E. S., Wolfson, B., Dubnansky, J., and Fitting, G. M., Jr.: Placental transfer of methoxyflurane. Brit. J. Anaesth. *40:* 588, 1968.

62. Sinclair, R. N.: Oesophageal cardia and regurgitation. Brit. J. Anaesth. *31:* 15, 1959.

63. Sykes, M. K., Young, W. E., and Robinson, B. E.: Oxygenation during anesthesia with controlled ventilation. Brit. J. Anaesth. *37:* 314, 1965.

64. Taylor, G., and Gerbode, F.: Observations on the circulatory effect of short duration positive pulmonary inflation. Surgery *30:* 316, 1948.

65. Theye, R. A., Moffitt, E. A., and Kirklin, J. W.: Anesthetic management during open intracardiac surgery. Anesthesiology *23:* 823, 1962.

66. Usubiaga, J. E., Iuppa, M. L., Moya, F., Wikinski, J. A., and Velazco, R.: Passage of procaine HCl and para-aminobenzoic acid across the human placenta. Amer. J. Obstet. Gynec. *100:* 918, 1968.

67. Watrous, W. G., Davis, R. E., and Anderson, B. M.: Manually assisted and controlled respiration; its use during inhalation anesthesia for the maintenance of a near-normal physiological state: a review. Anesthesiology *11:* 661, 1951.

23
Equine Anesthesia

L. W. HALL

Most of the special problems encountered in equine anesthesia are related to the size and weight of the animals or to the ease with which they become frightened. The difficulties experienced in handling and managing a horse are, of course, directly proportional to its size and strength, while its weight creates problems during general anesthesia. A large heavy horse cast by an inadequate or inexperienced casting team may sustain serious injuries when it falls and, once down, cannot be easily positioned for surgery. Furthermore, if a heavy horse is kept anesthetized or restrained in lateral recumbency for more than 1 to 2 hours, the weight of its body resting on the undermost limbs may produce ischemia of the muscles and nerve palsies. Horses have had to be killed because of palsies caused by prolonged recumbency in the lateral position. Difficulties are also encountered in horses which are particularly nervous and take fright when handled by strangers, approached suddenly, or placed in unfamiliar surroundings. Frightened horses take refuge in flight and will fight violently to escape from restraint. At such times the animal's behavior may cause serious injury to itself or to those attempting to control it.

A few horses are naturally so vicious or high spirited that they are difficult to manage at all times, but the majority of adult horses are quite amenable to handling provided that this is conducted in a quiet and gentle manner. However, the ease with which any horse can be controlled may be greatly increased by the judicious use of sedative and tranquilizing drugs, and for this reason considerable attention has been devoted to the study of these drugs in horses. While appropriate preanaesthetic medication may facilitate the induction of general anesthesia because medicated animals are less likely to be disturbed by rough or clumsy handling, sudden movements, and unfamiliar procedures, it must be remembered that sedation which interferes with the ability of the horse to remain standing may itself provoke excitement.

The recovery period after basal narcosis or general anesthesia also presents special problems. Panic may be seen if the animal discovers, when the effects of the agents used are declining, that it is unable to rise to its feet or is unable to maintain its balance once it has done so. It is, therefore, often necessary when working in confined spaces to restrain the animal until it is quite capable of standing unaided, or at least until the danger of a postanesthetic excitement phase has passed.

The choice of an anesthetic technique for a horse must involve consideration of all these special peculiarities in addition to the more general factors, such as the site and nature of the proposed operation or examination, together with the facilities, drugs, and assistance available. Some of the problems of equine anesthesia may be solved by the choice of local infiltration analgesia, regional nerve blocks, and mild sedation, but in this chapter consideration will only be given to basal narcosis and general anesthesia.

Respiratory and Cardiovascular Physiology in Relation to Anesthesia

Horses vary greatly in size and weight, and there is a corresponding variation in tidal and minute volumes of respiration and in anatomical dead space of the respiratory system. Tidal volumes of 7.5 to 12.0 liters with minute volumes of 36 to 96 liters have been recorded in anesthetized thoroughbreds weighing 460 to 600 kg.[44] These values are higher than those recorded by earlier workers[11, 23, 49] in horses other than thoroughbreds. Peak flow rates on expiration reach 1320 liters/minute, although for only a fraction of a second.[44] Spirometric tracings have shown gas flows of 190 to 990 liters/minute during approximately one-third of both inspiration and expiration. Clearly, observations such as these are very pertinent to the design of apparatus for inhalation anesthesia and will be referred to again later in this chapter.

Examination prior to Anesthesia

Once the risks which any patient carries with respect to both anesthesia and to the proposed operative procedure have been recognized, the anesthetic technique and the preoperative and postoperative treatment can be designed to prevent accidents and undesirable sequelae from occurring. Probably, in veterinary practice, most of the horses presented for anesthesia are normal, healthy, and young, while most of the operations are comparatively minor in nature. Nevertheless, if a supposedly healthy animal is dull or off its food, anesthesia should be postponed until the fitness of the animal is assured. Elderly or debilitated animals which are to undergo extensive surgical procedures may require very careful management if a successful outcome is to be obtained, and it is in such animals that a more detailed physical examination is needed to assess the risks involved.

The exact nature and scope of the preanesthetic examination are not easy to define. It should certainly not be too time consuming, nor in the majority of instances is it necessary for it to lead to an exact diagnosis. The anesthetist is more concerned with the general influence of any conditions present on the animal as a whole, rather than the exact nature of the conditions themselves. A procedure such as that outlined below is usually adequate, relatively easy to follow in most circumstances, and can be carried out without undue disturbance of the animal. During this examination an assessment of the animal's temperament can be made and this too may have a significant influence on the choice of anesthetic method and preoperative and postoperative management.

Some information regarding a horse's physical condition may be obtained from the owner or attendant in answer to questions relating to exercise tolerance. Respiratory distress on exercise may indicate either cardiac failure or respiratory disease. The presence of a soft moist cough is suggestive of airway secretions which may cause obstruction during anesthesia when the cough reflex is suppressed, or atelectasis afterwards. Tachycardia, as found in all febrile and many wasting diseases, usually means that the animal has decreased reserves to meet the circulatory stresses imposed by general anesthesia, and thus attention should always be paid to the pulse rate. Next, the examination should be directed toward the detection of cardiac thrills, the location of the apex beat of the heart, and an estimation of the jugular venous pressure.

A thrill over the heart indicates the presence of cardiovascular disease with, possibly, an increased anesthetic risk. Location of the apex beat is a useful guide both to the condition of the heart and the respiratory system. It may be displaced if there is a pleural effusion, pneumothorax, lung collapse, or a space-occupying lesion in the thorax. If there are no signs of pulmonary disorders, displacement of the apex beat indicates cardiac hypertrophy or dilation. Observation of the jugular venous pressure should be made with the horse in a normal standing position, its neck being at about 45° to the horizontal. In this position, the distention of the jugular vein should just be visible at the base of the neck. Venous distention above this level indicates obstruction of the anterior vena cava or a rise in right atrial pressure which may be due to right ventricular hypertrophy.

Diastolic murmurs always indicate the presence of heart disease; systolic murmurs may or may not. However, in the absence of other signs of heart disease, neither type of murmur is of much significance to the anesthetist, who needs to know more of the effective function of the heart rather than the exact nature of any cardiac lesion. Fitness for anesthesia is assessed on a knowledge of how the heart behaves at rest and during exercise, and on experience of how similarly affected animals have behaved in similar circumstances.

Auscultation of the lungs is also of very limited value. Rhonchi and crepitations indicate the presence of excessive amounts of sputum, while prolongation of the expiratory sound, especially when accompanied by high pitched rhonchi, is suggestive of emphysema or "broken wind" with its associated bronchospasm.

It cannot be suggested that a shortened clinical examination such as this is ideal, but it is often all that can be achieved. As in all clinical examinations, two factors operate: first, the thoroughness with which even the limited examination is carried out; and, second, the ability of the anesthetist to recognize the significance or insignificance of the findings.

Preparation for Anesthesia

Unless an operation is one of great urgency there is seldom any excuse for submitting an unfit horse to anesthesia. The majority of the conditions detected on even a simple clinical examination are amenable to treatment, and the fitness of a horse classified as a "poor risk" in the light of the findings of this examination can usually be greatly improved before the anesthetic is administered. The proper preparation of such animals may take time, but it is more important than the selection of any particular method or technique of anesthesia in minimizing the anesthetic mortality and morbidity rates.

Many of the hazards associated with the induction of general anesthesia can also be avoided by careful planning of the whole procedure. To avoid regurgitation of stomach contents or rupture of the stomach as the animal falls to the ground, the stomach must be empty when anesthesia is induced. All horses should be deprived of food for 6 to 12 hours prior to anesthesia, and it may be necessary to muzzle the horse during this period to prevent it from eating its bedding. Starvation for longer periods should be avoided as this depletes liver glycogen stores and reduces the ability of the liver to detoxicate anesthetic agents. Water should be allowed until about 2 hours before the induction of anesthesia. Whenever possible, racehorses should be taken out of training for at least 1 week before anesthesia, and shoes should be removed or covered with adhesive plaster bandages. If the horse is to be anesthetized in the open, a relatively large area of ground should be chosen to minimize the danger of the animal injuring itself during induction or recovery. If the induction of anesthesia is to be conducted indoors and a tilting table is not used, it is most important to insure that the bed on which the animal is to lie is adequately padded. Further protection against injury is afforded by the use of a rug and head gear padded with foam rubber (Fig. 23.1).

Premedication

Premedication must be regarded as part of the whole anesthetic procedure, specially tailored in each individual case and never given merely as a routine. In the majority of cases it is given to insure a quiet recovery from anesthesia which has been induced with a barbiturate drug

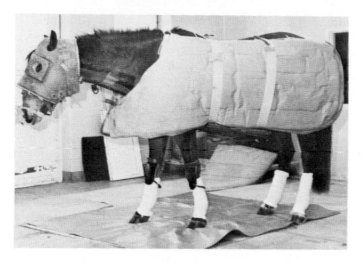

FIG. 23.1. Protective clothing. Horse blanket split along back and joined with quick release lacing. Padding of 3-inch-thick foam rubber.

administered by intravenous injection, and there is no need to produce heavy preanesthetic sedation, because the animal is normally docile enough for the accurate injection of a drug such as a barbiturate to be made without difficulty. In vicious or excitable horses, on the other hand, heavy preanesthetic sedation may be necessary if the induction of anesthesia is to be accomplished smoothly and safely. Heavy sedation may also be essential if the horse is to be restrained close alongside the vertically positioned top of an operating table.

There are three groups of drugs used for premedication in horses, namely: (a) parasympathetic antagonists; (b) analgesics; and (c) ataractics or tranquilizers.

PARASYMPATHETIC ANTAGONISTS

Both atropine and hyoscine may be used to reduce salivary and bronchial secretions produced in response to irritation of the upper respiratory tract by agents such as diethyl ether. In equine anesthesia, the anesthetic agents in common use do not increase the secretions in the airway, and thus these drying agents are only used when for some reason diethyl ether is to be administered. Hyoscine may give rise to excitement in horses and atropine is probably the agent of choice.

When diethyl ether is to be used, atropine should be given in doses of up to 65 mg about 20 minutes before anesthesia. Doses of this order are unlikely to afford any protection from disturbances of cardiac rhythm caused by impulses in the vagus nerves.[56]

ANALGESICS

Preanesthetic sedation of horses with analgesic drugs was popular before the introduction of the ataractic drugs and is still used today in animals which are actually in pain before an operation. Because morphine is such a powerful analgesic, some anesthetists consider that its use for premedication helps in the relief of postoperative pain, but there is little doubt that this is best controlled by the intravenous injection of an analgesic at the end of anesthesia.

Although morphine seldom exhibits undesirable effects in horses which are actually suffering from painful conditions, it may give rise to excitement in normal horses, and, for this reason, it is unwise to use morphine for premedication in fit, healthy animals. A combination of chloral hydrate (1 to 2 g/50 kg) and morphine (0.1 to 0.2 g/animal) is said to produce sedation with less risk of excitement.[64]

Methadone is popular in some European countries and is often administered with an ataractic (propionyl promazine) which potentiates its sedative action. Although methadone acts like morphine, it is said to be less likely to give rise to excitement in doses of less than 0.3 mg/kg.[39] It is usually given by intramuscular injection in doses of 50 to 150 mg (0.2 mg/kg).[64]

The opiate most commonly used in premedication is meperidine hydrochloride. It sedates nervous animals, making them easier to handle, and its analgesic properties are of value in certain painful conditions.[2] Meperidine hydrochloride is administered by intramuscular injection in doses of 0.5 mg/kg about ¾ hour before the induction of anesthesia. It may also be given by intravenous injection during or immediately after anesthesia to alleviate postoperative pain.

All the analgesic drugs cause respiratory depression, and, if given in large doses before the administration of an inhalation agent, they will slow down the induction of anesthesia.

ATARACTICS OR TRANQUILIZERS

These drugs depress the central nervous system, probably by interference with the functioning of the reticular activating system.[6, 7] They produce a degree of sedation not necessarily accompanied by lethargy or sleep and, usually, a reduction in spontaneous motor activity. At the moment, all the useful compounds of this type used in horses are phenothiazine derivatives. Following their use, the horse, when left alone, quiet and undisturbed, looks sleepy. Its head and upper eyelids droop, while the membrana nictitans is more obvious than usual and, in males, the penis hangs limply from the prepuce. However, the effects seem to be most marked in quiet horses, for vicious or excitable animals may show but little sedation. Even horses which appear well sedated can easily be aroused by noise, sudden movements, or rough handling. Occasionally the administration of one of these compounds to a horse results in the production of excitement which may be manifest for several hours.[17, 41] Heart block has

been known to follow the intravenous injection of these compounds.

It is clear that these compounds are not very useful as sedatives for horses. Attempts to increase the degree of sedation produced by increasing the dose have been unsuccessful. While the degree of sedation cannot apparently be increased by the administration of more than a minimum effective dose, the incidence of side effects increases sharply as the dose is raised. The widespread use of these compounds in horses is probably related more to the ease with which they may be administered rather than to the certainty or reliability with which they produce sedation. The choice of a particular compound on any occasion is usually dictated by the personal preference and experience of the administrator, although there are some indications that certain of these drugs are more reliable than others.

As far as premedication is concerned, the use of any of these phenothiazine derivatives will insure a quiet recovery after general anesthesia in which barbiturate drugs have been employed. It would seem likely that as other drugs are developed as general sedatives for horses, the use of the phenothiazine compounds will become restricted to this purpose alone.

Promethazine hydrochloride was introduced into horse practice as an antihistamine and was probably the first of the phenothiazine compounds to be used for premedication. Its solution is irritant to the tissues, and large swellings may occur at the sites of intramuscular injections. Largely for this reason, it is now seldom used in horses.

Chlorpromazine hydrochloride is another compound which is no longer used in horses since it is associated with a high incidence of undesirable effects. Its administration is not infrequently followed by violent excitement. Because its intravenous injection results in a fall in blood pressure, and because excitement is seen most frequently after intravenous administration, it was suggested that the two phenomena were connected. However, it has been demonstrated that the excitement seen in an experimental pony was not associated with hypotension[17] and it is more likely that excitement is precipitated by the onset of muscle weakness.[41] When excitement occurs it is both alarming and dangerous. The animal sinks on its haunches and then plunges forward in a panic-stricken manner. It is possible that this excitement is associated with overdose since it is not seen when only very small doses of chlorpromazine are given.[26]

Promazine hydrochloride is another compound which has been widely used in horses. It is not a very obvious sedative when given in the recommended doses of 0.5 to 1.0 mg/kg. It has been administered by intramuscular and intravenous injection, and, by the latter route, produces less fall in blood pressure than does chlorpromazine. Its intravenous injection has apparently been followed in a few horses by death, and this route of administration is no longer recommended. It has been claimed that promazine is safe, easy to administer, and quick acting, with a shorter period of activity than that of chlorpromazine.[8] It has failed to subdue horses which are difficult to manage, and many horses under its influence were easily upset by noise.[31] A fatality after the intravenous injection of 400 mg of promazine and one case of excitement in 100 horses given the compound have been reported.[15, 52]

Trimeprazine tartrate was used extensively for premedication by the intravenous injection of 0.5 mg/lb.[59] However, trimeprazine is a potent antihistamine and is now used mainly for this purpose.

Perphenazine has given rise to excitement in horses and an overdose produced convulsive siezures and disturbed muscular co-ordination.[65]

Pecazine produces no sedation at all in horses unless given in very heavy doses and is not used as a premedicant.

Propionylpromazine is quite widely used in some European countries and in Scandinavia. It produces a degree of sedation comparable with that produced by chlorpromazine although it is claimed to have more hypnotic action. Its administration seldom gives rise to excitement, and when excitement is seen, it is said to be short lived and less severe than that seen after chlorpromazine. At a dose rate of 0.15 mg/kg intravenously or 0.25 mg/kg intramuscularly, this compound produces drowsiness and sedation. It seems that it should be used with methadone to reduce the risk of excitement after its administration.[64] The dose is then 0.1 mg/kg together with a total dose of 50 to 100 mg of methadone. Its effects were found, in 180 horses, to be more predictable after intravenous rather than intramuscular administration.[28] Its action was more pronounced in elderly, sick, and very young horses, and while it proved useful for quieting frightened animals, it was ineffective in bad tempered animals.

Acepromazine is a potent phenothiazine derivative effective in very small doses. It has now been used extensively in Great Britain and North America and its efficacy as a tranquilizer, sedative, and premedicant drug has been demonstrated in large numbers of horses. The onset of action is seen about 5 minutes after its intramuscular injection.[43] There seem to be very few reports of undesirable actions associated with this compound, and of five phenothiazine compounds compared in a trial, only acepromazine and promazine did not produce any undesirable side effects.[27] This, together with the regularity of effect produced, probably makes acepromazine the ataractic of choice for horses—at least as far as any phenothiazine compound can be said to be a drug of choice. The dose used ranges from 0.05 to 0.1 mg/kg, depending on the type of animal and the effect to be produced. It is probable that, as with many other of this group of compounds, the doses recommended when it was first introduced were excessive. No adverse effects with a dose of 0.1 mg/kg have been reported, but larger doses could produce excitement.[40] Doses greater than 0.3 mg/kg produced ataxia.[53]

Comparison of the various phenothiazine derivatives is a very difficult task as they can really only be assessed by the individual anesthetist according to what is required on any particular occasion. Provided the horse is handled quietly, most of them will facilitate the induction of anesthesia, for horses under their influence will stand still while an intravenous injection is performed, thereby reducing the risk of perivascular injection of irritant drugs. They all enhance the effect of anesthetic agents so that the total amount of anesthetic administered over a period of time is reduced, although the initial rapidly injected dose of a barbiturate used for induction of anesthesia is not affected. They all prolong recovery from general anesthesia but render the recovery period smooth and free from excitement.

Although other compounds (such as the butyrophenones) have been tried in horses, only one, 5, 6-dihydro-4H-1, 3-thiazine [Xylazine, Rompun (Bayer, Germany)], has proved to be a better sedative than acepromazine. Although not devoid of undesirable attributes, this compound seems to possess certain properties which make it a better sedative for horses than any other compound currently used. Intramuscular injection of 2 to 3 mg/kg is followed by deep sedation which is apparent after 15 to 20 minutes and lasts about 30 minutes, after which recovery is rapid. While it is possible to arouse the sedated animal, such arousal seems never to be associated with excitement as it can be in animals sedated with phenothiazine derivatives. Sedation may be accompanied by analgesia, but this is difficult to assess. Intramuscular injection of clinically useful sedative doses has a negligible effect on the cardiovascular and respiratory systems. Intravenous injection of 0.5 to 1.0 mg/kg produces almost immediate sedation but is associated with bradycardia and a fall in cardiac output. Although these unwanted effects are transient and cardiovascular stability is rapidly regained, the intravenous injection of this compound may be a risk. Any attempt to produce deep states of anesthesia with large doses seems unjustified due to the likelihood of there being a protracted recovery period.

Basal Narcosis

Narcotic drugs are used in anesthesia to produce degrees of depression of the central nervous system varying from light sedation to deep anesthesia. Basal narcosis borders on general anesthesia and may be described as the stage of central nervous depression at which the animal is unconscious, but still responds to painful stimuli by moving.

Basal narcosis is often used in conjunction with local analgesia. Operating conditions are improved since restraint of the narcotized animal is relatively easy, and the animal is less likely to move suddenly during the operation, making it easier to carry out aseptic surgery. Under conditions of general practice, this combination of basal narcosis and local analgesia may offer distinct advantages over general anesthesia, since it may be employed by the surgeon operating alone without the assistance of an anesthetist, and recovery is usually more rapid than after general anesthesia.

Chloral hydrate $(Cl_3CH(OH)_2)$, the best basal narcotic for horses, has been used in veterinary practice for many years. Introduced into medicine in 1869, its use in the horse was first described in 1875 by Humbert.[25] It can be administered into the stomach by drenching or by stomach tube, but it must be given very dilute (1 part of chloral hydrate in 20 parts of water) and can be made still less irritant to the gastric mucosa by mixing with syrup, treacle, or mucilage. It may also be given by rectum, the dose being dissolved in about 4 liters of water and deposited high into the colon. When given by mouth or by rectum, incoordination develops rapidly and a sleepy state supervenes. It is usual to apply hobbles and cast the horse when obvious signs of sedation appear. There is no danger of excitement during the induction of narcosis and recovery is similarly free from trouble. Passage of the drug across the blood-brain barrier is slow, and it takes an appreciable time for the full effects of a dose to become apparent. As narcosis deepens, breathing becomes shallower and myocardial depression produces a fall in blood pressure.

Chloral hydrate may be given intravenously. It is usually administered as a 10% solution into the jugular vein of the standing or recumbent animal. In the standing animal, the needle is removed from the vein when incoordination develops and before the animal falls or is cast with ropes. Care must be taken to insure that the solution is not injected outside the vein and that the animal falls onto a soft bed. If the drug is to be administered to the recumbent animal, the horse must first be cast and restrained. Casting the fully conscious horse with ropes and hobbles is often more upsetting for the horse and may entail more danger of injury than the administration of the agent to the standing animal.

Great care must be taken to see that the needle is maintained in the correct position throughout the injection, and it is probably always safer to use a plastic intravenous cannula rather than a simple needle. The dose for the production of basal narcosis in a heavy horse is about 4.0 to 4.5 g/50 kg, and in a light horse, 5.0 to 6.0 g/50 kg of body weight.[66] Following basal narcotic doses of chloral hydrate, a horse should be able to rise to its feet and remain standing within 1 hour of administration of the drug. Recovery is usually quiet but hobbles should be left on until the animal makes obvious attempts to rise.

When longer periods of basal narcosis are needed, the administration of supplementary doses of chloral hydrate is unwise. Pentobarbital sodium can be used to prolong narcosis which has been induced with chloral hydrate. Supplementation of chloral hydrate narcosis in this way does not unduly prolong the recovery period. The pentobarbital sodium is administered by slow intravenous injection "to effect," and usually not more than 1 to 2 g are required to extend the period of basal narcosis to cover the duration of most of the operations commonly carried out on horses.

Intravenous Anesthesia

METHODS OF ADMINISTRATION

In the horse, intravenous injections are usually made into the jugular vein about half-way down the neck where the vein is, in most animals, easily located in its furrow. It is important that the horse is quietly and gently handled whenever venipuncture is to be performed, and the use of a twitch is not often helpful or necessary. Most horses will stand quite still while venipuncture is performed if the skin through which the intravenous needle is to be passed is first infiltrated with local analgesic solution. Since the accurate placing of a needle or cannula in the vein is extremely important when irritant solutions such as chloral hydrate or thiopental sodium are to be injected, time spent in the preliminary injection of local analgesic is not wasted. One or two milliliters of 2% lidocaine solution (preferably without adrenaline, since vasoconstrictors have been blamed for gray hairs at sites of injection) are deposited in the skin itself and in the underlying tissues over the vein, using a very fine needle. When local analgesia has developed, a stout needle is pushed through the skin, its point being directed towards the head. The vein is distended by thumb pressure just below the site of venipuncture, and the needle is advanced into the lumen of the vessel. Neck ropes should not be used to distend the vein since they tend to move the skin over the site. When the neck rope is released and the skin moves back into its normal position, it may pull the needle from the vein because horse skin, being thick, grips the intravenous needle tightly.

It is most important that the point of the needle is well within the lumen of the vein before the injection of irritant anesthetics such as thiopental sodium or methohexital sodium, for these compounds may cause extensive tissue damage if deposited outside the vein in the jugular furrow. A free flow of blood from the needle, or blood sucked easily back into a syringe, indicates correct positioning of the intravenous needle. During the injection, the hub of the needle should be held against the horse's neck in order to minimize the risk of it becoming dislodged if the horse moves suddenly. Stout needles 6 to 7 cm long with a bore of 2.5 to 3 mm are suitable for this type of work, the wide bore allowing injections to be made relatively quickly.

Syringes of more than 50-ml capacity are too unwieldy for convenience, so that the injection of large volumes of solution is accomplished by attaching an infusion apparatus to the intravenous needle and allowing the injection to proceed under gravity. For absolute safety when injecting irritant solutions, particularly when very rapid injection is to be made, the use of a plastic intravenous cannula of any one of the various patterns now on the market is to be thoroughly recommended. These cannulas may be introduced 6 to 8 inches along the lumen of the vessel and are most unlikely to be easily dislodged from the vein during the injection process (see Chapter 19).

If an irritant solution is accidentally injected perivascularly, 0.5 to 1.0 liter of normal saline should be injected into the area to dilute the irritant drug. The enzyme hyaluronidase may be added to this saline to cause dispersion of the agent through the tissues, or procaine hydrochloride may be added to promote vasodilation in that area and speed the removal of the irritant from the site. Further local treatment is not required, and poulticing may produce tissue necrosis.

THIOPENTAL SODIUM

Thiopental sodium, a thiobarbiturate, has an important place in equine anesthesia although it has only become acceptable since the introduction of the phenothiazine derivatives. By abolishing the postanesthetic excitement which is such an objectionable feature of thiopental in horses, these drugs have opened up a wide field of application for its use in equine

practice. Induction of anesthesia with this agent is now an acceptable, desirable,and widely practiced technique. It is rapid and does not necessitate the casting of the horse with ropes and hobbles, so that the anesthetist needs only the minimum of assistance. The assistance required is merely adequate and competent restraint of the horse's head to prevent movement of the animal while the very rapid injection is being made.

After the rapid intravenous injection of 1 g/90 kg, the animal falls to the ground, unconscious and relaxed, within 30 to 40 seconds, depending on the neck-brain circulation time. Most animals fall quietly but occasionally one will rear up after the injection has been made and fall heavily, which is dangerous and no better for the animal than being cast with ropes and hobbles. The attendant at the head of the horse should always be instructed to be on the alert and to back the horse one or two paces immediately if it shows any inclination to rear. A brief period of apnea follows transient respiratory stimulation, and there is a short lived fall in the blood pressure with a rise in the pulse rate. The period of surgical anesthesia is brief but is quite adequate for short surgical procedures such as castration. Consciousness returns rapidly and in horses which have not received premedication, the recovery period is usually characterized by violent struggling, great excitement, and muscular incoordination. During this time, the horse may make repeated and ineffectual attempts to rise and may sustain serious injuries. Because of this, horses which have not received premedication should be given a small dose of a phenothiazine derivative by intravenous injection towards the end of the period of anesthesia.

The dose of thiopental is computed from the body weight, and it is not always possible to weigh animals before anesthesia. In these circumstances, the weight may be assessed with sufficient accuracy from the formula:

Body weight in pounds =
$$\frac{\text{girth (in inches)}^2 \times \text{length (in inches)}}{300}$$

where the girth is measured just behind

the elbow and the length is the distance from the point of the shoulder to the buttock.

Rapid injection results in the brain being exposed to a high concentration of the agent and the development of an initial high concentration in the gray matter. Thiopental sodium crosses the blood-brain barrier very rapidly, and if the dose is correctly calculated and injected quickly enough, the initial concentration achieved in the gray matter will be high enough to produce surgical anesthesia. Immediately after this, the concentration of the agent in the blood starts to fall as the drug is removed into the "aqueous" tissues of the body.[4, 5, 34, 42, 47, 50] The blood returning to the brain therefore has a steadily declining concentration of thiopental, so that as soon as the concentration in the brain exceeds that in the perfusing blood, the agent will begin to disappear from the brain tissue with a consequent progressive lightening of anesthesia (see Chapter 11).

Failure to achieve induction of anesthesia may be due to incorrect estimation of the dose, injecting the dose too slowly, or perivascular administration. If the dose was too small, or was given too slowly, a repeat injection should be made immediately. If the first dose was too small, a slightly larger dose may be given in this repeat injection, but this is seldom necessary since the residual effects of the first injection will augment the second dose. Perivascular injection necessitates immediate attention to the injection site as described above, and while a second dose of thiopental may be injected on the other side of the neck, it is better, if there is no urgency about the operation, to postpone the interference for about a week.

As soon as the horse falls to the ground after the injection of the thiopental sodium, the assistant should apply his weight to the neck to prevent the horse from attempting to rise as anesthesia lightens. Hobbles should be applied as soon as the horse becomes recumbent unless the operation is to be of very short duration. The intravenous injection of a muscle relaxant such as succinylcholine chloride given immediately after the injection of the barbiturate facilitates endotracheal intubation when this is to be performed, and, in addition, makes restraint of the horse easier. When succinylcholine chloride is used in this manner, care should be taken to avoid handling the legs until the muscle contractions and fasciculations cease, when it will be found that the application of hobbles is very easy. Provided that only small doses of succinylcholine of the order of 0.1 mg/kg are employed, respiratory arrest does not occur, but it is always wise to have facilities for endotracheal intubation and intermittent positive pressure ventilation of the lungs available for immediate use.

Induction of anesthesia in horses with thiopental and succinylcholine subsequent to premedication is a safe and easy technique which is widely used under both field and hospital conditions. In hospitals, some workers prefer to use an operating table with a tilting top to which the standing animal is tied and which is then used to lower the horse into a horizontal position as it becomes unconscious, rather than let it fall to the ground before positioning it on the table (Figs. 23.2 and 23.3). When the tilting table is used, the table top is raised to the vertical position and the horse brought up alongside it. Straps are passed around the horse's body and, as the animal sinks after the injection of the thiopental, these straps are tightened while the table top is returned to the horizontal position. Opinions are divided over the merits of this technique. There is no doubt that the use of a tilting table in this manner is, theoretically, safer than merely allowing the unconscious horse to fall to the ground and then positioning it on a table top which has been lowered to ground level. However, it is often difficult to get a horse to submit to being tied, even very loosely, to the table top unless heavy preanesthetic sedation is employed. Very heavy sedation is most undesirable because it prolongs recovery from anesthesia, and provided the surface is suitably padded, anesthetized horses do not appear to come to any harm falling onto the ground or a horizontal table top at

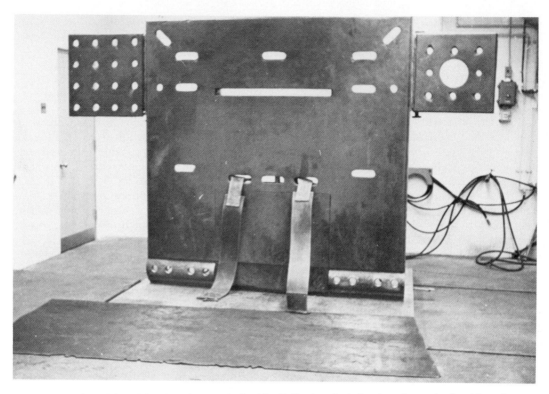

FIG. 23.2. A multi-positional equine surgical table. Following the induction of anesthesia with an intravenous barbiturate, the table is placed in a horizontal position. The table is rolled into the surgical area after anesthetization with an inhalation agent and surgical preparation.

ground level. Certainly, tilting tables are much more difficult and expensive to construct, and it has not yet been demonstrated in a convincing manner that this extra expense and trouble are indeed justified.

It is, of course, possible to prolong anesthesia by the administration of further doses of thiopental. This, however, has the disadvantage of delaying recovery, since the repeated doses lead to a gradual accumulation of thiopental on the body tissues so that redistribution within the body, upon which a reasonably rapid recovery depends, cannot occur. It is better to prolong anesthesia, when this is necessary, by the administration of an inhalation anesthetic.

METHOHEXITAL SODIUM

Methiohexital sodium is an oxybarbiturate which appears to possess some advantages over thiopental sodium in equine anesthesia. So far, it has been used to a relatively limited extent in Britain,[36] but it may come to replace the thiobarbiturates for routine anesthesia if its price becomes more competitive. Like thiopental, it is injected rapidly into the jugular vein, but it seems to be about twice as potent and the dose given is, consequently, of the order of 1 g/180 kg. The period of surgical anesthesia following the injection of one dose is approximately the same as after thiopental, but the recovery is more rapid. The animal which has received methohexital appears to be more alert and co-ordinated on regaining consciousness than the animal which has had thiopental, and seems to be remarkably free from "hangover." So far results from the use of this compound have been good, and while it is less irritant and there is not as much danger of tissue necrosis following

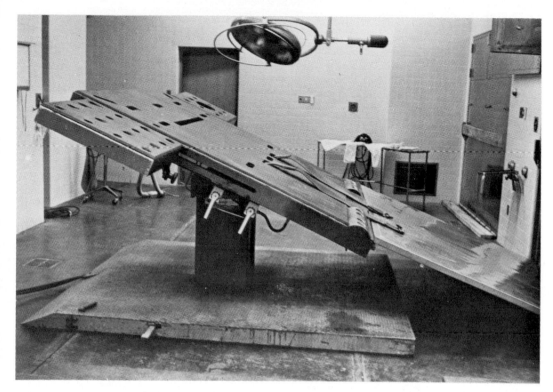

Fig. 23.3. The positional table is locked in place with the recovery stall doors; thus enabling a large animal to be pulled into the recovery area.

perivascular injection, approximate precautions to prevent this mishap should still be taken.

THIAMYLAL SODIUM

Thiamylal sodium is an untrashort acting thiobarbiturate which has attained more popularity in the United States than in Britain. It closely resembles thiopental, although it is rather more potent and has a slightly less cumulative effect. It would seem that, given in equipotent doses, this agent may be used instead of thiopental or methohexital sodium.

PENTOBARBITAL SODIUM

Pentobarbital sodium has been used in equine anesthesia but, except for reinforcement of chloral hydrate basal narcosis, it has no place in this field.

Chloral hydrate may be given into the stomach or into a vein to produce basal narcosis as already described, but it is also sometimes used to produce full general anesthesia. However, chloral hydrate is not a very good anesthetic agent, since recovery after the administration of full anesthetic doses takes at least 1½ to 2 hours and has been known to take 6 to 8 hours.

Mixture of chloral hydrate and magnesium sulfate or chloral hydrate, magnesium sulfate, and pentobarbital have recieved little attention in Europe but have been used with reported successful results by workers in the United States. Millenbruck and Wallinga[35] reported on the use of the mixture containing all three substances and state that after the induction of full surgical anesthesia (cessation of eye movements), the total period of recumbency lasts about 1 to 1½ hours.

Inhalation Anesthesia

The classification of methods for the administration of inhalation anesthetic agents is difficult,[18] but for equine anesthesia, there are two methods in common use today.

THE SEMIOPEN METHOD

This term may be used to describe the use of a face mask strapped over the horse's nostrils (sometimes over the mouth and nostrils), into which is placed a pad or sponge soaked with a volatile anesthetic agent. The well designed mask allows free air entry and prevents rebreathing. Chloroform is the only anesthetic agent which can satisfactorily be administered with such a mask, since diethyl ether is not sufficiently potent to produce anesthesia in a reasonable length of time, and the use of halothane in such a system is extremely expensive.

The semiopen system of administration has the advantages of reasonable safety and simplicity of equipment (which is inexpensive and portable), but it is a wasteful system and difficult to use in such a manner than smooth anesthesia is produced. As anesthesia lightens, and the tidal volume increases, the extra air drawn through the mask dilutes the anesthetic vapor so that the alveolar tension of the agent decreases and anesthesia continues to lighten. Conversely, as anesthesia becomes deeper and the tidal volume decreases, the inspired concentration rises with a consequent increase in alveolar tension and progression towards death. The animal may be able to decrease the alveolar tension by uptake of the anesthetic into the tissues, but deepening anesthesia is usually associated with a decreasing cardiac output so that the uptake is often reduced. Factors such as these make the semiopen administration of an inhalation agent a complicated method to understand.

Perhaps the main disadvantages of the semiopen method are: first, that it makes no provision whereby the oxygen content of the inspired air can be increased; and second, it does not allow control or assistance of the horse's breathing.

THE CLOSED OR PARTIALLY CLOSED METHOD

In recent years, several workers have devised anesthetic circuits for large animal use in which oxygen from cylinders is used to transport anesthetic vapors to the animal and in which the expired gases are partially or totally rebreathed after removal of carbon dioxide.[1, 10, 12, 13, 14, 46, 48, 51, 60, 61, 63, 67, 68] The introduction of this type of apparatus into horse anesthesia has enabled the horse to benefit from some of the more recent methods of anesthesia which have proved so successful in man and in small animals. The scope of surgery in horses has been extended because horses can now be kept safely anesthetized for long period of time, thus making complicated and lengthy surgical procedures a possibility. These methods are economical, oxygenation of the animal during anesthesia is improved, and respiration can be controlled or assisted when necessary.

There are two types of circuit in use, the "to and fro" circuit and the "circle system" (Figs. 23.4 to 23.8). Both incorporate a soda lime canister for carbon dioxide absorption and a rebreathing, or reservoir, bag. Where a vaporizer is included in the circuit, it is placed either in the fresh gas inflow line (e.g., Weaver type circle and most to and fro systems) or in series with the soda lime canister (Fisher-Jennings and Wynn Jones circle absorbers). Apparatus constructed for horses is designed with reference to equipment used in man. If the airway diameter is sufficiently large, flow will be laminar, but extra resistance to breathing may well produce turbulence. During deep rapid breathing, the gas flow generated by the animal can produce such great fluctuations in airway pressure that the patient's respiratory and cardiovascular systems may become severely embarassed. High resistance to breathing is tolerated by healthy animals for short periods, but resistance to expiration leads to raised mean intrathoracic pressures, impedes venous return, and reduces cardiac output and the circulating blood volume. If the circulating blood volume is already reduced, circulatory collapse may follow. Resistance to inspiration produces a greater negative pressure within the chest

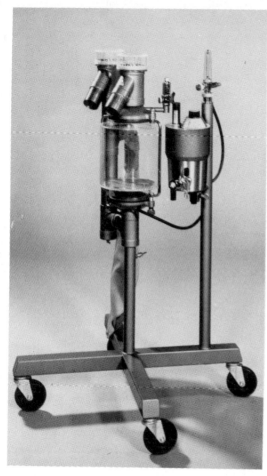

FIG. 23.4 North American Dräger equine anesthesia machine. To the right is a Vapor$^{(R)}$ halothane vaporizer and an oxygen flow meter. A nitrous oxide flow meter can be added. Courtesy of North American Dräger, Telford, Penna.

which can result in pulmonary edema and postanesthetic complications.

Resistance to breathing is affected by the shape and size of the soda lime canister, the length and diameter of the tubing, the endotracheal connector, and the diameter of all the apertures between masks, canisters, and bags. As long ago as 1946, Longuidice and Aranes discovered that anesthetic circuits designed for human patients were unsuitable for large animal patients.[32] In medical apparatus, the average airway diameter is 2.5 cm, and this produces a high resistance to

breathing at the gas flow rates generated by large animals. Nevertheless, Schebitz also used a closed circle type of apparatus with an airway of 2.5 cm, and in 1957 Fisher and Jennings produced a circle apparatus with 3.75-cm airways, using the argument that this was the average tracheal diameter of a large horse.[12, 48] In 1957 Reed, Allen, Glasser, and Keefe described a to and fro circuit with 7.5-cm airways, while in 1958 Hansson and Johannisson described a circle system designed for horses constructed with 5-cm diameter tubing. Hansson and Johannisson calculated the minimum airway diameter required by comparing tidal volumes and gas flow rates in man and the horse, and it was on this basis that they decided on the 5-cm diameter airway. A 5-cm diameter airway is now used by most workers. Four large animal anesthetic circuits in use in Great Britain were compared with respect to resistance to breathing, efficiency of carbon dioxide absorption, and apparatus dead space. The four circuits tested were (a) the Fisher-Jennings apparatus; (b) a modified Weaver-type circle system as used at the Cambridge School; (c) the to and fro absorber described by Wright and Hall in 1961; and (d) the vertical canister to and fro absorber manufactured by the British Oxygen Company Limited.[45]

All these circuits have been used successfully to maintain anesthesia for long periods of time in large numbers of horses. On investigation, the circuits were all found to maintain similar inspired carbon dioxide concentrations of below 3%, although because of the smaller soda lime canister in the Fisher-Jennings apparatus, this was not maintained for as long in this apparatus as in the others. Dead space, as was expected, remained constant in the circle systems but increased progressively in the to and fro circuits. Resistance offered to breathing was higher in the Fisher-Jennings apparatus than in the other pieces of apparatus.

From the anesthetic apparatus the gases and vapors are delivered to the animal using either a well fitting face mask

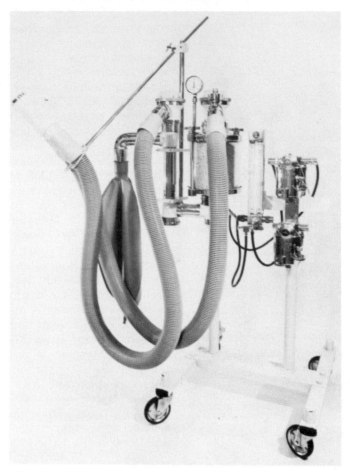

Fig. 23.5. Frazer Sweatman, equine anesthesia machine. The halothane vaporizer is a Fluotec Mark III. Nitrous oxide can also be added to the oxygen flow meter. Courtesy of Frazer Sweatmen, Lancaster, New York.

or an endotracheal tube. Face masks are rather cumbersome, and it is often difficult to obtain an airtight fit between the mask and the face, making controlled administration of the anesthetic almost impossible. For these resons, and because endotracheal intubation is very easy to perform in horses, endotracheal administration is usually preferred.

ENDOTRACHEAL INTUBATION

The endotracheal tube used should be of the greatest diameter which will pass easily through the larynx. It is impossible to recommend exactly what size of tube should be passed in any particular animal and there is, as yet, no standardization of tube sizes. An attempt is being made in Great Britain to reach some agreement over dimensions of endotracheal tubes for horses, and the range of sizes proposed is 18, 20, 25, 30, and 40 mm, internal diameter, with a wall thickness of 3.5 to 4.0 mm. Unlike tubes manufactured on the continent of Europe, all British ones are curved like Magill tubes designed for the human subject and are much easier to introduce because of this curve. The incorporation of an inflatable cuff makes it possible to obtain an airtight seal between the tracheal wall and the tube, so that all respired gases must pass through the lumen of the tube, and thus the anesthetic can be administered in a controlled manner.

The straight tubes manufactured in Europe are more difficult to introduce, but the British tubes are readily passed by blind manipulation through the mouth. There are various techniques which may be employed, but a very simple and successful one is as follows.

The anesthetized horse is placed on its side with its head moderately extended on the neck. The tube, coated with a suitable lubricant, is introduced into the mouth with the concavity of its curve directed towards the hard palate. Introduction into the mouth is made easier if a mouth gag is used, and care must be taken to insure that the thin wall of the cuff is not damaged by contact with the molar teeth. The tube is advanced until its tip lies in the pharynx and is then rotated through 180°. Rotation of the tube in this manner deflects the epiglottis forward so that it does not become impacted in the larynx and prevent the passage of the tube. The tube is manipulated to bring its tip exactly into the midline, and at the next inspiration is pushed rapidly into the trachea. Failure to enter the trachea indicates either incor-

rect alignment of the head on the neck or that the tip of the tube was not in the midline (see Chapter 17).

Transnasal intubation may also be carried out, but the size of tube which can be accommodated by the nostril is usually so small that it offers considerable resistance to air flow.

It is most important that all connectors between the endotracheal tube and anesthetic apparatus are well designed in order to avoid turbulence which greatly increases the resistance to breathing. Poorly designed endotracheal tube connectors offered more resistance to breathing than was encountered in the whole of the remainder of the anesthetic circuit.[45]

VAPORIZERS

The type of vaporizer used depends to some extent on the nature of the liquid to be vaporized, but in equine anesthesia, very fine control of the vapor concentration is seldom indicated. In clinical practice all that the anesthetist really needs to know about the vaporizer is that it behaves as expected when the control is ad-

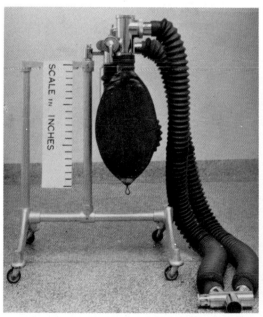
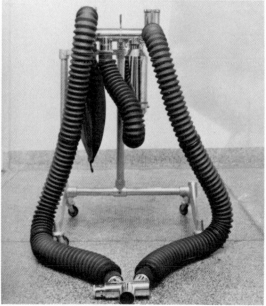

FIG. 23.6. British Oxygen Co. Large Animal Circle front and side view. Anesthetic vapors and oxygen are delivered to the circle from a standard anesthesia machine. Courtesy of Barbara M. Q. Weaver, University of Bristol.

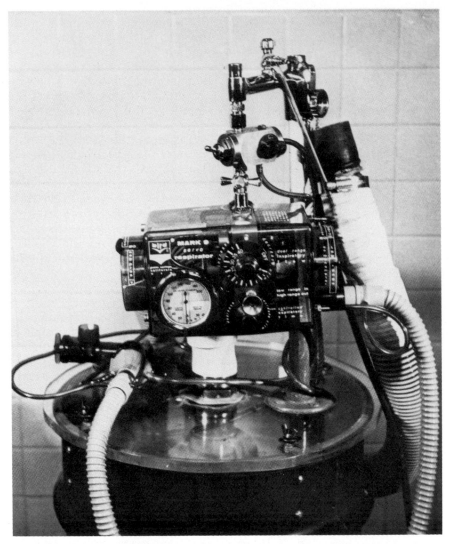

FIG. 23.7. An intermittent positive pressure apparatus constructed for large animal anesthesia. The equipment consists of Mark 9 Bird ventilator and a 30 liter bag placed in a hermetically sealed steel drum. This drum and bag replaces the rebreathing bag on the anesthesia machine. Courtesy of L. R. Soma, University of Pennsylvania.

justed. In other words, setting the control to a higher value should result in the emergence of a higher vapor concentration, and the concentration emerging should decrease when the control is moved in the opposite direction. Not all vaporizers have these characteristics at all gas flow rates.

In to and fro systems the vaporizer is nearly always placed in the fresh gas supply line outside the breathing circuit. In circle systems the vaporizer may also be inside the breathing circuit so that the horse's inspirations and/or expirations pass through it. The influence of the location of the vaporizer on the inspired tension of the anesthetic agent has been considered in some detail by workers in Cardiff who concluded that each position of the vaporizer has its own advantages and disadvantages.[33, 37] In the hands of an experienced anesthetist, either arrangement is equally safe (or unsafe). The inexperienced anesthetist, on the other hand, is perhaps best advised to use a vaporizer placed outside the breathing circuit, especially when potent agents are involved. However, relatively weak agents such as diethyl ether and agents with low vapor tensions such as methoxyflurane can only be administered effectively to horses from a vaporizer situated in the breathing circuit.

CHLOROFORM

The use of chloroform in horses was recorded by Percival in 1848, and since that time it has been one of the most widely

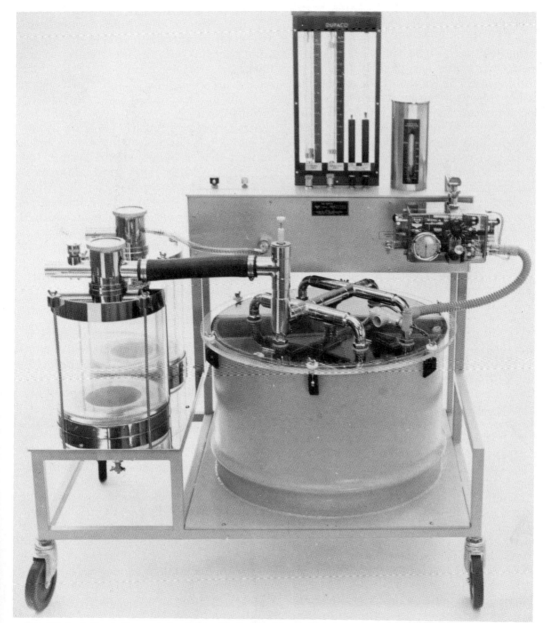

FIG. 23.8. A Davis Large Animal Anesthesia Machine, which incorporates a Bird ventilator and a series of rebreathing bags hermetically sealed in a large drum. This enables the administration of intermittent positive pressure ventilation during inhalation anesthesia. Courtesy of Dupaco Company, Arcadia, California.

used agents in equine anesthesia. It is both very potent and inexpensive so that it may be given by semiopen methods of administration. A very common technique using a simple face mask has been described.[14] For small horses and ponies, the mask is strapped to the standing animal and 30 to 60 ml or more of liquid chloroform are placed on a sponge located at the lower end of the mask. The animal is controlled by two men holding ropes attached to the head collar who stand about 5 or 6 feet from its side and slightly behind its head. When the animal loses consciousness, it falls to the ground where it is hobbled and restrained. The induction stage is often accompanied by considerable excitement and larger animals may be very difficult to control. For this reason, large horses are usually cast by ropes and hobbles before the mask is applied. It is certain that in the past asphyxia contributed to the speed of induction of anesthesia, but today most anesthetists use larger quantities of chloroform on the sponge and allow a free flow of air through the mask at all times. Once anesthesia has been induced, it is maintained by applying further quantities of liquid chloroform to the sponge as required.

Chloroform is also used in closed and semiclosed systems, and, in these, the liquid is vaporized in a stream of oxygen and delivered to the animal through a close fitting face mask or an endotracheal tube.

There can be no doubt that chloroform still has a place in equine anesthesia, since it is a potent, nonexplosive agent which is reasonably safe if used with care. Experience in its use suggests that prolonged administration should be avoided; that induction of anesthesia should be carried out in the premedicated horse with an intravenous agent; that deep anesthesia should be avoided; and that hypoxia and hypercapnia should never be tolerated. Hypoxia and hypercapnia increase the risk of cardiac arrhythmias occurring during anesthesia and the likelihood of liver damage becoming apparent later, while the administration of an overdose of chloroform produces almost simultaneous respiratory and circulatory failure so that resuscitation is not easy. Indeed, it is probably true to say that with chloroform more than with any other anesthetic agent, the results achieved are more a reflection of the skill of the anesthetist than the properties of the particular agent.

HALOTHANE

Today, this nonflammable, nonexplosive volatile anesthetic plays an important part in equine anesthesia. When closed or semiclosed methods of administration are available, it is often the agent of choice on account of its great potency and low toxicity.

After casting, anesthesia can be induced with halothane using a face mask connected to a closed circuit system. Induction is smooth, most horses do not object to being made to breathe the vapor, and the stage of excitement or delerium is short. The inspired concentration should be restricted to below 7% because there is danger of cardiac arrest if a very high concentration is inspired suddenly.

Induction of anesthesia with an intravenous barbiturate is preferred in most cases, since it does away with the need for casting with ropes and hobbles and is both more economical and quicker. However, induction of anesthesia with an intravenous barbiturate drug after premedication with a phenothiazine derivative may produce so much respiratory depression that the uptake of halothane is seriously hindered. This difficulty is usually overcome by excluding the soda lime canister from the breathing circuit until stable halothane anesthesia has been produced.

Good muscle relaxation can only be produced in the deeper planes of anesthesia where the blood pressure may be very low,[16] and in light anesthesia surgical stimulation may produce reflex movements, tachycardia, and, possibly, cardiac arrhythmias.[62, 69]

Recovery from anesthesia is reasonably rapid, and most horses can regain their feet without difficulty about 45 minutes after the administration of halothane has been stopped. When recovery is to take place in a confined space, some workers apply hobbles and forcibly restrain the horse for the first 30 minutes of the recovery period. Others leave the animal entirely alone on a deep soft bed in a field, or in a loose box with well padded walls, and claim that horses recovering from halothane anesthesia will not attempt to rise until they are quite in control of their limbs provided they are not disturbed in any way.

DIETHYL ETHER

Maintenance of anesthesia with diethyl ether still has a place in equine practice, because this agent is inexpensive, stimulates breathing, and is relatively nontoxic. The only practicable semiopen method of administration is that of Henkels[24] in which the horse breathes through a vaporizer which is surrounded by a warm water jacket. However, semiopen administration is undesirable since it gives rise to a concentration of vapor in the air which is unpleasant for the surgical team and which may be dangerous because of risk of fires. Administration by closed or semiclosed methods is more acceptable.[12, 46] Induction of anesthesia with diethyl ether is not really practicable, and even when given by closed and semiclosed methods, large quantities of the agent are used for maintenance. It is not too difficult to obtain a sufficiently high concentration of vapor in the inspired gases when the vaporizer is incorporated in the breathing circuit, but when the vaporizer is outside the circuit it must be surrounded by a warm water jacket or volatilization will be insufficient.

METHOXYFLURANE

Although this agent has been used to anesthetize horses,[9] its use would seem to be only of academic interest to the practical anesthetist. Induction of anesthesia is very slow; changes in the depth of anesthesia can only be achieved very gradually, and recovery is slow.

CYCLOPROPANE

Unless used in a completely closed circuit, this is an expensive agent, but it has a definite place in equine anesthesia. It is relatively insoluble in blood and body tissues so that induction and recovery from cyclopropane anesthesia are rapid; adjustments of tension in the brain can be achieved quickly, and thus it is possible to bring about rapid changes in the depth of anesthesia.

Like halothane, it may be given to the cast and restrained horse, or it may be given after induction with an intravenous barbiturate drug. At first, a mixture of equal parts of cyclopropane and oxygen is run into the circuit, but when the desired depth of anesthesia is reached, anesthesia may be maintained by the administration of about 20% gas with 80% oxygen.

Unless anesthesia is very prolonged, recovery from cyclopropane anesthesia is rapid, 50% of the gas in the body being eliminated within 10 minutes of stopping administration. After prolonged anesthesia, the cyclopropane which has accumulated in the fatty tissues of the body will be released slowly because of the relatively poor blood supply of the fatty tissues, and recovery will be slower but is usually complete within an hour.

Disadvantages of cyclopropane in horses include the production of respiratory depression or even apnea. However, respiratory arrest occurs long before circulatory failure and there is thus a wide safety margin. Apnea is usually produced by attempts to induce anesthesia too rapidly with the administration of high concentrations of cyclopropane. When this is attempted, apnea usually occurs before the onset of muscle relaxation. Under cyclopropane anesthesia, cardiac arrest does not occur suddenly but is preceded by arrhythmia. It has been found that a high concentration of the agent in the presence of hypoxia or hypercapnia is most likely to produce arrhythmias in horses and that these cardiac irregularities disappear if the ventilation is assisted. Factors such as these mean that a certain degree of skill and good apparatus are essential if the best results are to be obtained with cyclo-propane in horse practice.

NITROUS OXIDE

This weak gaseous anesthetic can be used in equine anesthesia to supplement volatile agents such as chloroform or halo-thane, and thus reduce the amount of vol-atile agent required. When this is done, care must be taken to insure that the oxy-gen concentration in the inspired gas mix-ture never falls below 30%, or hypoxia may occur due to the respiratory depres-sion caused by the volatile agent. There is always the danger of hypoxia whenever nitrous oxide is used, and the gas should never be admitted to a completely closed circuit of any type. It is always wise to use it with a relatively high total gas flow rate in a circuit with a deliberate leak.

In order to get the maximum effect from nitrous oxide, it is necessary to deni-trogenate the animal. This is an almost impossible task in horses because of the very large volumes of fresh inspired gases which are required, but partial denitro-genation is possible if the expiratory valve is left open and high total gas flow rates are used.

An anesthetic technique which is exten-sively used in man and which has been reported in small animals, involves the use of nitrous oxide-oxygen mixtures ad-ministered by intermittent positive pres-sure ventilation of the lungs. The patient is usually rendered unconscious with a barbiturate drug, paralyzed with a relax-ant, and ventilated with a nitrous oxide-oxygen mixture to maintain unconscious-ness throughout the operation. This method produces very good operating conditions, particularly for thoracic and abdominal surgery, recovery from anes-thesia is very rapid, and the necessity to use the more toxic volatile or intravenous agents is avoided. The use of this method in horses has not been fully explored. Hansson and Johannisson[23] designed and built a ventilator for horses but decided that this type of anesthesia did not pro-duce good results and had no place in equine practice. It is possible that their poor results were due to inadequate venti-lation, and in view of the usefulness of the method in other species of animal, it is probable that its use in horses warrants further assessment.

The Use of Muscle Relaxants in Equine Anesthesia

Among the relaxants which have been used in horses are *d*-tubocurarine, galla-mine triethiodide, succinylcholine (suxame-thonium, succinyldicholine), and guiacol glycerine ether (see also Chapter 12).

d-TUBOCURARINE

d-Tubocurarine was given to conscious horses and to horses under chloral hydrate narcosis in an attempt to discover whether it could be used to prevent motor response to stimulation and enable sur-gery to be carried out under light nar-cosis.[3] However, there is no dose which is effective for this purpose yet leaves the activity of the respiratory muscles unim-paired. Doses of 0.2 mg/kg will cause res-piratory paralysis in anesthetized horses and may be used for this purpose when apparatus for efficient intermittent posi-tive pressure ventilation of the lungs is available.

GALLAMINE TRIETHIODIDE

Gallamine has been used in horses at a dose rate of 0.11 to 0.22 mg/kg to give complete muscle relaxation and respira-tory arrest of 10 to 20 minutes' duration. Neostigmine has proved to be an effective antidote when administered in doses of the order of 10 mg (preceded with 30 to 60 mg of atropine) toward the end of the pe-riod of action of the gallamine. At present, except in experimental surgery, there are few indications for the use of this relaxant in horses. Unlike *d*-tubocurarine, which in doses sufficient to produce complete re-laxation causes a slight fall in blood pres-sure, gallamine produces a rise in blood pressure with some tachycardia. Pulse rates of 80 to 100 are not uncommon in horses under the influence of gallamine.

SUCCINYLCHOLINE CHLORIDE

Succinylcholine has been used quite extensively in horses[29]. Because horses have high cholinesterase levels in the plasma and tissues, succinylcholine is hydrolyzed quite rapidly so that the neuromuscular block produced by this agent is of short duration. It is also possible to select a dose which will paralyze the limb muscles for 2 or 3 minutes without having a marked effect on the respiratory muscles.

The intravenous injection of succinylcholine causes a rise in blood pressure, tachycardia, and cardiac arrhythmia. The onset of relaxation is preceded by muscle fasciculations which, in conscious human volunteers, have been found to be very painful. The dose which will produce paralysis of the limb muscles without causing serious respiratory embarrassment is 0.12 to 0.15 mg/kg. The drug should be used with caution in animals suffering from liver disease, cachexia, or malnutrition, since in such animals there may be a deficiency of pseudocholinesterase which will delay hydrolysis and prolong the action of the drug. Abnormal effects may also be encountered in conditions which give rise to electrolyte imbalance, and the organophosphorus anthelmintics will also prolong the action of succinylcholine.

The magnitude of undesirable effects such as the rise in blood pressure and muscle fasciculation is minimized by general anesthesia, and succinylcholine has proved to be a most useful drug in equine practice. It may be used to produce muscle relaxation during general anesthesia by the intermittent intravenous injection of 0.1 mg/kg whenever relaxation is particularly required by the surgeon, or it may be given by the continuous slow intravenous infusion of a dilute solution. Doses of 0.1 mg/kg do not produce respiratory arrest and, as well as being useful in the production of relaxation whenever this is required, they may be injected at any time if anesthesia appears to be getting out of control and the horse starts to move or kick. Dilute solutions are infused at the rate of about 0.03 mg/minute/kg of body weight, and careful watch is kept on the respiratory activity. The infusion is speeded up if greater relaxation is required and slowed or stopped if respiratory difficulty becomes apparent.

GUIACOL GLYCERINE ETHER

Guiacol ether is a compound of the mephanesin group which has achieved a degree of popularity in Germany where it is used for casting, to facilitate endotracheal intubation, and to produce relaxation during operative procedures carried out under general anesthesia or local analgesia. The practice of operating under local analgesia can, perhaps, be countenanced since this compound, unlike other muscle relaxants, has a central depressant action and causes drowsiness. Westhues and Fritsch[64] recommend its use together with a thiobarbiturate to induce light general anesthesia and its administration during chloral hydrate narcosis to produce relaxation. Administered by intravenous injection to the standing horse, the dose required for casting is approximately 0.08 to 0.1 g/kg; i.e., a 500-kg horse will require about 1 liter of a 5% solution of the drug. The duration of action after intravenous injection is 10 to 15 minutes, the safety margin is wide, and it is claimed that relaxation of the main skeletal muscles can be produced without abolishing respiratory movements.

INDICATIONS FOR THE USE OF RELAXANTS

The indications for the use of muscle relaxants in equine anesthesia are: (a) to facilitate endotracheal intubation, although the use of a muscle relaxant is by no means essential for endotracheal intubation in horses; (b) to facilitate the induction of inhalation anesthesia after unconsciousness has been produced with a barbiturate drug—a dose of suxamethonium chloride given immediately after the barbiturate ensures paralysis of the limb muscles, thus stopping the horse from moving or kicking during the uptake of the inhalation agent; (c) to control a horse which is moving in response to surgical stimulation under light anesthesia; (d) to produce muscle relaxation whenever it is required during an operation under general anesthesia.

CONTRAINDICATIONS TO THE USE OF RELAXANTS

a. Muscle relaxants should never be used where there are no facilities which will enable efficient artificial ventilation of the lungs to be carried out. Horses cannot be ventilated efficiently for any length of time by the intermittent application of pressure to the chest wall, nor can a large horse be ventilated adequately by any person blowing down an endotracheal tube.

b. Muscle relaxants should never be used if there is any doubt about the animal being conscious or unconscious. It is not humane to carry out any surgical procedure on a horse which is paralyzed but not unconscious. The effectiveness of local analgesia cannot be assessed in paralyzed horses, and it must be emphasized that the muscle relaxants do not, themselves, produce analgesia or anesthesia.

THE CASTING OF HORSES WITH SUCCINYLCHOLINE CHLORIDE

The relatively transient action of succinylcholine, and the possibility of injecting a dose which will paralyze limb muscles without at the same time giving rise to prolonged respiratory arrest, suggested its use as a means of immobilizing a horse when only the minimum of assistance was available. Trials in the United States, Scandinavia, and Australia soon showed the potential value of the method, and it was claimed to be safer than forcibly casting a conscious horse with ropes and hobbles.

The dose of succinylcholine given for restraint of horses is 0.18 mg/kg administered by rapid intravenous injection. After a period which depends on the circulation time but is usually of the order of 20 seconds, injection is followed by drooping of the head and leg weakness. The horse then collapses gently to the ground. Muscle fasciculations may be violent, and there is a period of respiratory arrest which may last for 1 to 2 minutes. Respiratory movements then start to return and there is a short period of vigorous hyperventilation. The period of relaxation lasts 4 to 8 minutes and, when the neuromuscular block wears off, the horse rises to its feet without ataxia.[19-22, 30, 38, 57]

Advocates of this technique claim that it is probably no less humane than casting fully conscious horses with ropes and hobbles and is less likely to lead to injury, while it also has the advantage that it enables a horse to be controlled with only the minimum of assistance. However, it appears that the method is not without risk to the life of even healthy horses. Irregularities in the electrocardiogram have been ascribed to anoxia during the period of respiratory arrest.[57] The heart rate accelerates a few seconds after the horse collapses to the ground and this is followed by bradycardia, cardiac irregularities, and cardiac arrest.[38, 58] Tachycardia which followed then persisted well into the phase of respiratory hyperactivity. Endocardial hemorrhages were found in 10 out of 15 horses which were postmortemed following succinylcholine administration.[30] Experimental studies have shown that succinylcholine may cause a rise in blood pressure and tachycardia even in anesthetized horses in the absence of hypoxia or hypercapnia. It has been suggested that this compound behaves in horses as in other animals, stimulating postganglionic nerve fibers and causing the release of adrenaline from the adrenal medulla.[55] Any agent which causes these effects may be expected to give rise to cardiac irregularities. In addition, in dogs, succinylcholine produces a significant rise in serum potassium levels, and, if this is also true in horses, a raised serum potassium level may contribute to the embarrassment of cardiac function.[54]

The Recovery Period after General Anesthesia

One of the greatest problems facing the anesthetist is to insure that recovery from general anesthesia is rapid, pain-free, and unaccompanied by postanesthetic excitement. A prolonged recovery, such as may follow the administration of full anesthetic doses of chloral hydrate, is fraught with danger, yet a very rapid recovery associated with violent excitement is equally undesirable. Prolonged recovery necessitates that the animal be kept under close observation, be restrained to prevent it from injuring itself by struggling, and be turned over at regular intervals to avoid pulmonary complications and muscle cramps. Rapid partial recovery may result in the horse attempting to stand long before it is able to maintain the standing position, so that it becomes frightened and makes violent uncoordinated movements, plunging about in a most alarming manner. It is essential that horses which have only partially recovered from a general anesthetic be left undisturbed, or alternatively, be kept adequately restrained, until they are capable of standing unaided.

The hazards associated with recovery from anesthesia are not nearly as great in small ponies as in thoroughbreds and heavy hunters. Small ponies usually make a quiet recovery if left alone in a loose box or paddock. In the thoroughbred and hunter, there are two methods used to insure that recovery is accomplished without injury to the animal. The first method is to restrain the animal with ropes and hobbles until it is certain that it is capable of standing unaided. This usually means that restraint must be maintained for about 1 hour after anesthesia. The second method is to leave the animal quite unrestrained and undisturbed in a darkened, well padded loose box, or in a field well away from hedges and fences.

Some anesthetics are particularly associated with a violent recovery period. Adequate medication with a phenothiazine derivative does improve the situation by reducing this tendency towards excitement, but it does, at the same time, increase the length of the recovery period. The administration of pain-relieving drugs such as meperidine hydrochloride helps towards the achievement of a quiet, smooth recovery if considerable pain follows the surgical intervention. It is probable that in veterinary anesthesia generally, too little attention is paid to the relief of pain in the postanesthetic and postoperative periods, and the use of analgesics in these periods warrants further study.

REFERENCES

1. Amman, K., and Suter, P.: Erfahrungen mit der Malolhannarkose beim Pferd. Berlin Munchen Tieraerztl. Wschr. 77: 1, 1964.
2. Archer, R. K.: Pethidine in veterinary practice. Vet. Rec. 59: 401, 1947.
3. Booth, N. H., and Rankin, A. D.: Studies on the pharmacodynamics of curare in the horse. I. Dosage and physiological activity of d-tubocurarine chloride. II. Curare as an adjunct to chloral hydrate anesthesia. Amer. J. Vet. Res. 14: 51 and 56, 1953.
4. Brodie, B. B., Bernstein, E., and Mark, L. C.: Role of body fat in limiting duration of action of thiopental. J. Pharmacol. Exp. Ther. 105: 421, 1952.
5. Brodie, B. B., Papper, E. M., Lief, P. A., Bernstein, E., and Rovenstein, E. A.: Fate of thiopental in man and method for its estimation in biological material. J. Pharmacol. Exp. Ther. 98: 85, 1950.
6. Buxton Hopkin, D. A.: Some suggestion for the neural basis of the anesthetic state. Brit. J. Anesth. 33: 114, 1961.
7. Buxton Hopkin, D. A., and Brown, D.: The reticular system and chlorpromazine. Anesthesia 13: 306, 1958.
8. Cunningham, J. A.: A report on the use of promazine hydrochloride in equine practice. Vet. Rec. 71: 395, 1959.
9. Douglas, T. A., Jennings, S., Longstreeth, J., and Weaver, D. A.: Methoxyflurane anaesthesia in horses and cattle. Vet. Rec. 76: 615, 1964.
10. Dozza, G.: Sull'uso di un apparecchio per la respirazione controllata nel cavallo. Atti Soc. Ital. Sci. Vet. 6: 232, 1952.
11. Dukes, H. H.: The Physiology of Domestic Animals, 7th ed. Bailliere, Tindall and Cox, London, 1955.
12. Fisher, E. W., and Jennings, S.: A closed circuit anesthetic apparatus for adult cattle and for horses. Vet. Rec. 69: 769, 1957.
13. Fowler, M. E., Parker, E. E., McLaughlin, R. F., and Tyler, W. S.: An inhalation anesthetic apparatus for large animals. J. Amer. Vet. Med. Ass. 143: 272, 1963.
14. Fowler, G. R.: General anesthesia in large animals. J. Amer. Vet. Med. Ass. 96: 210, 1940.
15. Gorman, T. N.: Promazine hydrochloride in equine practice. J. Amer. Vet. Med. Ass. 134: 464, 1959.

16. Hall, L. W.: Bromochlorotrifluoroethane ("Fluothane"): a new volatile anaesthetic agent. Vet. Rec. 69: 615, 1957.
17. Hall, L. W.: The effect of chlorpromazine on the cardiovascular system of the conscious horse. Vet. Rec. 72: 85, 1960.
18. Hall, L. W.: Wright's Anaesthesia. Bailliere, Tindall & Cassell, Ltd., London, 1966.
19. Hansson, C. H.: Succinylcholine iodine as a muscular relaxant in veterinary surgery. J. Amer. Vet. Med. Ass. 128: 287, 1956.
20. Hansson, C. H.: Clinical observations on casting horses and cows with succinylcholine. Nord. Vet. Med. 9: 753, 1957.
21. Hansson, C. H.: Studies on the effect of succinylcholine in domestic animals. Nord. Vet. Med. 10: 201, 1958.
22. Hansson, C. H., and Edlund, H.: Experimentella undersökningar och Kliniska erfarenheter av succinylcholinjodid (celocevin) ur veterinarmedicins synpunkt. Nord. Vet. Med. 6: 671, 1954.
23. Hansson, C. H., and Johannisson, D.: Inhalation anaesthesia with automatic artificial respiration during succinylcholine relaxation in large animals. Nord. Vet. Med. 10: 469, 1958.
24. Henkels, P.: Die zur Zeit optimale Technik der reflexlosen, leicht steuerbaren Pferdenarkose fur Klinik und Aussenpraxia. Deutsch. Tieraerztl. Wschr. 46: 801, 1938.
25. Humbert (1875): Quoted in Marcenac and Lemetayer: Contribution a l'etude de l'anesthesia a l'hydrate de chlorale par core veineuse, chez les equides. Bull. Acad. Vet. France 3: 141, 1930.
26. Jennings, S.: Personal communication, 1963.
27. Jones, R. S.: Methylamphetamine as an antagonist of some tranquillising drugs in the horse. Vet. Rec. 75: 1157, 1963.
28. Keller, H.: Erfahrungen mit Combelen (Propyonel-Promazin) Bayer beim Pferd. Schweiz. Arch. Tierheilk. 104: 468, 1962.
29. Larsen, L. H.: Recent developments in anaesthetics and muscular relaxants. New Zeal. Vet. J. 6: 61, 1958.
30. Larsen, L. H., Loomis, L. N., and Steel, J. D.: Muscular relaxants and cardio-vascular damage with special references to succinyl-choline chloride. Aust. Vet. J. 35: 269, 1959.
31. Limont, A. G.: Clinical observations on the use of promazine hydrochloride in horse practice. Vet. Rec. 73: 691, 1961.
32. Loguidice, C. N., and Aranes, G. M.: Universidad Nacional de La Plata, Facultad de Med. Vet, 1946. Cited by Westhues and Fritsch.[64]
33. Mapleson, W. W.: The concentration of anesthetics in closed circuits, with special reference to halothane. I. Theoretical study. Brit. J. Anaesth. 32: 298, 1960.
34. Mark, L. C., Burns, J. J., Campomanes, C. I., Ngai, S. H., Trousof, N., Papper, E. M., and Brodie, B. B.: Passage of thiopental and other barbiturates into brain. Fed. Proc. 14: 366, 1955.

35. Millenbruck, E. W., and Wallinga, M. H.: A newly developed anesthetic for horses. J. Amer. Vet. Med. Ass. 108: 148, 1946.
36. Monahan, C. M.: The use of methohexitone for induction of anaesthesia in large animals. Vet. Rec. 76: 1333, 1964.
37. Mushin, W. W., and Galloon, S.: The concentration of anesthetics in closed circuits with special reference to halothane. II. Clinical aspects. Brit. J. Anaesth. 32: 324, 1960.
38. Neal, P. A., and Wright, J. G.: The use of succinylcholine chloride as a casting agent in the horse prior to the induction of general anesthesia. Vet. Rec. 71: 731, 1959.
39. Noeggerath, N.: Dissertation, Hannover, 1953. Cited by Westhues and Fritsch.[64]
40. Nordström, G., Orstadius, K., and Lannek, N.: Plegicil—etl nytt sedativum i veterinar medicinsk praklik. (Plegicil—a new sedative in veterinary practice.) Medlemsbl. Sver. Vet-Förb. 10: 345, 1958.
41. Owen, L. N., and Neal, P. A.: Sedation with chlorpromazine in the horse. Vet. Rec. 69: 413, 1957.
42. Price, H. L., Kovnat, P. J., Safer, J. N., Conner, E. H., and Price, M. L.: The uptake of thiopental by body tissues and its relation to the duration of narcosis. Clin. Pharmacol. Ther. 1: 16, 1960.
43. Pugh, D. M.: Acepromazine in veterinary use. Vet. Rec. 76: 439, 1964.
44. Purchase, I. F. H.: Some respiratory parameters in horses and cattle. Vet. Rec. 77: 859, 1965.
45. Purchase, I. F. H.: Function tests on four large-animal anaesthetic circuits. Vet. Rec. 77: 913, 1965.
46. Reed, W. C., Allen, C., Glasser, M. E., and Keefe, E. R.: Ether anesthesia in horses. Vet. Med. 52: 474, 1957.
47. Richards, R. K., and Taylor, J. D.: Some factors influencing distribution metabolism and action of barbiturates. Anesthesiology 17: 414, 1956.
48. Schebitz, H.: Zur Narkose beim Pferd unter besonderer Benicksichtigung der Narkose im geschlossenen System. Mh. Veterinaermed. 10: 503, 1955.
49. Scheunert, A., and Trautmann, A.: Lehrbuch der Veterinar Physiologie. Paul Parey, Berlin, 1951.
50. Shideman, F. E., Gould, T. C., Winters, W. D., Peterson, R. C., and Wilner, W. K.: Distribution and in vivo rate of metabolism of thiopentol. J. Pharmacol. Exp. Ther. 107: 368, 1953.
51. Smith, M.: Anaestesi af hest og kvoeg. To and Fro—apparat til store husdyr. Nord. Vet. Med. 16: 140, 1964.
52. Sommerville, G. F.: Death of horse after administration of promazine. New Zeal. Vet. J. 8: 126, 1960.
53. Sonnichsen, H. V.: Plegicil (acepromazine): clinical use in horses. Medlemsbl. Danske Dyrlaegeforen. 43: 657, 1960.

54. Stevenson, D. E.: Changes in the blood electrolytes of anaesthetized dogs caused by suxamethonium. Brit. J. Anaesth. *32:* 364, 1960.

55. Stevenson, D. E., and Hall, L. W.: Pharmacological effects of suxamethonium. Vet. Rec. *71:* 818, 1959.

56. Stewart, H. C.: *General Anaesthesia*, edited by F. T. Evans and T. C. Gray, vol. 1. Butterworth & Co. (Publishers) Ltd., London, 1965.

57. Stowe, C. M.: The curariform effect of succinyl choline in equine and bovine species—a preliminary report. Cornell Vet. *45:* 193, 1955.

58. Tavernor, W. D.: The use of succinyl choline chloride as a casting agent in the horse. Vet. Rec. *71:* 774, 1959.

59. Tavernor, W. D.: Clinical observations on the use of trimeprazine tartrate as a sedative and premedicant in horses, cattle, pigs and dogs. Vet. Rec. *72:* 317, 1960.

60. Tavernor, W. D.: A simple apparatus for inhalation anaesthesia in adult cattle and horses. Vet. Rec. *73:* 545, 1961.

61. Tavernor, W. D.: Recent trends in equine anaesthesia. Vet. Rec. *74:* 595, 1962.

62. Vasko, K. A.: Preliminary report on the effects of halothane on cardiac action and blood pressure in the horse. Amer. J. Vet. Res. *23:* 248, 1962.

63. Weaver, B. M. Q.: An apparatus for inhalation anaesthesia in large animals. Vet. Rec. *72:* 1121, 1960.

64. Westhues, M., and Fritsch, R.: *Die Narkose der Tiere*, Band II: Allgemeinarkose. Paul Parey, Berlin, 1961. (English translation: *Animal Anaesthesia*, vol. 2. Oliver and Boyd, London, 1964.)

65. Williams, R. C., and Young, J. E.: Professional and therapeutic rationale of tranquilizers. Vet. Med. *53:* 127, 1958.

66. Wright, J. G.: *Veterinary Anaesthesia*, 1st ed. Bailliere, Tindall and Cox, London, 1941.

67. Wright, J. G., and Hall, L. W.: *Veterinary Anaesthesia and Analgesia*, 5th ed. Bailliere, Tindall and Cox, London, 1961.

68. Wynn Jones, E.: Equine anesthesia—maintenance by inhalation techniques. J. Amer. Vet. Med. Ass. *139:* 785, 1961.

69. Wynn Jones, E., Vasko, K. A., Hamm, D., and Griffith, R. W.: Equine general anesthesia—use of halothane for maintenance. J. Amer. Vet. Med. Ass. *140:* 148, 1962.

24
General Anesthesia of Ruminants and Swine

SYDNEY JENNINGS

General Anesthesia in Cattle

Because of the differences in anatomy and physiology of ruminants as compared with other species, cattle require special attention when general anesthesia is being considered. Within hours after birth until death cattle never lie in lateral recumbency. Animals like those of the equine, porcine, and canine species which commonly lie in lateral recumbency have flattened sides, and man who lies in the prone position is flattened dorsoventrally. Cattle are barrel-shaped so that when placed in lateral recumbency on a flat surface, one side of the abdomen is forced inwards causing intra-abdominal pressure and pressure on the diaphragm. All anesthetic agents depress the respiratory center to some extent, and therefore during the period when cattle are anesthetized and are in lateral recumbency pressure on the diaphragm is an additional hazard.

The collection of gas in the rumen of cattle when in lateral recumbency and the frequency of regurgitation of rumen contents in deep anesthesia are also hazards. Another complicating factor during general anesthesia is that the copious flow of saliva is not completely controlled by atropine. The inability of calves under 4 months of age to eliminate barbiturates rapidly and the fact that they remain anesthetized for prolonged periods when these agents are used are important species differences.

INTRA-ABDOMINAL PRESSURE

Intra-abdominal pressure and therefore pressure on the diaphragm during lateral recumbency may be reduced by placing an inflated rubber ring under the animal so that the weight of the animal is placed on the rib cage, lateral processes of lumbar vertebrae, pelvis, and hind limb. The bulging abdomen is allowed to sink into the central hollow of the ring. The inflated. rubber ring can be attached by straps to the animal before anesthesia is commenced and while the patient is still standing (Fig. 24.1). The upper abdominal wall will be flaccid due to the reduction of intra-abdominal pressure.

RUMENAL TYMPANY AND REGURGITATION

While some degree of rumenal tympany cannot be prevented in all cases, serious tympany can be prevented by eliminating food intake for at least 18 hours. Cows which are not restricted in diet regurgitate during halothane and ether anesthesia, whereas cows starved for 18 or 24 hours do not.[4] Water should be withheld for about 6 hours.

The risk of regurgitation may also be

344

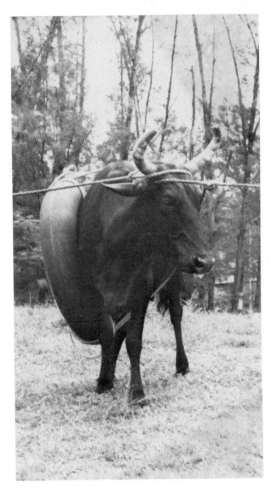

FIG. 24.1. Inflated rubber ring attached to cow before anesthesia.

reduced by placing a large firm cushion under the neck of the laterally recumbent animal so that the first part of the esophagus is higher than the cardiac sphincter. The head should be allowed to hang with the muzzle downwards to allow saliva to flow from the mouth (Fig. 24.2). In spite of the foregoing precautions, regurgitation of rumenal contents always remains a hazard, and the trachea should be intubated. Once the tube is in position, the animal may regurgitate with less hazard. If the animal has regurgitated during anesthesia, the endotracheal tube should be allowed to remain in position during recovery until there are free movements of the mandible. The endotracheal tube should

be withdrawn from the trachea with the cuff at least partially inflated so that any ingesta or saliva that has entered the first part of the trachea will be drawn into the pharynx.

SALIVATION

Saliva continues to flow in considerable quantities during general anesthesia in cattle.[1] Suppression of salivation in the dog and the human does occur under halothane anesthesia.[2, 12] However, in cattle a flow of up to 24 ml/minute has been measured during halothane anesthesia, as have flows up to 78 ml with ether and 33.9 ml with chloroform. Antisialagogues do not reduce salivation but make the secretion more viscid in nature.[6] Inhalation of saliva can be minimized by proper head placement and endotracheal intubation.

PREANESTHETIC MEDICATION AND SEDATION

Physical restraint can be used to control most cattle for the induction of anesthesia, if such restraint does not distress them unduly. Cattle recover from general anesthesia without excitement, and the use of tranquilizers usually is not indicated, although occasionally they might be used in order to facilitate induction of anesthesia in a fractious bull or cow. Cattle are sometimes so unmanageable through nervousness or ferocity that it is virtually impossible to make a venipuncture. Such animals are usually under ranch or semiranch conditions or are wild bovidae in zoological parks. If too much physical restraint is used to control them, they may go into shock and die. Severe fatigue and respiratory distress increase the hazard of anesthesia, so that it is better to sedate such animals before anesthesia.

Chlorpromazine, Promazine Hydrochloride, and Trimeprazine Tartrate. In spite of the disadvantages of chlorpromazine as a tranquilizer in horses, the drug produces satisfactory results in cattle. It is given by intramuscular injection of 1 mg/kg, and the effect can be expected 30 to 60 minutes later. If used before general anesthesia, the drug prolongs the recovery

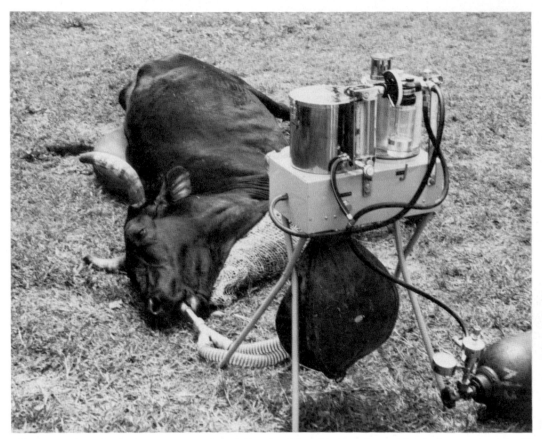

FIG. 24.2. Anesthetized cow supported on inflated rubber ring to reduce abdominal pressure and with cushion to raise esophagus and allow head to slope downwards.

period but not to the extent that the animal cannot be placed in sternal recumbency. If the drug is being used for purposes other than preanesthetic medication, the dose can be increased to 1.5 mg/kg. When used at either dose level, cattle are unable to rise for 1 or 2 hours.

Promazine and trimeprazine can also be used for sedation in cattle, but even in doses twice that of chlorpromazine the effects are not nearly so pronounced.

Chloral Hydrate. In cases where cattle cannot even be approached and where a captive weapon is not available, chloral hydrate can be used to sedate the animal. Water is withheld for 24 hours, and then 8 liters of water containing 100 to 150 g of chloral hydrate are made available. The effect of the drug can be expected in 30 minutes.

INHALATION ANESTHESIA

A most convenient method of inducing anesthesia prior to maintenance by volatile or gaseous anesthetic agents is that of administering soluble barbiturates intravenously (see below). The method has the outstanding advantage that the stage of excitement which figured so much in the anesthetic methods of the past can be eliminated. Anesthesia may also be induced by volatile or gaseous anesthetic agents. In this instance, a face mask can be fitted to the animal's muzzle and the mask connected to the anesthesia apparatus.[5, 14, 15] Using a mask for the induction of anesthesia with an inhalation anesthetic, the animal may pass through the excitement stage with a longer induction period. Once anesthesia has been induced, the continued use of the face mask eliminates in large measure the advantages of closed circuit anesthesia, especially in cattle. A perfect mask fit can not be attained on the face of the animal, especially because of the layer of hair between the mask and the skin, and dilution with room air will occur. This decreases the efficiency of the system. If it becomes necessary to use artificial respiration by compression on the rebreathing bag, gases will be forced down the esophagus instead of into the lungs. Regurgitation is not uncommon in cattle with the great danger of aspiration of not only regurgitated material, but saliva.

Those types of apparatus described as suitable for horses (see Chapters 17 and 26) are suitable for adult cattle and heifers. Apparatus suitable for human use or for large dogs is appropriate for cattle under 5 months of age.

Halothane Anesthesia. Halothane is a particularly useful anesthetic agent in cattle because of its wide margin of safety. Because it is comparatively costly, it should be administered in a closed circuit in order to be used more economically. When standard sizes of simple glass vaporizers are used, there are times when it is necessary to allow the carrier gas to bubble through the liquid halothane in order to build up a sufficient concentration of vapor for the induction of anesthesia. As in the horse, the precision vaporizers calibrated to higher concentrations can be effectively used and advised (see Chapter 16). Concentrations of halothane and fresh gas flows described for the horse are applicable for cattle.

Stage 3, planes 2 and 3 of anesthesia can be judged by slow regular excursions of the rebreathing bag, by the presence of a slight palpebral reflex, and presence of the anal reflex. The eye will be in a normal position and have a pupil of moderate size (Fig. 24.3).

Before stage 3 is reached, the eye is rotated downward so that the pupil is hidden by the lower eyelid (Fig. 24.4). If the animal has been in plane 2 or 3 of stage 3 and later the eye is found to be rotated downwards, it is a certain sign that anesthesia is lightening and that the patient is passing to stage 2 and is an indication for the further administration of anesthetic agent.

Ether Anesthesia. When anesthesia by

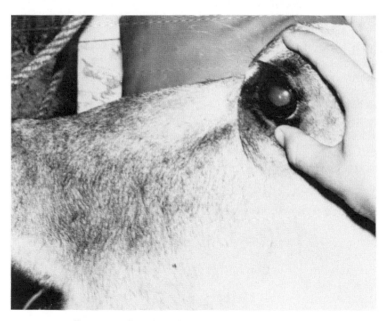

FIG. 24.3. Position of eye in stage 3, planes 2 and 3.

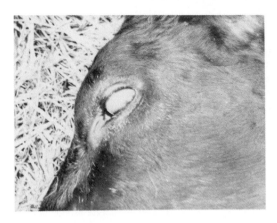

FIG. 24.4. Position of eye in stage 3, plane 1.

volatile agents was induced in both human and animal patients by use of various types of face masks, it was found impossible to anesthetize cattle with ether because a sufficient vapor concentration did not develop. Attempts have been made to increase the concentration of ether vapor in rebreathing methods of administration to large animals by using water baths to surround the vaporizer.[7]

When using the rebreathing apparatus, it is still highly unsatisfactory to attempt to vaporize sufficient ether by passing the required flow of oxygen through ether even when hot water is used to surround the vaporizer. If, however, a circle system is used in which all of the inspired air is drawn through an in the circuit vaporizer (Fig. 24.5), then satisfactory vaporization can be achieved. In this apparatus, there is conservation of heat and the combined effect of the warm expired air of the animal, together with the heat generated by the reaction of CO_2 and soda lime, is sufficient to vaporize ether adequately. With this form of apparatus it is possible to induce and maintain anesthesia in cattle when temperatures are below freezing.

Ether is a safe and satisfactory anesthetic in cattle of all ages. There is a greater excretion of saliva than there is with halothane, and the induction and the recovery periods are longer.

Methoxyflurane Anesthesia. Methoxyflurane is not readily vaporized, because of its low volatility, in sufficient concentration for anesthesia in cattle when va-

porizers external to a circuit are used. When an apparatus is used where the inspired gases are drawn through the agent, however, vaporization is adequate.[3] Although induction with this agent can be attained, it is more satisfactory when used to maintain anesthesia after induction with a barbiturate.

Cyclopropane Anesthesia. Cyclopropane used in a closed circuit is a satisfactory agent in cattle of all ages. By virtue of the fact that cyclopropane is a gas at atmospheric pressure, problems associated with vaporization of liquids are eliminated. The only disadvantages associated with the agent are its expense and explosive nature.

Chloroform Anesthesia. The potency of chloroform is such that it can be administered to cattle in a simple face mask both for induction and maintenance of anesthesia. The low cost of the agent makes it economically practical to use in this manner. There are, however, two outstanding disadvantages in using it in this manner. First, in order to administer a sufficient concentration it is necessary to restrict the air intake also, and the animal is made to suffer a degree of anoxia; second, the crude method of administration prevents a careful control of depths of anesthesia.

Chloroform is readily volatilized in simple vaporizers or by precision vaporizers by passing the normal requirement of oxygen through or over the liquid; when these gases are passed into the rebreathing system, chloroform gives satisfactory and easily controlled anesthesia in cattle. The past history of chloroform is its worst attribute. Deaths during induction and postanesthetic toxicity in various species have dominated the literature. Such history was collected at a time when chloroform was administered in a crude manner. The bias against chloroform is great, but there is a need for reassessment of the usefulness of chloroform when administered in modern apparatus.

INTRAVENOUS AGENTS

The use of barbiturates to produce surgical anesthesia for long periods cannot be

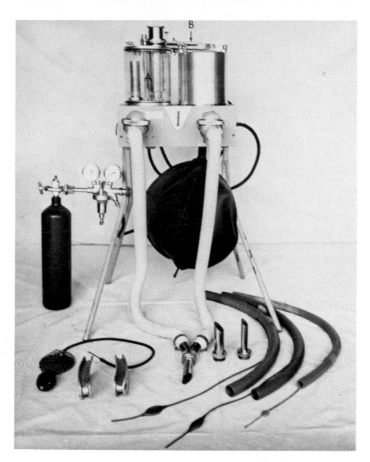

FIG. 24.5. The in the circuit vaporizer (A) of the Fisher-Jennings anesthesia apparatus can be used for ether or methoxyflurane. The bracket (B) can be used to mount out of the circuit vaporizers.

recommended. They have to be broken down in the liver or excreted by the urinary system and therefore, unlike volatile and gaseous agents, they cannot be quickly removed. Without doubt the most valuable use of barbiturates is to produce light anesthesia of short duration for purposes of endotracheal intubation prior to maintenance of surgical anesthesia by volatile or gaseous agents. They may also be used with safety for operations that can be performed within a few minutes because, unlike horses, cattle do not recover with excitement.

Various dose levels of barbiturates have been given by different authors, but the variation depends entirely on the speed of administration. When given slowly, a much higher dose level is required and the recovery from anesthesia is greatly re-

tarded. A dose level can be calculated only when the whole amount is to be injected within a few seconds.

Calves under 4 months of age are exceptional in their recovery from barbiturates as compared with adults, and even after anesthesia with so-called short acting barbiturates, they may not be able to stand for periods of up to 24 hours.

Thiopental Sodium. At the present time, thiopental sodium is the most popular anesthetic agent for induction of anesthesia in cattle, especially prior to endotracheal intubation and maintenance of anesthesia by volatile agents. For rapid intravenous injection into the jugular vein, the dose level is 1 g/100 kg of body weight. In horses it is not important if the estimation of the body weight, within reasonable limits, is not exact, and the same applies to cattle. In cattle, however, it is most desirable that the animal be not placed into too deep a plane of anesthesia so that regurgitation of rumenal contents occurs before endotracheal intubation has been completed. Therefore, a conservative estimation of the weight of the animal should always be made. It is convenient to dissolve each gram of thiopental sodium in 5 ml of sterile water so that an average dose can be contained within a 20-cc syringe.

Pentobarbital Sodium. The method of administering pentobarbital sodium and the dose level are the same as those for thiopental sodium. Following anesthesia there is a recovery period of about twice that following thiopental sodium. It therefore has disadvantages when used for induction of anesthesia prior to the use of volatile anesthetics, but when used as the only anesthetic for minor surgical operations, the delayed recovery period has some advantage.

Thialbarbital Sodium. The use of thialbarbital sodium is similar to that of thiopental sodium except that for cattle, the dose level is twice that of thiopental. The uses of both are similar.

BASAL NARCOSIS-CHLORAL HYDRATE

Although many of the pharmacological actions of chloral hydrate in large animal species were known toward the end of the last century and in the early part of the present century, it was not until around 1945 that increasing members of veterinary clinicians in many parts of the world began to use the drug for what was then described as an anesthetic agent. The popularity of this agent increased enormously up to within recent years, but is now rapidly declining with the advent of safe means of anesthetizing large animals. Chloral hydrate should never be used for surgical anesthesia as it is then exceedingly dangerous. In order to place the agent in its proper perspective, it is better described as a hypnotic or a drug to produce a basal narcosis; when used for this purpose it is still the drug of choice in adult cattle. Since a large proportion of

cattle can be restrained and cast to the ground without undue excitement on the part of the animal and without undue human effort, intravenous administration is to be preferred, especially as the complicated digestive system of cattle causes irregular absorption of the drug when given in water by mouth or by stomach tube. Range cattle and bulls are the exception in regard to handling, however, and they should first be tranquilized.

A useful concentration of chloral hydrate is 10% in a sterile water solution which provides a convenient volume of fluid and simplifies the calculation of a correct dose level of 10 to 12 g/100 kg. Because of the irritant effects of the drug on perivascular tissue and because movements of the animal are liable to dislodge a hypodermic needle, it is preferable to use a large bore needle with a polyethylene catheter or at least a long needle which has been well seated. A slow injection is made by gravitation. The maximum dose level will be placed in the flask, but the exact amount to be administered will be judged by the reflexes of the animal as it passes into deep sedation. No attempt should be made to produce anesthesia deeper than stage 3, plane 1. Palpebral and anal reflexes are still present and the pupils are still rotated downwards and are not centrally fixed. Respiratory and cardiac inadequacy are liable to occur in deeper planes of anesthesia before adequate analgesia occurs. Complete analgesia should be produced in the surgical area by regional or local analgesia.

Various combinations of chloral hydrate and magnesium sulfate and chloral hydrate and pentobarbital have been suggested by various workers, but the combinations do not appear to have any advantages over chloral hydrate alone nor are they safer in producing true surgical anesthesia.

General Anesthesia in Sheep and Goats

INHALATION ANESTHESIA

It is convenient to describe anesthesia in sheep and goats as if they were one species using the word sheep only because there is virtually no difference in the pattern of anesthesia. Whereas regurgitation of rumenal contents in anesthesia is common in cattle, it is far less frequent in sheep. Thus this hazard of cattle anesthesia is less of a problem in sheep. Furthermore, as compared with cattle, sheep do not salivate as excessively during induction of anesthesia and this is not as serious a problem in the smaller ruminants.[9]

Any form of circle absorber apparatus suitable for human use or apparatus suitable for large dogs is appropriate for sheep. A 3- to 5-liter rebreathing bag is adequate.

Although induction of anesthesia in sheep may be attained by the use of barbiturates administered intravenously, it is convenient, safe, and easy to induce with the same volatile or gaseous agent that is to be used for maintenance of anesthesia. A face mask made of hard rubber, or one which has a seal of rubber latex around the periphery can be used. The animal is restrained either in sternal or lateral recumbency, the face mask fitted, and a mixture of oxygen and the anesthetic administered.

Oxygen or nitrous oxide-oxygen in combination with halothane or methoxyflurane can be used. The induction concentration for halothane anesthesia is 2.5 to 3.5% and for methoxyflurane, 1.5 to 2%. Maintenance levels for the respective agents are between 1.5 and 2% for halothane and 0.5 to 1% for methoxyflurane. The concentrations for induction and maintenance of anesthesia generally are similar for all species (see Chapter 17).

A correct plane of anesthesia is judged by regular slow excursions of the rebreathing bag and by the continual presence of a slight palpebral reflex. Swallowing movements or movements of the eye or eyelids indicate that anesthesia is too light. If the interdigital integument of a forefoot is squeezed between an index finger and thumb nail, a reflex may be provoked. If the reflex is slight the animal will be in stage 3, plane 2, but if the

squeezing provokes a strong movement of the limb the animal will probably be in plane 1.

The foregoing pattern of anesthesia is sometimes complicated slightly by apnea which is common in sheep during the induction of anesthesia. This hypoventilation during the induction of anesthesia prevents the animal from taking in sufficient anesthetic agent, and the animal may respond to surgical stimulation. In this event it may be necessary to make a few rhythmical manual compressions of the rebreathing bag to assist ventilation. When no barbiturate has been used for induction, recovery from anesthesia is rapid, and even after prolonged anesthesia, sheep are sometimes standing within 10 to 20 minutes after being disconnected from the apparatus. Some animals, however, may take up to 1 hour, depending upon the duration of surgical anesthesia and the anesthetic agent used.

Halothane is by far the inhalation anesthetic of choice; its nonflammability, general lack of irritating properties, ease of induction, and rapid recovery are its major attributes. Ether has been used successfully in sheep as in other animals.[6, 14] Chloroform can be used to supplement nitrous oxide-oxygen anesthesia.[6] Methoxyflurane anesthesia has many of the virtues of halothane, but the longer induction and recovery period are a disadvantage in sheep as in other animals.

INTRAVENOUS ANESTHESIA

Most workers use the jugular vein for intravenous injections in sheep with the animal held in a sitting position or in lateral recumbency with the head extended fully. The jugular vein is large and easy to locate, but it has the disadvantage that, in most breeds, a large amount of wool must be removed.

The cephalic vein lies on the mediolateral aspect of the foreleg above the carpus. An assistant may sit the animal on its haunches, and in most cases it is sufficient if he encircles the upper part of the leg with finger and thumb to cause the vein to fill, or alternatively rubber tubing may be used as a tourniquet until the vein is located by sight or palpation. The process is made easier if the hair (or wool in some breeds) is carefully clipped and the area cleaned with alcohol. (Fig. 24.6).

For right dominant persons, the right leg of the animal is used and the left hand grasps the upper foreleg. After the venipuncture is made, the syringe is grasped with the left hand while it is still holding the leg. From then on the right hand is used only to withdraw the plunger to make sure there is a flow of blood into the syringe and to depress the plunger to make the injection. By this means, if the animal should move the limb, the syringe also moves with the limb and the needle remains in the vein.

The sodium salts of pentobarbital and thiopental are suitable and fairly safe anesthetic agents for the small ruminants especially for surgical interventions that require general anesthesia for no longer than 10 to 15 minutes, or for induction of anesthesia prior to endotracheal intubation and maintenance of anesthesia by volatile and gaseous agents. They cannot be described as safe agents for prolonged anesthesia. The two agents may be classed together because the recovery from either is approximately the same after an initial injection sufficient to produce surgical anesthesia. Young ruminants take longer to recover from barbiturate anesthesia. Adult small ruminants can be standing within 15 to 20 minutes after a single dose. As with these agents in other species, it is difficult to assess either the exact dose or the recovery period as both factors depend entirely on the amount administered and the rapidity with which the agents are given.

Caution should be used in administering the whole of a precalculated dose rapidly since sheep are notoriously prone to liver damage from parasites, and fatty infiltration of the liver is common in late pregnancy and in postpartum. Wide variations of dose levels of pentobarbital have been suggested, and in large measure this variation is related in part to the speed of injection. It is convenient to use pentobar-bital or thiopental as a 2.5 or 5% solution for small animals and as a 10% solution for large rams and ewes; thus the difficulty of using a syringe greater than 20 cc is avoided. The average dose is about 30 mg/kg, but is it convenient to take up 40 mg/kg into the syringe. A quarter of the dose is injected rapidly followed by a pause of 30 seconds; from then on small quantities are injected at 30-second intervals until the required stage of anesthesia is reached. If longer anesthesia is required, it is well to administer the agent over a period of 10 minutes. If a short period of anesthesia is necessary, for example, to intubate an animal, the total amount injected should be less and of a shorter duration.

Commercially available solutions of pentobarbital sodium containing propylene glycol may cause hemolysis and hematuria in goats.[10] A correct plane of anesthesia can be judged in the same way as that described under anesthesia with volatile and gaseous agents.

After a single dose of barbiturate, even when administered slowly, it is unlikely that a sheep will remain anesthetized for more than ½ hour. The administration of further doses is fraught with dangers unless given under ideal hospital conditions. When an endotracheal tube is not being used in an anesthetized sheep, the neck should be raised to reduce the risk of regurgitation, but the head should be allowed to hang with the muzzle downwards so that saliva may flow from the mouth. On no account should the hind quarters be raised higher than the rest of the body or pressure brought to bear on the abdomen.

General Anesthesia in Swine

The use of volatile and gaseous anesthetic agents administered in a rebreathing system is undoubtedly the safest and most satisfactory form of general anesthesia for swine. Induction with barbiturates and endotracheal intubation are difficult in this species. The sparsity of superficial veins and the temperament of swine make intravenous injection diffi-

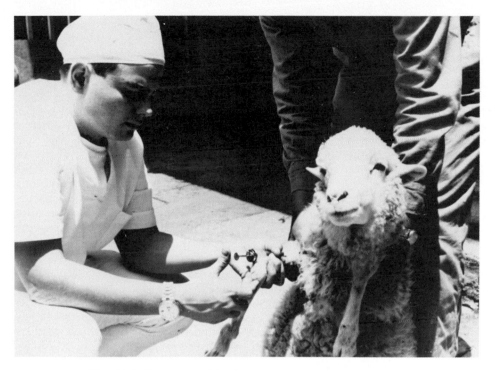

Fɪɢ. 24.6. Intravenous injection in sheep using cephalic vein.

cult. Once intubation is completed, however, and the animal is connected to the apparatus, the maintenance of anesthesia is as simple and safe in the pig as it is in other species. It is fortunate that the demands for general anesthesia in swine in the field are not frequent but at the same time it is also unfortunate that the worker in the field does not have regular practice with the particular techniques required. Those who do not have practice in such techniques would be well advised not to attempt intubation unless absolutely necessary. Fortunately, nature has provided the pig with a snout that lends itself to the fitting of a face mask. The pig rarely vomits and salivation is not a major problem.

INDUCTION OF ANESTHESIA

In order to perform endotracheal intubation, it is necessary to have the pig in light plane of anesthesia. A short acting barbiturate such as thiopental sodium given fairly rapidly can be used, or inhalation anesthesia can be induced with a tightly fitting snout mask. The mask is used until sufficient depth is attained for intubation of the trachea.

Fairly safe and satisfactory anesthesia can be maintained in pigs with a snout mask, thereby eliminating the difficulties associated with endotracheal intubation. The mask is connected to a rebreathing system. The closer fit of the snout mask insures less dilution of the inhaled anesthetic with room air. Nevertheless, it is far from ideal because there is no guarantee of constant clear airway and there is at the best some leakage of gases. Swine are being used increasingly as experimental animals, and thus in institutes, laboratories, and veterinary hospitals where the demand for general anesthesia is greater, the rebreathing system of administering inhalation agents with endotracheal intubation is commonly employed.

The types of rebreathing systems (circle or to and fro) used for dogs are suitable for pigs up to 70 kg provided a rebreathing bag of 5-liter capacity is used. For adult pigs it is necessary to use apparatus designed for large animal species. Maintenance of anesthesia is similar to other species. If a relaxant drug has been used to prevent laryngeal spasm, then artificial respiration is necessary until spontaneous respirations have returned.

Signs of surgical anesthesia in the pig have no species characteristics and stage 3, plane 3 is judged by relaxed musculature, slow regular respirations, slight palpebral and anal reflexes, and a relaxed jaw.

Halothane Anesthesia. Halothane has all the advantages in swine that it has in other species and is an excellent anesthetic agent for pigs. Because of its potency it is particularly useful for induction of anesthesia by administration with a snout mask prior to intubation. A considerable amount is required for induction in an adult animal, however, and in view of its relative cost, this has to be taken into consideration. Where halothane has been used for induction and maintenance, recovery is rapid even after prolonged anesthesia.

Other Inhalation Agents. Ether is a safe anesthetic agent for pigs provided that it is used for maintenance only and is administered through an endotracheal tube. Ether provokes copious salivation and bronchial secretion and it should not be administered through a tightly fitting snout mask for this reason.

Chloroform as an anesthetic agent for pigs has for many years been considered a fairly safe agent even when administered by entirely open methods. When used in closed and semiclosed circuits with ample oxygen, it gives a smooth anesthesia not unlike that with halothane. With modern equipment there is room for reappraisal of this agent for not unduly prolonged anesthesia in pigs.

Cyclopropane gives satisfactory anesthesia in swine, but for maintenance it should be given in a completely closed circuit.[8, 13] It can be used for induction by means of a semiclosed circuit, using a snout mask, but the expense of the agent has to be considered.

Methoxyflurane can be used as described for other species, but a longer induction and recovery should be anticipated.

INTRAVENOUS ANESTHESIA

There are not many readily detectable superficial veins in the pig, and virtually the only veins that can be used for intravenous injections are those of the ear (Fig. (24.7). They can be seen readily but they are of small caliber and are not suitable for injections of large volumes of fluid. Small pigs may be held in the arms of an assistant who grasps the opposite ear to prevent head shaking. The largest vein is selected, the sparse hair clipped, and the ear wiped with ether on cotton wool to remove the grease and thus allow the color of the vein to be seen more readily. The vein is made to fill by pressure from another assistant's thumb placed distally to the point of injection, or a rubber band may be tied at the base of the ear. A needle of 1-mm bore, not more than 3 cm long, and preferably with a short bevel point is used. When the needle appears to have entered the vein the thumb pressure or rubber band is released and a small quantity of the anesthetic liquid is injected. If the color of the vein changes by the fluid forcing the blood down the vein, it is obvious that the vein has been entered correctly. If the color does not change and a small extravascular swelling appears, a further attempt to enter the vein must be made or another vein selected. A 40-cm length of 1-mm-bore polythene tubing can be used to join the needle and syringe to allow flexibility of movement.[13] Such devices are particularly useful in pigs because of their attempts to shake the head.

Thiopental Sodium Anesthesia. Thiopental is an excellent drug for induction of anesthesia prior to intubation and maintenance of anesthesia by other agents. As with all other species the dose level will be directly proportional to the rate at which it is administered. Thiopental should be administered as quickly as possible. The

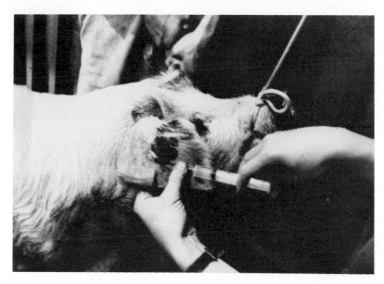

Fig. 24.7. Intravenous injection in the pig using the ear vein.

small ear vein will not permit the rapid injection of large volumes of fluid such as can be achieved in other farm animals when using, for example, the jugular vein. With this limitation and with some guidance as to the approximate dose level, half of the estimated dose should be given rapidly and portions of the remainder given without undue delay until the required depth of anesthesia is attained. Approximately 29 mg/kg for small pigs, and 24 mg/kg for large pigs as a 5 or 10% solution is a guide. After the first half is given there should be a lapse of 30 seconds and intervals of 15 seconds between the succeeding portions. With the foregoing dose level and timing there might well be a considerable amount of unused solution left over. The animal is likely to be immobile with light anesthesia for a period of 10 minutes.

Pentobarbital Sodium Anesthesia. Pentobarbital may be used for the induction of light anesthesia for intubation when administered in the same dose level and in a manner described for thiopental. At higher dose levels (35 mg/kg), the duration of anesthesia will be between 30 and 40 minutes. A quarter is given as rapidly as the pig ear vein will allow, and the further amount required for surgical anes-thesia given over a period of 5 minutes. Continual administration of small amounts at further intervals in order to prolong anesthesia cannot be recommended.

INTRAPERITONEAL INJECTIONS

The intraperitoneal route for the administration of anesthetic agents in pigs is far from ideal, particularly because there are individual variations in response even after careful weighing of the animal and computing of dose levels. There may, however, be circumstances where lack of assistance, lack of equipment, and primitive conditions leave no option. An assistant should suspend the pig by the hind legs and a short beveled needle should be inserted between the umbilicus and pubis, 2 to 5 cm from the midline.[14] Food should be withheld for 24 hours to reduce bowel volume.

Thiopental can also be used, but is not highly recommended.[6] A dose level for pigs up to 20 kg is 30 mg/kg, and for those between 20 and 30 kg is 24 mg/kg.

Chloral hydrate as a 5% solution may also be administered intraperitoneally at a dose level of 0.3 g/kg. The irritant properties of chloral hydrate do not appear to cause much harm. With both the foregoing agents, the maximum effect can be expected after approximately 30 minutes and lasts for about 1 hour.

Endotracheal Intubation

CATTLE

Several methods are suggested for intubation in cattle. A hand is passed through the animal's mouth to the pharynx, and the endotracheal tube is fed along the side of the operator's arm. The tube is manipulated by the fingers over the epiglottis and through the larynx.

An alternative method is the passage of a rubber stomach tube into the trachea. The endotracheal tube is then threaded over the first tube which acts as a guide for the endotracheal tube as it is pushed into the larynx and trachea.[11] A long laryngoscope with illumination can be used

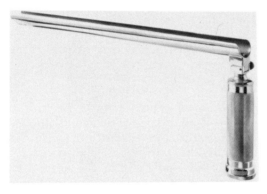

FIG. 24.8. Rowson type of laryngoscope suitable for cattle and swine. (Courtesy of Longworth Scientific Instrument Co., Berks, England.)

and intubation carried out by direct vision (Fig. 24.8). The intubation in calves is similar to techniques employed in sheep and goats. Sizes for various animals are shown in Table 24.1.

It is always advisable to use a mouth gag in cattle because in light anesthesia there may be movements of the mandible, and the sharp edges of bovine molar teeth can damage the endotracheal tube. The types of gags which are wedge-shaped with side flanges to cover the edges of the molar teeth are most suitable (Figs. 24.9 and 24.10).

SHEEP

The animal is placed on its back so that the soft palate will fall away from the larynx and the head will be extended as far as possible. The tongue is taken between index finger and thumb of one hand and pressed against the mandible so that the mouth is forced open. Before experience is gained, it is convenient to have an assist-

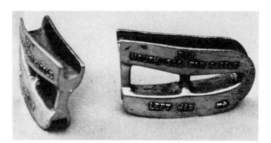

FIG. 24.9. Left and right pair of Drinkwater cattle mouth gags.

TABLE 24.1

Endotracheal tube sizes for ruminants

Animal	Internal Diameter	Approximate External Diameter	Length
	mm	*mm*	*cm*
Large bulls	30	38	100
Average cows	25	31	80
Yearling cattle	20	26	80
Calves, 6 months	18	22.5	60
Calves, 3 months	16	19.5	60
Large sheep	16	19.5	60
Medium size sheep	14	17	50
Lambs	12	15	40

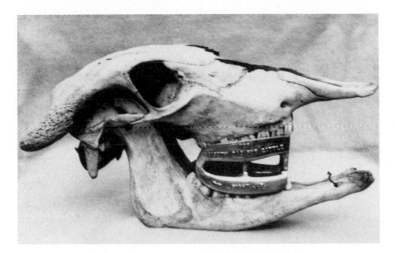

FIG. 24.10. Mouth gags covering both edges of all molar teeth.

ant with an index finger pressing on the hard palate to prevent the head from rising. The endotracheal tube is taken between finger and thumb of the other hand, the end passed through the mouth into the pharynx, and then, with a quick light thrust, the tube is slipped blindly through the open larynx. If the animal is breathing, the thrust should be made to coincide with inspiration. If the tube has passed correctly through the larynx, the passing of the end of the tube over the tracheal rings will be appreciated, and the expiration of air through the tube will be heard. If apnea is present, it will be necessary to make a sudden pressure with the hand on the animal's thorax to force air through the tube. It cannot be emphasized too strongly that on no account should the tube be grasped by the whole hand and forcibly pushed against the larynx; the thrust, although rapid, is of the gentlest nature with finger and thumb only. There will be no resistance to the passing of the tube if it is correctly directed. It may be necessary to alter the angle of the head a little if the tube is obviously coming against an obstruction.

With the animal also on its back intubation may be performed with the aid of an illuminated laryngoscope but the method is not as easy as it is, for example, in the dog, where the jaw can open more widely than in sheep. An extension can be

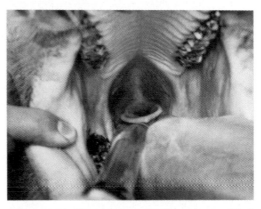

FIG. 24.11. Placement of the laryngoscope blade in the pig, showing the apex of epiglottis when the tongue is depressed by the blade. (Courtsey of Hill and Perry.[8])

added to the blade to facilitate its use. Laryngoscope blades are designed for human use where the blade can sink into a broad soft tongue base. The high and hard dorsum of the sheep's tongue tends to jump to one side or the other of the blade. Once intubation is completed, the cuff of the endotracheal tube should be inflated and the tube should be secured in place by tying a narrow bandage around the tube and around the mandible just behind the incisor teeth.

SWINE

There are a number of reasons why intubation is not easy in the pig. The animal has a relatively small larynx, the mouth is elongated, the mouth cannot be opened widely, the sides of the cricoid cartilage bend convexly into the orifice of the larynx, and there is a ventral slope from the larynx into the trachea. For a pig of 50 kg, an oral cuffed tube of 9-mm internal diameter is suitable and for an adult sow, one of 12 mm is suitable. The readily available tubes of these calibers used for humans or dog are not long enough for large pigs. They should be approximately 30 and 50 cm long, respectively. A malleable metal rod passed into the tube is useful to stiffen the tube and create a slight bend at the tip of the tube to aid in insertion of the tube into the larynx. A mouth gag of the type that has two knobs and not bars is convenient. A laryngoscope with a blade 510 mm long for adult pigs and one 405 mm long for small pigs is recommended (Fig. 24.8).[13]

The anesthetized pig is placed on its back or sternum or in lateral recumbency, provided that in each position the head is extended. The jaw is opened as far as possible with the mouth gag, the tongue is pulled forward by an assistant, and the laryngoscope is placed at the base of the tongue or the tip of the larynx and depressed for viewing of the larynx (Fig. 24.11). An alternative method is to depress the tip of the epiglottis with the laryngoscope blade to expose the laryngeal opening. A long pair of forceps grasping a tampon of gauze should be available to remove mucus from the larynx if any difficulty in intubation is encountered.

REFERENCES

1. Berra Sanvicente, H.: Cuantificacion del flujo salival en bovinos con anestesia intubada en circuito cerrado usando bromoclorot-rifluoretano, cloroformo y éter. Professional thesis. Universidad Nacional Autonoma de Mexico, Mexico City, Mexico, 1967.
2. Brennan, H. J., Hunter, A. R., and Johnstone, M.: Halothane: A clinical assessment. Lancet 2: 453, 1957.
3. Douglas, T. A., Jennings, S., Longstreeth, J., and Weaver, A. D.: Methoxyflurane anesthesia in horses and cattle. Vet. Rec. 76: 615, 1964.
4. Fernández Fernández, A.: Estudio de la regurgitación de contenido ruminal en anesthesia general en bovinos y métodos de eliminación de este fenómeno. Professional thesis. Universidad Nacional Autonoma de Mexico, Mexico City, Mexico, 1967.
5. Fisher, E. W., and Jennings, S.: The use of Fluothane in horses and cattle. Vet. Rec. 70: 567, 1958.
6. Hall, L. W.: *Wright's Veterinary Anesthesia and Analgesia*, 6th ed., pp. 162, 267, 362, and 369. Bailliere, Tindall & Cassell, Ltd., London, 1966.
7. Henkels, P.: Die zur Zeit optimale Technik de refexlosen, leicht steuerbaren Pferdenarkose für Klinik und Aussenpraxis. Deutsch. Tieraerztl. Wschr. 46: 801, 1938.
8. Hill, K. J., and Perry, J. S.: A method of closed-circuit anesthesia in the pig. Vet. Rec. 71: 269, 1959.
9. Jennings, S.: The use of volatile anesthetic agents in horses and farm animals. Canad. Vet. J. 4: 86, 1963.
10. Linzell, J. L.: Some observations on general and regional anesthesia in goats. In *Small Animal Anesthesia*, edited by O. Graham-Jones, p. 168. Pergamon Press, New York, 1964.
11. Messervy, A., and Wynn Jones, W.: Endotracheal intubation in cattle. Vet. Rec. 68: 32, 1956.
12. Raventos, J.: The action of fluothane: a new volatile anesthetic. Brit. J. Pharmacol. 11: 394, 1956.
13. Rowson, L. E. A.: Endotracheal intubation in the pig. Vet. Rec. 77: 1495, 1965.
14. Westhues, M., and Fritsch, R.: *Animal Anaesthesia*, vol. 2, pp. 249, 321, and 224. Oliver and Boyd, London, 1964.
15. Wynn Jones, E.: The administration of general anesthesia to the horse and ox. J. Amer Vet. Med. Ass. 127:484, 1955.

25
Avian Anesthesia

JOHN SANFORD

The techniques employed in the general anesthesia of birds have been developed from those used for mammals. In spite of marked anatomical and physiological differences, the response to general anesthetics is essentially similar in both classes of vertebrate. Birds, however, may not experience pain as readily as mammals.[33] For instance, caponization produces little overt response after the initial incision, although the operation involves manipulations which would be extremely painful in mammals. Pigeons show no evidence of pain to the incision and manipulations needed to insert intracardiac catheters via the jugular veins.[11] Many operations, including suturing a torn crop, removal of a superficial tumor, or evisceration cause little response in birds.[3] In parakeets, however, there are areas of the body where painful sensations are readily provoked including the head, scaled parts of the legs, digits, limb joints, and vent. Cutting the skin of these birds apparently is less painful than manipulation and stretching. In spite of these differences, anesthesia should be used for birds to the same extent as is considered necessary in mammals.

Stages of Depression

LIGHT NARCOSIS

The bird is sedated and lethargic, and the eyelids tend to droop.

MEDIUM NARCOSIS

The feathers become ruffled and the head is lowered. The bird can be roused easily but only struggles a little if picked up.

DEEP NARCOSIS

There is little or no response to sounds. Fluttering is provoked by painful stimuli, and there may be shrill cries, particularly with barbiturate narcosis. If the bird is placed on its back, there is some attempt at co-ordinated movement. Respirations are usually fairly rapid, regular, and deep but may become irregular after stimulation.

ANESTHESIA

Light. Reflex responses are present, but there are no voluntary movements and no response to vibration or postural changes.

Medium. The palpebral reflex is lost, and pedal and corneal reflexes are sluggish. Respirations are slow, deep, and regular.

Deep. Reflex responses are absent. Respirations are very slow but usually regular.

Signs of General Anesthesia

The most commonly used tests of reflex responses have been pinching of comb and wattles, pinching of the interdigital web, and touching the cornea. The corneal reflex, as in other animals, is not a reliable indicator of the depth of anesthesia.[18] It appears and disappears during urethane anesthesia irrespective of the depth of anesthesia,[23] and it is lost in very deep anesthesia, which was usually irreversible.[21] In the anesthesia of poultry, the comb reflex is the most useful guide, while the toe reflex is less reliable, and the corneal reflex is unreliable.[33] The depth of halothane anesthesia in hens and turkeys can be assessed by the absence of response to pinching of the skin in the region of the cloaca, the interdigital web, and comb and wattles. Responses disappear in that order as anesthesia is deepened.

Respiratory rate is sometimes useful as a guide to the depth of anesthesia[9]; an increase in rate usually signifies a lightening of anesthesia, while deep anesthesia is accompanied by a progressive slowing of respirations.[26] During induction and in light anesthesia there may be movements of the head, wings, or legs. This may occur if the bird is stimulated, and the response to a skin incision may be exaggerated.[3] Stimulation of the larynx during intubation may give rise to movement of the head and wings.

Although it is possible to assess the depth of anesthesia in a bird by its response to various stimuli, such tests are not always satisfactory, and some have concluded that lack of any response during surgery is the only reliable guide.[5, 14, 23, 34]

Inhalation Anesthesia

Volatile anesthetics for general anesthesia have been considered to be dangerous because of the nature of the avian respiratory system.[8, 35] Difficulties have been associated with control of the concentration of anesthetic administered so as to prevent overdose. Renewed interest in the use of inhalation anesthetics in domestic animals has stimulated the development of more refined techniques and improvements in anesthetic equipment.

It is difficult to administer respiratory assistance in birds when an overdose has been given. The areas for gaseous exchange in the avian lungs do not terminate in blind sacs as in mammals, but communicate with the large air sacs. This allows a double passage of respiratory gases and inhalation agents through the lungs, on the way to the air sacs during inspiration, and again through the lungs on leaving the air sacs during expiration.

Experimental studies of air flow in the respiratory system of the hen indicate that the major portion of gaseous interchange takes place during expiration as gases leave the air sacs via the recurrent bronchi.[15] At the end of inspiration, the carbon dioxide content of the anterior sacs is greater than that of the posterior sacs which more closely resembles that of the inspired air. This is due to the dissimilar communications of the anterior and posterior air sacs. The anterior air sacs receive air which has passed through the dorsal, para, and ventral bronchi, whereas the posterior air sacs receive inspired air directly through the mesobronchi.[32] Pressure changes in the lungs and air sacs are synchronous so that there is no evidence that thoracic and abdominal respiratory movements are antagonistic.[32] In spite of several experimental investigations, it is still not entirely clear how air circulates in the respiratory system of the bird. It is more likely that some form of circulation occurs other than a simple to and fro oscillation.[4] This double period of gaseous exchange may make control of the concentrations of inhalation anesthetics more difficult.[26] If apnea occurs, suction may be as necessary as forced ventilation to reduce the concentration of anesthetic in the air sacs. Recent success with inhalation anesthesia in birds suggests that the safe use of inhalation anesthesia is governed by the same factors that operate in mammals, and that failure is more likely to be due to poor techniques than to some inherent difference in avian respiration.

METHODS OF ADMINISTERING VOLATILE ANESTHETICS

In the simplest method, volatile anesthetics are sprayed directly into the nostrils of small birds with a syringe and fine needle.[12] Although this method apparently is satisfactory, it is generally considered inadvisable to bring high concentrations of irritant solutions such as ether into direct contact with the sensitive nasal mucosa. Small birds may be placed in a box or jar containing a pad of cotton wool onto which the anesthetic liquid is poured. This simple method of induction has been used satisfactorily in many cases, but a glass or transparent plastic container should be used so that the bird can be observed at all times. A simple modification of this method for inducing anesthesia in parakeets has been used. It consists of a glass tube, 20 cm long by 2.2 cm in diameter, with a pad of cotton wool placed at one end. The tube is passed over the head and down to the level of the wings with the bird lying on its back.[16]

Similar tube-type masks connected to the delivery hose of an anesthetic machine can be used.[1, 19] As a substantial oxygen flow may be delivered from an anesthetic machine, it is essential that the mask is loose fitting, since an airtight system may cause damage from overinflation of the respiratory tract. A cat mask (Hall's type) has been used to administer a halothane-oxygen mixture to turkeys, ducks, and chickens (Fig. 25.1).[36] This is a semiopen Magill circuit. Rebreathing is prevented by maintaining a high rate of gas flow. A transparent plastic bag can be wrapped around the mask and head of the bird to prevent dilution with room air during inspiration (Fig. 25.2).

Anesthesia can be induced by a nonvolatile agent and maintained with an inhalation agent using a semiclosed or closed circuit system. Intubation of the trachea is quite easy in the hen, although anatomical differences make it somewhat more difficult in the cock.[17] The lower jaw is depressed, and the tongue is drawn forward. The opening of the larynx can then be seen and a suitably sized tube inserted without difficulty. Movement may occur when the tube is inserted into the larynx. For young birds (1- to 2-week-old chicks) a

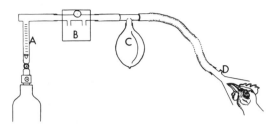

FIG. 25.1. Apparatus for administration of inhalation agents to poultry. *A*, flowmeter; *B*, vaporizer; *C*, rebreathing bag; *D*, expiratory valve. (Courtesy of R. S. Jones.)

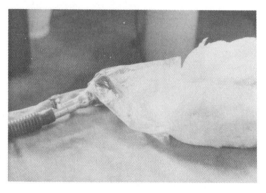

FIG. 25.2. Cat mask with polyethylene bag attached to form a head mask for poultry. (Courtesy of R. S. Jones.)

cannula having an external diameter of 1 mm and an internal diameter of 0.5 mm can be used. For older birds (3 to 4 weeks), the dimensions are increased to 1.27 mm, external diameter, and 0.97 mm, internal diameter. The Cole pediatric tubes can be used for various size birds. The endotracheal tube can be secured with tape or gauze to the maxilla.

A "to and fro" system with a soda lime carbon dioxide absorber and a polyethylene rebreathing bag has been employed for inhalation anesthesia in fowl (Fig. 25.3).[17] The rebreathing bag is 22.5 cm long by 7.5 cm wide with a capacity of 250 ml. The absorber is 14.0 cm long and 3.0 cm in diameter and contains 25 g of soda lime. The cuffed endotracheal tubes have an internal diameter of 7.0 mm and are 25 cm long.

A simple unidirectional air flow system to provide artificial respiration in birds has been described.[2] With the bird lying

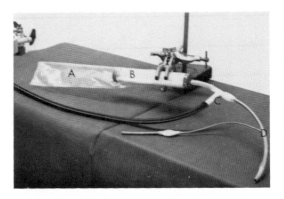

FIG. 25.3. A to and fro apparatus for administration of inhalation anesthetics. *A*, rebreathing bag; *B*, soda lime container. *C*, T-piece; *D*, cuffed endotracheal tube. (Courtesy of K. J. Hill and D. E. Noakes.)

on its side, a 15-gauge, 6.5 cm hypodermic needle attached to rubber tubing is inserted between the last two ribs on the dorsal flank to enter the post-thoracic air sac. After the needle is pushed through the body wall, it is taped in position. The tube is then connected to an air or oxygen supply and a continuous stream (1 liter/minute for an adult cock) is passed through the respiratory tract. For abdominal surgery, air is passed in the same manner through an endotracheal tube. This method produces complete apnea, but oxygenation is adequate. Although this method provides a simple means of introducing volatile anesthetics, it is very difficult to control, and careful regulation of anesthetic vapor concentrations is necessary. On the other hand, it has the advantage that respiratory efficiency, during anesthesia, does not depend on the maintenance of adequate respiratory movements.

ANESTHETIC AGENTS

Inhalation anesthesia in birds is most frequently carried out with one of four agents: ether, cyclopropane, halothane, or methoxyflurane. Nitrous oxide-oxygen anesthesia has been used in hens, and as with mammals, only light narcosis is achieved.[21] Nitrous oxide-oxygen in combination with other inhalation anesthetics such as halothane can be used in fowl.

Ether. Both ether and ethyl chloride have been used satisfactorily in the fowl.[33] Ether has a hypotensive action in the fowl, producing a fall of 30 to 50 mm Hg in arterial blood pressure, followed by partial or complete recovery within a few minutes.[33] When using the cone-type mask, ether anesthesia can be achieved within 30 to 60 seconds with 2 ml of ether. Vomiting occasionally occurs during recovery from ether anesthesia in the parakeet. Ether can be administered with a simple mask to chickens and deep surgical anesthesia maintained.[21] Fatalities may result from improper control of ether concentration.

Cyclopropane. This compound has been used successfully in fowl in a closed circuit system.[17] Birds should be fasted for 9 to 12 hours to minimize the risk of regurgitation. Anesthesia is first induced with intravenous pentobarbital, and an endotracheal tube is connected to a to and fro closed circuit system for the maintenance of cyclopropane anesthesia (Fig. 25.3). A mixture of 1 part cyclopropane to 4 parts oxygen is given until the rebreathbag is moderately distended, and then the initial flow rate (100 to 200 ml of oxygen per minute) is reduced. Anesthesia was successfully maintained in 20 birds weighing 2.0 to 4.5 kg for periods of 0.5 to 3 hours. On cessation of anesthesia, recovery occurred in 10 to 20 minutes. Apnea due to an excessive concentration of cyclopropane can be corrected by flushing out the apparatus with oxygen. Anesthesia can be induced with cyclopropane, avoiding the use of barbiturates.

Halothane. Halothane has been used in various species of birds using different techniques.[16, 20, 25] A total of 0.25 ml on a cotton wool pad induces anesthesia within 15 to 30 seconds in parakeets, and 3rd-stage anesthesia can be maintained for 5 minutes.[16] Anesthesia can be induced in small birds (parakeets and canaries) by placing them in a small chamber connected to the anesthetic apparatus.[20] Anesthesia is maintained by using the end of the flexible tubing as a "mask." Concentrations of halothane required range from 0.5 to 1.5%. Halothane anesthesia has been used successfully in larger birds, i.e., chickens, ducks, and turkeys, and is administered to chickens at a concentration of 2 to 4% in 200 to 400 ml of oxygen per minute, using a nonrebreathing system.[25, 26] Surgical anesthesia is reached in less than 5 minutes, and the concentration of halothane can be reduced to 1 to 2% after 1 hour. Recovery of consciousness occurs within 5 to 20 minutes after withdrawal of the anesthetic. Similar methods can be used for turkeys and ducks, although the duck may require a longer induction time and higher concentration of halothane.

Methoxyflurane. This drug has been used successfully in parakeets.[6] The bird's head is inserted into a small bottle containing anesthetic and cotton. There is serious risk of overdose, probably due to the relatively crude technique. Methoxyflurane also can be administered by techniques described for other inhalation agents.

If used with care under well controlled conditions, there is little doubt that methoxyflurane can be a useful volatile anesthetic for birds. At the present time there is little evidence to suggest that methoxyflurane is more advantageous than other anesthetic agents such as halothane or cyclopropane.

It must be stressed that with all volatile anesthetics, apnea may result from accumulation in the air sacs unless an adequate flow of oxygen is maintained during both anesthesia and recovery periods. In contrast to mammals, the possibility of respiratory arrest is more likely in the recovery period because of the accumulation of the anesthetic in the air sacs. This is not due to absorption from the sacs, but recirculation and gas exchange via the recurrent bronchi. This can be prevented by the continued administration of oxygen during the initial recovery period.

Injectable Agents

Whenever practical, anesthetic agents should be administered by careful intravenous injection. The depth of anesthesia can be controlled as can the duration of the induction period. In large birds such as fowl or duck, injections may readily be made into the brachial vein using a fine bore needle 1 to 2 cm in length. Where the volume of solution to be injected is small, a 1-ml tuberculin syringe should be used and, in any case, the syringe used should never be larger than is required for the computed dose.

To enter the brachial vein, the bird should be placed on its back with one wing extended. The vein is then clearly visible crossing the humerus and can be entered without difficulty. Puncture of the wall of the vessel may result in leakage of blood which makes further use of the vein impossible. The jugular vein can be used in small birds.[22]

Intraperitoneal injection is very convenient for birds of all sizes, but care is needed to avoid puncture of the abdominal air sacs. The needle should be inserted in the midline, midway between the cloaca and sternum. It should be directed anteriorly and maintained almost parallel to the abdominal wall.[20]

Intramuscular injections may be made into the pectoral muscles. There is some risk of puncturing a venous plexus in the muscle, and it is advisable to withdraw the plunger of the syringe slightly to insure that a blood vessel has not been entered. For parakeets, the volume of the intramuscular injection should not exceed 0.5 ml. If a larger volume is required it can be given as two injections, one on either side.[20] The temperature of the solution for injection should be warmed to 38 C. A short fine needle should be used and directed at an angle of 15° from the horizontal.

BARBITURATES

The use of barbiturates in mammalian anesthesia is well established, and several drugs of this group have been used successfully in birds. Sodium pentobarbital can be used, either intramuscularly or intravenously, and for anesthesia of longer duration, phenobarbital has been employed. Thiopental has not been used extensively in poultry, since when given intravenously anesthesia lasts for only a few minutes followed by a recovery period of

75 to 110 minutes.[21, 23] Also, there is a strong tendency for this compound to produce apnea and should be given with care. Short acting barbiturates have value for the induction of anesthesia in birds followed by an inhalation agent.

Sodium pentobarbital has been used both as a single anesthetic agent in birds and also preliminary to the induction of inhalation anesthesia. It should be given by slow intravenous injection when possible, so that the effects can be assessed as the injection proceeds. A standard solution of sodium pentobarbital containing 60 mg/ml should be diluted sufficiently to permit slow continuous injection. The actual dilution employed depends upon the weight of the bird and the apparatus available. If a 1-ml tuberculin syringe is used, accurate control of the rate of the injection may be possible in large birds without dilution of the standard solution.

The dose in poultry and other birds is very variable, and doses of 16 to 60 mg/kg may be needed to produce surgical anesthesia (Table 25.1). In all species of birds, the duration of surgical anesthesia is short when compared to mammals. The safety margin with pentobarbital is small, but it is possible to avoid overdose if injection is made slowly and carefully.

Pentobarbital may also be given by intramuscular injection particularly in small birds such as canaries and parakeets. Solutions ranging in strength from 0.5 to 7.5 mg/ml have been used in doses of 7.5 to 50 mg/kg. As with intravenous pentobarbital, the dose varies a great deal. Anesthesia is induced in 5 to 10 minutes and lasts for up to 30 minutes. Pentobarbital can be given in doses of 30 to 40 mg/kg to anesthetize small cage birds.[20] A solution containing 3 mg/ml is recommended. The dose of pentobarbital given intramuscularly in hens is 45 mg/kg.[15] The intraperitoneal dose in pigeons is 40 mg/kg.[31] A dilute solution containing 3.0 mg/ml should be used.

Although intramuscular injection may be necessary in small cage birds, it is advisable to give sodium pentobarbital intravenously whenever possible. The hypotensive and respiratory depressant effects of this drug are as marked in birds as they are in mammals, so that slow administration is desirable. The relatively short duration of action of sodium pentobarbital in birds is thought to be due to the rapid metabolism of the drug, although the recovery period may last for more than 12 hours. Using the intramuscular route, it is necessary to compute the required dose from the weight of the bird. A computed dose may sometimes be grossly inaccurate, as in the case of a small bird with a large tumor. There is considerable variation in the recommended doses of sodium pentobarbital. This variation is of particular importance when attempting to compute a dose for intramuscular or intraperitoneal injection, and it is suggested that a low dose should be selected in the first instance.

Sodium phenobarbital has been given to poultry by intramuscular or intraperitoneal injection in doses of 180 mg/kg.[33] Although this dose has produced adequate anesthesia for experimental studies, the delayed induction (up to 1 hour) and uncertain effect make this anesthetic unsatisfactory for surgical operations.[21] Recovery is prolonged and may take up to 24

TABLE 25.1

Intravenous pentobarbital in larger birds

Bird	Dose	Duration of Surgical Anesthesia	Recovery Time	Reference
	mg/kg	*Min*	*hr*	
Hens	31-59	12-60	10	Author
Chickens	5-21	10		Hill and Noakes,[17] Sykes[33]
Pigeons	12-16	10		Lee[254]
Ducks	16-28	10		Lee[24]

hours. A mixture of 3 parts sodium pentobarbital and 1 part sodium thiopental has been used.[8, 30] When used by the author, however, this mixture proved to be inferior to sodium pentobarbital in regard to its duration of action.[21]

CHLORAL HYDRATE

A 10% aqueous solution of chloral hydrate (2 to 4 ml) can be given intravenously to fowls weighing 1.4 to 1.6 kg. This produces anesthesia within 0.5 to 2 minutes, persisting for 18 to 60 minutes. Larger doses affect respirations, and 6 ml of the solution invariably is lethal. Chloral hydrate orally in doses of 0.17 to 0.33 g/kg for fowls, 0.26 to 0.33 g/kg for ducks, and 0.22 to 0.33 g/kg for geese produces anesthesia within 30 minutes which persists for 0.5 hour in geese, 2.5 hours in ducks, and 4.5 hours in fowls.[24]

CHLORAL HYDRATE, MAGNESIUM SULFATE, AND PENTOBARBITAL MIXTURE

A proprietary mixture of these three compounds known as "Equithesin" was developed for intravenous anesthesia in horses and has been used in birds. The mixture has the following composition: chloral hydrate, 4.26%; magnesium sulfate, 2.12%; and sodium pentobarbital, 0.96% in an aqueous solution containing 20% propylene glycol with 9.5% ethanol. Given intramuscularly (2.5 to 3.0 ml/kg), it is a satisfactory general anesthetic for the fowl but there are variations in the duration of anesthesia.[13, 30] The reliability is greatly improved if anesthesia is induced intravenously with sodium pentobarbital and a combination of 17.4% chloral hydrate and 8.48% magnesium sulfate, given intramuscularly. A dose of 1.65 ml/kg of this mixture is sufficient to produce deep anesthesia for a mean period of 59 minutes (Fig. 25.4). The induction dose of sodium pentobarbital is 11.0 to 38.0 mg/kg administered over a 10-minute period. This combination of drugs is undoubtedly capable of producing a long period of surgical anesthesia with a fair degree of safety. Recovery from anesthesia is prolonged, and in some birds

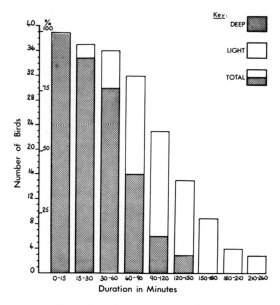

FIG. 25.4. Duration of anesthesia, in 39 hens given a chloral hydrate-magnesium sulfate mixture and sodium pentobarbital. (From Jordan et al.[21])

may take more than 24 hours. The intramuscular injection of this irritant solution can produce muscle damage, but this appears to be temporary and poultry are not noticeably affected by it.[21, 30] Muscle damage may be of more significance in flying birds but there have been no reports to suggest that it is of serious consequence.

This mixture (Equithesin) has also been used in parakeets and canaries. A dose of 2.5 ml/kg is given through a 26-gauge, ¼-inch needle into the pectoral muscles. Anesthesia is induced in 5 to 10 minutes and lasts for 30 to 60 minutes.[12]

URETHANE

This compound has been employed to produce anesthesia of long duration in birds which are used in nonsurvival experiments, and generally it causes less respiratory depression than barbiturates. Both respiratory rate and tidal volume are reduced by approximately 50% during anesthesia.[31]

It has cytotoxic actions and is unsuitable for clinical use. A 43% aqueous solution is injected intravenously in three stages, the total dose being computed as 1.5 g/kg.[23] The first third of the calculated dose is given rapidly to induce light anesthesia. The injection is continued slowly for 10 to 15 minutes until medium depth of surgical anesthesia is attained. About two-thirds of the total calculated dose is required to reach this stage, and further quantities are given as needed. Anesthesia can be maintained for periods of up to 9 hours.

Urethane (300 mg/kg) has also been used in pigeons intraperitoneally. A 25% solution is recommended. It is apparently quite satisfactory for anesthesia in experiments of long duration and probably is more reliable than a long acting barbiturate for this purpose.

OTHER COMPOUNDS

The steroid anesthetic hydroxydione has been given intravenously to hens. Anesthesia lasts for only 10 minutes.[33] Glutethimide also was given intravenously, the anesthesia lasting for less than 5 minutes. This drug was not considered satisfactory except possibly for induction of anesthesia.

Premedicants and Depressants

Several preanesthetic tranquilizers and depressants have been used in mammals to facilitate the induction of anesthesia in difficult to handle animals. A few of these drugs have been tested in birds, although in many cases the results have not been encouraging. Chlorpromazine was found to be unsatisfactory in parakeets and fowl.[16, 21] Thiambutene in small doses produced only mild sedation while larger doses produced spasms and fatal convulsions.[16] A combination of dehydrobenzperidol (0.1 mg) and fentanyl citrate (0.002 mg) has been used successfully to tranquilize parakeets.[37] Within 3 to 15 minutes of administration, the birds became easier to handle and flying was reduced, although the ability to fly was not impaired. Twice the dose resulted in tranquilization with impaired flying ability.

Larger doses produced loss of the righting reflex, rigidity, tremors, and convulsions.

Reserpine has been used as a tranquilizer for young wild turkeys during transport from the hatchery to the releasing ground.[10] A dose of 0.2 mg/kg intramuscularly prevented deaths which had previously occurred during transport, but the effective dose range appears to be very narrow. A new hypnotic agent, R7315 (Janssen Pharmaceuticals, Saunderton, High Wycombe, England) has been used intramuscularly in several species of birds.[27] A dose range of 5 to 20 mg/kg (1% aqueous solution) produces a stage of depression which was described in the following terms: "No response to sound stimuli. The bird is completely ataxic and only a slight fluttering is observed when painful stimuli are applied."[27] Analgesia was augmented by the local application of ethyl chloride before surgery was performed.

α-Chloralose given orally may be used to stupefy wild birds.[29] Wheat or maize bait containing chloralose produces narcosis in 15 to 30 minutes after ingestion with the effect lasting for 10 to 20 hours. Bait containing 11.5% chloralose by weight was most effective, but had a mortality rate of slightly less than 50%. The oral LD_{50} for feral pigeons is 131 mg/kg. The action of chloralose in capsules is much slower but, because of the more accurate dosage, it is safer than when applied to flour or grain. α-Chloralose in concentrations of 1.5% on cereal or pea baits has been used in several species of birds, but the mortality was more than 50% in small birds and 19% in wood pigeons.[28]

Local Analgesia

It is generally agreed that because of toxicity, the commonly used local anesthetic drugs are unsuitable for use in birds. Attempts to produce infiltration anesthesia in parakeets using lidocaine or procaine result in death, and it has not been possible to establish an effective safe dose. A spray containing ethyl aminobenzoate, butyl aminobenzoate, and tetracaine HCl has been recommended for local anesthesia.[12] This preparation apparently has a longer duration of action than ethyl chloride.

Causes of Death and Resuscitatory Measures

It is usually considered desirable to fast birds for some hours before administration of anesthesia in order to reduce the possibility of inhalation of food following regurgitation from the crop. Although poultry may conveniently be fasted overnight, withholding of food for more than 6 hours may be harmful to small cage birds.[12] In such birds, where metabolic activity is high, the fasting period should be limited to 2 to 3 hours.

Apart from the more obvious causes of death directly associated with overdose or toxic properties of the anesthetic agent, several other factors must be considered for safe anesthesia. These are of particular importance in small cage birds and are as follows.

COOLING

This may result from feather removal, excessive flow of anesthetic gases from a mask, too liberal application of alcohol or other volatile antiseptics, matting of plumage, and anesthesia of long duration.[3]

POSTURE

Birds fixed on their backs with wings outstretched may suffer trauma to the brachial plexus if attempts are made to flap the wings.[20]

HEMORRHAGE

This is obviously of particular importance in cage birds where the permissible blood loss during surgery is very small.

OBESITY

This is linked with fatty changes in the parenchymatous organs.

FLUID

Accumulation of fluid in the air sacs may lead to asphyxia.

Apnea may be more rapidly fatal in birds than in mammals, and small cage birds are particularly vulnerable. It has been suggested that in parakeets, a period of apnea lasting for more than 5 seconds is an indication to begin artificial respiration.[12] This is effected by applying digital pressure to the thorax at a rate of 2/second together with administration of oxygen.

When inhalation anesthetics are used, it is important to clear the anesthetic from the air sacs if respirations become weak. It may be of value to apply gentle suction at expiration as well as forced inspiration. The use of oxygen during the recovery period has been described by several workers.[17, 20, 26]

In larger birds artificial respiration may be applied by endotracheal intubation and manual pressure on a rebreathing bag or by a mechanical respirator. Cannulation of an abdominal air sac will allow a one-way flow system of ventilation either from the air sac to the trachea or in the opposite direction. This method appears to be more efficient than when the flow is from trachea to air sac.[7]

An environmental temperature of 70 to 80 F should be maintained during the recovery period. This period can also be shortened if the recovery cage is well lighted.[20]

There have been few reports of the use of central nervous system stimulants to aid resuscitation. Intramuscular injection of bemegride has been used, a suitable dose for parakeets being 0.2 ml of a solution containing 3.5 mg/ml.[12]

REFERENCES

1. Arnall, L.: Some common surgical conditions of the budgerigar. Vet. Rec. 72: 888, 1960.
2. Arnall, L.: Anesthesia and surgery in cage and aviary birds (1). Vet. Rec. 73: 139, 1961.
3. Arnall, L.: Aspects of anesthesia in cage birds. In Small Animal Anesthesia, edited by O. G. Jones, p. 137. Pergamon Press, New York, 1964.
4. Biggs, P. M., and King, A. S.: A new experimental approach to the problem of the air pathway within the avian lung. J. Physiol. 138: 282, 1957.

5. Blount, W. P.: *Disease of Poultry*, p. 318. Bailliere, Tindall and Cox, London, 1947.
6. Brinkman, D. C., and Burch, G. R.: Metofane (methoxyflurane) anesthesia in a variety of animal species. Allied Vet. *36:* 36, 1964.
7. Burger, R. E., and Lorenz, F. W.: Artificial respiration in birds by unidirectional air flow. Poult. Sci. *39:* 236, 1960.
8. Church, L. E.: Combuthal anesthesia for baby chicks. Poult. Sci. *36:* 788, 1957.
9. Cragg, B. G., Evans, D. H. L., and Hamlyn, L. H.: Optic tectum of *Gallus domesticus:* a correlation of the electrical responses with the histological structure. J. Anat. *88:* 292, 1954.
10. Earl, A. E.: Reserpine (Serpasil) in veterinary practice. J. Amer. Vet. Med. Ass. *129:* 227, 1956.
11. Eliassen, E.: A method for measuring the heart rate and stroke/pulse pressures in birds in normal flight. Abok for Universitetet i Bergen, No. 12, 3, 1960.
12. Friedburg, K. M.: Anesthesia of parakeets and canaries. J. Amer. Vet. Med. Ass. *141:* 1157, 1962.
13. Gandal, C. P.: Satisfactory general anesthesia in birds. J. Amer. Vet. Med. Ass. *128:* 332, 1956.
14. Gordeuk, S., and Grundy, M. L.: Observations on circulation in the avian kidney. Amer. J. Vet. Res. *11:* 256, 1950.
15. Graham, J. D. P.: The air stream in the lung of the fowl. J. Physiol. *97:* 133, 1939.
16. Grono, L. R.: Anesthesia of budgerigars. Aust. Vet. J. *37:* 463, 1961.
17. Hill, K. J., and Noakes, D. L.: Cyclopropane anesthesia in the fowl. In *Small Animal Anesthesia*, edited by O. G. Jones, p. 123. Pergamon Press, New York, 1964.
18. Hole, N.: Chloral hydrate as a general anesthetic for the fowl. J. Comp. Path. *46:* 47, 1933.
19. Jones, O. G.: In Arnall, L.: Discussion of some surgical conditions of the budgerigar. Vet. Rec. *72:* 888, 1960.
20. Jones, O. G.: Restraint and anesthesia of small cage birds. J. Small Anim. Pract. *6:* 31, 1965.
21. Jordan, F. T. W., Sanford, J. and Wright, A.: Anesthesia in the fowl. J. Comp. Path. *70:* 437, 1960.
22. Kerlin, R. E.: Venipuncture of small birds. J. Amer. Vet. Med. Ass. *144:* 870, 1964.
23. King, A. S., and Biggs, P. M.: General anesthesia in *Gallus domesticus* for non-survival laboratory experiments. Poult. Sci. *36:* 490, 1957.
24. Lee, C. C.: Experimental studies on the actions of several anesthetics in domestic fowls. Poult. Sci. *32:* 624, 1953.
25. Marley, E., and Payne, J. P.: A method of anesthesia with halothane suitable for newborn animals. Brit. J. Anaesth. *34:* 776, 1962.
26. Marley, E., and Payne, J. P.: Halothane anesthesia in the fowl. In *Small Animal Anesthesia*, edited by O. G. Jones, p. 127. Pergamon Press, New York, 1964.
27. Marsboom, R.: R7315—A new hypnotic agent in birds. Int. Zool. Year Book *5:* 200, 1965.
28. Murton, R. K., Isaacson, A. J., and Westwood, N. J.: The use of baits treated with alpha-chloralose to catch wood-pigeons. Ann. Appl. Biol. *52:* 271, 1963.
29. Ridpath, M. G., Theale, R. J. P., McCowan, D., and Jones, F. J. S.: Experiments on the value of stupefying and lethal substances in the control of harmful birds. Ann. Appl. Biol. *49:* 77, 1961.
30. Sanger, V. L., and Smith, H. R.: General anesthesia in birds. J. Amer. Vet. Med. Ass. *131:* 52, 1957.
31. Sinha, M. P.: Vagal control of respiration as studied in the pigeon. Helv. Physiol. Pharmacol. Acta *16:* 58, 1958.
32. Sturkie, P. D.: *Avian Physiology*, p. 89. Comstock Publishing Associates, Ithaca, N.Y., 1954.
33. Sykes, A. H.: Some aspects of anesthesia in the adult fowl. In *Small Animal Anesthesia*, edited by O. G. Jones, p. 117. Pergamon Press, New York, 1964.
34. Warren, D. C., and Scott, H. M.: The time factor in egg formation. Poult. Sci. *14:* 195, 1935.
35. Wright, J. G.: *Veterinary Anesthesia*, 2nd ed., p. 207. Bailliere, Tindall and Cox, London, 1952.
36. Wright, J. G., and Hall, L. W.: *Veterinary Anesthesia*, 3rd ed., p. 250. Bailliere, Tindall and Cox, London, 1961.
37. Yelnosky, J., and Field, W. E.: A preliminary report on the use of a combination of droperidol and fentanyl citrate. Vet. Res. *25:* 1751, 1964.

26
Restraint and Anesthesia of Small Laboratory Animals

DONALD CLIFFORD

Mice

Mice are used for studies in many areas of biological research. The advantages of these animals lie in genetic similarities of inbred strains, size, and reproductive capabilities.

HANDLING

Elaborate equipment and facilities are not required to manipulate mice. They can be handled simply by picking them up by the tail or grasping them over the shoulders. Some strains, feral mice, or those that have been injected with infectious agents may be handled more easily and safely with forceps. Albino strains of mice are easier to handle and have been used more extensively than others.

ANESTHETIC AGENTS AND TECHNIQUES

Pentobarbital sodium is a satisfactory anesthetic agent for most short surgical procedures in mice. The most common routes are intraperitoneal or intravenous. For intraperitoneal administration, the mouse is grasped over the neck and back with the left hand and rotated to expose the abdomen. The tail may be bent back between the small and ring fingers. The abdomen is moistened with alcohol and the injection is made superficially into the caudal quarter of the peritoneal cavity to avoid the liver and kidneys. A tuberculin syringe and 25-gauge needle is used.

The intraperitoneal administration of pentobarbital, although the most frequent route of injection, has serious disadvantages because of the wide variation in response of mice.[29] Following the administration of 80 mg/kg, 30% of the mice were anesthetized while 20% mortality was experienced with 90 mg/kg (Table 26.1). In an effort to obtain surgical anesthesia without a high mortality, chlorpromazine has been used prior to barbiturate anesthesia in mice (Table 26.2). Large doses of chlorpromazine, 50 to 60 mg/kg, were necessary. There was increased granularity of the cytoplasm and poorer staining with hemotoxylin and eosin in the livers of animals that received the chlorpromazine and pentobarbital combinations.

Generally the very young, the fat, and older mice are poorer anesthetic risks. One method that can be used to lower mortality when the intraperitoneal route is used is to supplement light pentobarbital anesthesia with inhalant anesthetics. This is particularly helpful in procedures where there may be considerable loss of blood. The blood volume of an adult mouse (20 g) is approximately 2 ml.

In contrast to male rats, male mice sleep longer than females following intraperitoneal administration of pentobarbital (Figs. 26.1 and 26.2). Regardless of the route of administration, dilution of 1 part commercial preparations (50, 60, and 65

TABLE 26.1

Duration of surgical anesthesia and survival of female albino mice (Harlan) after intraperitoneal injection of 0.5% pentobarbital sodium*

Group†	Pentobarbital	Surgical Anesthesia	Survivors	Duration of Surgical Anesthesia in Survivors
	(mg/kg)	*(%)*	*(%)*	*(min)*
1	65	20	90	3.6 (0-8)
2	80	30	100	3.6 (0-19)
3	90	80	80	6.0 (0-20)
4	100	100	70	111.0 (109-115)
5	110	100	40	124.0 (84-168)
6	120	100	20	127.0 (123-132)

* Courtesy of Dolowy, W. C., Mombelloni, P., and Hesse, A. L.: Chlorpromazine premedication with pentobarbital anesthesia in a mouse. Amer. J. Vet. Res. *21:* 156, 1960.

† Ten animals were used in each group.

TABLE 26.2.

Duration of surgical anesthesia and survival rates in female albino mice (Harlan) after injection of chlorpromazine hydrochloride intramuscularly, followed by pentobarbital sodium intraperitoneally 30 minutes later*

Group	No. of Animals	Chlorpro- mazine	Pento- barbital	Surgical Anesthesia	Survivors	Duration of Surgical Anesthesia in Survivors
		(mg/kg)	*(mg/kg)*	*(%)*	*(%)*	*(min)*
7	5	25	40	40	80	82 (0-95)
8	5	50	40	20	80	95 (0-95)
9	30	50	50	80	87	22 (0-51)
10	10	60	50	50	10	17 (0-56)
11	10	60	60	100	80	78 (67-99)

* Courtesy of Dolowy, W. C., Mombelloni, P., and Hesse, A. L.: Chlorpromazine premedication with pentobarbital anesthesia in the mouse. Amer. J. Vet. Res. *21:* 156, 1960.

mg/kg) with 9 parts sterile water or physiological saline is recommended.

The intravenous injection of anesthetic agents in mice through the lateral vein of the tail is difficult, and considerable practice is required to become proficient.[15] Essential to successful venipuncture is a holding device for the animal. Commercial models similar to that described for rats are available (Fig. 26.3). Hand-made models fashioned from large plastic syringes or metal can be used.[32] Once the mouse is secured in the holder, the tail may be immersed in hot water. Another technique that produces a longer period of vasodilation consists of confining the mouse in a plastic cage with a wire top and heating the animal with a 100-W bulb for 10 to 15 minutes. After the dorsolateral

veins of the tail are visible, the tail is bent over the index finger and held with the thumb (Fig. 26.4). A 1-ml tuberculin syringe with a 25- to 27-gauge needle is used for venipuncture. No attempt to aspirate blood into the syringe is made, and care should be taken not to inject air into the animal. Injection of 0.1 ml of air may kill the mouse. The tail is held firmly over the site of injection after administration to prevent extravasation of blood.

Another method for intravenous injections is the placement of the mouse in hardware cloth. The lingual and metatarsal veins also can be used as a site for intravenous injection (Fig. 26.5).

Introduction of general anesthesia with an ether jar and maintenance with a small nose cone have been routine anesthetic

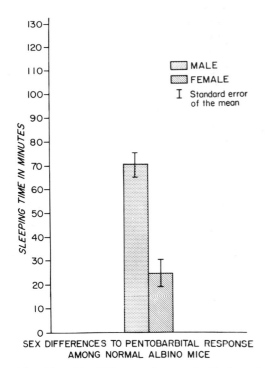

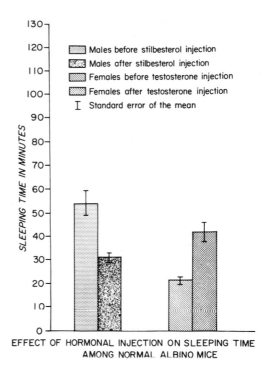

SEX DIFFERENCES TO PENTOBARBITAL RESPONSE
AMONG NORMAL ALBINO MICE

EFFECT OF HORMONAL INJECTION ON SLEEPING TIME
AMONG NORMAL ALBINO MICE

FIG. 26.1. Sex differences in pentobarbital sensitivity indicated by longer sleeping time in male mice (44 animals) compared to females (50 animals). (Courtesy of Westfall, B. A., Boulos, G. M., Shield, F. L., and Garo, S.: Sex differences in pentobarbital sensitivity in mice. Proc. Soc. Exp. Biol. Med. *115:* 509, 1964.)

FIG. 26.2. Male mice (10 animals) pretreated with stilbestrol slept less than control males (10 animals). Female mice (10 animals) pretreated with testosterone slept longer than control females (10 animals). (Courtesy of Westfall, B. A., Boulos, G. M., Shield, F. L., and Garo, S.: Sex differences in pentobarbitol sensitivity in mice. Proc. Soc. Exp. Biol. Med. *115:* 509, 1964.)

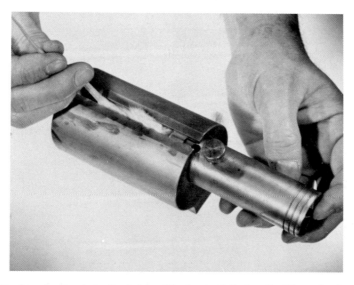

FIG. 26.3. Positioning of a mouse in the holder. The top is slotted so that the animal can be placed in the cylinder quickly and easily. The setscrew in the nosepiece is tightened when the animal is in position. (Courtesy of Stoner, R. D., Brookhaven National Laboratory, Upton, Long Island, N.Y.)

techniques for mice in many laboratories.[1] Mortalities as high as 50% can be expected when major surgery is performed following this type of anesthesia. Mice salivate profusely when exposed to ether. Endotracheal intubation can be performed in mice, but the rat or guinea pig usually is preferred for procedures which necessitate artificial ventilation.

Marked differences have been noted in response to anesthetic agents between inbred strains of mice,[8] and certain

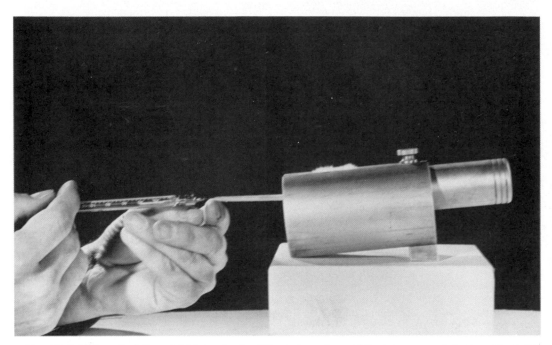

FIG. 26.4. Either the left or right lateral vein of the tail can be used for intravenous injection. The tail is bent over the index finger to facilitate insertion of a 25-, 26-, or 27-gauge needle. (Courtesy of Stoner, R. D., Brookhaven National Laboratory.)

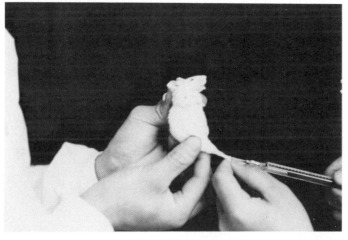

FIG. 26.5. Techniques of intravenous injection via the metatarsal vein of the mouse. (Courtesy of Nobunaga, T., Nabamura, K., and Imamichi, T.: A method for intravenous injection and collection of blood from rats without restraint and anesthesia. Lab. Anim. Care 16: 40, 1966.)

strains (C_3H, C_cHf, A, HR) were more susceptible to accidental exposure to chloroform.[18] Cyclopropane, halothane, chloroform, ether trichlorethylene, and carbon dioxide in addition to pentobarbital and tribromethanol have been used for general anesthesia in mice.[16]

Methoxyflurane has been used in small rodents. A small gauze sponge is placed in a surgical dressing jar and ¼ to ½ ml of methoxyflurane is applied to the sponge. The animal is removed from the jar after the induction of anesthesia and maintained with a small nose cone. The source of methoxyflurane can also be a standard vaporizer with a carrier gas such as oxygen. Small rodents should be kept warm during and following general anesthesia.

Changes in body temperature will also affect the anesthetic and LD_{50} of pentobarbital in mice.[27] In one study, the sleep dose at 20 C was 90 mg/kg and 105 mg/kg at 30 C. The LD_{50} was 160 mg/kg at 20 C and 234 mg/kg at 30 C in the same study.[44] Injections were given intraperitoneally.

Guinea Pigs

Guinea pigs are clean and easy to handle; however, they are not an ideal animal for anesthetic and surgical studies due to the inaccessibility of superficial veins and their peculiar reactions to certain anesthetic drugs.

HANDLING

Special precautions must be taken to insure that guinea pigs are provided with ample vitamin C. This is provided by adding vitaminc C to the drinking water as well as providing fresh vegetables such as lettuce and cabbage. Animals which are deficient in vitamin C are more susceptible to the effects of anesthetic agents.[6] Guinea pigs are active, alert, and will usually run to the opposite corner when one tries to pick them up. They are picked up by grasping them over the back of the neck with one hand while the other hand is used to support the abdomen and hindquarters (Fig. 26.6). Guinea pigs are one of the more docile laboratory animals.

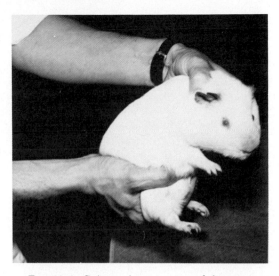

FIG. 26.6. Guinea pigs are removed from a cage or container by grasping them over the back of the neck while the other hand supports the body.

Occasionally older males may bite, and their nails can be long and sharp. Guinea pigs also can be immobilized by rolling them in a towel or placing them in a plastic holder.

CHOICE OF AGENT AND TECHNIQUE

Both volatile and injectable anesthetic agents have been used in guinea pigs.[5] Pentobarbital is probably the most common anesthetic agent in this species.[12] The lack of accessible superficial veins makes it difficult to inject this drug intravenously; however, the marginal vein of the ear and pudic vein in the male have been used (Fig. 26.7).[37]

Pentobarbital is usually administered intraperitoneally. The preferred site of injection is the lower abdomen, using a ½-inch, 24-gauge needle. Dilution of the 6% solutions with an equal quantity of physiological saline is recommended. The inadvertent injection of pentobarbital into the liver, spleen, intestinal tract, bladder, or abdominal fat will result in altered induction or postanesthetic complications. In order to prevent this, the animal should be held in a "head down position."

The anesthetic dose of pentobarbital by the intraperitoneal route varies from 28 to 40 mg/kg.[41] Pentobarbital given intra-

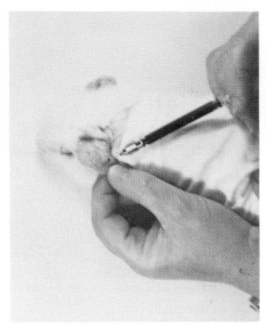

FIG. 26.7. The aural vein can be used as a route for administering anesthetic agents. (Courtesy of Dr. D. Going, Dental Branch, University of Texas, Houston, Texas.)

peritoneally at 37 mg/kg induced anesthesia within 15 minutes and lasted an average of 21 minutes.[19]

The duration of surgical anesthesia was lengthened when chlorpromazine (25 mg/kg) was administered intramuscularly prior to the intraperitoneal injection of pentobarbital (30 mg/kg).[19] The induction time remained the same, but the duration of surgical anesthesia was increased to 49.6 minutes. Smaller doses of either chlorpromazine (10 mg/kg) or pentobarbital (25 mg/kg) did not significantly change the duration of surgical anesthesia. Meperidine was also found to increase the sleeping time induced by pentobarbital in guinea pigs.[41]

The lethal dose of pentobarbital intraperitoneally in guinea pigs varies from 45 to 70 mg/kg.[11, 41] Young animals are less sensitive to the toxic effects of pentobarbital than older animals.[11] The use of pentobarbital, 28 and 40 mg/kg, for cesarean sections in pregnant guinea pigs resulted in postnatal apnea, and a number of the newborn required resuscitation following delivery.[4] Neurological sequelae such as piloerection, incoordinate gait, delayed righting, etc. were observed in the neonates. They recovered within a week, and survivors after this time were comparable to young that were born from placebo-injected mothers. Newborn young which were heavily anesthetized shortly after birth exhibited signs that were similar to changes observed in cesarian deliveries under pentobarbital. The neurological manifestations closely resembled guinea pigs in which the umbilical or uterine vessels were occluded prior to delivery.[3]

Ether stimulates a copious secretion in this species and necessitates the prior administration of atropine. The dose of atropine (0.25 mg) is higher than that recommended for most species. Following premedication, anesthesia can be induced in an ether jar or by the use of a face mask. A peculiar "squirming" movement is sometimes encountered in animals which have been anesthetized with volatile agents. It does not signify return of consciousness and additional anesthetic should not be administered. The trachea in guinea pigs, as in other rodents, is not easy to intubate.

Inhalation anesthetic agents such as nitrous oxide, halothane, and trichlorethylene have been used in guinea pigs. Inhalant anesthetic agents require no preanesthetic medication.[37] Animals do not appear unduly excited during the induction of anesthesia with halothane or methoxyflurane, and there is minimal salivation. The inhalation agents can be delivered to a small face mask from a vaporizer. Recovery occurs in 30 to 40 minutes after cessation of administration. When open chest surgery is performed, the trachea may be exposed or artificial respiration administered through an endotracheal tube.

Techniques using pediatric anesthesia equipment which have been described for smaller pet animals can also be adopted for use in laboratory mammals (see Chapter 17).

Carbon dioxide can be used to provide short periods of anesthesia for cardiac puncture and inoculation.[39] General anesthesia is induced in 10 to 15 seconds and lasts for about 45 seconds. Carbon dioxide also increases the yield of blood which can be obtained.[47]

Rats

Rats are extremely important laboratory animals, and have been used in almost every field of biomedical research. Rats adapt rapidly to a new environment and are very prolific.[33]

Black and cotton rats are generally more excitable or even aggressive, and must be handled with special care, while other, e.g., Sprague-Dawley or Wistar strains, are usually docile. Rats should not be picked up by their tails, but may be immobilized by the tail and picked up by grasping them by the shoulders. Some prefer to place the thumb under the animal's chin. They may be further examined and manipulated by rolling them in a towel or placing them in a transparent plastic restraining device. Gloves are not necessary to handle albino rats with the occasional exception of older male animals.

ANESTHETIC AGENTS AND TECHNIQUES

Pentobarbital sodium, ether, and other inhalation agents have been used successfully in rats. The method of administration of these and other agents will vary depending on the nature of the studies

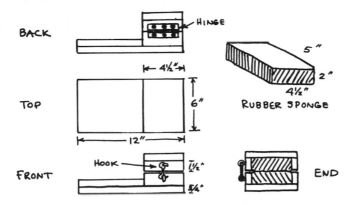

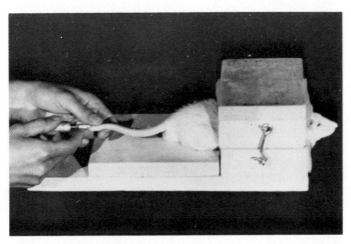

FIG. 26.8. Specifications for construction of a rat-holding device. (Courtesy of Abildgaard, C. F.: A simple apparatus for holding rats. Lab. Anim. Care *14:* 235, 1964.)

which are being undertaken, the previous experience of the investigator, and equipment available.

The intraperitoneal and intravenous routes are the most common for pentobarbital. The technique of intraperitoneal administration is similar to that recommended for guinea pigs. Anesthesia ensues in 5 to 15 minutes and is effective for 45 minutes. If the initial intraperitoneal dose is inadequate, ¼ of the original calculated dose can be administered in 45 minutes. The dose of pentobarbital, for both intravenous and intraperitoneal administration, is 30 mg/kg for light anesthesia and 40 mg/kg for longer and deeper anesthesia. Strain differences should always be considered, and the above recommendations should only be used as guidelines. Doses of 25 to 60 mg/kg have been used. Lethal doses (LD_{50}) have ranged from 48 to 75 mg/kg in one study,[34] and 90 to 100 mg/kg in another study.[17] The variation is probably due to age, weight, sex, and strain differences.

The long tail veins of the rat provide an excellent route for administration of intravenous anesthetics. The rat may be immobilized by rolling it in a towel. Plastic, metal, or wooden restraining devices can also be used (Fig. 26.8). Routes for the intravenous administration of drugs are shown in Figure 26.9, A, B, and C.

Immersing the tail or foot in warm water or holding it near a heat lamp will dilate the vessels and aid insertion of needle. A 20-gauge syringe needle may be inserted into the caudal vein without difficulty. A thin walled 19-gauge needle can be used to aid in the placement of an indwelling polyethylene catheter. The catheter can be sutured in place to prevent dislodging. Premedication with chlorpromazine will prolong pentobarbital anesthesia in the rat.[20]

Inhalation techniques and agents described for the guinea pig can also be used for the rat. Endotracheal intubation can be performed in the rat with the aid of balloon-shaped stainless steel oval speculum to facilitate the visualization of the larynx (Fig. 26.10).[40]

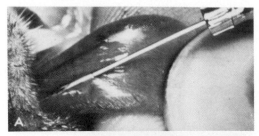
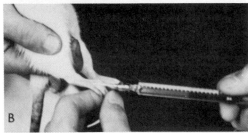
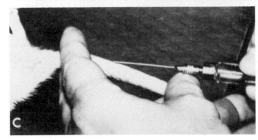

FIG. 26.9. Injection via the lingual vein (A), metatarsal vein (B), and caudal vein (C). (Courtesy of Nobunaga, T., Nabamura, K., and Imamichi, T.: A method for intravenous injection and collection of blood from rats without restraint and anesthesia. Lab. Anim. Care 16: 40, 1966.)

Rabbits

Rabbits are docile and easy to restrain, although they are not an ideal species for anesthetic or surgical research. The dose of intravenous anesthetic agents varies from one rabbit to another and in the same rabbit at different times.[30] The margin of safety between the anesthetic and lethal doses of pentobarbital or thiopental for this species is less than for other rodents and carnivores. Maintaining the animal in a lighter plane of anesthesia with the aid of narcotic analgesics or volatile agents may reduce the mortality.

RESTRAINT

Rabbits are gentle animals; however, if they are not restrained properly the han-

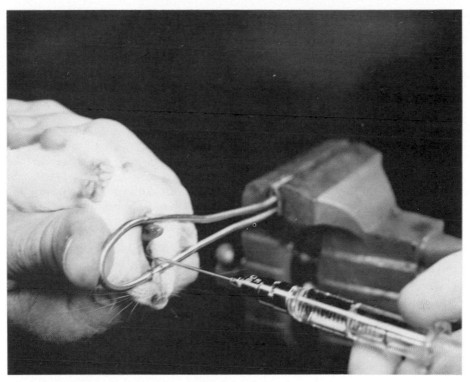

FIG. 26.10. A stainless steel wire firmly held in a vise can be used as an oral speculum to facilitate endotracheal intubation. The animal is moved laterally toward the wide part of the loop to obtain better exposure of the oral pharynx. (Courtesy of Kessel.[40])

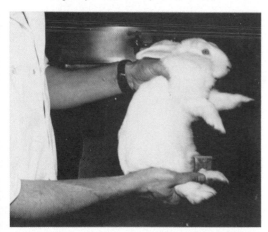

FIG. 26.11. A convenient method of transporting rabbits without the risk of injury to the animal or attendant consists of stabilizing the body with one hand around the shoulders while the other hand is used to support the body.

dler can be badly scratched by the powerful hind legs. A convenient method of removing rabbits is to grasp the animal over the shoulders with one hand while the other hand is used to support the hind legs and body (Fig. 26.13). Small rabbits can be immobilized and lifted by grasping them over the back caudal to the diaphragm with the palm of the hand pressed against the fur. Large rabbits may be lifted by placing the hands under the abdomen from opposite sides. The rabbit should not be lifted by the ears.

Rabbits may be placed in a somnolent state which resembles hypnosis by a manipulative and vocal procedure.[43] This is done by rhythmically stroking the abdomen and speaking in a low soothing monotone (Fig. 26.12).

ANESTHETIC AGENTS AND TECHNIQUES

There is no completely satisfactory method of anesthetizing rabbits. The margin of safety or difference between the anesthetic dose and the dose producing respiratory arrest appears very small in

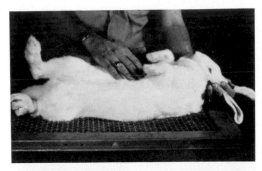

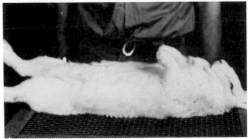

FIG. 26.12. The rabbit is "hypnotized" by rhythmically stroking the abdomen and speaking in a low soothing monotone. When the rabbit is in the somnolent state, it is relaxed and remains motionless without restraint. Procedures such as subcutaneous, intravenous, or intramuscular injections may be carried out without evidence of pain or need for further restraint. (Courtesy of Rapson.[43])

some animals and these two endpoints seem to be reached simultaneously.

The most common anesthetic agent for general anesthesia in rabbits is pentobarbital, although the thiobarbiturates or certain volatile agents are undoubtedly superior. The large superficial ear vein is plainly visible, and one person can anesthetize the animal without assistance when it is confined in an appropriate holding or restraint box (Fig. 26.13). These boxes are available from commercial sources or can be easily constructed. Feline restraint boxes or bags are also satisfactory. Equipment that allows the rabbit to be removed before it is completely anesthetized is more serviceable since it is difficult to evaluate the depth of anesthesia in restraining devices. Metal equipment can be sanitized easily. Many mechanical means of restraint do not prevent the rabbit from shaking its head so that if the first attempt is unsuccessful, it will

become increasingly difficult to induce anesthesia by the intravenous route. The application of xylene results in venous dilation facilitating venipuncture. Quiet handling of the rabbit, dilution of the barbiturate to a 2 to 3% solution, use of 22- to 25-gauge needles, and a slow induction after the initial relaxing dose are recommended for successful anesthesia. Pressure should be applied over the vein following withdrawal of the needle. Accidental perivascular injection of a barbiturate should be followed by infiltration with procaine hydrochloride or saline.

The cephalic vein of the foreleg has been used to inject barbiturates by the intravenous route in a manner similar to that used for dogs and cats. A 22- to 25-gauge needle, depending on the size of the rabbit, is used. Standard digital and palpebral reflexes along with rate and depth of respiration are employed to evaluate the depth of anesthesia. There are subtle differences in those signs between rabbits and other species. The depth and rate of respiration are the most reliable means of predicting impending difficulties. The duration of surgical anesthesia following the intravenous administration of thiamylal is approximately 10 minutes.[30] Prolongation of the anesthetic period can be effected by increasing the induction time. The anesthetic period following the intra-

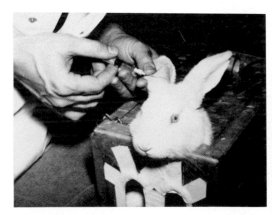

FIG. 26.13. Intravenous injection of a barbiturate via the ear vein. A holding or restraining box that is demountable or permits removal of the animal will facilitate the final evaluation of the level of anesthesia.

venous injection of pentobarbital may be too short for many surgical procedures, and it will be necessary to administer additional pentobarbital or inhalant anesthetic.

The anesthetic and lethal intravenous doses of pentobarbital for rabbits are approximately 30 to 35 mg/kg and 60 to 70 mg/kg, respectively. There is a marked variability in the response to pentobarbital, and one author found the intravenous anesthetic dose to vary from 7 to 83 mg/kg with an average of 45 mg/kg.[42] The technique of intraperitoneal injection into the caudal quadrant of the peritoneal cavity resembles that described for the guinea pig and other small rodents. This route cannot be recommended as the sole means of administration of anesthetic due to the great variation in dose required by rabbits. Atropine (0.5 mg) should be given for premedication.

The ultra short acting intravenous barbiturates (thiamylal or thiopental) should be given slowly and to effect. If given carefully with constant observation of changes in heart rate, respiration, and degree of relaxation, a high degree of success can be achieved. A calculated amount of any barbiturate should not be administered to rabbits and doses established in one laboratory for a given strain should be used only as a guideline.

Pentobarbital results in a short anesthetic period, and, because of this, other agents have been investigated. The anesthetic doses of urethane in the rabbit, as in the dog and cat, are approximately 750 mg/kg intravenously and 1500 mg/kg intraperitoneally.[11, 25, 33] Variation in the required dose is great but less than with the barbiturates. The lethal dose of urethane by intravenous injection in rabbits is approximately 2000 mg/kg.[26] It is thought that urethane has a wider margin of safety than pentobarbital in rabbits,[9] but due to the long recovery period, 36 hours or more, delayed deaths due to postanesthetic complications occur.

Ether anesthesia has been used in rabbits for many years, but it does not appear to be the anesthetic of choice. Rabbits metabolize atropine more rapidly than other animals, and doses are required at more frequent intervals.[31] The rabbit's trachea has been intubated using the technique similar to that reported in rats, mice, and guinea pigs, but this is not easily accomplished. Methoxyflurane, halothane, and trichlorethylene with nitrous oxide have been used with success in rabbits.[45] The preanesthetic dose of chlorpromazine in the rabbit is 1 to 5 mg/kg.

Hamsters

Hamsters, namely Chinese and Syrian, are newcomers to the laboratory, and they are used primarily in studies of infectious agents. Hamsters are not always docile laboratory animals. To avoid being bitten, one seizes the animal firmly by the back of the neck. Subcutaneous or intramuscular injections can be made with the opposite hand. Intraperitoneal injection is accomplished by holding the animal by the loose dorsal skin with the left hand so that the abdominal skin is tense and facing the needle. The site of injection is ½ to 1 cm above the pubis in the lateral abdominal wall.

Following the administration of morphine to hamsters, analgesia is present without apparent narcosis or respiratory depression.[14, 38] These species appear unique in this regard.

CHOICE OF AGENT AND TECHNIQUE

Ether alone or following ethyl chloride has been used in hamsters.[48] Prior to anesthesia with injectable or volatile anesthetics, atropine, 0.1 to 0.25 mg/lb is recommended. Methods described for the administration of inhalation agents in other small laboratory animals can be used for the hamster.

If surgery is performed, one should remember that penicillin will produce delayed illness and death in hamsters.[29] In guinea pigs, similar deaths are thought to be due to proliferation of gram-negative bacteria in the intestinal tract.[23]

Chinchillas

Chinchillas, small rodents from the Andes, have been raised in large numbers

for their pelts and are exceptionally valuable for breeding purposes. Their use as a
laboratory animal has been limited. Chinchillas are delicate animals and do not
appear to sustain diseases or the stresses
of the laboratory as well as other rodents.
They are very docile but some animals
will bite if the opportunity is provided.
One method of handling chinchillas is to
grasp the animal at the base of the tail
and pull the animal while the other hand
is maneuvered behind the head.

CHOICE OF AGENT AND TECHNIQUE

Ether produces salivation which may
result in postoperative respiratory complications and death, if not preceded by
atropine. The intravenous dose of pentobarbital is 30 mg/kg but may have to be
decreased or increased depending on the
physical status of the animal. Chinchillas
recover rapidly from pentobarbital and
usually do not remain under surgical
anesthesia for more than 30 minutes. The
intraperitoneal route of administering
pentobarbital is not as reliable but has
been used.

Meperidine, 10 to 15 mg by intramuscular injection, can be used as a preanesthetic agent in chinchillas. For short periods of anesthesia, thiopental has been
employed.

Mink

Mink are not domestic animals and
should be respected for their nervousness,
speed, and viciousness. Mink cages are
constructed so that the animal can be
forced from the nest box into a carrying
box, wire cage, or metal tube with a minimum of physical restraint. In some instances, a box trap is placed in the pen.
This may be constructed so that a gloved
hand can be inserted to grasp the animal
(Fig. 26.14). Mink can be forced from the
nest box into carrying cages by blowing
into the animal's face or lured out by
scratching on the side of the nest box. The
gloves or mittens usually consist of an
outer leather or heavy cloth cover. The
inner glove or mitten is made of soft cloth
which permits greater flexibility.

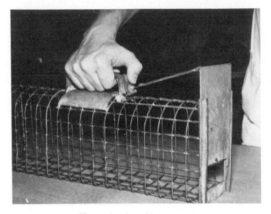

FIG. 26.14. Trap for handling mink. The door of
the trap can be opened and closed remotely from the
handle.

An alternate method is to run the animal from the nest box into a tapered
sleeve which is about 2 feet in length. A
metal tube with one end covered with wire
or a metal funnel has been used for inhalation anesthesia, vaginal smears, and
other techniques. Sacs and other devices
have been designed for special examination.[10] Some mink breeders employ specially designed cages or boxes which are
provided with an adjustable bottom and
allow the animal to be squeezed against
the top to facilitate manipulation or
the administration of drugs.

CHOICE OF AGENT AND TECHNIQUE

The intraperitoneal dose of pentobarbital is 36 mg/kg in young vigorous animals.
The actual injection can be made while
the animal is held by an assistant or
pressed against the wire of the cage. Low
doses of pentobarbital (10 mg for a 1- to 2-
lb mink) can be given intraperitoneally for
sedation.[28] This can be followed by additional injections or inhalation anesthesia.
Subcutaneous injection of pentobarbital,
22 mg/kg, has been used to facilitate examination and artificial insemination of
mink.[28] Small bore plastic artificial insemination tubes can be used to inject
liquid preparations into the stomach.
Sedatives and hypnotics could be administered in this manner. Mink can be anesthetized with inhalation agents by forcing

the muzzle into a small face mask or by placing them in an anesthetization chamber.

Weasels, martens, wolverine, fishers, badgers, and other mustelids behave similarly to mink.[36] The larger fisher, wolverine, and bader requires special techniques for handling due to their greater strength and capacity to inflict damage. Intraperitoneal injection of pentobarbital, intramuscular injections of sedative drugs, through the bars of a squeeze cage or administration of volatile agents by means of an anesthetization chamber as outlined for undomesticated cats is recommended for these mammals rather than manual restraint (see Chapter 30).

Skunks

Skunks are one of the most easily domesticated wild animals. They are naturally friendly, easy to tame, affectionate, and playful. Although they are not commonly used as a laboratory animal, many are kept as pets. Patience and knowledge of these animals is necessary to handle, restrain, and anesthetize them without becoming scented.

RESTRAINT

At 5 to 6 weeks of age, skunks can be handled and anesthetized with little danger of scenting the surgeon or the environs. It is probable that their defensive mechanisms are not fully developed until after weaning. Scenting fluid is present but it does not appear as tenacious, and young skunks can be handled without ejecting. Fluid from young skunks is similar to that of older animals but can be removed easily with soap and water, while the fluid of older animals can be removed only with great effort.

In older animals that have not been descented, handling requires infinitely more alertness and finesse. Ordinarily they will not scent unless frightened, cornered, or rapidly approached. The effective range which an adult skunk can spray varies between 10 and 20 feet, and they are exceedingly accurate within this distance. They must be "set" to express their scent glands, and if they can be kept moving or picked up by the tail, they can be prevented from ejecting their scent. Once the animal is suspended by its tail it is unable to eject.

CHOICE OF AGENT AND TECHNIQUE

Pentobarbital can be administered intraperitoneally in dilute solution. The veins are difficult to find, and the hazard of being scented is too great to use the intravenous route. The dosage is approximately 30 mg/kg as for other small carnivores. Some animals may require supplemental anesthesia. A 22- to 25-gauge needle is advised, and the preferred site is the lower abdomen to avoid intrahepatic or intrasplenic injection. The onset of action is rapid and full effect can be expected in 20 minutes, but in some animals the action is more rapid. Pentobarbital may be included in the food, but 1 or 2 hours may elapse before the full effect is manifest; there is greater danger of vomiting with this method than in the fasted animal, and it is difficult to control the depth of anesthesia. A greater mortality can be anticipated in young skunks 4 to 5 weeks old.

Preanesthetic medication consisting of promazine (4.4 mg/kg) and meperidine (10 mg/kg) produces sedation in the skunk. Although animals with this premedication are easier to handle, they can be aroused. Succinylcholine (0.20 to 0.26 mg/kg) has been administered successfully to skunks.[22]

Ferrets

Ferrets become very tame if they are handled frequently and leather gloves or tongs usually are not necessary. The preferred method is to grasp them firmly about the neck with one hand while the other hand is used to support the abdomen and pelvic limbs. Another technique is to grasp and remove the ferret from its cage by the tail. It is then placed on top of the cage where it will pull in the opposite direction. The animal then can be grasped around the neck with the opposite hand.

CHOICE OF AGENT AND TECHNIQUE

The intraperitoneal dose of pentobarbital varies from 35 to 58 mg/kg.[27] The lesser dose is adequate in most instances.[21] The duration of anesthesia is 30 to 45 minutes followed by a recovery period of 3 to 4 hours. The margin of safety is reported to be small. The cephalic or recurrent tarsal vein can be used for intravenous administration.

Inhalation anesthetic agents have been used in this species, utilizing techniques previously described for other laboratory mammals (see Chapter 17).

Foxes

In general, foxes are fearful and nonaggressive toward man and can be handled easily. Most mature foxes, e.g., red, black, silver, or Arctic, weigh from 10 to 12 pounds and can be caught with or without the use of leather gloves by grasping and swinging them off the ground by the tail with one hand while they are seized by the neck with other hand. A fox which is suspended in the air by its tail is comparatively helpless and ordinarily will not curl up and bite. Restraining the fox by the neck enables a general examination. Obviously this free hand technique should be practiced only by those familiar with foxes. An alternate method of restraint consists of grasping the fox by the neck with tongs or snare.[24] However, the animal may bite the wood or metal and injure its mouth. Leather gloves are helpful in handling young pups. Once the fox is held by the neck, it is not difficult to induce anesthesia via the intravenous route or inhalation anesthesia with a cone or mask. Muzzling may be necessary with some animals. Larger doses of preanesthetic agents are required to produce sedation or tranquility in wild animals than in their domestic cousins. Morphine may be used although unfavorable responses have been observed.[32] Sedation can be obtained in 20 to 30 minutes following the intramuscular administration of 1 to 4 mg/kg of promazine in feral foxes.[7]

The intravenous barbiturates are administered to the fox in a manner and dose similar to the dog, and techniques for inhalation anesthesia used in the dog can be applied to foxes.

Exotic Animals

The need for restraint and anesthesia in Canidae other than the dog and fox (e.g., wolf, dingo, coyote, jackal, and wild dog) and in Hyaenidae (e.g., hyena and aardwolf) arises primarily in zoos. Adult animals are larger and more vicious than foxes, so that methods outlined for these species do not apply. The use of a squeeze cage is most helpful. Narcotics or tranquilizers in doses slightly in excess of those recommended for dogs are advised; this is to minimize injury to the animals and hazards to attending personnel. Anesthetic methods and agents discussed for dogs, bears, and undomesticated cats should be consulted for details. Some members of the marsupial group such as the Tasmanian devil and Tasmanian wolf can be handled in a manner similar to the Canidae.

Chlorpromazine (100 mg) has been used prior to inducing anesthesia in a kangaroo with nitrous oxide-ether and oxygen. Promazine (4.4 mg/kg) by intravenous route has been used to quiet a wallaby.[35] Intravenous administration of pentobarbital via the recurrent tarsal vein has also been used for kangaroos and wallabies. The coccygeal vein on the lateral aspects of the tail may be used as a route of injection. Quokkas have been anesthetized by intraperitoneal injection of pentobarbital (80 to 100 mg/kg) and amobarbital (90 mg/kg).

Two other families, the Viverridae (e.g., civet cat, palm civet, genet, binturong, and mongoose) and the Procyonidae (e.g., raccoon, kinkajou, cacomistle, coati, and raccoon-like dog) are handled in a manner similar to that of the Mustelidae and are described under "Mink."

Raccoons can be sedated with ataractic agents such as chlorpromazine or promazine. They can be administered intramuscularly or subcutaneously and are relatively safe if the dose does not exceed 5 mg/kg. Meperidine (11 mg/kg) can also be used safely in raccoons. Small doses of phencyclidine, 1 to 2 mg/kg, produce calmness while larger doses approaching 4 mg/kg will produce marked sedation.[46] Unpremedicated raccoons require about the same amount (30 to 35 mg/kg) of pentobarbital as dogs. Supplement injection via veins in the limbs may be used to reach a deeper plane of anesthesia.

Wild rodents vary from small squirrels, chipmunks, prairie dogs, muskrats, gerbils, agouti, and gophers to the larger beaver, capybara, nutria, paca, and porcupine. It is difficult to find any detailed information on the anesthesia of these animals and, presumably, they can be handled like other wild animals, the specific method used depending upon size.

The armadillo represents the edentates which include the anteater, aardvark, pangolin, and sloth.[2] Ether, pentobarbital, and thiopental have been employed as anesthetic agents in these species.[13]

REFERENCES

1. Ambrus, J. L., Ambrus, C. M., Harrison, P. W. E., Moser, C. E., and Cravitz, H.: Comparison of methods for obtaining blood from mice. Amer. J. Pharm. 123: 100, 1951
2. Anderson, J. M., and Benirschke, K.: The armadillo, Dasypus novemcinctus in experimental biology. Lab. Anim. Care 16: 202, 1966.
3. Becker, R. F., and Donnell, W.: Learning behavior in guinea pigs subjected to asphyxia at birth. J. Comp. Physiol. Psychol. 45: 153, 1952.
4. Becker, R. F., Flannagan, E., and King, J. E.: The fate of offspring from mothers receiving sodium pentobarbital before delivery. A study in the guinea pig. Neurology (Minneap.) 8: 776, 1958.
5. Bernstein, I. L., and Agee, J.: Successful lobectomy in the guinea pig. Lab. Anim. Care 14: 519, 1964.
6. Beyer, K. H., Stutzman, J. W., and Hafford, B.: The relation of vitamin C to anesthesia. Surg. Gynec. Obstet. 79: 49, 1944.
7. Blackmore, D. K.: Problems encountered in attempting to anesthetize and sedate British wild foxes (Vulpes vulpes). In Small Animal Anesthesia, p. 191. The Macmillan Company, New York, 1964.
8. Borselleca, J. F., and Manthei, R. W.: Factors influencing pentobarbital sleeping time in mice. Arch. Int. Pharmacodyn. 111: 296, 1957.
9. Bree, M., and Cohen, B.: Effects of urethane anesthesia on blood and blood vessels in rabbits. Lab. Anim. Care 15: 254, 1965.
10. Campbell, R. S.: Artificial breeding of mink. Amer. Fur Breeder 12: 25, 1940.
11. Carmichael, E. B., and Posey, L. C.: Nembutal anesthesia. I. Toxicity of Nembutal (pentobarbital sodium) for guinea pigs. Anesth. Analg. (Cleveland) 16: 156, 1937.
12. Carmichael, E. B., and Posey, L. C.: Nembutal anesthesia. II. Some observations on the effect of repeated administration of Nembutal (pentobarbital sodium) in guinea pigs. Anesth. Analg. (Cleveland) 16: 199, 1937.
13. Chambers, E. E.: Anesthesia and surgery in the monkey and ant-eater. North Amer. Vet. 26: 731, 1945.
14. Chen, K. K., Powel, C. E., and Maze, N.: The response of the hamster to drugs. J. Pharmacol. Exp. Ther. 85: 348, 1945.
15. Croft, P. G.: An Introduction to the Anesthesia of Laboratory Animals. Universities Federation for Animal Welfare, London, 1960.
16. Davey, D. G.: The use of pathogen-free animals. Proc. Roy. Soc. Med. 55: 256, 1962.
17. DeBoer, B.: Effects of thiamine hydrochloride upon pentobarbital sodium ("Nembutal") hypnosis and mortality in normal, castrated and fasting rats. J. Amer. Pharm. Ass. 37: 302, 1948.
18. Deringer, M. K., Dunn, T. B., and Heston, W. E.: Results of exposure of strain C_3H mice to chloroform. Proc. Soc. Exp. Biol. Med. 83: 474, 1953.
19. Dolowy, W. C., and Hesse, A. L.: Chlorpromazine premedication with pentobarbital anesthesia in guinea pig. Illinois Vet. 3: 112, 1960.
20. Dolowy, W. C., Thompson, I. D., and Hesse, A. L.: Chlorpromazine premedication with pentobarbital anesthesia in the rat. Lab. Anim. Care 9: 93, 1959.
21. Donovan, B. T.: Anesthesia of the ferret. In Small Animal Anesthesia, p. 185. The Macmillan Company, New York, 1964.
22. Dyson, R. F.: Experience with succinyl choline chloride in zoo animals. Int. Zool. Year Book 5: 205, 1965.
23. Farrar, W. E., Jr., and Kent, T. H.: Enteritis and coliform bacteremia in guinea pigs given penicillin. Amer. J. Path. 47: 629, 1965.
24. Fitch, J. A.: Care and handling of the fox. North Amer. Vet. 19: 17, 1938.
25. Florey, H., and Marvin, H. M.: The blood-pressure reflexes of the rabbit under urethane anesthesia. J. Physiol. 64: 318, 1927.
26. Flury, F.: Abderhalden's Handbuch. Cited by Spector, W. S.: Handbook of Toxicology, vol. I. W. B. Saunders Company, Philadelphia, 1956.
27. Fuhrman, F. A.: The effect of body temperature on the duration of barbiturate anesthesia in mice. Science 105: 387, 1947.
28. Fuhrman, F. A., and Stuhr, E. T.: Pentobarbi-

tal sodium as an anesthetic for minks. J. Amer. Vet. Med. Ass. *98:* 43, 1941.

29. Gage, J. C.: The variation in the susceptibility of mice to certain anesthetics. Quart. J. Pharm. Pharmacol. *6:* 418, 1933.

30. Gardner, A.: The development of general anesthesia in the albino rabbit for surgical procedures. Lab. Anim. Care *14:* 214, 1964.

31. Godeaux, J., and Tonnesen, M.: Investigations into atropine metabolism in animal organism. Acta Pharmacol. (Kobenhavn) *5:* 95, 1949.

32. Grice, H. C.: Methods for obtaining blood and for intravenous injections in laboratory animals. Lab. Anim. Care *14:* 483, 1964.

33. Griffith, J. I., and Farris, E. J.: *The Rat in Laboratory Investigation.* J. B. Lippincott Company, Philadelphia, 1942.

34. Gruber, C. M., Ellis, F. W., and Freedman, G.: A toxicological and pharmacological investigation of sodium sec-butyl ethyl barbituric acid (Butisol sodium). J. Pharmacol. Exp. Ther. *81:* 254, 1944.

35. Heuschele, W. P.: Experiences with promazine in captive wild animals. Biochem. Rev. *29:* 3, 1959.

36. Heuschele, W. P., and Gandal, C. P.: Handling and treatment of common exotic mammal pets. J. Amer. Vet. Med. Ass. *138:* 608, 1961.

37. Hoar, R. M.: Anesthetic technics of the rat and guinea pig. In *Experimental Animal Anesthesiology,* p. 325. U.S.Air Force School of Aerospace Medicine, Aerospace Medical Division (AFSC), Brooks Air Force Base, San Antonio, Texas, July 1965.

38. Houchin, O. B.: Toxin levels of morphine for the hamster. Proc. Soc. Exp. Biol. Med. *54:* 339, 1943.

39. Hyde, J. L.: The use of solid carbon dioxide for producing short periods of anesthesia in guinea pigs. Amer. J. Vet. Res. *23:* 684, 1962.

40. Kessel, H.: A simple aid in the intubation of small animals. Lab. Anim. Care *14:* 499, 1964.

41. Maykut, M. O.: The combined action of pentobarbital and meperidine and of procaine and meperidine in guinea pigs. Canad. Anaesth. Soc. J. *5:* 161, 1958.

42. Pinschmidt, N. W., Ramsey, H., and Haag, H. B.: Studies on the antagonism of sodium succinate to barbiturate depression. J. Pharmacol. Exp. Ther. *83:* 45, 1945.

43. Rapson, W. S., and Jones, T. C.: Restraint of rabbits by hypnosis. Lab. Anim. Care *14:* 131, 1964.

44. Raventos, J.: The influence of room temperatures on the action of barbiturates. J. Pharmacol. Exp. Ther. *64:* 355, 1938.

45. Stevenson, D. E.: Inhalation anesthesia in rabbits, guinea pigs and hamsters. In *Small Animal Anesthesia,* p. 109. The Macmillan Company, New York, 1964.

46. Stoliker, H. E.: The physiological and pharmacological effects of Sernylan: a review. In *Experimental Animal Anesthesiology.* U.S. Air Force School of Aerospace Medicine, Aerospace Medical Division (AFSC), Brooks Air Force Base, San Antonio, Texas, July 1965.

47. Stone, W. S., Amirian, K., Duell, C., and Schadler, C.: Carbon dioxide anesthetization of guinea pigs to increase yields of blood and serum. Lab. Anim. Care *11:* 299, 1961.

48. Worden, A. N., and Lane-Petter, W.: *The UFAW Handbook on the Care and Management of Laboratory Animals.* Universities Federation for Animal Welfare, London, 1957.

27
Restraint and Anesthesia of Subhuman Primates

DONALD CLIFFORD

Restraint and sedation of primates are grouped arbitrarily under the headings of (a) small monkeys that can be handled with gloves and (b) large primates such as baboons and chimpanzees which weigh more than 10 kg and usually require special facilities and techniques.

There are many aspects of the care and management of monkeys that set them apart from other animals. Small monkeys are often timid and must be handled carefully. The macaques and other old world monkeys appear to be resistant to the stress of handling, usually reproduce in captivity, and adapt better to a new diet and environment. Large baboons, chimpanzees, and the rhesus are potentially dangerous primates, and at least two people should be present when they are removed from their cages, treated, or handled in any manner. A squeeze cage may be necessary to manage these larger animals. Attempts should be made to handle primates gently and quietly with as few people as are necessary to accomplish the task. Familiar surroundings and faces are less apt to excite these animals. Protective clothing, specialized equipment, and trained personnel are required.

The viral diseases of subhuman primates are particularly important since these animals are reservoirs of several agents which are pathogenic for man; pox virus, B virus, enteroviruses, adenoviruses, and the virus of infectious hepatitis of chimpanzees are notable examples. Whenever monkeys or apes are kept in close proximity to man, tuberculosis must be considered and proper facilities maintained for isolation, testing and acclimatization of new arrivals to the colony.

Before undertaking an investigation in which medium sized monkeys are required, an investigator should consider whether it might be advantageous to use the more expensive but docile stump-tailed macaques (*Macaca speciosa*) rather than the cheaper rhesus monkeys. Physiologically these two species are very similar,[15] but it should be remembered that the gentle stump-tailed macaques become more difficult to handle as they become older. Information is available on the comparative anatomy and physiology of the various subhuman primates.[14, 26, 31, 34]

Physical Restraint

There is great variation and, understandingly, some overlapping in the preanesthetic sedation and methods needed for restraint in various subhuman primates, depending on species, size, age, and sex.

Small monkeys can be manipulated by one person with gloves while the anthropoid apes require special holding devices, ancillary equipment, and possibly drugs

385

for sedation. Young gorillas, for example, although approximately the same size as a chimpanzee, are often very affectionate and can be handled easily while an adult male chimpanzee is a potentially dangerous animal. Dominant males in a gang cage and nursing females often will resist when restrained. Certain macaques and baboons, as well as other species, are untrustworthy and vicious. These individuals should not be included in chronic experiments. Some species (e.g., Vervet) rarely attack humans if grasped by the tail, whereas this would be an invitation to disaster in some other species.

Owners, keepers, or attendants can furnish valuable insight as to the personality of primates under their care. Before attempting to handle an animal, it is often helpful to clean the quarters in a routine manner, removing food and other items. It is most important that everything be well planned in advance. If there is a delay on the part of an untrained handler, escape of the primate or injury to personnel may occur. Monkeys are difficult to outwit on the second occasion and are masters at removing bolts, opening latches, and finding other ways to freedom. Observation of the animal for alertness, general condition, and review of records may reveal information pertinent to disposition and habits. Physical restraint by direct contact may be considered undesirable, and, with proper equipment, e.g., squeeze cages and anesthetization chambers, subhuman primates can be restrained and anesthetized without physical contact.[12] Cages with restraining or squeeze devices are available from several manufacturers.

SMALL MONKEYS

Small monkeys have become common pets as well as one of the most desirable laboratory animals. The basic handling does not vary essentially between the pet and laboratory specimen once they have been confined by the owner or animal attendant. Frequently owners or laboratory attendants place collars about the neck or abdomen to control these small primates. People responsible for these animals have usually gained their confidence through feeding and general care so that they may be able to restrain them easily. In many instances they can be made to extend an arm for a venipuncture or intramuscular injection, but, more commonly, greater physical restraint may be necessary. Both arms can be held behind the back with one hand (elbow lock) while the hind leg and tail are held with the other hand (Fig. 27.1). An alternate technique is to hold both arms together in extension while the legs and tail are also extended with the other hand. The lumbar pin or grasping the animal about the waist, the neck grip, and the arm catch with use of gloved hand have been used for initial restraint of small monkeys.[13]

The types of gloves which are used include (a) the Fort Detrick glove—a leather glove with a heavy fiber cuff extending to the elbow, (b) a long cuffed leather glove,

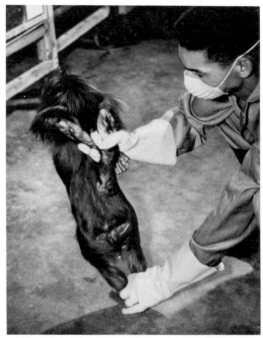

FIG. 27.1. One hand firmly grasps the arms of the animal while the handler's other hand restrains the legs. Relaxation of either hold will be met with an explosive attempt to escape. (Courtesy of Palmer, A. E.: Restraint of monkeys. Maryland Vet. 7: 4. 1965.)

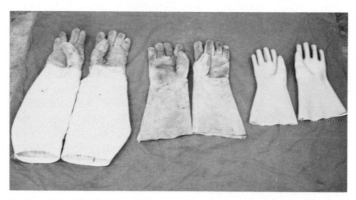

FIG. 27.2. *Left*, the Fort Detrick glove; *middle*, a long cuffed leather glove; and *right*, a long cuffed cloth-lined rubber glove. (Courtesy of Palmer, A. E.: Restraint of monkeys. Maryland Vet. 7: 4, 1965.)

(c) a long cuffed cloth-lined rubber glove, and (d) the elk hide glove (Fig. 27.2). The elk hide glove has snap-on outer shell consisting of a reinforced palm, thumb, and index finger (Fig. 27.3). Gloves protect the handler from bites but reduce tactile sensitivity and increase the possibility of escape.

In zoos or gang cages, where several individuals are housed together, small monkeys can be caught with a wide mouthed net. Care must be exercised to prevent the animal from being injured by the rim of the net. Once the animals are in the net, it can be twisted to prevent escape. If burlap rather than a net is used, there is greater risk for the handler since the monkey can see out more easily than the handler can see in. When several monkeys are confined in a large cage or room which has a door on the opposite side, the animals may be herded through the door into a squeeze cage. In the absence of a door, a canvas partition or curtain with a hole in the middle which leads to a small cage may be used.

One must be cautious in entering a gang cage where several monkeys are housed. Size is not always a dependable means of measuring aggressiveness as exemplified by Capuchins, which are often defiant and offensive. Two or more males of some species are apt to charge one person. Females with young or young animals will usually attempt to escape unless cornered. The keeper or attendant

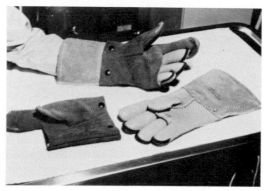

FIG. 27.3. An elk hide glove with snap-on outer shell.

is often able to predict the movements of individuals in his care, and one should always be quiet and cautious when handling monkeys. Another means of grasping small monkeys is with the use of tongs or a snare. Great care must be taken to avoid injuring the animal when these devices are used, and they are not recommended for routine use.

Another device, the clam or NIH monkey net, permits capture of a small monkey which is free or in a cage.[11] This holding net is simply constructed, requires little space, and can be autoclaved or sterilized. The net is most effective for removing monkeys from cages by covering the entire cage front. They can be constructed to fit the particular cage in use (Fig. 27.4). Special cages with squeeze panels facilitate capture and routine care (Fig. 27.5).

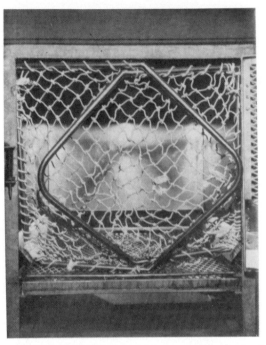

FIG. 27.4. The net placed in one of the standard monkey cages. The dimensions of the net must correspond closely to the inside of the cage. (Courtesy of Gay.[11])

Once a monkey has been caught in a net or by a gloved handler, bare handed restraint affords better control.

Many transport cages, squeeze cages, special devices, and chains have been developed to handle or restrain unanesthetized monkeys.[3, 6, 8, 10, 19, 20, 27, 28]

LARGE PRIMATES

The larger primates (over 10 kg), e.g., adult male rhesus, baboon, mangabay, drill, mandrill, and the larger anthropoid apes, usually require squeeze cages for safe handling. Some squeeze cages are constructed of aluminum with wheels or handles so that they can serve for transportation as well as restraint. The technique whereby plywood partitions are progressively moved toward one end of the cage by sliding them between the bars, thus confining the animal, is a good means of restraint. More elaborate squeeze cages have been designed for handling and treatment of various sized animals (Figs. 27.6 and 27.7).[2, 29]

Adult anthropoid apes must always be considered dangerous animals, and special facilities such as squeeze cages and anesthetization chambers should be constructed as part of the housing unit. If this equipment is part of their natural environment or can be placed so that they will unsuspectingly enter, much time and effort will be saved. Young chimpanzees many times can be trained to take medication voluntarily, or drugs can be administered by various routes without difficulty.[9] Water hoses, electric prods, and tear gas guns may be required when refractory animals cannot be lured into the restraining device, but these methods are not advocated for routine use.

Sedating Drugs

Sedating drugs are not necessarily essential for the management of smaller primates, but are indicated as in other species prior to general anesthesia. The effect of narcotics and tranquilizers given in combination is very marked in small primates. Meperidine (11 mg/kg) and promazine (4.4 mg/kg) will permit extensive handling of small as well as larger species. Often surgery can be performed by the additional infiltration of a local anesthetic agent following the above regimen.

Another combination of a narcotic (fentanyl, 0.4 mg/ml) and tranquilizer (droperidol, 20 mg/ml) has been used in subhuman primates. The term neuroleptanalgesia has been introduced to describe the state of analgesia and central nervous system depression produced by a tranquilizer and a potent narcotic. Effective sedation and analgesia has been described in gorillas and chimpanzees when 2.5 mg/kg of droperidal were given intramuscularly followed by 0.01 to 0.02 mg/kg of fentanyl intravenously.[23, 25] The fentanyl-droperidol mixture (Innovar-Vet) has been administered intramuscularly to baboons at a dose of 1 ml/9 kg. When given to smaller primates such as the squirrel monkey, a microliter syringe should be used. The dose for the squirrel monkey is 0.05 ml/kg. The narcotic fentanyl can produce a bradycardia when

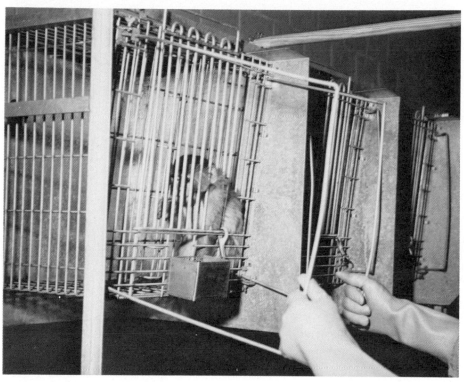

FIG. 27.5. Intramuscular medication can be accomplished without handling. This type of equipment also facilitates removing a monkey from its cage. (Courtesy of Palmer, A. E.: Restraint of monkeys. Maryland Vet. 7: 4, 1965.)

given in the generally recommended doses and should be preceded with atropine. If the vagotonic actions of fentanyl are noted, they can be reversed by the intravenous injection of atropine. Oral administration of the mixture is also effective. Depending on the dose of the fentanyl-droperidol combination used, varying degrees of sedation can be produced: slight sedation to aid in restraining the animal to marked sedation and analgesia enabling minor surgical procedures with local anesthetic infiltration. The depressant effects of the narcotic component (fentanyl) can be reversed with narcotic antagonists. This is especially important if an excessive amount is given and profound depression occurs, or if a rapid recovery is desired following a short procedure. Other narcotics such as meperidine and/or other tranquilizers can also be employed advantageously in subhuman primates. Many other drugs such as chlor-

promazine, perphenazine, proprionyl promazine, reserpine, bulbocapine, meprobamate, and chlordiazepoxide have been used in primates.[1, 5, 21, 22]

Phencyclidine is a valuable drug for the production of sedation and immobility in primates. Phencyclidine acts primarily on the central nervous system producing depression at low doses and hyperexcitability and convusions at high doses. In monkeys, calming and sedation occur at 0.3 to 0.5 mg/kg, and a "cataleptoid-like" state and immobilization occur at 0.8 to 1.5 mg/kg. The larger doses can produce convulsions and death.[5, 24, 32]

During the stage of immobilization, the degree of depression somewhat resembles the lighter planes of general anesthesia. The animal does not respond to noxious stimuli, but the corneal, pupillary, and patellar reflexes are still present. An increase in muscle tone occurs; muscle tremors and involuntary twitching of fa-

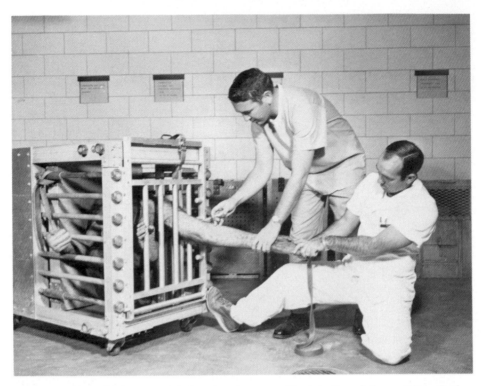

Fig. 27.6. A 120-lb male chimpanzee being given intramuscular injection of phencyclidine. Both arms are restrained and the animal is pressed toward one end of the cage. (Courtesy of Day.[7])

cial muscles and limbs are noted. The administration of drugs which produce general anesthesia will abolish the tremors and produce muscle relaxation. Phencyclidine, like other depressants, reduces the quantity of the intravenous or inhalation anesthetic needed to produce general anesthesia.

The smaller active monkeys such as squirrel monkeys require a larger dose (1 to 2 mg/kg) to obtain the same effect as in the larger animals. Smaller doses are required by the intravenous route, and atropine is indicated prior to administration of phencyclidine to prevent excessive salivation.[18] Increasing the dose does not result in better relaxation but may evoke convulsions.[4]

Phencyclidine is an excellent drug to produce sedation in anthropoid apes. A dose of 0.5 mg/kg intravenously immobilizes a chimpanzee without apparently causing electrocardiographic, cardiovascular, or respiratory changes that would obscure the physiological effects of an experimental drug.[16] Poor skeletal relaxation, hippus, and occasional nystagmus are observed.

Other preanesthetic agents have also been employed in the anthropoid apes to facilitate restraint. Comparitively large doses (1 to 3 mg/kg) of morphine must be used in chimpanzees to induce drowsiness and sluggishness.[30] The fact that large doses are necessary to produce "chemical restraint" may be the reason why this drug has been thought to be ineffective.

Perphenazine (1.25 to 4.4 mg/kg) added to canned pineapple juice takes effect in 3 hours and persists for 6 to 7 hours.[33] Laboratory procuedures which ordinarily require much effort can be accomplished easily.

General Anesthesia

INTRAVENOUS AGENTS

The barbiturates, particularly pentobarbital and thiopental, are very common anesthetic agents in subhuman primates.

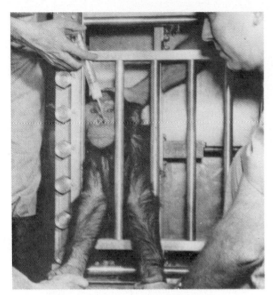

FIG. 27.7. Squeeze cage used for restraint of a small chimpanzee. (Courtesy of Britz et al.[2])

The intravenous route is preferred since it affords better control of the induction of anesthesia. The cephalic, saphenous, femoral, or tail vein can be used. The dose of pentobarbital is approximately 30 mg/kg by intravenous route, but consideration must be given to differences caused by age, preanesthetic medication, and the presence of disease. Recovery usually takes place in 4 to 5 hours. Thiopental and thiamylal are valuable agents for short periods of anesthesia and for the induction of anesthesia prior to inhalation anesthesia.

The anesthetic agents and techniques used in large monkeys and apes are not basically different from those used in small monkeys. The prime differences are in restraint and induction. A squeeze cage and proper preanesthetic medication are essential. The strength, cunning, and offensive capabilities of large primates are phenomenal, and people should not attempt to house, treat, or conduct research with these animals without carefully considering the hazards of their care and management.

In general, oral medication with barbiturates is not highly successful, but chimpanzees can be trained to drink grape juice with quinine which is then replaced with pentobarbital. Other medication can also be given by careful training and by masking the taste of the drug.

INHALATION ANESTHESIA

It is relatively easy to administer volatile agents to small monkeys; anesthesia may be induced in an anesthetization chamber, by a face mask, or with an intravenous thiobarbiturate. Anesthesia is then maintained with open, semiclosed, or closed technique, depending upon the equipment available and personal preference of the anesthetist.

In larger primates which are difficult to handle, phencyclidine or other drugs can be administered for restraint, and inhalation anesthesia then induced via a face mask (Fig. 27.8) or intravenous barbiturates. Inhalation anesthesia can be maintained with the face mask or preferably through an endotracheal tube. Large anesthesia chambers for inhalation agents have been constructed of plexiglass and are a good means of producing unconsciousness to facilitate initial restraint.[17] Nitrous oxide can be used for this purpose, but when used, the anesthetic state borders on anoxia, and it therefore should be administered only until unconsciousness occurs. Emergence is rapid and restraint by other means is necessary. Nitrous oxide and oxygen (75% nitrous oxide and 25% oxygen) can be continued via a mask but must be supplemented with thiobarbiturates or volatile anesthetic agents such as halothane or methoxyflurane. The description of techniques and equipment used for inhalation anesthesia would be redundant at this time; the management of inhalation anesthesia of primates is similar to that used in other species.

For the smaller squirrel monkeys, the semiopen and nonrebreathing methods used in the cats and small dogs are applicable, and the same principles apply. For the larger monkeys and apes, the rebreathing systems used in larger dogs and adult man are the methods of choice. The advantages, hazards, and technique of intubation of the trachea are similar. For

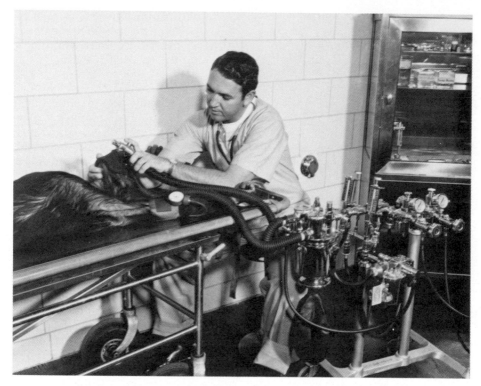

Fig. 27.8. Induction of anesthesia with halothane in a Heidbrink field model anesthesia machine with a Fluotec Mark II vaporizer. A human face mask will fit the facial contours of a chimpanzee. (Courtesy of Day.[7])

more specific information the reader is referred to Chapters 17 and 18.

REFERENCES

1. Bolz, W.: Neuroleptica und potenzierte Narkose speziell bei Zootieren. Proceedings of the Fourth International Symposium on Diseases of Zoo-Animals. Nord. Vet. Med. *14:* (suppl. 1), 17, 1962.
2. Britz, W. E., Fineg, J., Cook, J. E., and Miksch, E. D.: Restraint and treatment of young chimpanzees. J. Amer. Vet. Med. Ass. *138:* 653, 1961.
3. Carmichael, M., and MacLean, P. D.: Use of squirrel monkey for brain research with description of restraining chair. Electroenceph. Clin. Neurophysiol. *13:* 128, 1961.
4. Chen, G., Ensor, C. R., Russel, D., and Bohner, B.: The pharmacology of 1-(1-phenyl-cyclohexyl)piperidine HCl. J. Pharmacol. Exp. Ther. *127:* 241, 1959.
5. Chen, G. M., and Weston, J. K.: The analgesic and anesthetic effect of 1-(1-phenylcyclohexyl) piperidine HCl on the monkey. Anesth. Analg. (Cleveland) *39:* 132, 1960.
6. Cohen, B. J.: An improved trap-transport cage for monkeys. J. Lab. Clin. Med. *38:* 495, 1951.

7. Day, P. W.: Anesthetic technics for the chimpanzee. In *Experimental Animal Anesthesiology*. U.S. Air Force School of Aerospace Medicine, Aerospace Medical Division (AFSC), Brooks Air Force Base, San Antonio, Texas, July 1965.
8. Dolowy, W. C., and Hesse, A. L.: A combination restraint table and cassette holder for routine chest radiography in unanesthetized monkeys. J. Amer. Vet. Med. Ass. *133:* 124, 1958.
9. Elder, J. H.: Methods of anesthetizing chimpanzees. J. Pharmacol. Exp. Ther. *60:* 347, 1937.
10. Ellison, T., Gill, C. A., and Riddle, W. C.: A restraining table for small laboratory primates. Amer. J. Vet. Res. *25:* 872, 1964.
11. Gay, W. I.: A net designed for capturing caged monkeys. Lab. Anim. Care *10:* 75, 1960.
12. Graham-Jones, O.: Notes on the restraint and anesthesia of primates. Proceedings of the Fourth International Symposium on Diseases of Zoo-Animals. Nord. Vet. Med. *14:* (suppl. 1), 76, 1962.
13. Greer, W. E.: "Safety" in the non-human primate colony operation. Presented at the 16th Annual Meetings of the Animal Care Panel, Philadelphia, 1965.

14. Hartman, C. G., and Straus, W. L., Jr.: The anatomy of the rhesus monkey, *Macaca mulatta*. Hafner Publishing Company, New York, 1961.

15. Hensley, J. C., and Langham, W. H.: Comparative fundamental physiological parameters of *Macaca mulatta* and *Macaca speciosa*. Lab. Anim. Care *14:* 105, 1964.

16. Joffe, M. H.: An anesthetic for the chimpanzee: 1-(1-phenylcyclohexyl)piperidine HCl. Anesth. Analg. (Cleveland) *43:* 221, 1964.

17. Kinard, R., and McPHerson, C. W.: The use of trichlorethylene and halothane anesthesia in the restraint of laboratory primates. Amer. J. Vet. Res. *21:* 385, 1960.

18. Kroll, W. R.: Experience with sernylan in zoo animals. Int. Zool. Year Book *4:* 131, 1962.

19. Landolt, R. E., Peters, D. C., and Davenport, P.: A device to facilitate the restraint of laboratory animals. Lab. Anim. Care *12:* 121, 1962.

20. Lilly, J. C.: Development of a double-table-chair method of restraining monkeys for physiological and psychological research. J. Appl. Physiol. *12:* 134, 1958.

21. Marsboom, R., and Mortelmans, J.: Some pharmacological aspects of analgesics and neuroleptics and their use for neuroleptanalgesia in primates and lower monkeys. In *Small Animal Anesthesia*. The Macmillan Company, New York, 1964.

22. Marsboom, R., Mortelmans, J., and Vercruysse, J.: Neuroleptanalgesia in monkeys. Vet. Rec. *75:* 132, 1963.

23. Marsboom, R., Mortelmans, J., Vercruysse, J., and Thienpont, D.: Effective sedation and anesthesia in gorillas and chimpanzees. International Symposium on Diseases of Zoo-Animals. Nord. Vet. Med. *14:* Proceedings of the Fourth (suppl. 1), 95, 1962.

24. Melby, E. C., and Baker, H. J.: Phencyclidine for analgesia and anesthesia in simian primates. J. Amer. Vet. Med. Ass. *147:* 1068, 1965.

25. Mortelmans, J.: Sedation and anesthesia in anthropoid apes. Int. Zool. Year Book *3:* 119, 1961.

26. Pickering, D. E., and Kao, T. T.: Fluid and electrolyte therapy for monkeys. J. Amer. Vet. Med. Ass. *138:* 527, 1961.

27. Pinkerton, J. O.: A restraining device for unanesthetized monkeys. J. Lab. Clin. Med. *23:* 1085, 1938.

28. Rahlmann, D. F., Hanson, J. T., Pace, N., Barnstein, N. J., and Cannon, M. T.: Handling procedures and equipment for physiological studies on the pig-tailed monkey (*Macaca nemestrina*). Lab. Anim. Care *14:* 125, 1964.

29. Rich, S. T., and Cohen, B. J.: A restraint unit for large monkeys. Lab. Anim. Care *12:* 113, 1962.

30. Spragg, S. D. S.: Morphine addiction in chimpanzees. Comparative Psychological Monograph 15, 1940. Cited by Yerkes, R. M.: *Chimpanzees: A Laboratory Colony*. Yale University Press, New Haven, 1943.

31. Srikantia, S. G., and Gopalan, C.: Some biochemical and physiological features of normal monkeys (*Macaca radiata*). J. Appl. Physiol. *18:* 1231, 1963.

32. Vondruska, J. F.: Phencyclidine anesthesia in baboons. J. Amer. Vet. Med. Ass. *147:* 1073, 1965.

33. Wallace, G. D., Foder, A. R., and Barton, L. H.: Restraint of chimpanzees with perphenazine. J. Amer. Vet. Med. Ass. *136:* 222, 1960.

34. Wiener, A. S., and Moor-Jankowski, J.: Blood groups in anthropoid apes and baboons. Science *142:* 67, 1963.

28
Anesthesia of the Porpoise

S. H. RIDGWAY AND J. G. McCORMICK

Porpoises (or dolphins) are small toothed whales and are mammals which have developed a completely aquatic life. Respiratory, thermoregulating, circulatory, and renal physiology have adjusted, and changes are reflected in some anatomical variations.

Cetaceans have large, highly convoluted, well developed brains. The Atlantic bottlenose porpoise (*Tursiops truncatus*) is especially impressive in its cerebral development and its apparent intelligence.[3, 16, 27] In addition, these porpoises have a very sophisticated underwater "sonar" system[5, 8, 12, 20, 32, 37] and highly sensitive hearing over a wide range of frequencies.[8] These characteristics, in addition to the physiological, anatomical, and behavioral adaptations to an aquatic environment, have made this group of animals very interesting and important for scientific study. The maintenance of comprehensive medical care for such valuable laboratory animals and the need to study various aspects of physiology, including audition, dictated the development of anesthetic procedures suitable for major surgery in porpoises.

The physiological and anatomical specializations which have resulted from the adaptation of cetaceans to aquatic life have required the development of specific procedures for producing safe, surgical anesthesia. Apneustic breathing, apparently complicated central nervous system control of respiration, specialized thermoregulation, and structure and functioning of the larynx have necessitated some alteration of standard equipment and procedures.

Anatomy and Respiratory Mechanics

Porpoises breathe through a modified nasal orifice called the blowhole. It is located on the dorsum of the head just anterior to the cranial vault. The migration of the nasal orifice from the end of the rostrum (the usual position in land mammals) to the highest point on the forehead provides a distinct advantage to an animal who must spend his life under water and surface to breathe while swimming. A porpoise can complete the respiratory cycle (inspiration and expiration) in 0.3 seconds.[13] With a tidal volume of 5 to 10 liters of air,[7] the flow rates through the air passages range from approximately 30 to 70 liters/second during expiration and inspiration. Bottlenose porpoises breathe on an average of two to three times each minute. After inspiration, the animal holds an apneustic plateau for 20 or 30 seconds, then very rapidly exhales and inhales again.

In porpoises, the blowhole appears on the surface as a single transversely crescentic opening with concavity facing forward. It is closed by a muscular nasal plug. The blowhole is naturally closed except when the muscles of the forehead contract to open the orifice. The vestibular and tubular air sacs are located ventral to the blowhole and relate directly to paired nares which begin a few centimeters down the respiratory passage. The septum that divides the nares begins as a cartilage covered by mucous membrane and continues for 10 to 20 cm as a bony partition. The respiratory passage becomes single again just above the intra-narial insertion of the glottis.

The larynx is very specialized, forming an arytenoepiglottal tube to give a direct route between the internal nares and the lungs, allowing the animal to breathe through the blowhole only. The arytenoid and epiglottal cartilages are elongated to form a tubular spout-like organ projecting 8 to 10 cm up from the floor of the naso-pharynx with the upper end held in the internal nares by a muscular sphincter formed of palatopharyngeal musculature (Fig. 28.1).

The trachea is short with numerous heavy rings, many of which anastomose. This arrangement seems to provide for maximum elasticity for a free and rapid movement of air. The trachea gives off a separate right bronchus 10 cm or so from the base of the larynx and then bifurcates into two main bronchi about 5 cm caudad. It is important that the endotracheal tube extends no more than about 20 cm past the proximal tip of the glottis to prevent blockage of the separate right bronchus.

The lungs are large and elongated, extending forward to a point 6 to 8 cm in front of the first ribs and as far posterior as the second or third lumbar vertebra. The bulk of the lung tissue is in the dorsal aspect of the thorax as the sternal margins are very thin. The lungs show little or no external lobulation and are somewhat

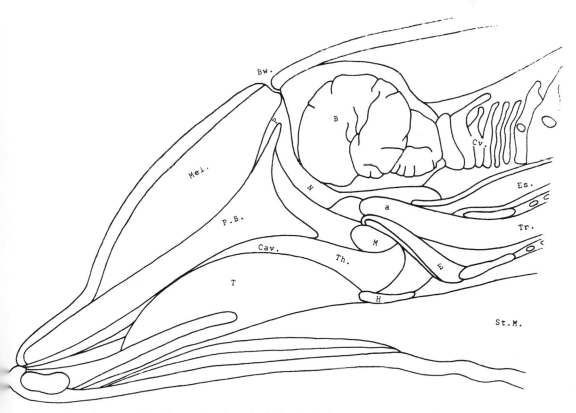

FIG. 28.1. Line drawing of a section through the head of a bottlenose porpoise outlining major anatomical points of interest in anesthesia. *B*, brain; *N*, nares; *A*, arytenoid; *E*, epiglottal; *M*, muscle; *H*, hyoid; *T*, tongue; *Bw.*, blowhole; *Cv.*, cervical vertebra; *Mel.*, melon; *P*, premaxillary sacs; *Cav.*, cavity of mouth; *Th.*, throat; *P.B.*, premaxillary bone; *Tr.*, trachea; *Es*, esophagus; *St.M.*, sternohyoideus muscle.

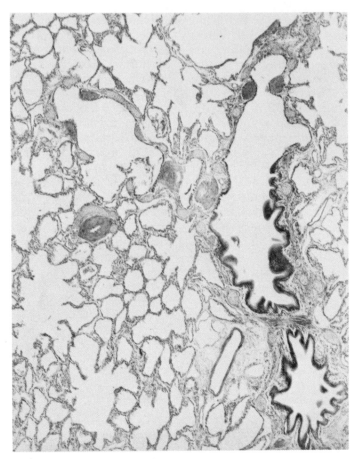

FIG. 28.2. Photomicrograph of porpoise lung. ×40.

asymmetrical in conformation, possibly due to the separate right bronchus. The main bronchi, the stem bronchi, and the bronchioles are supported by an extensive network of cartilage rings which anastomose at irregular intervals. These cartilages produce a strong, resilient bronchial tree, which aids in rapid, effective ventilation and the adjustment to pressure changes. The lungs as a whole are highly elastic and the pleura is very thick and also contains elastic tissue. In each bronchiole, myoelastic valves produce from 6 to 18 compartments. There are also muscular sphincters at the junction of the terminal bronchioles and the alveolar sacs. Thus, in the porpoise lung, there is a great deal of smooth muscle, myoelastic tissue, and hyaline cartilage (Fig. 28.2).

In view of the above anatomical consid-erations, it is interesting to note that expiration in the pilot whale has been observed to be totally passive with elastic recoil as the driving force.[24a]

Furthermore, preliminary studies indicate that during anesthesia, controlled respiration with an apneustic plateau is necessary for proper expansion and inflation of the alveoli of the porpoise lung. Respiration without an apneustic plateau leads to a deterioration of the preparation as evidenced by blood gas values and heart rate changes.

The alveolar walls are thick, and there is a sheet of fibroelastic tissue which divides the septum between the alveoli. The respiratory capillary bed is doubled so that the alveolar capillaries are in contact with only one alveolus. In other mammals there is a single layer of capillaries which are in contact with two alveoli. The gross and microscopic anatomy of the lungs of several species of cetaceans has been studied.[1, 6, 24, 35, 38]

Sleep in Porpoises

It is not known whether porpoises lose consciousness during sleep, and if so, whether they awake for each breath. The behavior of porpoises during what is apparently natural sleep has been reported.[14, 16, 18, 19] A passive surface sleep has been described during which the porpoise hangs near the surface with the head and trunk almost parallel to the water surface and the tail dangling down somewhat. Both eyes are closed. In the absence of a water current, the animal rests almost motionless. About twice each minute the tail will stroke slowly, lifting the animal to the surface for a breath. Long periods of sleep (1 hour or so) are always of the surface sleep variety. The porpoise's surface sleep respiration has been attributed to a reflex mechanism involving the stroking of the tail flukes and exposure of the blowhole to air.[36]

A second type of sleep referred to as "cat napping" or "bottom sleep" has also been described.[18] In this type of sleep, the animal rests near or on the bottom, coming up periodically to breathe. This napping may last as long as 4 minutes before the animal comes to the surface to breathe, after which it may or may not resume the nap. A similar type of sleep behavior has been noted in which the animal makes a few rapid swimming strokes and then coasts around the tank as its eyes droop.

Some observers believe that porpoises do not sleep in any way similar to sleep that occurs in other mammals and that only one-half of the brain sleeps at any one time, allowing the animal to actively surface under conscious volition for each breath during sleep periods.[14, 15] These special theories were examined in detail,[19] with the conclusion that respiration in the porpoise can be automatic or can be brought under voluntary control, just as in other mammals.

It is our opinion that *Tursiops truncatus* and *Lagenorhynchos obliquidens* do sleep somewhat as other mammals do and that control of the large specialized larynx, the muscles of the blowhole, and the stroking of the tail fluke to surface are reflux mechanisms which are most important to prevent drowning during sleep. These animals do appear to have central nervous system centers that are similar to terrestial mammals in their responsiveness to carbon dioxide or oxygen arterial tensions.[19, 30] An extreme tolerance to blood CO_2 buildup has been reported in marine mammals in general.[4, 7, 33]

History of Anesthesia in Porpoises

Porpoises have never been successfully anesthetized without complete respiratory control and positive pressure ventilation.[11] The first known attempt to anesthetize a porpoise was in 1932. Ether was administered by a cone held over the blowhole. The porpoise did not survive. In 1955 a group of researchers attempted to use pentobarbital anesthesia for electroneurological recordings of the brain of *Tursiops truncatus*.[14] The sodium pentobarbital was administered intraperitoneally, and the dosages for a series of five animals ranged from 10 mg/kg to 30 mg/kg. In each case there was reported loss of respiratory control before other signs of anesthesia, and all of the animals died.[14]

Intravenous thiopental sodium was administered in three porpoises for euthanasia and produced a rapid onset of anesthesia with loss of reflexes. After injection of only about 6 mg/kg, the porpoise seemed to lose control of the blowhole, and it fluttered flaccidly as the animal inspired. The drug was continued to effect until lid and gag reflexes were lost. The dosage ranged from 15 to 25 mg/kg. Respiratory arrest occurred soon after completion of the administration of the thiopental. After administration of the anesthetic, the heart beat was rapid, 140 to 160 beats/minute, and steady. The bradycardia arrhythmia[7, 9, 26] disappeared as soon as the anesthetic was administered. None of these animals took a breath after the drug had been completely administered, and it seemed apparent that death had resulted from asphyxia.

It is obvious that control of respiration is essential to obtain deep planes of anesthesia. An apneustic plateau control unit (Bird Corporation, Palm Springs, Calif.) compatible with the Bird Mark 9 large animal respirator, was developed in 1964. This unit effectively imitates the natural respiration of the porpoise in inflating the lungs rapidly, holding an apneustic plateau for a variable period, and then deflating and rapidly filling the lungs again.

The Bird equipment was used in an attempt to produce barbituate anesthesia in a porpoise. Unfortunately, the methohexital sodium (5 mg/kg) and thiopental sodium (13 mg/kg) were given intraperitoneally and an anesthetic death resulted.[22] Subsequent to this trial, 50 to 70% nitrous oxide with oxygen was used for anesthesia. Nitrous oxide-oxygen anesthesia with succinylcholine chloride to produce muscle relaxation has also been used for major surgery in porpoises.[23]

Endotracheal Intubation

Endotracheal intubation in a large porpoise can be accomplished when the animal is awake (in emergencies) or following moderate doses of thiopental sodium. Rusch-modified equine endotracheal tubes (24 to 30 mm) with inflatable cuffs can be used. As an assistant holds the mouth open with soft towels, the hand is inserted into the pharynx. The larynx (Fig. 28.1) is grasped and pulled from its intranarial position, two fingers are inserted into the glottis, and the tube guided in through the palm of the hand. Thiopental sodium (10 mg/kg of body weight), when injected into the veins of the tail flukes, will relax the animal safely and quickly, thereby facilitating intubation.[29] Some very small species are difficult to intubate in this manner, and a smaller tube can be introduced through the blowhole in such species as the *Delphinus delphis* and the *Stenella styx*.[31]

The removal of the endotracheal tube is a most critical procedure in a porpoise. The tube must not be removed or positive pressure ventilation terminated until spontaneous ventilation is adequate. This will be manifested by movements of the animal's blowhole, movements of the thorax, struggling during inspiratory and expiratory cycles, and "tube bucking" or applying back pressure against the respirator. When these signs have become clearly evident, the endotracheal tube is removed and the larynx replaced into its normal intranarial position. If the animal does not blow within 3 minutes or so, or if the heart rate falls below about 60 beats/minute, the tube is reinserted and positive pressure ventilation is resumed.

Nitrous Oxide Anesthesia

The use of succinylcholine as an adjunct to nitrous oxide-oxygen anesthesia precludes assessment of the depth of anesthesia by the use of reflex signs because of the attendant muscle relaxation. To determine the depth of anesthesia during nitrous oxide-oxygen anesthesia, the following reflexes were assessed: (a) eyelid reflex, contraction or closure of the eyelid induced by tapping on the medial canthus of the eye; (b) gag reflex, contraction of the throat muscles when the hand is inserted into the pharynx; (c) swimming reflex, movements of the tail up and down in a swimming motion; (d) pectoral scratch reflex, movements of the pectoral flippers in response to a pinprick or scratch of the chest or axillary region; and (e) blowhole reflex, movements of the blowhole when the finger is inserted into the nares of the vestibular sacs.

A Bird Mark 9 respirator with porpoise apneustic plateau control unit was used as an open system. The animals were intubated before the induction of anesthesia, and a mixture of 60% N_2O and 40% O_2 was administered. This concentration of nitrous oxide produced no loss of reflexes, and the animal's eyes could still follow a finger moving near the head. An increase of the concentration of nitrous oxide to 80%, balance oxygen, produced cynosis in 6 minutes. With this concentration, only an anal reflex could be elicited. With a reduction of the concentration of nitrous oxide to 70%, the cynosis cleared, and the animal rapidly became active again. All of the reflexes returned and the animals attempted voluntary inspiration through the blowhole.

In a second series of animals, 1 hour of 80% nitrous oxide, balance oxygen, slightly raised the threshold for the "pinprick pectoral reflex"; however, all of the other animal's reflexes were present. No cyanosis occurred. The cyanosis noted in the first series was eliminated in the second by the increase in airway pressure during the apneustic plateau.

It is our impression that nitrous oxide, unsupplemented, is inadequate for major surgery in the porpoise. This follows the findings in other species in that nitrous oxide unsupplemented, with thiobarbiturates, narcotics, or other depressants, in most cases does not produce sufficient analgesia for surgery.

Workers have reported the absence of plasma cholinesterases in the *Tursiops truncatus*,[23] which probably contraindicates the use of succinylcholine chloride in this species.

Halothane Anesthesia

Probably the most important single consideration in the choice of a general anesthetic, so far as porpoises are concerned, is rapid recovery with minimal aftereffects. Porpoises are slightly negatively bouyant but their overall bouyancy is near neutral. Thus in their aquatic environment they are suspended in a condition of semiweightlessness. When out of water, the animal is subject to several stresses, including the necessity to breathe and maintain circulation against the weight of its own body. This makes it important to get the animal back into the water as soon as possible after a surgical procedure.

Halothane anesthesia is advantageous for the following reasons. (a) It is a potent agent. (b) It provides rapid induction and rapid recovery. (c) Halothane is not spasmogenic to the larynx and bronchi. (d) It is relatively nonirritating to mucous membranes. (e) It can be combined with nitrous oxide. (f) It is nonflammable.

The main disadvantage, especially with the open system, is expense. Halothane is delivered with the Fluotec Mark III vaporizer in conjunction with the Bird Mark 9 respirator, equipped with an apneustic plateau control mechanism.

The percentage of halothane to be used for induction and maintenance was determined somewhat by trial and error but generally coincided with concentrations necessary in other animals. Administration of 1.5% halothane in oxygen resulted in a half-hour induction period before the loss of "tube bucking" and the proper depression of reflexes; administration of 2.5% gave a smooth induction in 15 minutes. The induction period for 3.5% halothane ranged from 5 to 15 minutes, and 0.75 to 1.0% halothane was sufficient to maintain surgical anesthesia. Occasionally an animal might require a slightly higher concentration of halothane for maintenance. The concentration of halothane could be lowered to 2.0% when thiopental was given for intubation of the trachea. Swimming movements of the free tail flukes similar to those observed in surface sleep were found to be a reliable indication of depth of anesthesia. When these movements disappeared, the animal was sufficiently anesthetized for surgery to begin. During induction, the swimming movements disappeared just after the loss of the eyelid reflex. Anesthesia was maintained with the lowest concentration of halothane necessary to inhibit movement of the tail fluke. The lid reflex was the next most dependable criteria for assessing the depth of anesthesia. All other reflexes (except anal reflex) were not prominent during periods of surgical anesthesia.

Animals which are allowed to recover on 60% ambient air and 40% oxygen recover all reflexes in 10 to 15 minutes, except for the blowhole reflex. Depending on the duration of anesthesia, the blowhole reflex returns approximately 15 to 45 minutes after the start of the recovery period. At this time, extubation can be performed safely.

The swimming reflex cannot be easily observed if the porpoise is restricted with rigid wooden retainers.[22] The animal can be effectively restrained with seat belts over the anterior and thoracic regions, which do not impair the movement of the tail fluke (Fig. 28.3).

Measures of gases and the pH of blood samples taken from the tail fluke artery during anesthetization correlate well with corresponding adjustments of pulmonary ventilation. Because the central artery of the tail fluke is surrounded by a venous plexus, venous and arterial blood might occasionally intermingle during puncture of an artery or vein.

During recent studies of auditory physiology of the porpoises,[20] four *Tursiops truncatus* and one *Lagenorhynchus obliquidens* were maintained under halothane anesthesia for periods ranging from 11 to 24 hours. No pathology that could be attributed to the prolonged periods of halothane anesthesia were noted. Serum transaminase (serum glutamic okalacetic transaminase and serum glutamic pyruvic transaminase), ornathine carbamyl transferase, and lactic dehydrogenase levels did not vary significantly from values found in unanesthetized controls.[21] The mean arterial blood pressure monitored from the caudal artery of the tail stock averaged 115 mm Hg. Before anesthesia, mean arterial blood pressure usually ranged from 120 to 130 mm Hg in the *Tursiops truncatus*, although in one animal it was 140 mm Hg. The *Lagenorhynchus obliquidens* averaged 145 mm Hg prior to anesthesia and 130 mm Hg during anesthesia. Blood pressure in pelagic odontocetes such as *Lagenorhynchus obliquidens* is normally higher than in *Tursiops truncatus*. This is probably due in part to the higher hematocrit and higher total blood volume.[24, 28]

Thiopental Sodium Anesthesia

Six animals (*Lagenorhynchus obliquidens* and *Tursiops truncatus*) were anesthetized with thiopental only. In each case the drug was administered via a tail fluke

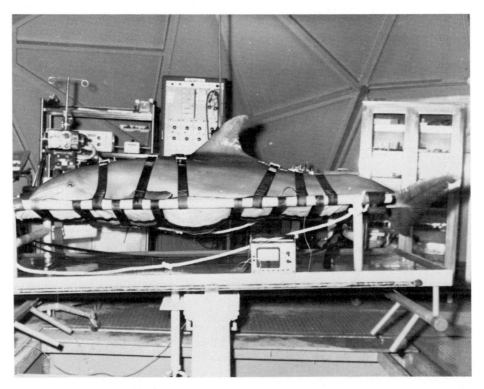

FIG. 28.3. Restraint of porpoise with seat belts during surgery to allow movement of tail fluke. This reflex movement is an index of the level of anesthesia.

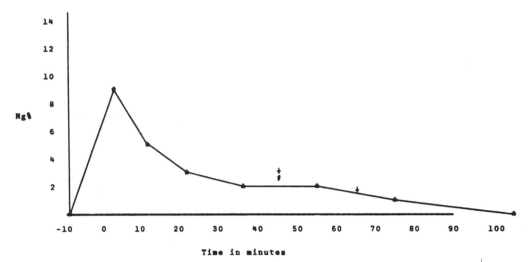

FIG. 28.4. Blood level of thiopental sodium from a 65-kg *L. obliquidens* given 650 mg of drug. ⬇, signs of voluntary respiration start; ↓, animal off respirator.

vein, and positive pressure ventilation was initiated as described. A dosage of 10 mg/kg of body weight resulted in 10 to 15 minutes of very light anesthesia. During this period, only the most minor procedures could be performed and all reflexes were present except the blowhole reflex. However, signs of voluntary respirations evidenced by "tube bucking" and movements of the blowhole did not begin to appear until 45 minutes after the initial injection. Blood levels of thiopental were 2.0 mg % (Fig. 28.4). The endotracheal tube could not be safely removed until 1 hour after the administration of thiopental.

Dosage of 15 to 25 mg/kg produced periods of surgical anesthesia ranging from 10 to 25 minutes. Recovery of respiration, however, required 1 to 2½ hours. In general, the *Lagenorhynchus obliquidens* required a slightly larger dosage than did the *Tursiops truncatus*. In each of the six cases, the animals recovered completely from the anesthesia. These preliminary observations indicate that barbituate anesthesia can be safely employed in porpoises, but the animal must be on positive pressure ventilation, and the body temperature must be kept within normal range.

Tranquilization

Administration of several tranquilizers in dosages approaching those of land mammals results in death. When very small dosages are used, no noticeable change in behavior is observed. A large female *Tursiops truncatus*, after the administration of trifluromeprozine intramuscularly, lapsed into a state that appeared to be behaviorally identical with the surface sleep described earlier. This state was observed for about 6 hours, and 18 to 20 hours after injection, she was awake and swimming normally. Trifluromeprozine was given to a highly trained male of the same species. On 3 successive days, the animal was given 20 mg orally, but no change in behavior was noted. Late on the evening of the 3rd day, 40 mg was given orally. The porpoise was observed periodically from 8 A.M. to 6 P.M. on the following day. The animal spent much of the time in a state identical with surface sleep. He could be awakened by a loud splash against the water and would seem to startle briefly upon awakening. When awakened, the porpoise would take food, although he was somewhat lethargic about eating. When not asleep, he would often be seen to roll over and over lazily as the current carried him around the tank. By 24 hours after the administration of the drug, the animal was fully awake and active, showing no signs of drowsiness. The respiratory pattern in each case was much more regular during sleep than the active and awake pattern. Breaths occurred regularly at 30-second intervals. Paraldehyde has been used to orally sedate excited male porpoises.[17]

Subsequent experimentation with phenothiazine-derived tranquilizers, including trifluromeprazine HCl and acepromazine maleate, demonstrated that temperature regulation is a primary factor in porpoise deaths that have occurred after tranquilizer administration. The phenothiazine-derived tranquilizers such as the two just mentioned, chloropromazine HCl, and promazine HCl cause hypothalamic depression and peripherial vasodilation. Thus, the important heat-conserving peripheral vascular mechanisms[2, 34] are blocked by these agents. We have measured deep rectal temperatures as low as 82 F only 45 minutes after the administration of 20 mg of acepromazine maleate to a 70-kg white striped porpoise. This animal was placed on a respirator and kept moist with warm water and survived. Loss of respiratory control was probably related to the extreme lowering of body temperature.

When the use of a tranquilizer is indicated, chlordiazepoxide HCl and/or diazepam should be employed. These agents do not cause marked hypothalamic depression, ganglionic blocking, or peripheral vasodilation with the resulting loss of body heat that can occur from the use of phenothiazine-derived tranquilizers. Human dosages of chloriazepoxide HCl have been employed in bottlenose porpoises with satisfactory results.

REFERENCES

1. Belanger, L. F.: A study of the histological structures of the respiratory portions of the aquatic mammals. Amer. J. Anat. 67: 437, 1940.
2. Bel'Kovich, V. M.: Characteristics of thermal control in an aquatic environment (English translation). Bionika 35: 125, 1965.
3. Brethnach, A. S.: The cetacean central nervous system. Biol. Rev. 35: 187, 1960.
4. Elsner, R., Franklin, D. L., Van Citters, R. L., and Kenny, D. W.: Cardiovascular defense against asphyxia. Science 153: 941, 1966.
5. Evans, W. E., and Powell, B. A.: Discrimination of different metallic plates by an echolocating delphinid. In Animal Sonar Systems, edited by R. G. Busnel, vol. 1, pp. 363–383. Laboratoire de Physiologie Acoustique, Jouy-en-Josas, France, 1966.
6. Fiebiger, J.: Uber Ergentumlichkeiten im Aufbau der Delphinlunge und ihre physiologische Bedeutung. Anat. Anz. Bd. 48: 640, 1916.
7. Irving, L., Scholander, P. F., and Grinnell, S. W.: The respiration of the porpoise, Tursiops truncatus. J. Comp. Physiol. Psychol. 17: 145, 1941.
8. Johnson, C. S.: Auditory Thresholds in a Bottlenose Dolphin, Naval Ordinance Test Station Technical Report, 1966.
9. Kanwisher, J., and Sundnes, G.: Physiology of a small cetacean. Hvalradets. Skr. 48: 45, 1966.
10. Kellog, W. N.: Auditory scanning in the dolphin. Psychol. Rec. 10: 25, 1960.
11. Langworthy, O. R.: A description of the central nervous system of the porpoise (Tursiops truncatus). J. Comp. Neurol. 54: 437, 1932.
12. Lawrence, B., and Schevill, W. E.: Tursiops as an experimental subject. J. Mammal. 35: 225, 1954.
13. Lawrence, B., and Schevill, W. E.: The functional anatomy of the delphinid nose. Bull. Mus. Comp. Zool. Harvard Univ. 114: 103, 1956.
14. Lilly, J. C.: Man and Dolphin, pp. 48. Doubleday, New York, 1961.
15. Lilly, J. C.: Animals in aquatic environments: adaptation of mammals to the ocean. In Handbook of Physiology—Environment, Am. Physiol. Soc. pp. 741, 1964.
16. McBride, A. F., and Hebb, D. O.: Behavior of the captive bottlenose dolphin, Tursiops truncatus. J. Comp. Physiol. Psychol. 41: 111, 1948.
17. McBride, A. F., and Kritzler, H.: Observations on pregnancy, parturition, and postnatal behavior in the bottlenose dolphin. J. Mammal. 32: 251, 1951.
18. McCormick, J. G.: The behavior and physiology of sleep and anesthesia in the Atlantic bottlenose dolphin, Tursiops truncatus. Master's thesis. Princeton University, Princeton, N.J., 1967.
19. McCormick, J. G.: Relationship of sleep, respiration, and anesthesia in the porpoise: a preliminary report. Proc. Nat. Acad. Sci. U.S.A. 62: 697, 1969.
20. McCormick, J. G., Wever, E. G., Ridgway, S. H., and Palin, J.: Function of the porpoise ear as shown by its electrical potentials. (abst.) J. Acoust. Soc. Amer. January 1970.
21. Medway, Wm., McCormick, J. G. Ridgway, S. H., and Crump, J. F.: Effects of prolonged halothane anesthesia in some cetaceans. J. Amer. Vet. Med. Assn. 157: 576, 1970.
22. Nagel, E. L., Morgane, P. J., and McFarland, W. L.: Anesthesia for the bottlenose dolphin. Science 146: 1591, 1964.
23. Nagel, E. L., Morgane, P. J., and McFarland, W. L.: Anesthesia for the bottlenose dolphin. Also Author's Addendum. Sm. Anim. Clin. 61: 233, 1965.
24. Neuville, H.: Recherches sur genre steno et remarques sur quelques sutres cetaces. Arch. Mus. Paris (No. 6, Serie 3), 176, 1928.

24a. Olson, C. R., Elsner, R., Hale, F. C., and Kenney, D. W.: Blow of the pilot whale. Science *163:* 953, 1969.

25. Ridgway, S. H.: Medical care of marine mammals. J. Amer. Vet. Med. Ass. *147:* 1055, 1965.

26. Ridgway, S. H.: The bottlenose dolphin in biomedical research. In *Methods of Animal Experimentation*, edited by W. I. Gay, vol. 10, pp. 387–446. New York, Academic Press, 1968.

27. Ridgway, S. H., Flanigan, N. J. and McCormick, J. G.: Brain to spinal cord ratios in porpoises: possible correlation with intelligence and ecology. Psychonom. Sci. *6:* 491, 1966.

28. Ridgway, S. H., and Johnston, D. G.: Blood oxygen and ecology of porpoises of three genera. Science *151:* 456, 1966.

29. Ridgway, S. H., and McCormick, J. G.: Anesthetization of porpoises for major surgery. Science *158:* 510, 1967.

30. Ridgway, S. H., Scronce, B. L., and Kanwisher, J.: Respiration and deep diving in a bottlenose porpoise. Science *166:* 1650, 1969.

31. Rieu, M., and Gautheron, B.: Preliminary observations concerning a method for introduction of a tube for anesthesia in small delphinids. Vol. 78. Laboratoire d'Acoustique Animals, Lab. Pub Jouy-en-Josas, France, 1968.

32. Scheville, W. E., and McBride, A. F.: Evidence for echolocation by cetaceans. Deep-Sea Res. Oceanogr. Abstr. *3:* 153, 1956.

33. Scholander, P. F.: Experimental investigations on the respiratory functions of diving mammals and birds. Hvalrad. Skr. *22:* 1, 1940.

34. Scholander, P. F., and Schevill, W. E.: Counter current heat exchange in the fins of whales. J. Appl. Physiol. *8:* 333, 1955.

35. Simpson, J. G., and Gardner, M.: Microscopic anatomy. In *Mammals of the Sea: Biology and Medicine*, edited by S. H. Ridgway. Charles C Thomas, Publisher, Springfield, Ill. In press (1970).

36. Tomilin, A. G. "On the Behavior and Communication of cetaceans." Trans. Inst. Ocean. Acad. Sci. USSR, *18:* 2, 1955.

37. Turner, R. N., and Norris, K. S.: Discriminative echolocation in a porpoise. J. Exp. Anal Behav. *9:* 535, 1966.

38. Wislocki, G. B.: On the structure of the lungs of the porpoise (*Tursiops truncatus*). Amer. J. Anat. *44:* 47, 1929.

29
The Capture and Restraint of Wild Animals

A. M. HARTHOORN

The term wild animals is used here to mean wild, free living animals. When wild animals in cages are discussed they are referred to as captive animals. Domesticated or semidomesticated wild animals (such as eland ranched with cattle) fall into the categories of wild or domestic stock according to their degree of tractability.

The term tranquilizer or ataractic is used for those compounds, which when given in optimum quantities, alter the demeanor of the animal while causing no or minimal incapacitation. The administration of tranquilizing agents (such as the phenothiazines) to wild animals newly caught in nets will reduce mortality. This does not mean, however, that these animals would be easier to catch if released, make less effort to escape if pursued, or will not defend themselves if seized. The term tranquilization implies a subjective feeling, one which cannot be expressed in animals. Wild animals cannot be captured with tranquilizers unless these are given in quantities to induce a state bordering on narcosis or anesthesia.

Narcotics can be used for immobilization and capture of some animals. They induce a state of sedation so that animals will no longer respond to normal stimuli or avoidance objects. When the narcotics are mixed with tranquilizers, a degree of sedation is produced which more nearly approaches a "tranquil state," i.e., it will not try to escape or attack and will submit to completely foreign and normally highly disturbing procedures such as being led or ridden. This neuroleptic condition was termed "neuroleptic narcosis" and commonly termed "neuroleptanalgesia." This state of "deep sedation" has been the basis of all work on immobilization of ungulates since 1960. It is a state from which the animal can be disturbed by normal rousing stimuli. Anesthesia can be superimposed on this state of deep sedation.

Indications for the Restraint of Wild Animals

The need for immobilization and capture of free living animals has increased because of a greater awareness of the importance of conservation, and the value of wild animals as a natural resource has stimulated research into their habits, performance, and physiology.[9]

For many study projects the need arises to capture animals for measurements and markings as well as blood sampling, collection of ectoparasites, and weighing (Fig. 29.1). The marking and measuring of live animals is required for studies such as growth and incremental rates, recruitment and longevity, and the study of migration and movement patterns. Physiological measurements of increasing sophistication are performed with growing frequency as the methods of handling free living fauna improve.[6, 17, 23, 24, 26, 41]

The rising value and increasing rarity of certain species militate against their extermination whenever they conflict with expanding human settlement or intensified agricultural practices. The capture of adult animals by established trapping techniques is prohibitively expensive or is of questionable humaneness and is often fatal to high proportions of the victims caught. Teams have now been trained to relocate the animals with the use of modern drug immobilizing techniques.[29] The converse of the problem arises where the animals become too numerous in one reserve and dispersal of the population is indicated rather than destruction. Public conscience will no longer tolerate the wholesale massacre of animals subjected to a natural or artificial catastrophe. Large scale rescue operations have been set into action to remove animals when exposed to such catastrophies.[40] The techniques of restraint of wild animals are being increasingly used to render assistance to those animals caught in traps or snares set by poachers. Under these circumstances of restraint, a diagnosis of the severity of injuries can be made and assistance rendered to those animals which are amenable to surgical or medical treatment.

Projectile Syringe

The injection of drugs to the unrestricted and even the paddocked animal is performed with a projectile syringe.[73, 74] The syringe is designed to inject its contents after the needle has penetrated the tissue either instantaneously through the agency of an explosive cap and striker mechanism incorporated behind the plunger, or more slowly through the pressure exerted by a spring. Compressed gas or gas evolved from chemical action has also been used. The needle is usually barbed or collared to insure its retention during the extrusion of the syringe contents.

The projectile syringes, like the projectors, are currently of several types. The original type of projection and syringe

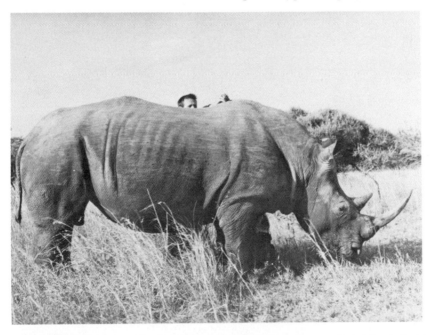

Fig. 29.1. Measurements may, with advantage, be carried out on the standing animal. A white bull rhinoceros, 2000 kg of body weight, has just risen after an injection of nalorphine.

(Palmer Chemical and Equipment Company, Douglasville, Georgia) evolved for small syringes proved unsuitable for the much larger syringe needed initially for African conditions. The mechanism also was not suited to projection over long distances or to withstand the increased impact resulting from other than the CO_2-powered projector.[37]

The various problems were overcome by a modified acid-carbonate activating mechanism which could be hand-made in a work shop. This mechanism (Fig. 29.2) has certain advantages also over the explosive cap discharge mechanism currently supplied with the Palmer projectile syringe. On smaller animals, the latter is prone to cause considerable bruising and tissue damage, with likelihood of secondary effects. Under the force exerted by the detonation of the percussion cap, the ejected fluid stream contents act like a solid rod, penetrating tissue to a remarkable depth with subsequent, often extensive formation of hematomas. The speed of injection and consequent wide distribu-

tion of the syringe contents usually hasten absorption. Extensive and fatal trauma may be caused by injection into the thoracic or peritoneal cavities. Except for special circumstances such as the injection of elephant who are adept in the rapid removal of the syringe, the shower method of injection is to be preferred. Compressed air mechanisms are incorporated in the Paxarms (Paxarms Ltd., Timaru, New Zealand) and Yeoman (Jack the Yeoman Ltd., London, England) syringes.

In general, 2- or 3-ml capacity syringes that can be fitted with needles of different sizes are used. They should empty within seconds of penetration, and the force should be adequate to push the plunger fully home even if the needle is partially blocked. To minimize tissue damage from impact, the maximum range of the projectile and the distance separating the projector from the animal at the time of firing should be so compounded that the syringe strikes at the latter part of its trajectory. This becomes less important

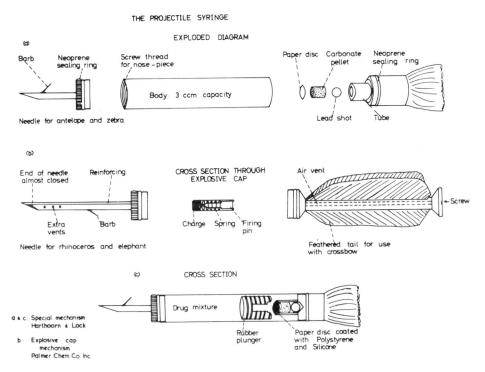

FIG. 29.2. The projectile syringe.

with gas guns and especially the gas pistols designed for close range. When powder charge guns or powerful cross bows are used, the animal and syringe may be damaged. The syringe may enter the abdominal cavity or sink from sight in a muscle mass, or else mushroom and fail to inject. When striking too hard, syringes will tend to bounce off in spite of barbs and collars on the needles. Curiously enough, an animal that suffers severely from bruising is the pachyderm.

Large bore needles should terminate in a cone and possess holes in the shaft to permit egress of the injection fluid. A core of skin may block large needles. Irritant solutions must be avoided as their administration under nonsterile conditions may produce an abscess. Large and proportionately heavy syringes and needles are no longer indicated with the general use of more potent drugs. If used they cause considerable trauma, as the oscillations of the syringe are transmitted to the usually reinforced needle as the animal runs off. The use of light small syringes and needles is advised when possible. Thin needles that bend in response to the muscle movements will inflict minimal damage on thick skinned animals in which long needles are required. The barbs on these needles should be placed far enough back so that it engages the skin rather than the muscle tissue.

The shortest needle commensurate with penetration of the skin should be used. Collared needles are seldom satisfactory and tend to allow back flow of the injection fluid through the hole in the skin caused by passage of the collar. To remove a needle, a small incision can be made over the site of the barb, causing less trauma than the manipulation necessary to extract the barb through the original penetration.

Where simple precautions are routinely observed, untoward reaction at the site of injection is rare in spite of the conditions under which the injection is made. Valuable animals may be given precautionary injection of antibiotics, and the wounds should be treated also to minimize attraction to flies and predators.

Captive Animals versus Free Ranging Animals

A large and growing number of reports are available in the literature on the chemical restraint of captive wild animals. The restraint of captive animals by chemical compounds ranges from the reduction of aggressive reaction through the use of tranquilizing drugs to actual anesthesia or paralysis.[45] The control of captive animals offers a number of advantages as compared to the capture of wild animals in their natural environment which is mainly related to the relative ease of drug administration. For comparison, the principal advantages associated with chemical restraint of captive as compared to wild animals may be listed as follows: (a) the ability to incorporate tranquilizers or sedatives into the food; (b) the relatively long time usually available to allow these compounds to act; (c) the advantages associated with the increasing effectiveness of tranquilizers when administered repeatedly over long periods; (d) the advantage of using preanesthetic medication; and (e) administering a computed restraining dose over several injections.

The gradations between captive animals that can be handled like domestic stock such as tame lion that can be easily injected through animals such as hyena that readily take anesthetic compounds in meat, to virtually wild animals such as nervous antelope or zebra in large grazing paddocks, are almost infinite. Methods used for truly captive animals are already well documented, and many of the methods evolved for the tranquilization of domestic hoofed animals are fairly readily applicable to related wild captive animals of similar size.[57]

Broadly speaking, the capture of the wild animal as compared to the captured species is a more difficult operation for the following reasons. (a) The body weight has to be estimated under fleeting and very difficult conditions. (b) The injection is often made at extreme range. (c) Large doses have to be used to insure rapid immobilization to minimize the chances of escape into cover and also minimize risk to personnel who may have to search for them in the thicket. (d) The entire dose has to be incorporated in one projectile syringe. (e) The animal has to be followed to keep it in sight which is tantamount to chasing, so that the pejorative effect of a strong sympathetic discharge constitutes an added hazard to survival. (f) Aid such as artificial respiration is normally precluded if the animal becomes temporarily lost in vegation.

The restraint of captive animals will not be dealt with, bearing in mind that the methods and drugs described for wild animals may be applied with suitable modification to captive zoo animals (see Chapter 30).

Neuromuscular Blocking Drugs

Neuromuscular blocking agents have been used extensively for the capture of wild animals in a number of countries including America, Europe, and Africa. The principal substances which have been used are nicotine alkaloids,[2, 18, 22, 44, 60] succinylcholine (Tables 29.1 and 29.2), gallamine triethiodide[50] (Table 29.3), and benzodioxane.[63]

Most reports on the use of neuromuscular blocking agents for animal capture indicate a 10% mortality. Under certain conditions they have been used with great success.[8, 16, 64, 65, 67] In these cases the capture has usually been restricted to one age group and sex in one particular species in a certain area. With the exception of benzodioxane, the safety margin by paralyzing drugs is small and tends to be insufficient to balance inaccuracies in judging body weight under field conditions.

Animals immobilized with neuromuscular blocking agents are fully conscious and sight and hearing are apparently unimpaired, a fact not always appreciated by those using these drugs for animal capture. One of the main disadvantages of their use under some field conditions is death from respiratory paralysis before the animals can be found. Regurgitation is a common problem in the ruminant. In other than field conditions, gallamine has been used in cattle when methods to prevent regurgitation are available.[30]

Succinylcholine has been used successfully in ungulates when a prolonged study has necessitated the frequent capture of a large number of a particular species.

TABLE 29.1
Doses of succinylcholine chloride used for the capture of wild animals

Species	Number	Generic Name	Dose Range	Mean Dose
			mg/kg	*mg/kg*
Deer	21	Odocoileus	0.02-0.11	0.06
Red deer	4	Cervus elaphus	0.18-0.61	0.51
Mule deer	3	Odocoileus hemionus	0.22-0.33	0.26
African lion	2	Felis leo	0.22-0.85	0.47
Bush pig	2		0.56-0.6	0.58
Deer, fallow	2	Dama dama	0.16-0.22	0.19
Deer, axis	2	Axis axis	0.13-0.13	0.13
Deer, sika	3	Cervus nippon	0.09-0.22	0.15
Deer, bharasignha	5	Cervus dubauceli	0.004-0.07	0.05
Wildebeest	15	Gorgon taurinus	0.075-0.45	0.15
Wildebeest	79	Comochaetis taurinus albojubatus	0.62-0.63	0.06
Wildebeest, young	79	Comochaetis taurinus albojubatus	0.07-0.08	0.08
Wildebeest, adults	10	Comochaetis taurinus albojubatus	0.05-0.07	0.06
Domestic goat	5	Capra prisca	0.55-1.40	0.80
Himalayan goat	2	Hemitragus jamianious	0.23-0.29	0.26
Sheep, Barbary	1	Ammotragus lervia	0.22	
Antelope, pronghorn	1	Antelope capra	0.22	

TABLE 29.2

Doses of succinylcholine chloride used for the capture of wild animals

Species	Number	Generic Name	Dose Range	Mean Dose
			mg/kg	*mg/kg*
Wapiti (elk)	3	Cervus canadinsis	0.046-0.07	0.06
Bison	1	Bison bison		0.09
Eland	2	Taurotragus oryx o.	0.05-0.06	0.05
Tiger	1	Felis tigris	0.76	
Sumatran tiger	3	Pathera t. Sumatrae	0.25-0.28	0.29
California sea lion	2	Zalophus Californianus	0.19-0.97	0.59
Springbok	1	Antidorcas marsupialis		0.29
American black bear	3	Euaractos americanus	0.73-0.31	0.66
Alaskan brown bear	1	Ursus Middendorffi		0.22
Aoudad	1	Ammotragus lervia		0.38
Spider monkey	3	Ateles geoffroyi	2.20-8.80	5.06
Nilgai	3	Boselaphus tragocamelus	0.24-0.28	0.25
Uganda kob	46	Adenota kob thomasi	0.28-0.54	0.36
Gray seals	25	Helichoerus grypus	120-150*	135*
Puku	6	Adenota vardonii v.	0.48-1.30	0.50
Buffalo	4	Syncerus caffer c.	8.0-10.0*	9.3*
Burchell's zebra	20	Equus Burchelli	0.64 (ineffective)-0.93 (lethal)	0.79
Grant's gazelle	9	Gazella granti	0.22 (ineffective)-0.33 (lethal)	0.28
Giraffe	6	Giraffa camelopardalis	0.05 (ineffective)-0.55 (lethal)	
Impala	2	Aepyceros melampus m.		0.40
Thompson's gazelle	14	Gazella thomsoni	0.46 (ineffective)-0.62 (lethal)	0.55
Topi	6	Damiliscus corrigum	0.15 (ineffective)-0.19 (lethal)	0.19
Hippopotamus	21	Hippopotamus amphibius	0.11-0.13	0.14

* Total dose (milligrams).

Under these circumstances a standard dose is used which is varied only as young animals grow. The dosage of succinylcholine has been reported as varying widely at different times of the year, presumably as a result of variations in nutritional states. As a new group of animals is approached, even in a related species, the doses must be established by trial.[56]

Under field conditions an injection may be made into relatively avascular tissue. When using a short acting substance such as succinylcholine, part of the absorbed dose may be metabolized before the total dose has been absorbed. This results in an insufficient blood level for immobilization to occur. The small safety margin is a deterrent to further injections being made. An advantage of succinylcholine is its rapid onset of action, short duration in most species, and apparent lack of long term effects. Its main disadvantage is the lack of an effective antagonist, and a number of deaths have been reported possibly associated with respiratory and cardiac disturbances.[48, 55, 76, 81, 82]

Competitive neuromuscular blocks such as gallamine and curare[69] have been used successfully on many wild animals (Table 29.3). The dose rate of gallamine may be reduced if given in combination with suitable tranquilizers.[42] The onset of respiratory paralysis is slower, and an effective and rapidly acting antagonist is available. Lower doses can be given to produce muscle weakness in large animals, preferably after the prior administration of tranquilizers. This method has been used with success for the implantation of sensors under local anesthesia in captive African buffalo restrained in a crush.

For competitive neuromuscular blockers, prostigmine is an effective antagonist when given intravenously. The rapid res-

TABLE 29.3

Doses of flaxedil used for the capture of large animals

Species	Number	Generic Name	Dose Range	Mean Dose
			mg/kg	mg/kg
Elephant	3	Loxodonta africana	1.76-1.98	0.83
Burchell's zebra	9	Equus burchelli bohmi	2.86 (ineffective)-3.10 (lethal)	
Bush pig	3	Potomachoerus porcus dae-monis	8.8-11.0	9.90
Cape buffalo		Syncerus caffer c.	2.86-2.86	2.86
Giraffe	5	Giraffa camelopardalis	2.64-4.4	3.48
Grant's gazelle	3	Gazella granti g.	2.90 (ineffective)-3.52	3.41
Spotted hyena	1	Crocuta crotcuta	3.08-3.94 (lethal)	
Thomson's gazelle	4	Gazella thomsonii t.	2.86-3.30	3.08
Topi	3	Damaliscus korigum topi	2.57-3.30	2.85
Wildebeest, calves	27	Connochaetus taurinus albo-jubatus	3.30-7.48	3.74
Wildebeest, adults	28	Connochaetus taurinus albo-jubatus	2.42-4.18	2.94
Hippopotamus	2	Hippopotamus amphibius		3.96
Buffalo	6	Syncerus caffer c.	2.64-2.86	2.75
Giraffe	8	Giraffa camelopardalis	1.92-5.50	3.72
Rhinoceros	10	Diceros bicornis b.	1.32-1.98	1.68
Elephant	7	Loxodonta africana	1.98-3.52	2.97
Rhinoceros	8	Diceros bicornis b.	0.14-0.87	0.25
Giraffe	3	Giraffa camelopardalis	0.55-0.88	0.73

toration of full muscle power in large animals with an undiminished aggressive drive can result in considerable damage to equipment; unfortunately, many recurrences of paralysis after release have been reported. Effective and safe use of prostigmine and related compounds requires considerable skill and pharmacological knowledge, and the attempted capture of animals such as giraffe by nonspecialized personnel has resulted in heavy mortality, although the dose rates of gallamine used were demonstratively safe when used under expert guidance.

Nicotine alkaloids have been used for the capture of wild animals. On the whole the degree of distress caused to animals, the unpredictability of reaction, and the danger of handling such a poisonous substance has discouraged the use of nicotine. When neuromuscular blocking agents are indicated, the newer drugs with fewer side reactions are the agents of choice.

Under field conditions artificial respiration may usually be given effectively to animals weighing about 50 to 100 kg. Even here, however, failure has been registered presumably due to insufficient ventilation. Respiration given to animals the size of zebra (300 kg) is usually ineffective due to the large dead space and strong rib cage. Also, a proportion of animals appear to undergo spasm of the glottis which renders manual respiration impossible. A small oxygen cylinder with reduction valve, pressure tube, and large bore needle or trochar for insertion through the wall of the trachea may be the most effective way of administering oxygen to large animals under field conditions.

Phencyclidine

The advent of phencyclidine (Sernylan) has provided a substance that is speedily absorbed and effective at low dose levels. It was found very suitable for monkeys,[72, 75] goats,[86] pigs,[83] cats,[32] and zoo animals.[53] Unfortunately, its use in wild animals such as buffalo and eland was reportedly fatal, with the animals dying of bloat or regurgitation of ruminal contents and subsequent asphyxiation.[77] Experimental injection into cattle resulted in tremors, spasms, and prolonged sedation, but not a high proportion of fatalities.[78] It has been used in the rhino.[11]

Phencyclidine induces a taming effect at low dosages and, at slightly higher dosages, a cataleptoid state.[13] With further increase an "anesthetic-like" state supervenes, but with the corneal and pupillary reflexes unimpaired. Clonic convulsions tend to occur at higher dosage levels.

For the *Felidae* and other carnivores, the compound phencyclidine has proved safe and effective (see Chapters 13 and 30). It has been used to capture wild lion and to anesthetize captive lion at weekly intervals. It has been used on a number of leopard to remove them from snares, and also on trapped hyena. Experimentally, a large overdose may be given to domestic cats without fatality.[32] The dose rates used for the wild *Felidae* have been 0.75 mg/kg of body weight with minor variations on either side of this dosage (Table 29.4).

Clonic spasms of varying severity are usually experienced, and these may be controlled by thiobarbiturates if required and reduced with the phenothiazine tranquilizers. Atropine may be given to control the frothing that may result from the persistent lip and jaw movements. Chlorpromazine and scopolamine may be combined with the phencyclidine in one projectile syringe.[10] Lion and leopards usually commence to recover in about 1 hour and hyena, given about 5 mg/kg, have shown considerable recovery in 2 to 3 hours. It is remarkable that the wild *Felidae* such as lion and leopard fail to regain their normal aggressive instincts and fight reaction for some time during the recovery stage and may be restrained by hand while sitting or after they have begun to walk.

Phencyclidine is rapidly absorbed through the mucous membranes of the mouth, and refractory animals including lion, hyena, and smaller carnivores such as mongoose have been rapidly sedated by squirting a small amount at strengths of 100 to 200 mg/ml into the mouth of the animal as the animal snarled or tried to bite. Under these circumstances, an effect is usually seen in 5 minutes, and the animal becomes sufficiently tractable to enable an intramuscular injection within 10 minutes. Overdose results in delayed recovery so that the state of marked depression may last for 12 to 24 hours with resulting demands on staff for nursing, but with little apparent ill effect on the subject if the necessary attention is given during this period.

Hippopotamus have been given small quantities (0.25 to 0.3 mg/kg), which is sufficient to render them delirious; they surface and move about aimlessly.[66] This enables young specimens to be netted.

Narcotic-Tranquilizer Combinations

THIAMBUTENE

Prior to 1960 centrally acting compounds were generally not used for capture of wild animals except for limited use of phencyclidine. Experiments oriented toward finding a safe and reversible system for the capture of highly valuable

TABLE 29.4
Doses of phencyclidine used for restraint

Species	Number	Generic Name	Dose Range
			mg/kg
Cat	9	Domestic	0.02-0.27
Giraffe	4	Giraffa camelopardalis	0.006-0.014
Impala	3	Aepyceros melampus	0.006-0.01
Hippopotamus	3	Hippopotamus amphibius	0.003-0.007
Buffalo	2	Syncerus caffer c.	0.007-0.009
Baboon	1	Papio ursinus Orientalis	0.11
Goat	9	Domestic	0.5-16.0

and rare large wild animals showed that domestic ungulates could be restrained with morphine-tranquilizer-scopolamine mixtures. The effectiveness of this mixture appeared to rest on the counteraction of the excitatory effects of morphine by the tranquilizer. While the administration of morphine alone causes predominantly a state of locomotor activity, the mixture induced standing, or sternal recumbency with little evidence of excitement. The scopolamine was added to control salivation. On reversal of the morphine action the animal was able to rise, walk normally, and, in general, exhibit only a tranquilized or sedated state. The mixture proved highly successful for capture and relocation of the white (square lipped) rhinoceros.[31, 43, 68] The mean dose in a large series of captures was 4.0 mg/kg (Fig. 29.3).

The diethylthiambutene hydrochloride

(Themalon, Burroughs Wellcome and Company, London) mixtures were used to capture hippopotamus, several species of of antelope,[70] young elephants, and buffalo. The virtues of this mixture rested primarily on its low mortality and reversibility. Furthermore, the immobilizing effect of the thiambutene could be reduced gradually, in contradistinction to the reversal of muscle relaxants which, on intravenous injection of the antagonist, often cause a rapid and occasionally temporary reversal, during which the animal might break loose and damage vehicles and personnel. This enables the reversal of the immobilized state to be carried out in stages commensurate with the dictates of the circumstances, e.g., a small amount of antidote is given on finding the animal; a slightly larger amount is given on arrival of the capture party and this is finally combined with the administration of tran-

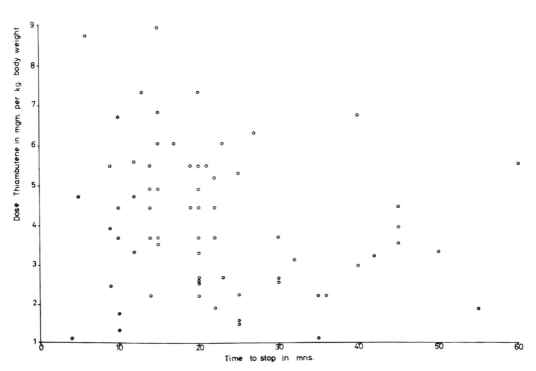

FIG. 29.3. Doses of thiambutene used for the capture of white (square lipped) rhinoceros.

quilizer such as chlorpromazine and tying of the hind legs to prevent walking away. Lastly, when the large vehicle and crate arrive, a full dose of antidote can be given with or without tranquilizer.

The disadvantage of the thiambutene mixture was its large bulk and consequent slow absorption (Fig. 29.3). This precluded its use on animals larger than subadult rhinoceros or young elephant owing to the problem of ballistics in projecting the very large syringes, and it was unsuitable for most of the small animals who tended to get lost during the time interval during injection and the onset of immobilization.

Tranquilizers

Chlorpromazine has been extensively used but recently has been replaced by the more active acetylpromazine. The latter has the advantage of higher activity and also the field advantage of rendering the narcotic M.99 (Etorphine) more soluble and thus less likely to be precipitated by the addition of the scopolamine solution.[21] There is now a tendency to use the more active fluorophenothiazine derivatives,[66] and undoubtedly there is much scope for experimentation with different tranquilizers which act synergistically and are physically compatible with the M.99 series of compounds. The physical compatibility is increased by the use of solvents other than water such as propylene glycol or dimethyl sulfoxide, which enable M.99 to be used at higher concentration. The relative activities of various phenothiazine derivatives in the inhibition of conditioned avoidance response in rats have been listed[46] in which fluphenazine was found to have a very high order of activity, with trifluoperazine, triflupromazine, and chlorpromazine in decreasing order. At the present method of use, the tranquilizers are used primarily as adjuncts to the narcotics, especially the M.99 series, or after the reversal of the narcotic effect. More recently, the phenothiazine tranquilizers have fallen into disfavor following deaths due to hyperthermia in hot areas.

ETORPHINE (M.99)

The principal disadvantages of the thiambutene mixture were overcome in 1963 with the availability of oripavine derivatives later to be known as the M series of compounds. In this series, endoethenotetrahydrothebaine* (M.99) proved to be as effective as thiambutene while greatly reducing the quantity of mixture that need be injected and also the time for absorption.

Chemistry. M.99 and M.183 are two of a new series of potent narcotics derived from thebaine.[4, 5] Thebaine is an alkaloid present in opium (0.2 to 0.8%) and has formally been regarded as a therapeutically useless by-product of morphine and codeine manufacture. It has no analgesic activity and acts as a nervous system stimulant. The structure of these substances is similar to that of morphine but is characterized by the addition of an extra ring structure and side chains (Figs. 29.4 and 29.5). The ketonic adducts of thebaine were found to have analgesic actions similar to those of morphine. Primary and secondary alcohols produced by the reaction of grignard reagents on these were found to possess greater analgesic activities further increased by O-demethylation of the thebaine derivative to the corresponding oripavines. Included in this series are those having the code number M.99 and M.183 (Fig. 29.5).[5]

The bases of these compounds have

---

* Several variations of this formula have subsequently come into being, namely:

6:14 Endoetheno-7-α(-2-hydroxy-2-pentyl)-tetrahy-drooripavine hydrochloride
  Reckitt & Sons Ltd., Hull, England
      or
7,8-Dihydro-7α-(1(R)-hydroxy-1-methylbutyl)-O⁶-methyl-6,14-endoethenomorphine
  British Pharmacopoeia Commission
      or
1,2,3,3a,8,9-Hexahydro-5-hydroxy-2α-(1(R)-hydroxy-1-methylbutyl)-3-methoxy-12-methyl-3,9a-etheno-9,9b-iminoethanophenanthro (4,5-bcd) furan
  (Recently used in U.S. publications)
14. M.183
3-Acetyl-6:14-endoetheno-7α-(2-hydroxy-2-pentyl)-tetrahydro-oripavine hydrochloride
  Reckitt & Sons Ltd., Hull, England

analgesic activities up to almost 10,000 times greater than that of morphine when determined by the subcutaneous route in rats (tail pressure method); high activities have also been shown in other mammals.[5]

Pharmacology. In general, these compounds have a pharmacological profile similar to that of morphine in that they produce analgesia, depression of respiration, inhibition of gastrointestinal motility, and stimulatory or depressant effects on the central nervous system. These central nervous system effects, however, differ among the different species of domestic hoofed animals.[36] In wild animals the effect of M.99 and M.183 given alone ranges from virtually purely depressant effects seen in the large animals such as elephants, to a state of excitement manifested by intense locomotor activity in some antelope such as nyala. The locomotor activity is expressed by a characteristic high stepping or hackney gait and circulating movements. The head tends to be held high, and cerebral depression is manifested by an inability to circumvent normally insignificant obstacles.

M.99 has been used for animal capture rather than the acetyl derivative M.183 which tends to be slower acting and less potent. The effects of M.99 on domestic animals such as the horse include tachy-

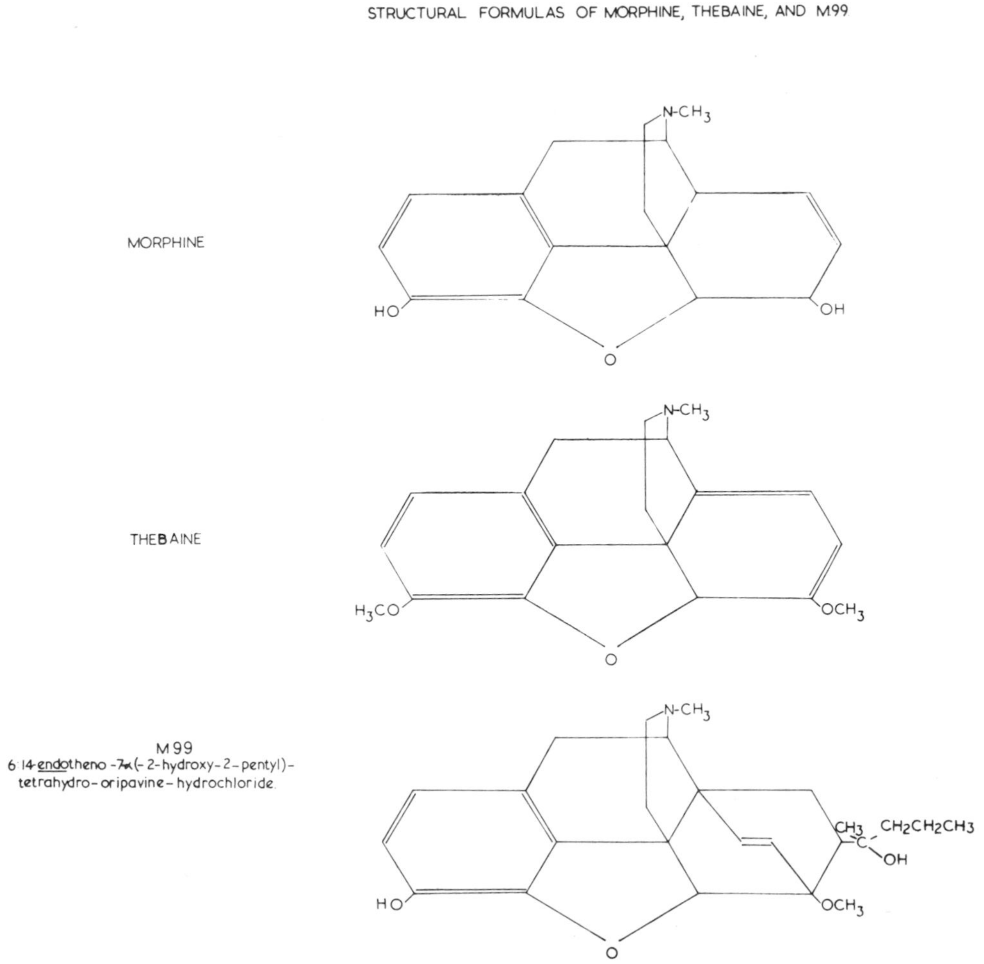

STRUCTURAL FORMULAS OF MORPHINE, THEBAINE, AND M99

FIG. 29.4. Structural formulas of morphine, thebaine, and M.99.

STRUCTURAL FORMULAS OF M.183 AND M.285.

M.183

3-acetyl-6 14-endotheno-7α-(2-hydroxy-2 pentyl)-tetrahydro-oripavine hydrochloride

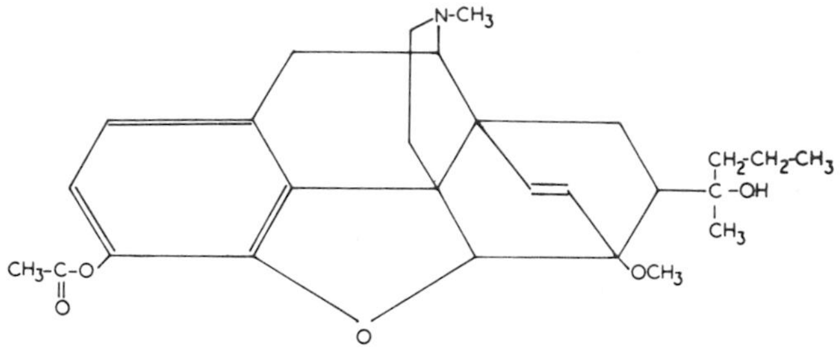

M.285

N-cyclopropylmethyl-6,4-endotheno-7-(2-hydroxy-2-propyl)-tetrhydro-nororipavine hydrochloride

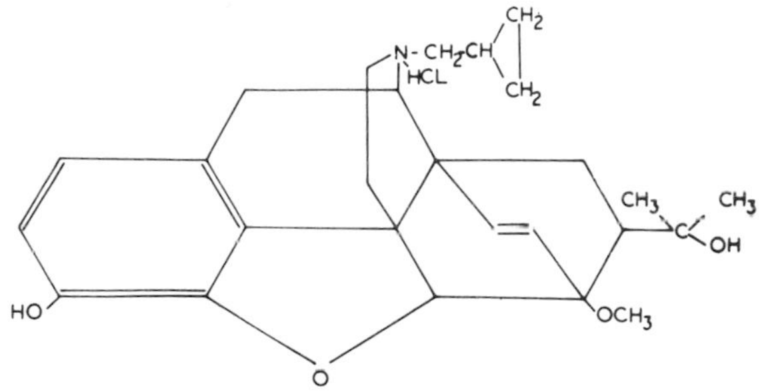

FIG. 29.5. Structural formulas of M.183 and M.285.

cardia and a rise in blood pressure which has not been noticeable in other animals such as the goat. There appears to be a cessation of ruminal activity.

The injection of M.99† into most standing animals resulted in rapid collapse. Intramuscular injection into goats induced collapse in about 6 minutes, and intravenous, within 20 to 260 seconds (Table 29.5). Intravenous injection into donkeys caused collapse within 36 to 90 seconds. The time interval between injection and falling did not always reflect the time taken to become incapacitated. All animals would on occasion become rigid but remain standing. In that position they are incapable of resistance or coordinated movement.

Low dose rates administered to goats (0.2 mg and below) produced failure of the postural, but retention of the righting reflexes. Head and neck would be held rather rigidly upright; the position of sternal recumbency could be assumed at will. Steers would collapse, but often in dog-sitting position with the forelegs

† M.99 and the antidote M.285 have now been marketed as Immobilon-Revivon by the manufacturers, Messrs. Reckitt & Colman Pharmaceutical Division, P. O. Box 114, Hull HU8 7EL.

TABLE 29.5

The effect of M.99 on pulse and respiration of conscious castrated male goats

Number	Total Dose	Route	Pulse Rate		Respiration Rate		Nalorphine
			Before	After	Before	After	
	µg/kg		beats/min		frequency/min		mg
1	0.5	I/V*	72	72	20	20	
2	0.5	I/V	80	80	15	12	
3	1.0	I/V	80	82	16	12	
4	2.5	I/M†	80	82	12	18	40
5	5	I/M	82	76	16	14	40
6	10	I/M	78	84	12	15	40
7	25	I/V	64	96	13	8	14
8	50	I/V	61	59	12	16	40
9	100	I/M	80	76	20	16	
10	150	I/M	76	80	18	9	
11	200	I/M	96	78	22	9	
12	200	I/M	96	78	22	9	
13	250	I/V	84	100	21	7	

* I/V, intravenous.
† I/M, intramuscular.

TABLE 29.6

The effects of intravenous M.99 on the pulse and respiration of conscious donkeys (270 kg)

Number	Sex	Total Dose	Pulse Rate		Respiration Rate		Nalorphine
			Before	After	Before	After	
		mg	beats/min		frequency/min		mg
1	M	0.5	42	128	23	12	60
2	F	0.5	56	104	24	8	100
3	F	0.5	56	114	66	9	100
4	M	1.0	41	120	28	9	
5	F	1.0	72	152	34	10	60
6	F	1.0	78	139	45	14	60
7	F	2.0	59	128	16	8	100
8	M	2.0	52	136	17	8	100
9	F	2.0	52	120	11	7	100
10	F	3.0	58	84	11	7	100
11	M	4.0	44	108	12	4	200
12	F	5.0	49	140	16	10	200

straight out, head and neck stiff, and tongue protruding. Donkeys would hold the neck and forelegs stiffly, but also the hind legs and back muscles would exhibit rigidity at high dosages.

The frequency of respiration was reduced in all animals but particularly in the donkey (Table 29.6). The impression was gained that this decrease was due less to the central depression than to difficulty induced by rigidity of the neck and chest muscles. Breathing was stertorous, in steers often of a "sobbing" pattern. On several occasions the breathing improved after the administration of chlorpromazine, which also induced relaxation of the neck allowing the head to lower. Delay in respiratory rhythm was enhanced by breath holding and prolonged exhalations through partly closed glottis.

The pulse rate in the goat showed no increase or fall (Table 29.5). That of the donkey showed a sharp rise (Table 29.6). The rise may, in part, have been due to the muscular effort resulting from muscle rigidity, but its continuation past the nalorphine recovery stage suggests a specific effect by M.99 on the heart. Nalorphine has little effect on reducing the heart rate, but then it also does not affect the convulsant action of the narcotics. Horses show a steep rise in the blood pressure which can be minimized with phenothiazine tranquilizers. These do not, however, reduce the tachycardia.

Recordings made of intraruminal pressures in the goat and the sheep showed that ruminal contractions remained in complete abeyance from the time of collapse to the time of recovery. Ruminal movements recommenced about the time the subject was able to return to his normal stance.

The donkey usually showed signs of recovery after 20 to 30 minutes, especially at the lower dosages. Goats similarly started to regain consciousness after 30 minutes when sufficient amounts had been administered to produce relaxation and unconsciousness. Only one donkey was permitted to recover completely without the benefit of nalorphine, and none of the horses were. Spontaneous recovery in donkeys and horses results in an undesirable excitement phase with rapid locomotory movements which were best curtailed with nalorphine. This phenomenon was not seen in the goat, and those with the highest dose rates were left to recover unaided. Donkeys receiving chlorpromazine remained in a state of stupor for some time, but those without additional tranquilizer settled down to graze after a short period of excitement exhibited by walking about.

The effect of intravenous injection of M.99 on the donkey, the horse, and, to a lesser extent, on the ox, was an abolition of postural reflexes so that the animal fell to the ground. Tenseness of musculature of the legs and neck remains. The head was usually held high and the forelegs stiffly extended. The spastic condition appears to be exaggerated in the horse, and convulsive movements were exhibited. These are of a spasmodic but predominantly tonic convulsive nature, alternating with clonic locomotory movements. In order of intensity they are exhibited in horses, donkeys, steers, sheep, and goats, with goats exhibiting almost none of these reactions, only depression. In steers, no excitement was seen at medium to high dose rates, but much excitement may be exhibited if the M.99 was reversed by an insufficient quantity of nalorphine. This may be reduced by mixing the injection of nalorphine with approximately 100 to 150 mg of chlorpromazine and injecting these together. A dose of 0.25 mg of M.99 to a 300-kg steer resulted in excitement manifested by trotting around the periphery of the wire enclosure with raised head and protruding tongue for nearly 30 minutes.

Solubility. This compound is soluble in aqueous solution at 5 mg/ml, at which concentration it is generally used from large animals down to medium sized antelope. The water is best adjusted to a pH of 4.5 with hydrochloric acid. This appears to increase the keeping quality of the solution under field conditions and guards against a rise in pH due to alkalinity of the container. It should be noted that the solubility of M.99 was decreased from its initial value of 5 mg/ml to 1.3 mg/ml with the addition of scopolamine (hyoscine hydrobromide at 50 mg/ml) due to common ion effects, and to 1.2 mg/ml with scopolamine at 100 mg/ml at a temperature of 20 C.[19] The total amount under these conditions in the standard 2-ml quantity of mixture used was 2.7 mg of soluble M.99, although this rises to 5.3 mg if the temperature is raised to 40 C. With the addition of 20 mg of acetylpromazine, the solubility of the M.99 was raised to 2.5 mg/ml, the M.99 maleate being more soluble than the hydrochloride.[28] Scopolamine is now generally not used in the M.99-tranquilizer mixture.

For field work, it was found to be advantageous to introduce approximately 1 ml of the tranquilizer solution (50 mg of acetylpromazine) into the projectile syringe before adding the measured quantity of dissolved M.99. This guarded against precipitation of the M.99 from solution by contaminants or unsuitable lubricant inside the projectile syringe. More tranquilizer solution could be subsequently added to the limit of the syringe capacity.

The speed of absorption of M.99 is increased if dissolved in dimethylsulfoxide (DMSO). The solubility of the M.99 is increased, and also is its miscibility increased with certain tranquilizers. The DMSO solution has been used advantageously for the capture of elephant. The danger of inadvertent absorption through the human skin is greatly increased, and the use of M.99 in DMSO is not recommended except under the most rigorously controlled conditions. A somewhat safer method is to add DMSO to the M.99 solution only in the projectile syringe. In the latter case, the principal safeguards must be directed to the subsequent handling and cleaning of the syringes. The mixing of DMSO and a watery solution results in a considerable rise in temperature.

Immobilization of Wild Animals

Etorphine and also Fentanyl‡ (M.99) has been used successfully to immobilize wild animals of more than 20 different species.[6, 33, 34, 35, 39, 51] To date it has not been found unsuitable for any type of hoofed animal, although some species react more favorably than others. They are the only compounds to date that have been found suitable for all the wild ungulates.

The immediate response to injection depends primarily on the usual flight reaction of the species and the animals in the particular area; for instance, if intensive hunting occurs, disturbance will result in panic flight. To a certain extent, it

‡ Fentanyl (R-4263 citrate), also a morphine-like analgesic, is usually administered with butyrophenones such as Azaperone (R-1929) or Fluanizone (R-2028), Janssen Pharmaceutica, Beerse, Belgium.

will vary according to the impact of the syringe and its weight. The first effects are seen usually after a lapse of 2 to 6 minutes, depending upon the dose administered. The early changes are a subtle difference in the method of walking and a failure to react instantly to unevenness in the ground or an obstacle. Later, definite signs of ataxia will be evident, often accompanied by alterations in the carriage of the head, ears, or tail.

Subsequent effects differ according to the dose rate. Heavy dosage will result in early immobilization, often accompanied by prostration. Species differences are also seen, and wildebeest and zebra are readily immobilized completely to a stage of near anesthesia; other antelope such as oryx and nyala remain ambulant even after very large doses (Fig. 29.6). When complete immobilization does not occur, through light or medium dosage or species idiosyncrasy, characteristic behavior patterns are exhibited. These patterns will be dealt with fully in the next section. In short, the subject will show varying degrees of the following alterations of normal behavior depending on the species. Generally speaking, characteristic behavior patterns are as follows: (a) leaving the herd and moving off in a different direction; (b) a strong tendency to be attracted by unusual objects or noises; (c) circling movements, often with a definite point such as a motor vehicle as the center; (d) upward and backward carriage of the head (Fig. 29.2); and (d) a "hackney" gait.

Immobilization is an elastic concept and the degree of akinesia will depend on species and doses. With light to medium doses, all animals will remain on their feet with the exception of certain light antelope such as impala. Mostly, the animals will walk gently unless disturbed. When approached noisily, they will shy away and gallop for a short stretch of 20 to 50 meters before coming to a halt. Hearing seems to be unimpaired (possibly accentuated), but the eyesight is affected. Most animals will readily approach a person standing still, and many are caught in that manner. Other animals such as kudu,

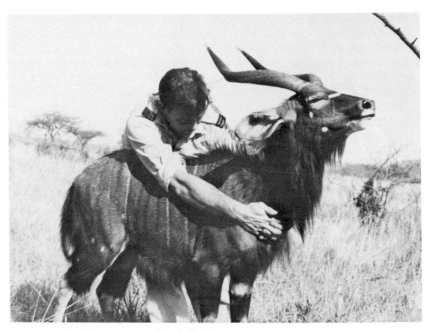

FIG. 29.6. The adult male nyala shows to exaggerated degree the impulse and characteristic of many animals under M.99 influence to move continually forward with head and neck raised.

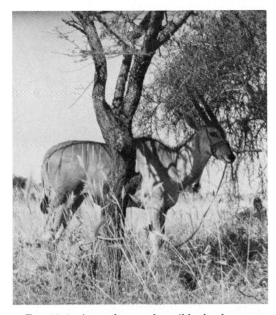

FIG. 29.7. A newly caught wild eland accepts being haltered and tied to a tree with no struggling for a period of 2 hours.

usually be surrounded or made to walk into a rope held between two scouts. They are then restrained manually (Fig. 29.6) by head or tail or by roping the hind legs. If prolonged restraint is required, the M.99 is partially replaced by tranquilizer, after which the urge to move forward disappears (Fig. 29.7), so that restraint becomes simplified.

The typical "hackney" gait is exhibited by giraffe and by most animals (including domestic cattle) under light dosage. Zebra show less excitement, and rhinoceros and elephant show almost none. Zebra and rhinoceros in particular, under light to medium dosage, tend to walk very slowly until they are stopped by a bush or fallen tree. Zebra have been seen to lean against a tree or droop over a fallen log. When animals remain stationary, the legs are often held very stiffly. Sometimes, if approached carelessly, the standing subject may break into an awkward gallop. Buffalo will rise from upright recumbency to make a half-hearted and ineffective rush forward when approached. The reaction to handling is usually mild. One man can usually restrain adequately large antelope such as wildebeest.

eland, nyala, and giraffe do not come to a halt, but continue to move at a high stepping trot. Progress is erratic, often in circles, and usually slow. The animals can

The reaction to ear tagging is a good criterion to the degree of analgesia. Ear tagging is usually resented intensely when attempted by manual restraint or in a semiparalyzed animal; however, multiple ear tags have been put into standing and completely unrestrained rhinoceros under M.99 without their appearing to notice or, in one case, without disrupting the grazing pattern. Fentanyl citrate is less suitable for the very large animals, owing to its lower activity (about one-fifteenth that of M99) and the larger quantities, therefore, required.

Giraffe are always lightly dosed, and these animals will show some distress at being handled. Marking procedure has therefore to be carried out speedily. If relocation is desired, a collar (with quick release fastening) and two side lines will enable a giraffe to be guided over a considerable distance to a holding enclosure.

Elephant are not easy to coerce, and for marking should be given a large enough dose to cast them on their side. Placement on their brisket hampers breathing[66] to an extent that will eventually prove fatal if they are not pulled over. For physiological experiments such as the measuring of the circulation to the ear, the standing elephant may be mounted with the help of a ladder (Fig. 29.8).[38]

Most animals will acquiesce to handling without real protest, the oryx being the one noted exception, while at the same time carrying the most formidable weapons. Most animals should, however, be handled with circumspection, but particularly those that normally tend to fight rather than flee such as the male buffalo. It may be noted that mature male giraffe have been seen to lash out with both front feet when approached while under light thiambutene dosage. Crating for reloca-

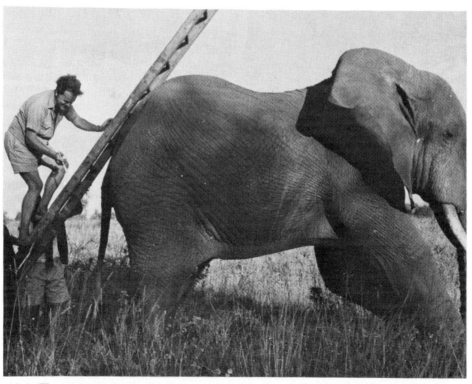

Fig. 29.8. The extent to which wild animals can be handled under the influence of chemical compounds is illustrated by the demeanor of this elephant. The wild African elephant is normally approached on foot only with extreme circumspection. The animal is being mounted for the double purpose of marking and to gain access to the blood vessels at the base of the ear.

tion is the object of a large portion of immobilizing exercises. For this purpose, small or medium antelope are readily caught by nets, spotlight, or after injection with succinylcholine, and subsequently tranquilized and moved in numbers. Centrally acting drugs are therefore used for the larger animals such as giraffe, eland, wildebeest, zebra, rhinoceros, and young elephant.

After immobilization, animals can usually be led into a crate (giraffe to a stockade) without difficulty. For crating, an antagonist to M.99 is usually given and more tranquilizer administered. It should be noted that occasional animals (including domestic cattle) display an urge to press forward. If this is seen in crated animals, immediate measures must be taken in the form of further antidote or tranquilizer, and, if possible, also a restraining chest band. Rhinoceros may die of heart failure due to the excessive exertions, and all animals suffer self-inflicted damage to the skin of the head and to the horns unless restrained. The type of damage normally encountered in animals caught by other means due mainly to fear and attempted escape is not seen in animals captured and tranquilized as described.

Reversal of Narcotic Immobilization

Immobilization by the narcotics thiambutene, morphine, or the M.99 series can be successfully reversed by all narcotic antagonists, e.g., nalorphine, lorphan, or other compounds of the M series of oripavine, e.g., M.285.§ Nalorphine and similar antagonists abolish most of the characteristic action of narcotics. Nalorphine is a derivative of morphine in which the N-methyl group of morphine is replaced by an N-allyl group[52] (see Chapter 13).

Nalorphine has been used exclusively in counteracting immobilization by thiambutene. It has been found effective in all medium and large antelope, zebra, buf-

falo, and sufficiently effective in rhinoceros to permit recovery even after large doses of thiambutene.

The amount of nalorphine necessary to counteract a given dose of a narcotic is not a constant relationship to the dose of narcotic. Pragmatically, for field use, the body weight of the subject can be used as a guide. For instance, a 200-kg zebra captured with 1 mg of M.99 can normally be restored to normal activity by the intravenous injection of 40 to 60 mg; a 2000-kg rhinoceros also immobilized with 1 mg of M.99 needs about 400 to 600 mg of nalorphine and frequently more. It has been apparent that very large doses of antagonists tended to exert some depressant effect. Where there has been no immediate response to the first injection of nalorphine, it has been necessary to proceed with caution. The use of large quantities of this substance has proved expensive and somewhat cumbersome to administer. It has not infrequently given rise to anxiety owing to its apparent depressant reaction when administered in large amounts to the very large ungulates. On elephants, it proved impossible to use for the reasons stated above, and with these animals, contrary to the results with other species, losses have occurred partly due to a lack of response and partly because the very large amounts needed were sometimes not available.

The effective and large scale immobilization of elephant has been possible with the use of the narcotic antagonist M.285. It is related to M.183 and M.99 in a manner similar to the relationship of nalorphine to morphine. It is soluble in water at 35 mg/ml at 20 C. Doses of M.285 up to 100 mg/kg have been administered subcutaneously to rats daily over a period of 21 days without ill effect; the median lethal dose for M.285 by the subcutaneous route is 560 mg/kg. M.285 was found to be a potent antagonist to morphine in the rat, approximately 35 times as effective as nalorphine and the duration of action 2 to 3 times as long.[7] M.285 has proved highly effective in counteracting M.99 depression in the elephant, and amounts of 40 to 50

§ Cyprenorphine, N-cyclopropylmethyl-6,4-endo-etheno-7-(2-hydroxy-2-propyl)-tetrahydro-nororipavine hydrochloride, Reckitt and Sons, Ltd., Hull, England.

mg administered intravenously were routinely effective in counteracting doses of 5 to 8 mg of M.99 in elephants weighing 3000 to 7000 kg.[66]

At the onset it should be appreciated that the reversal of a narcotic antagonist is not complete. The depressant effects of narcotics are almost completely removed, but the stimulant effects are not entirely alleviated. Furthermore, the antagonists themselves are not without some depressant effect, although mild in the dosage normally used.

Before the synthesis of M.285 in 1965, nalorphine was used exclusively, and, owing to its greater availability, it is still used primarily to reverse the effects of M.99 on small and medium sized animals. As, however, the amount administered bears a relationship to the weight of the animal, its use on the large beasts becomes prohibitively expensive. In cases where it was administered in very large quantities, it was felt that the response was not proportional to the amount injected. In elephants a complete lack of response has been reported on several occasions, and this may have been due to insufficient amounts, the intramuscular route of injection, or possibly a depressant effect exercised on this species by several grams of nalorphine.

Normally small and medium sized animals (200 to 300 kg) respond with alacrity to a full dose of nalorphine (60 to 100 mg), so that the subject rises from a lying position to gallop off usually no more than 30 to 45 seconds after an intravenous injection. No lack of response to nalorphine has been seen in any animal with the exception of elephant, although a slow response has occurred in the rhinoceros. The antagonist was always given intravenously (into the jugular or ear vein), except to standing elephant when the intramuscular route was employed. When small quantities of the antidote were injected to antagonize partially the immobilizing substance, a graded response may be obtained. This may be employed to induce an animal to rise so as to enable it to walk to another area for weighing or where

crating may be easier. In light animals and even zebra, the injection of even small quantities of 10 to 20 mg of nalorphine have rendered the animal sufficiently active to break loose. This was, however, rare, and with experience the amount needed in relation to the degree of the depression can be gauged.

It seems that the degree of tranquilization obtained following the alleviation of the morphine-like depression with an antagonist was somewhat greater than the degree of sedation induced by the tranquilizer alone. It seems to be a combination of the residual effects of M.99, the antagonist, and the tranquilizer.

The graded response to the small quantities of nalorphine, e.g., 60 mg intravenously to a 1000- to 1500-kg rhinoceros, enables effective aid to be given to these animals when immobilized in areas dangerous to the animal. Rhinoceros frequently become immobilized in streams, lacking the power to climb to the far bank. For this reason, those following on horseback or otherwise carry the antagonist. With the assistance of partial or graded antagonism of the immobilizer, the animals concerned have been able to extricate themselves and walk to a safe area while still being sufficiently controllable. Under light M.99 dosage and partial reversal, the animals may be induced to walk, in fact tend to walk forward, but are easily guided. This is an important aspect of the capture and of transporting wild animals. It should be noted that there is no other feasible way of moving an adult giraffe prior to teaming, owing to their shape and delicacy. It is also virtually impossible to get a freshly caught grown rhinoceros weighing some 2500 kg, or even less, into a suitably fitting crate unless the animal will walk into it voluntarily, or with only mild coercion. Earlier methods whereby the tied animal was winched on to a lorry were not conducive to survival, particularly as the journey out of the bush is apt to take half a day, and frequently longer.

The degree of tranquilization and reversal of narcosis in the rhinceros must be judged precisely. If the animal is too much under the influence of morphine-like substances, the stupor may be such that he will not recognize the end of the crate as a solid object and may attempt to push through, during which he may lose a horn or even die of exertion. If too lightly sedated, he may try to fight his way out constructively. Acetylpromazine at a dose range of 100 mg for a medium sized rhinoceros has been found effective. Medium sized antelope and zebra are usually given about 0.1 mg/kg of body weight, and more to smaller animals. The ideal state arrived at is one where the animal prefers to lie in sternal recumbency, but can rise at will, if necessary. The tranquilizer is usually administered intramuscularly. It may, however, be given intravenously and even mixed in one syringe with the nalorphine. It should be clearly understood that the administration of nalorphine and M.285 antagonize only the M.99 or a similar moiety and not the tranquilizer that may have been included. The nalorphine will therefore not restore the animal to normal, and the effect of the tranquilizer and scopolamine remains. In spite of this, most animals rise to their feet.

The demeanor of the animal after a full dose of antidote and no further tranquilizer is markedly different from that exhib-ited previously. An immediate awareness of human bystanders will be exhibited and movement will occasion instant flight. Horned antelope will frequently make a threatening pass as they canter away. If extensive handling of animals is required, further injection of tranquilizer should be given prior to or simultaneously with the antagonist.

Requirements of Various Species

RHINOCEROS, ELEPHANT, AND HIPPOPOTAMUS

The species comprising this first group of animals with some exceptions all tend to run when the injection has been perceived (Table 29.7). In geographical areas where these animals are undisturbed, the penetration of the needle may be felt but not associated with human agency. In that case, the sensation was ignored, or else (in the case of elephant) the syringe was removed. In areas where hunting occurs, all the animals will run until slowed by the drug effect. The running reaction will be particularly strong if the approach was observed through hearing, sight, or smell. Elephants may panic only when the human smell from the projectile syringe has been perceived after inspection with the trunk. Hippopotamus will head for water and should therefore be injected at

TABLE 29.7
General reactions of various species to M.99

Species	Reaction
White rhinoceros, elephant, black rhinoceros, hippopotamus, giraffe	No tranquilizer is needed to achieve a full immobilizing effect. Little or no excitement is evidenced.
Zebra, wildebeest, waterbuck, hartebeest, tsessebe, impala, buffalo	These animals may be captured with the use of M.99 alone if administered in large doses. Light and medium dosage tends to induce excitement and running. Normally these animals are caught with the use of medium doses together with a tranquilizer.
Eland, nyala, oryx, kudu	These animals cannot be immobilized by even very large doses of M.99 unless a sufficient amount of tranquilizing drugs is added. In these animals the stimulation is the most prominent feature, and the excitant effect of these compounds prevails over that of the depressant.

a suitable distance from the nearest river or lake. The reaction to injection is intensified if associated with the feeling of being hunted, and the problem of keeping them in sight may be formidable.

It is advised to attempt to follow the passage of the animal from a convenient vantage point with the aid of binoculars rather than trying to follow in thick vegetation where harm to vehicle and personnel can occur from the terrain or attack by the animal. All of these animals can be aggressive; for example, when pressed closely, the hippopotamus will attack, having at its disposal more formidable means of harm than the rhinoceros. The black rhinoceros may attack immediately on injection, but after that are rarely aggressive, and only if followed very closely. Elephants tend to charge rather ineffectively when molested, although occasionally if roused excessively may turn out to be very assiduous in their pursuit. It is one of the species against which a motor car body constitutes no defense. Lastly, the white rhinoceros attacks only very rarely, although if it does, it will follow much more effectively than a black rhinoceros and exhibit considerable skill in pursuit.

The dangers associated with handling the large African ungulates on their own ground are not materially greater than those of domestic animals in veterinary practice as long as the practicant is fully aware of the behavioral tendencies of the species, and indeed of the local group or race that he is dealing with.

Time Lapse between Injection and Capture. The time interval between the syringe penetrating the hide and the animal becoming sufficiently quiet to enable it to be handled will be referred to as the "time lapse." The time lapse depends first on the dosage and the speed of absorption, and also on the resistance of the subject.

The dose rates vary widely as a result of the difficulty in body weight estimation, especially with large animals of this group and those that live in thick cover. The problem is considerably accentuated when single animals are encountered and if they allow only a cursory estimation to be made before disappearing again from sight. Errors of over 100% are frequently made by experienced game rangers. On occasions, a syringe intended for one animal will find its mark in another owing to a sudden shift of position which may be occasioned by the disturbance caused by the projectile syringe.

The results of injections of drugs affecting the central nervous system by any route other than the intravenous are inclined to vary even under the best of conditions. It is therefore not surprising that a greater discrepancy is found resulting from intramuscular injections of wild animals. The time lapse is increased if the animals are excited, and particularly when chased. The animals continue to run until a condition of areflexia sets in.

Dosage Rate. This group of animals needs a relatively small dose of M.99 for immobilization, with the elephant being the lowest, requiring a minimum average dose rate of 0.56 μg/kg of body weight.[66] White rhinoceros are intermediate with an average dosage of 1.8 μg/kg, and 2.55 μg is the dose for the black rhinoceros.

The dose rates for the mature animals in this group are often surprisingly small (Tables 29.8 and 29.9). The rhinoceros in Figure 29.1 was captured with only 1 mg of M.99 and 100 mg of scopolamine, and the elephant in Figure 29.8 was captured with 4 mg of M.99 and 500 mg of hyoscine.

Large animals will tend to stop even when lightly dosed, and elephant in particular will stand "four square" and will not move under any coercion. In this they differ from the other groups, which usually remain ambulant. There are indications that young animals take higher dose rates and are more easily persuaded to move while under the influence of the immobilizing compound. There appears to be little difference in the dose rates for males and females with the use of thiambutene but considerable difference when M.99 is used. These figures may be influenced by the number of older bulls taken off farm land. Old bulls tend to keep on

TABLE 29.8
*Doses of M.99 for the capture of large hoofed wild animals
according to Pienaar[66] and Niekerk[61][62]*

Species	Generic Name	Dose of M.99	Dose of Acetyl-promazine or Trifluopromazine
		mg	mg
Red hartebeest	Alcephalus busephalus caama	1.0	10-15
Bontebuck	Damaliscus dorcas	1.0	10-15
Blesbock	Damaliscus dorcas phillipsi	1.0	10-15
Black wildebeest	Connochaetes gnu	1.5	15-20
Springbuck	Antidorcas Marsupialis m.	0.25-0.5	5
Impala*	Aecyperos malampus m.	0.25-0.5	5
Waterbuck, male*	Kobus ellipsiprymnus e.	3.0-3.5	20
Waterbuck, female†	Kobus ellipsiprymnus e.	2.0-2.5	20
Warthog	Phacochoerus	1.0-1.5	20
Blue wildebeest	Connochaetes taurinus t.	2.0	20
Zebra	Equus Burchellis	2.0	20
Tsessebe	Damaliscus lunatus l.	1.0	10-15
Buffalo, male	Syncerus caffer c.	1.0-5.0	40
Buffalo, female	Syncerus caffer c.	3.0-4.0	30
Elephant, large	Loxodonta africana	7.0-8.0	50-60
Elephant, small	Loxodonta africana	5.0-6.0	40-50
Roan antelope	Hippotragus equinus e.	2.0-3.0	20
Sable antelope	Hippotragus niger n.	2.0	
Oryx	Oryx gazella g.	2.0-3.0	15-20
Kudu	Tragelaphus strepsiceros s.	2.5-4.0	—‡
Eland	Taurotragus oryx o.	5.0	—‡

* Using a dose rate of 0.5 mg, narcotic antagonist must be injected within 30 minutes.
†Therapeutic index unfavorable and succinylcholine recommended.
‡With 50 mg of trifluopromazine and 75 to 100 mg of phencyclidine.

walking for longer periods but react badly to high dose rates. The capture of old bulls of any species is usually avoided where possible, as they have a limited life span and are difficult to dose effectively and handle.

The placement of the syringe is important in the pachydermatous animals. The needle must enter the skin at right angles if excessively long needles are to be avoided. Extra long needles (more than 3 inches) unbalance the syringe in flight and cause trauma when the muscles are moved subsequent to the needle's entry; the syringe and needle remain *in situ* until the animal stops. An area of thin skin must therefore be used to implant the syringe. An important factor which influences the speed of absorption are the layers of fascia that lie subcutaneously under the skin of the animals in this group, and particularly along the back. Bone must of course be avoided; when the rib cage is hit no tranquilizing effect is obtained and the loss of both animal and syringe may follow. This is one of the most frequent causes of failure when aiming at the shoulder muscle mass. The ear of the elephant is inclined to come back and can intercept the syringe. Rapid immobilization of elephant and rhinoceros usually follows an injection in the shoulder posterior to the region of the humerus or spine of the scapula, or else the posterior quadrant of the hind limb below the level of the acetabulum (Fig. 29.9). The body surfaces suitable for injection in this group of animals differ mark-

TABLE 29.9

Doses of M.99 for the capture of large hoofed wild animals

Species	Number	Generic Name	Dose Range	Mean Dose
			μg/kg	μg/kg
Elephant	12	Loxodonta africana	0.2-1.8	0.8
Elephant	3	Loxodonta africana	1.0-3.3	1.9
White rhino	50	Ceratotherium simum simum	0.5-11.8	1.8
Black rhino	5	Diceros bicornis	1.2*-1.5 mg*	1.3 mg*
Black rhino	7	Diceros bicornis	1.4-4.5	2.5
Giraffe	7	Giraffa camelopardalis	2.8-4.5	3.6
Zebra	8	Equus burchelli	2.6-2.8	2.3
Zebra	11	Equus burchelli	5.4-6.0	5.7
Zebra	12	Equus burchelli	1.1-9.7	9.9
Wildebeest	12	Connochaetes taurinus	1.5-7.7	5.7
Buffalo	3	Syncerus caffer caffer	3.0-3.3	3.2
Kudu	2	Tragelaphus strepsiceros S.	4.8-6.3	5.5
Impala	4	Aepyceros elampus e.	4.1-4.8	4.5
Waterbuck	1	Kobus elipsyprymnus e.		5.5

* Total dose.

edly from other groups, particularly in possessing no sheets of panniculus muscle which in other species render shallow injections feasible.

Lower doses can be employed successfully in areas where the animals are quiet and thus will not run or only run when injected. Higher dosages may have to be used in difficult terrain and thick bush where the following of the quarry presents a real problem. The long time lapses are largely due to the fact that an animal moving slowly in thick vegetation is not catchable due to the inevitable noise made by the captors, whereas similar conditions on the grassy plains permit easy capture.

Need for Adjuvants. The need for adjuvant compounds to assist the action of the main immobilizing drug and to protect the subject from excitement and struggling is minimal in this group of animals. Initially it appeared that tranquilizers would be unnecessary with M.99 in this group of animals. This seemed fortunate in that the amount needed for the larger animals would cause undue dilution of the immobilizing drug. Several untoward incidents occurring with M.99 alone indicated that there may have been undue

excitement, and use of acetylpromazine (30 to 60 mg) combined with M.99 is recommended. (On account of the dangers of hyperthermia (see above) other tranquilizing substances are being used with increasing frequency such as the powerful compound Rompun Va 1470 (Bayer) for capture and Diazepam (Roche Products, Ltd.) for transport.)

In the very early trials using morphine for immobilization, scopolamine or atropine was found beneficial for decreasing salivation and tracheal mucus. The scopolamine furthermore appeared to act synergistically with the depressant effects of morphine. It came to be used as a routine ingredient in all the immobilizing mixtures for most animals with the exception of the hippopotamus. The sweating mechanism of this animal is totally blocked by atropine and the immobilized animal will be threatened by death from hyperthermia. Large doses of narcotics are used in the hippopotamus to insure immobilization on land and to prevent the hippo from regaining his preferred watery environment. Where there is a high probability of hippopotamus reaching deep water before immobilization, M.99 should not be used, as drowning will result. In this case phencyclidine (0.3 to 0.4 mg/kg) and a phenothiazine derivative tranquilizer should be used. This produces delirium sufficient to allow a suitable sized hippopotamus to be netted.[66]

Behavioral Responses. This group of ungulates do not normally show excitement as a result of drug action except in a minor way after they have stopped. The effect of the drug mixture is to slow the recipient down until he either just ambles along, stands, or goes down. It should be made clear that the tendency for this group of animals to run is associated with injection and the desire to get away from the hunter. It is not an effect of the narcotic and is therefore in contrast to other animals which "run" as a behavioral response to the drug action.

Black rhinoceros tend to exhibit some excitement before immobilization, and, especially under the effect of thiambutene, show a tendency to crash through bushes and fall forward. With M.99 this excitement can be minimized through the capability of adding a greater quantity of acetylpromazine (100 mg). White rhinoceros, once halted, usually view the approach of their captors with unconcern. Only rarely is any resistance offered. The black rhino is somewhat more temperamental and if down tends to throw its head from side to side. This, however, is easily prevented and remedied by giving more tranquilizer and a little nalorphine to enable them to rise.

Hippopotamus are the only animals in this group that show definite extrapyramidal symptoms manifested mainly by vocal breathing and protrusion of the tongue. None of the animals in this group has shown the curious tendency to approach motor cars and other avoidance objects which is a marked trend in many other species, particularly zebra, wildebeest, eland, and nyala. The hippopotamus, if not properly incapacitated or thoroughly tranquilized, may swing sideways

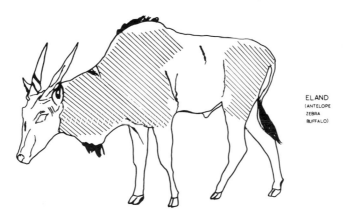

ELAND
(ANTELOPE
ZEBRA
BUFFALO)

SHADED AREAS REPRESENT PARTS SUITABLE FOR INJECTION BY PROJECTILE SYRINGE

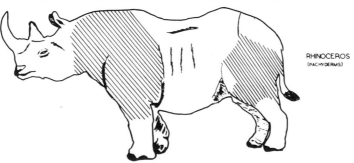

RHINOCEROS
(PACHYDERMS)

FIG. 29.9. Areas suitable for injection with the projectile syringe.

with open jaws at anyone approaching, and the front end is best avoided. Younger ones can be controlled by a noose thrown over the jaws. Elephants circle before coming to a half, as is also true in other species, but they appear either oblivious or disinterested in the sight or sound of motor vehicles once they have reached this stage of immobilization. They should, however, be approached with circumspection and their reactions tested by noise, etc. from a safe distance. Elephants put tremendous effort into keeping on their feet, especially the old bulls that do not normally lie down. They should not be allowed to lie on their briskets but should be pulled over with a rope, as in that position (on the brisket) they will readily become anoxic and die.[66]

These animals, even when standing, are usually unconcerned and show minor resentment only to people walking within a yard or two of the head. In that case they usually rumble and attempt to lift the trunk. As the drug effect begins to wear off the animal may show his displeasure by head movements and swaying. It must be remembered that the elephant's trunk is a highly dangerous weapon, and exceptional care should be taken not to approach too close if there are any signs of recovery. Young elephant (700 kg) can become very troublesome, swinging their trunk and taking short rushes forward. This can occur about 1 or 2 hours after initial immobilization as the drug's effects subside.

The reaction to nalorphine and M.285 differs somewhat among species. Routinely it is given intravenously, the only exceptions being those animals that are well on their way to recovery before antidote administration, particularly if they are to be released. The pattern of the recovery of the heavy ungulates is generally slow. The rhinoceros and elephant are often very reluctant to rise, even if clearly able to do so. This originally created a problem and caused some anxiety; it being apparent that the animals would be far better on their feet. It was soon found that repeated injections of nalorphine served little purpose. In some instances, an electric cattle prodder for the rhino and small doses of caffeine and sodiobenzoate for elephants were beneficial. Usually a large dose (60 mg) of M.285 will induce elephants to rise and walk off. The hippopotamus, unfortunately, has no easily accessible superficial veins and has to be injected intramuscularly.

GIRAFFE

The giraffe are considered separately owing to their special build rather than to any atypical reaction to immobilizing mixtures. The reaction of the giraffe to the impact of the projectile syringe is stereotyped; the giraffe invariably reacts by moving off at a slow center to a distance varying from 100 to 300 yards and then stopping to look back. It is not possible to approach a giraffe unobserved, and the injection is therefore associated with human agency. The subsequent behavior of the giraffe depends upon the degree of previous disturbance and the discretion of the capture party. More often than not the animal will remain standing until the drug mixture starts to take effect. Otherwise he will move along at a walking pace. The giraffe is one of the animals that will turn his head to sniff the syringe, and the human smell clinging to this may cause some alarm.

The time lapse between injection and capture is usually long because low dose rates are used and the giraffe is not easily captured while still fairly active. Fortunately, their wanderings are rather aimless, and they are very easy to keep in sight. Its response to narcotics resembles that of the larger antelope rather than that of the large ungulates just described. Ataxia in the giraffe is undesirable and casting can easily damage the giraffe's neck.

Animals that have not become immobilized with the suggested dose rate have usually been injected in the areas unfavorable for the quick absorption of the injected mixture (Tables 29.8 and 29.9). The area of the shoulder forms a large target where the results are usually good.

The hind quarters, approximately below the ischial tuberosities, may also be used. The long dorsal slope from the base of the neck to the tail is covered by very thick hide supported by avascular fascial layers, and absorption from injections placed in this area is slow.

Pienaar[66] suggests that M.183 is a safer compound to use for the capture of giraffe than the related, more potent, M.99. The onset of its reaction is more gradual than that of M.99 and its effect is less drastic on cardiac function and respiration. Acetylpromazine (20 mg) in combination with M.183 (2 mg) is recommended for the young giraffe (300 to 600 kg).

Behavioral Responses. The injected giraffe is usually caught either by natural objects or by a light rope held at breast height into which he is allowed to walk (Fig. 29.10). When caught in this way there is little attempt to struggle and the animals will mainly try to go forward as before. In this, giraffe show a similarity to such animals as the nyala (Fig. 29.6) which show a tendency to walk forward unless restrained.

Giraffe are easily cast down to their brisket for marking. Holding the animal's head down on the ground is unnecessary and indeed can be fatal, as regurgitation and aspiration of rumenal contents occur almost immediately. A cinch on the legs brings these animals down to sternal recumbency very quickly after which they can be restrained easily.

The giraffe caught for marking will rapidly ambulate from sternal recumbency after an intravenous dose of nalorphine. When animals are to be housed in an enclosure the nalorphine may be omitted or else a small intramuscular injection of nalorphine (20 mg) is given. After an injection of nalorphine, the giraffe seems to return to complete normality, in contrast to many other animals. This again may be associated with light dose rates of both the narcotic and tranquilizer.

ZEBRA, BUFFALO, AND WILDEBEEST

An interesting aspect of this group of animals (Table 29.7) is that it contains a

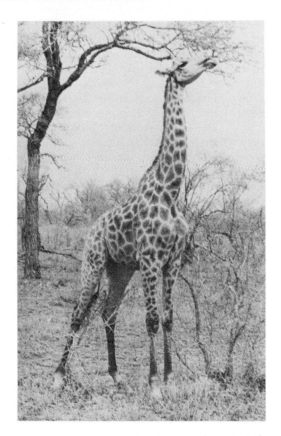

FIG. 29.10. Giraffe, showing the characteristic pose exhibited by this animal and also by most of the antelope. In this state the animal may be easily caught and is often stopped by a bush or low branch.

monogastric species as well as ruminants. Yet the reaction of, for instance, wildebeest has a much greater similarity to that of the zebra than to the antelope in the last group. Buffalo are also included in this group.

Most of the animals in this group are open plains game species which are inclined to be shy, and their flight distance tends to be great. Their safety lies in a limited flight which is designed to take them out of range but not out of sight. The plain is their home, and they cannot hide and are normally safe as long as the predator or hunter can be seen. Continued contact with these animals is therefore no problem.

These animals may sniff at a syringe in the shoulder or flank upon which they react by leaping in the air, jinking, or running for a short distance. The injected animal tends to return to the herd until the immobilizing mixture starts to take effect, when it usually wanders away on its own. The nonplains game such as buffalo will seek to hide in bush or long grass. This makes them difficult to follow. In areas where animals are not too numerous they may be tracked, as they seldom go far. This is a simple undertaking where impala and waterbuck are concerned, and the process is accelerated if a number of scouts can fan out to pick up first tracks on the subject's circles. With buffalo greater caution is usually exercised.

With correct dosage and proper injection, the time lapse is seldom long. A reaction is usually observed in 4 to 5 minutes, and it is rare to lose animals of this group once a reaction has commenced. If the animal has stopped, there is little need for haste. It is possible that it may have stopped without being incapacitated. In that case the flight of his herd mates or the sound of an approach may precipitate flight. It is customary, therefore, to let an apparently immobilized animal stand for a while before an approach is made, in particular if the animal is found in a clear area. Often the animal will stand under the drug effect while others of his kind are around, but will be roused if they leave. On occasions the time lapse on incapacitation and handling may be unexpectedly long when an animal stands still under the drug influence, but is just sufficiently awake to run away from an approaching footstep or evade seizure by horn or tail.

A superficial injection is usually quickly absorbed owing to the well developed sheets of panniculus muscle found in these animals, even if the syringes are not well placed.

Dosage Rate and Adjuvant Drugs. The dosage of the principal immobilizing drug is very similar for all the animals in this group. The dose for an impala weighing 50 kg is 0.2 mg of M.99, although 0.5 mg may be used with caution. Zebra and wildebeest weighing about 300 kg

need about 1.25 mg, although 1.5 mg is by no means excessive, and 2 mg may be used. The dose rate of tranquilizer is also not critical, and most of these animals may be caught without its use. The reaction is improved and hastened with the addition of about 40 or 50 mg of acetylpromazine; also, the final capture is made easier and excitement reduced.

It is required to strike a balance between the need for adequate tranquilizer and the undesirability of diluting excessively the principal drug and thus delaying absorption. Acetylpromazine at 40 to 50 mg/ml causes no excessive dilution. At the strength of 200 mg/ml the quantity of hyoscine needed is seldom more than 0.2 ml. The entire volume of the mixture can be held under 2 ml.

Many of the animals caught have been given suboptimal amounts of tranquilizer if the concentrated form of acetylpromazine is not readily procurable. Other tranquilizers such as triflupromazine may be used, and there are indications that they may be more effective for certain species. The dose rate is fairly constant in these animals as there is little difference in the body weights between individuals of the same species. An adult male hartebeest seldom differs more than a few kilograms from another adult male hartebeest in the same area and at that particular time of the year; also, they reach adult size in a short space of time. This is in marked contrast to animals previously described.

Behavioral Response to Drug Effect. The behavioral response to the drug effect in these animals is usually one of increasing sedation. A definite period of excitement is rarely seen, although hartebeest and tsessebe are more inclined this way than zebra, waterbuck, and wildebeest. No definite high head carriage is exhibited. Sometimes animals will trot with short steps and raised carpus, but only for a short while, and they soon come to a halt. Usually they will walk slowly with drooping head until they stop. Once halted they will stand or lean in a drowsy manner or go down.

Lightly dosed animals as those in which

absorption is delayed exhibit curiosity rather than excitement. Many animals would approach the car a number of times to within a few yards before jibbing. Some have approached so close that they could easily be caught by seizing a horn or an ear from the interior of the car. Once caught the animals in this group usually stand quietly. Compulsive trotting is rare, and if disturbed they will trot or canter for a short distance and then settle down to walking or standing. When they stand the head is usually dropped low, which contrasts with the previously discussed group of animals.

Sight appears to be impaired and those animals that walk are usually halted by solid objects in their path. Bushes are traversed rather than avoided, and capture may be effected as the animal pushes through with difficulty. When animals are lost to sight, their passage through undergrowth may be heard and the noise made is quite different from any made by a normal beast.

When large doses of the order of 1.5 to 2 mg of M.99 are injected, animals such as zebra tend to stop quickly and to go down. This is of advantage if either a large number of animals are to be captured quickly or the country tends to be thick. Even though the animals go down, they usually retain sternal recumbency. It has been the practice to monitor heart rates and respiration, and a special watch should be kept on recumbent animals.

Animals in this group generally acquiesce well to handling. When they are seized by horn or tail, little resistance is offered. Usually they stand still when forward progress is impeded. Mature buffalo, however, tend to be aggressive, and the immobilized animal should be approached with care until the extent of the incapitation is evident.

The reaction to intravenous nalorphine or M.285 is usually dramatic. If the animal is lying down it will rise precipitately within 30 seconds (Fig. 29.11). On regaining their feet, a short gallop is usually performed; often a degree of excitement is evident, particularly in zebra, and they will trot around and vocalize. Very small doses of nalorphine (15 mg) given to induce only partial recovery is usually sufficient to enable the subject to break away.

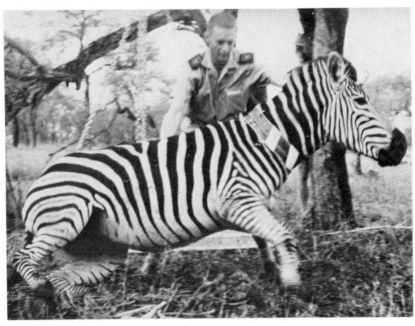

FIG. 29.11. On receiving an intravenous injection of nalorphine, most animals jump to their feet suddenly after an interval of 30 to 90 seconds.

Young buffalo given small amounts of nalorphine become very difficult to control and chlorpromazine (1 mg/kg) may be given to render them tractable.

To reduce excitement in the zebra on the injection of nalorphine, 10 mg of acetylpromazine should be given intravenously simultaneously. This obviates having to give two injections and the difficulty of synchronizing the action of the two compounds.

ELAND, NYALA, ORYX, AND KUDU

The animals in this group are wary and difficult to approach (Table 29.7). They either live in thick cover as does the kudu and nyala or else, like the oryx, tend to take flight if approached to a distance of less than 150 yards. On injection, these animals take flight and seek cover or else travel long distances before they are halted by the drug action. The nyala and kudu which live in dense cover have been injected when standing; eland and oryx only when running from a following vehicle, and these continued to run after the injection had been effected. The bush antelope move less far but are comparably difficult to find or follow.

The time lapse between injection and capture in these animals is long, which is due in part to their natural shyness, inducing a strong reaction to put the maximum distance between themselves and the hunter, and partly as a result of their reaction to narcotics which comprises excitement with very little depression. This, together with the response to injection, will induce a state of intense locomotary activity which may take them over long distances. Furthermore, the degree of incapacitation is often small so that avoiding action continues to be possible, thus further prolonging capture. The running reaction induces a rise in body temperature and eventual exhaustion. Capture of these animals is therefore undertaken in the cool times of the day only. Recent results indicate that higher dosages of M.99 and the use of tranquilizers render capture more efficacious.

Dose Rate. The dose rate for the animals in this group is relatively high. This is due to an *a priori* need for high dosage to immobilize these animals, but is also necessary to prevent them from getting out of sight and lost in thick cover. Animals in the previous groups described will slow up as a result of a very light dose, and a second injection can usually be administered without difficulty from an approach on foot. This group of animals will become excited by a subimmobilizing dose, and a second injection is difficult to effect. For this reason, also, a higher dose rate of M.99 is administered.

Using a high dosage of over 20 μg/kg, the nyala will go down rapidly and without struggling. Attempts were made to reduce the dose rate of M.99 by incorporating chlorpromazine at 3 mg/kg and varying doses of phenycyclidine, but with only partial success. Increasing the tranquilizer moiety rather than the M.99 so as to render the animals easier to handle on capture has been a more reliable method. As the animals in this group become excited as a result of M.99 administration, there is need for a tranquilizer to reduce the tendency for these animals to run. More important is the reduced struggling on capture when adequate amounts are administered with the narcotic. Rompun with M.99 or azaperone with fentanyl has also been used.

Behavioral Response to Drug Effect. The response of the animals in this group to narcotics is the typical pose reminiscent of the Straub-Hermann effect which is induced in certain laboratory animals by drugs with a morphine-like action. The gait becomes stilted and paces become rapid but shortened. The carpus is lifted high off the ground, the so-called hackney gait. The head and neck are curved backwards and the head is held horizontally. Their eyes are kept almost closed, the nostrils are predominantly dilated, and the tongue is often protruded. Breathing is stertorous and the noise made is positive snorting and vocalization as distinct from the snoring-type noise made by some animals such as elephant due to relaxation of the soft palate.

These animals tend to stay on their feet with all but the highest dosages. They also remain ambulant, and none of the eland, oryx, kudu, or male nyala become stationary for any length of time. All these animals remained wary and reacted instantly to a footstep or breaking twig, so that an approach on foot is precluded. Nyala will approach closely enough to be seized. The kudu were caught by surrounding them by a small group of men, preferably holding short lengths of rope between them. Eland are caught by running after them and seizing them by the tail. Oryx, owing to their aggressive disposition and lethal horns, are caught from a motor car by means of a rope dropped over the horns from a light pole. Considerable degrees of depression can be produced with large amounts of tranquilizers so that the rapid recovery pattern of the other groups of animals is not possible.

The response to an intravenously administered dose of the narcotic antagonist is similar to most species—a rapid increase in the awareness of the animal and stronger efforts to escape. The animals in this group were, however, usually standing or able to rise without the benefit of nalorphine. The change therefore resulting from the nalorphine injection is less clear-cut than in the previous group of animals, which were usually recumbent and responded by jumping to their feet.

Neuroleptic Narcosis and Behavior

The behavior of the wild animal under the influence of certain centrally acting substances has often been described as tranquil, and the substances used as tranquilizers. Tranquilizers are a group of substances that have been remarkably misnamed,[28] and the word as a general term is probably best avoided unless a meaning can be filtered out that can be meaningful to the scientist dealing with animals or that can denote a special attitude or behavior pattern in a closely designed set of circumstances (see Chapter 13).

The tranquilization (in the general meaning of the word) of free living wild animals and also domestic animals is not possible. States of delirium can be induced that render even very large animals such as the hippopotamus easy to catch with ropes. Alterations in the normal behavioral patterns can be induced by the modification and depression of certain reactions so that the animal is rendered abnormal. This is in contrast to the usual medical connotation in which patients are tranquilized to find relief from disability or anxiety,[49] and to liberate patients from the constraints of a locked ward.[47]

The clinical usefulness of tranquilizing drugs lies in their use to modify fear and anxiety. Fear as an emotion in wild animals probably does not occur unless the animal is subjected to an unnatural situation. It is a subjective term, and the word is used as a theoretical construct in the kind of situation in which the human subject would show fear.[1] The wild animal reacts to specific stimuli in his environment. Various situations such as the presence of a preditor will trigger the defense reaction, which is a graded behavioral response whose initial signs are alerting and which may culminate in the familiar signs of fright and flight.[1] Certain chemical compounds modify this behavior but do not suppress it. Chlorpromazine, for example, has the ability to affect animal behavior differentially by causing a marked reduction in aggression but an increase in flight.[12]

Recently acquired habits are thought to be more susceptible to modification through drug effects.[58] Also some chemical compounds produce a greater decrement in certain reactions such as the avoidance motivated by fear than in approach motivated by hunger.[3] It is, on this basis, easier to understand how certain animals under the influence of narcotic compounds will modify the reaction to certain avoidance objects such as motor vehicles, and even by apparently attracted by them insofar as they approach them repeatedly. At the same time, a footstep will send those animals galloping off, albeit for a short distance only, to return as the stimulus dies down. The effect of the chemical may be said to reduce the stimulus generalization in the fear-motivated habit of avoidance more than the curiosity-motivated habit of approach.

It is generally accepted that various drugs administered at the earliest moment when animals are caught in traps or nets will reduce the mortality for reasons other than self-inflicted injury. Amylobarbital sodium has been found useful in the therapy of combat neurosis of man.[27] In animals, fear, as distinct from normal flight reaction, seems to develop when an animal's normal behavior pattern is disrupted, such as through roping, netting, or capture. The fear-motivated reaction may be reduced by a variety of drugs that tend to restore the animal's normal activity, i.e., pattern of activity, feeding and drinking, and to reduce the fear-motivated behavior that results in aberrant physiological reactions leading frequently to sickness and death.

It is possible, however, that the fear complex apparently suffered by freshly caught animals is a combination of fear, a desire to escape, hunger due to food refusal, and frustration resulting from disruption of normal habits. Various drugs may affect different aspects of this complex, and as the science of psychopharmacology advances, a rational basis for alleviating the various aspects of this syndrome may be evolved. Meanwhile, drug mixtures rather than specific drugs are often preferential for both the capture and subsequent treatment of animals during captivity.

To a certain extent, the effect of mixtures must be a true potentiation, e.g., the action of mixtures of acetylpromazine, M.99, and scopalamine seems to produce an effect which is considerably in excess of that produced by any dose of the separate drugs. However, the function of phe-nothiazine derivatives when administered with the M series goes beyond this insofar as some animals cannot be caught with theoretically unlimited doses of M.99 or the phenothiazines, but respond to relatively small doses of the two administered together. In this case, the phenothiazines appear to have a specific depressant action on subcortical areas which are excited by the M compounds.

The effects of the narcotics depend upon dose and species. The motor areas of the cerebral cortex are only depressed by large doses of morphine. In general, morphine depresses multineuronal reflexes but augments two-neuron reflexes.[85] The M series of compounds appear to block incoming activity so that there is a lack of response rather than a depression of activity. The depression of the medulla is slight as evinced by reduction in respiration only after gross overdose, although eventually an anesthetic-like condition is achieved with loss of corneal reflex, but without muscle relaxation. In some species muscle tone is increased. It is probable that these compounds depress the function of the reticular activating system, which may be described as a monitor that regulates the intensity with which stimuli are appreciated.[47] The ultimate immobilizing effect is, however, in large part due to simpler motor retardation.

The species difference in reaction is marked so that wild ungulates may be divided into three main groups according to their reaction (Table 29.7). In describing the reaction of wild animals to psychoactive drugs, the conditions under which these were administered are qualifying factors. Experimentally, it has been demonstrated that totally different reactions to the injection of amylobarbital and amphetamine sulfate are obtained, depending on whether the test animals are in new environments.[71] In the same way, different reactions can be expected with injection of M.99-tranquilizer mixture, depending on whether the injected animal is aware that it is being hunted or not, whether it is in an area where it is normally hunted or in a sanctuary, or whether it is chased before and/or after injection. In other words, the degree of excitement or depression that follows injection depends to a large extent on the stage of excitement or tranquility of the animal during injection and whether the animal is pursued to effect injection, or subsequently so as to follow in close country. Under these circumstances the depressant effect of the injected compounds is likely to be delayed.

A common experience is that animals captured with centrally acting compounds are far easier to approach on subsequent days than those captured with neuromuscular blocking agents. The former are more responsive to captive conditions; whether this is due to reduced registration or retrieval is perhaps immaterial under the circumstances. The effect on conflict behavior during the initial days of captivity is possibly a long term effect of the phenothiazine tranquilizer, which probably affects behavior for several days subsequent to administration[59]; this initial period is all important in the rapid acceptance of food and captive conditions.

REFERENCES

1. Abrahams, V. C., Hilton, S. M., and Malcolm, J. L.: Sensory connexions to the hypothalamus and mid-brain, and their role in the reflex activation of the defence reaction. J. Physiol. (London) 164: 1, 1962.
2. Anderson, C. F.: Anaesthetising deer by arrow. J. Wildlife Manage. 25: 202, 1961.
3. Bailey, C. J., and Miller, N. E.: The effect of sodium amytal on an approach-avoidance conflict in cats. J. Comp. Physiol. Psychol. 45: 205, 1952.
4. Bentley, D. W., Boura, A. L. A., Lister, R. E., Fitzgerald, A. E., Hardy, D. G., McCoubrey, A., and Aikman, M. L.: Compounds containing morphine-antagonizing or powerful analgesic properties. Nature (London) 206: 102, 1965.
5. Bentley, D. W., and Hardy, D. G.: New potent analgesics in the morphine series. Proc. Chem. Soc. (London) 220, 1963.
6. Bligh, J., and Harthoorn, A. M.: Continuous radiotelemetric records of the deep body temperature of some unrestrained African mammals under near-natural conditions. J. Physiol. (London) 176: 145, 1965.
7. Boyd, R. J.: Succinylcholine chloride for immobilisation of Colorado mule deer. J. Wildlife Manage. 26: 332, 1962.
8. Buechner, H. K., Harthoorn, A. M., and Lock, J. A.: Immobilising Uganda kob with succinylcholine chloride. Canad. J. Comp. Med. 24: 317, 1960.
9. Buechner, H. K., Harthoorn, A. M., and Lock, J. A.: The immobilisation of African animals in the field with special reference to their transfer to other areas. Proc. Zool. Soc. London 135: 261, 1960.
10. Campbell, H., and Harthoorn, A. M.: The capture and anaesthesia of the African lion in his natural environment. Vet. Rec. 75: 275, 1963.
11. Carter, B. H.: Immobilisation of rhino with sernyl. Kenya Game Department Report. Typescript, July 1960.
12. Chance, M. R. A., and Silverman, A. P.: The structure of social behaviour and drug action. In Animal Behaviour and Drug Action, Ciba Foundation Symposium. J. & A. Churchill, Ltd., London, 1961.
13. Chen, G., Ensor, C. R., Russell, D., and Bohner, B.: The pharmacology of 1-(1-phenylcylohexyl) piperidine HCl. J. Pharmacol. Exp. Ther. 127: 241, 1959.
14. Child, G.: The capture of black rhinoceros on islands in Lake Kariba. Department of Wildlife Conservation, Rhodesia. Typescript, 1960.
15. Coetzee, H. G. T.: Report of the municipal veterinarian. Zoological Gardens, Bloemfontein, South Africa, Roneo. (Mimiograph), 1960.
16. Cowan, I. McT., Wood, A. J., and Nordan, H. C.: Studies in the tranquilisation and immobilisation of deer (Odocoileus). Canad. J. Comp. Med. 26: 57, 1962.
17. Craighead, F. C., Craighead, J. J., and Davies, R. S.: Radiotracking of grizzly bears and biotelemetry. Interdisciplinary conference on the use of telemetry in animal biology and physiology in relation to ecological problems, edited by Lloyd E. Slater, p. 133. Pergamon Press, Oxford, 1963.
18. Crockford, J. A., Hayes, F. A., Jenkins, J. H., and Feurt, S. D.: An automatic projectile type syringe. Vet. Med. 53: 115, 1958.
19. Daglish, C., and McDougall, J. I.: The solubility of M.99 in aqueous solutions of hyoscine hydrobromide and acepromazine. Report No. 974, Reckitt & Sons Ltd., Hull, England. Roneo (Mimeograph), 1965.
20. Dews, P. B., and Morse, W. H.: Behavioural pharmacology. Ann. Rev. Pharmacol. 1: 145, 1961.
21. Dietz, O., and Kuntze, A.: Die Anwendung der Muskelrelaxatien unter besonderer Beruecksichtigung der Zootiere. Nord. Vet. Med. 14: 30, 1962.
22. Feurt, S. D., Jenkins, J. H., Hayes, F. A., and Crockford, J. A.: Pharmacology and toxicology of nicotine with special reference to species variation. J. Sci. 127: 1054, 1958.

23. Fisher, E. W.: Arterial puncture in cattle. Vet. Rec. 68: 691, 1956.

24. Fisher, E. W.: Arterial puncture in horses. Vet. Rec. 71: 514, 1959.

25. Flook, D. R., Robertson, J. R., Hermanrude, O. R., and Buechner, H. K.: Succinylcholine chloride for immobilisation of North American elk. J. Wildlife Manage. 26: 334, 1962.

26. Goetz, R. H., and Budtz-Olsen, O.: Scientific safari—the circulation of the giraffe. South African Med. J. 29: 773, 1955.

27. Grinker, R. R., and Spiegel, J. P.: War Neurosis. Blakison, New York, 1945.

28. Hamilton, M.: Prediction of clinical response from animal data; a need for theoretical models. In Animal Behaviour and Drug Action, Ciba Foundation Symposium. J. & A. Churchill, Ltd., London, 1964.

29. Harthoorn, A. M.: Translocation as a means of preserving wild animals. J. Fauna Pres. Soc. (Oryx) 6: 215, 1961.

30. Harthoorn, A. M.: The use of neuromuscular blocking agents on domestic cattle. Vet. Rec. 74: 395, 1962.

31. Harthoorn, A. M.: Capture of the white (square lipped) rhinoceros ceratotherium simum simum (Burchell) with the use of drug immobilisation technique. Canad. J. Comp. Med. 26: 203, 1962.

32. Harthoorn, A. M.: On the use of phencyclidine for narcosis in the larger animals. Vet. Rec. 74: 410, 1962.

33. Harthoorn, A. M.: Neuroleptic narcosis; an approach to anaesthesia in large animals. Nature (London) 198: 1116, 1963.

34. Harthoorn, A. M.: The value of neuroleptic narcosis in restraint; compared with that of anaesthesia, sedation or paralysis. Proceedings of the Symposium on African Mammals, Zoological Society of South Africa, Salisbury, Rhodesia, September 1963.

35. Harthoorn, A. M.: The tranquilisation and handling of large animals. A field and laboratory study. Department of Physiology, University College, Nairobi. Roneo, 1965.

36. Harthoorn, A. M.: The use of a new oripavine derivative for restraint of domestic hoofed animals. J. South African Vet. Med. Ass. 36: 45, 1965.

37. Harthoorn, A. M.: Application of pharmacological and physiological principles in restraint of wild animals. Wildlife Monograph No. 14, Wildlife Society, Washington, D.C., 1965.

38. Harthoorn, A. M.: Large animal restraint. A prerequisite for conservation and research. Africana 2: 19, 1966.

39. Harthoorn, A. M., and Bligh, J.: The use of a new oripavine derivative with potent morphine-like activity for the restraint of hoofed wild animals. Res. Vet. Sci. 6: 290, 1965.

40. Harthoorn, A. M., and Lock, J. A.: The rescue of rhinoceros from Kariba Dam. J. Fauna Pres. Soc. 5: 352, 1960.

41. Harthoorn, A. M., and Luck, C. P.: Aspects of the circulation in the pinna of the African elephant (Loxodonta africana). J. Physiol. (London) 163: 52, 1962.

42. Harthoorn, A. M., and Luck, C. P.: The handling and marking of the wild East African elephant. Secondary preliminary report. Brit. Vet. J. 119: 526, 1962.

43. Harthoorn, A. M., and Player, I. C.: The narcosis of the white rhinoceros. A series of eighteen case histories. Proceedings of the Fifth International Symposium on Diseases of Zoo-Animals, Amsterdam, 1963. Cited by A. M. Harthoorn, 1965.

44. Hatch, R. D., Ferris, D. H., Link, R. P., and Calhoun, J.: Unsatisfactory results with nicotine immobilisation of a deer and brahma cossbred cattle. Two case reports. J. Amer. Vet. Med. Ass. 135: 92, 1959.

45. Heuschele, W. P.: Chlordiazepoxide for calming zoo animals. J. Amer. Vet. Med. Ass. 139: 996, 1961.

46. High, J. P., Hassert, G. L., Rubin, B., Piala, J. J., Burke, J. C., and Craver, B. N.: Pharmacology of fluphenazine (Prolixin). Toxic. Appl. Pharmacol. 2: 540, 1960.

47. Himwich, H. E.: Psychopharmacologic drugs. Science 127: 59, 1958.

48. Hofmeyr, C. F. B.: Some observations on the use of succinylcholine chloride (suxamethonium) in horses with reference to the effect on the heart. J. South American Vet. Med. Ass. 31: 251, 1960.

49. Hollister, L. E.: The present status of tranquilising drugs. Calif. Med. 89: 1, 1958.

50. Jewell, P. A., and Smith, E. A.: Immobilisation of grey seals. J. Wildlife Manage. 29: 316, 1965.

51. King, J. M., and Carter, B. H.: The use of the oripavine derivative M.99 for the immobilisation of the black rhinoceros, and its antagonism with the related compound M.285 or nalorphine. East African Wildlife J. 3: 19, 1965.

52. Klavano, P. A., and Johnson, V. L.: Nalorphine hydrochloride as a narcotic antagonist in dogs. J. Amer. Vet. Med. Ass. 154: 399, 1954.

53. Kroll, W. R.: Experience with Sernylan in zoo animals. Int. Zoo Year Book 4: 131, 1962.

54. Kruuk, H.: Seregeti research project. Personal communication, 1966.

55. Larsen, L. H., Loomis, L. N., and Steel, J. D.: Muscular relaxants and cardiovascular damage; with special reference to succinylcholine chloride. Aust. Vet. J. 35: 369, 1959.

56. Lock, J. A., and Harthoorn, A. M.: A note on the use of suxamethonium chloride (succinylcholine chloride) for the restraint of zebra. Vet. Rec. 71: 919, 1959.

57. Louw, G. N., Kemm, E. H., and Fourie, P. C.: Tranquilisation and premedication of pigs and sheep with the benzodiaserpine derivative R.O. 5-2807. Proceedings of the South African Society for Animal Production, No. 2, Pretoria, p. 136, 1963.

58. Masserman, J. H.: Behavior and Neurosis. Hafner Publishing Co., New York, 1943.

59. Miller, N. E.: Discussion of Marrazzi, A. S.:

Inhibition as a determinant of synaptic and behavioral patterns. Ann. N.Y. Acad. Sci. *92:* 1028, 1961.

60. Montgomery, G. G.: A modification of the nicotine dart capture method. J. Wildlife Manage. *25:* 101, 1961.

61. Niekerk, J. W. van and Pienaar, U. de V.: Adaptations of the immobilising technique to the capture, marking and translocation of game animals in the Kruger National Park. J. Sci. Res. National Parks South Africa (Koedoe) *5:* 137, 1962.

62. Niekerk, J. W. van, and Pienaar, U. de V.: A report on some immobilising drugs used in the capture of wild animals in Kruger National Park. J. Sci. Res. National Parks South Africa (Koedoe) *6:* 126, 1963.

63. Niekerk, J. W. van, Pienaar, U. de V., and Fairall, N.: A preliminary note on the use of Quiloflex (benzodioxane hydrochloride) in the immobilisation of game. J. Sci. National Parks South Africa (Koedoe) *6:* 109, 1963.

64. Orr, S. M., and Moore-Gilbert, D. J. C.: Field immobilisation of young wildebeest with succinylcholine chloride. East African Wildlife J. *11:* 60, 1964.

65. Oxenham, R.: Immobilisation experiments. Report of the Game Department, Chilanga, Zambia. Typescript and roneo, 1964.

66. Pienaar, U. de V.: Capture and immobilising techniques currently employed in Kruger National Park and other South African national parks and provinicial reserves. Kruger National Park, Skukuza. Ronco, 1966.

67. Piperno, E.: Effects of various paralyzers, tranquilisers and anaesthetics on white-tailed deer. Paper presented at Midwest Wildlife Conference. Roneo, 1965.

68. Player, I. C.: Report on the translocation of drugged square-lipped rhino to Kyle Dam Game Reserve, Rhodesia. National Park Game and Fish Preservation Board, Mtubatuba, Zululand. Roneo, 1966.

69. Post, G.: The use of curare and curare-like drugs on elk (wapiti). J. Wildlife Manag. *23:* 365, 1959.

70. Royal Veterinary College of East Africa Expedition: The use of a thiambutene/phencyclidine/hyoscine mixture for the immobilisation of the topi (Damliscus korrigum) and the hippopotamus (Hippopotamus amphibius). Vet. Rec. *75:* 630, 1963.

71. Rushton, R., and Steinberg, H.: Mutual potentiation of amphetamine and amylobarbitone measured by activity in rats. Brit. J. Pharmacol. *21:* 295, 1963.

72. Rutty, D. A., and Thurley, D. C.: Further observations on the use of phencyclidine in monkeys. Vet. Rec. *74:* 883, 1962.

73. Short, R. V.: A syringe projectile for use with a bow and arrow. Vet. Rec. *75:* 883, 1963.

74. Short, R. V., and King, J. W.: The design of a crossbow and dart for the immobilisation of wild animals. Vet. Rec. *76:* 628, 1964.

75. Spalding, V. T., and Heymann, C. S.: The value of phencyclidine in the anaesthesia of monkeys. Vet. Rec. *74:* 158, 1962.

76. Stevenson, D. E., and Hall, L. W.: Pharmacological effects of suxamethonium. Vet. Rec. *71:* 818, 1959.

77. Talbot, L. M.: Field immobilisation of large mammals. Serengeti-Mara Wildlife Research Project. Roneo, 1960.

78. Talbot, L. M.: Field immobilisation of some East African wild animals and cattle. 1. East African Agr. Forest J. *26:* 92, 1960.

79. Talbot, L. M., and Lamprey, H. F.: Immobilisation of free-ranging East African ungulates with succinylcholine chloride. J. Wildlife Manage. *25:* 303, 1961.

80. Talbot, L. M., and Talbot. M. H.: Flaxedil and other drugs in field immobilisation and translocation of large mammal in East Africa. Mammalology *43:* 76, 1962.

81. Tavernor, W. D.: The use of succinylcholine chloride as a casting agent in the horse. Vet. Rec. *71:* 774, 1959.

82. Tavernor, W. D.: The effect of succinylcholine chloride on the heart of the horse; clinical and pathological aspects. Vet. Rec. *72:* 569, 1960.

83. Tavernor, W. D.: A study of the effect of phencyclidine in the pig. Vet. Rec. *75:* 1377, 1963.

84. Taylor, R. H., and Magnussen, W. B.: Preliminary note on capture and marking of wild ungulates in New Zealand. New Zealand J. Sci. *28:* 2, 1965.

85. Wikler, A.: Sites and mechanism of action of morphine and related drugs in the central nervous system. Pharmacol. Rev. *2:* 435, 1950.

86. Wilkins, J. H.: The effect of a new analgesic induction agent on goats. Vet. Rec. *73:* 767, 1961.

30

Restraint and Anesthesia of Bears and Undomesticated Cats

DONALD CLIFFORD

Bears

The subject of ursine anesthesia is not confined to the administration of anesthetic agent, but must include means of approaching and restraining bears. Bears do not have retractile claws, so even a playful blow can produce a serious injury. Captive bears that are not crowded, annoyed, or placed in an unusual situation ordinarily will not seek to harm human beings. Grizzly and polar bears are notable exceptions.[8]

THE CAPTURE AND RESTRAINT OF FREE BEARS

The culvert trap and special steel traps with offset jaws have replaced the conventional steel bear traps as the method of capture. A bear may be immobilized and then anesthetized in these devices or transferred to a squeeze cage or placed in an airtight cage suitable for receiving a volatile agent.

The use of succinylcholine chloride or phencyclidine and the introduction of the Cap-Chur rifle*, first used as a means of immobilizing deer,[11, 13] permits accurate delivery of the agents at a distance of 25 yards and has facilitated the restraint of wild animals.[12, 18] Guns which employ powder as the propulsive charge, cross-

---

*Palmer Chemical and Equipment Co., Douglasville, Georgia.

bows, or syringes fastened on the tip of a pole may be used. Syringes with a collar rather than a barb are preferred, and the hind leg or hip regions are the best target site. Needles from 1 to 2 inches in length are used, depending on the size of the animal.

Succinylcholine in the intramuscular dose of 0.4 mg/kg (20 mg/100 pounds) has been found to be quite reliable for all bears.[4, 16] A common technique in the use of succinylcholine, when the weight of the animal is uncertain, is to use a small initial dose which can be increased if found to be inadequate. Intramuscular doses take effect in approximately 3 to 6 minutes and last about 4 to 10 minutes. Delay or insufficient immobilization results if the agent is deposited in a poorly vascularized area or if leakage occurs around the site of injection. Since excessive doses of succinylcholine may paralyze the respiratory muscles, means of artificial ventilation should be available. There is no antagonist for succinyl choline. Gallamine triethiodide, a "curarelike" muscle relaxant, has been used.[1] The advantage of this drug is that it can be reversed with neostigmine (see Chapter 12). Atropine should be administered first to control salivation. Once the free animal has been immobilized with gallamine, or succinylcholine or forcibly restrained, an

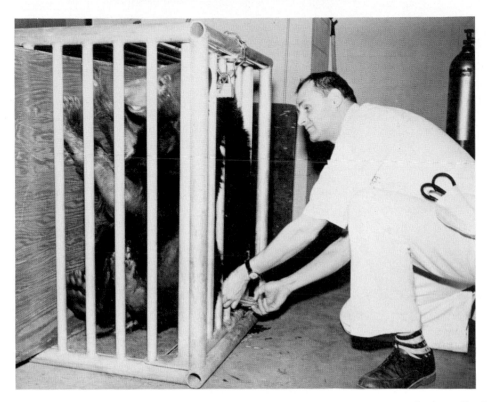

FIG. 30.1. The bear is squeezed into one end of the aluminum cage where preanesthetic medication is administered intramuscularly.

injectable or volatile agent can be administered (Figs. 30.1, 30.2, and 30.3).

Phencyclidine, which can be administered by means of the Cap-Chur rifle, will facilitate physical restraint of bears. It can be used with barbiturates and/or inhalation agents to produce surgical anesthesia. The intramuscular dosage required is not well established and varies from 0.6 to 2.2 mg/kg.[14] Other agents, such as nicotine alkaloids, have been used but are hazardous. (See Chapter 13 for other cyclohexamines.)

THE RESTRAINT AND IMMOBILIZATION OF CONFINED BEARS

In zoos, bears can be captured in squeeze cages or airtight boxes where a number of drugs can be administered. These cages vary from a bulky, fixed cage to a relatively simple mobile cage where plywood panels are used to confine the animal (Figs. 30.1 and 30.2).[4] The use of chloral hydrate, pentobarbital, or phencyclidine in syrup is usually ineffective, since bears detect the presence of such agents before sufficient amount is taken. Even if a considerable amount of these agents is ingested, the level of sedation may not be satisfactory.

Depressants are not as effective in bears as they are in certain other carnivores, although large doses of morphine (9.9 mg/kg) and promazine (4.8 mg/kg) or other tranquilizers can be used for preanesthetic medication.[1, 5, 15] Drugs should be administered by syringe to animals in a squeeze cage, since Cap-Chur guns are traumatic at short range. The veins in the limbs or tongue may be used after depression or immobilization by preanesthetic medication or succinylcholine for the injection of anesthetic agents. The veins of the legs are small in relation to the size of the animal, and embedded in fat; those of the hind limb are the most accessible.[3]

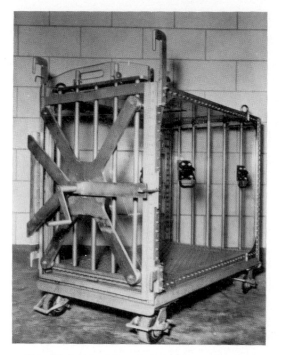

FIG. 30.2 Specially designed anesthetization chamber and squeeze cage. Anesthesia can be induced safely in bears by introducing an inhalation anesthetic into this chamber. (Courtesy of P. Day: Symposium on Experimental Animal Anesthesiology, Brooks Air Force Base, San Antonio, Texas, 1964.)

Sodium pentobarbital by intravenous injection has been used for general anesthesia in bears; other routes of administration decrease the margin of safety. The dose is approximately 31 to 35 mg/kg, but there is considerable species difference. Recovery can be expected in approximately 3 hours.

Airtight cages are used to facilitate induction of general anesthesia with volatile agents (Fig. 30.3). The administration of atropine and sedative drugs is indicated prior to anesthesia. Inhalation anesthesia can be maintained by endotracheal intubation and the use of the rebreathing system (see Chapter 17). A nose cone or mask has also been used for the induction of inhalation anesthesia. In laboratories and zoos where there is a wide range of anesthetic equipment, inhalation agents can be used. In the field, intravenous anesthesia is easier to employ.

Undomesticated Cats

Administration of parenteral depressants will result in some sedation of wild cats, but the oral route is generally unsatisfactory.

Large zoological *Felidae* usually can be

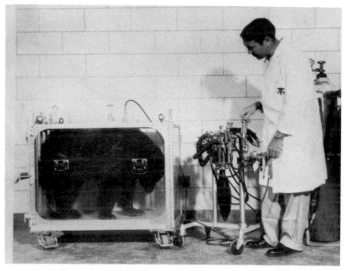

FIG. 30.3 Induction of anesthesia with nitrous oxide-oxygen, 1:1, and halothane, 4%. The rate of flow of 10 liters/minute was reduced to 6 liters/minute after the chamber was saturated. The bear was immobilized in 20 to 25 minutes. This technique was used to facilitate minor surgery. (Courtesy of P. Day: Symposium on Experimental Animal Anesthesiology, Brooks Air Force Base, San Antonio, Texas, 1964.)

trapped in squeeze or transport cages without difficulty. When properly placed in a squeeze cage, inspection, palpation, auscultation, and other procedures are not as difficult or hazardous as might be anticipated.

DRUGS FOR PREANESTHETIC MEDICATION AND SEDATION

In undomesticated and also domesticated cats, promazine (4.4 mg/kg) and meperidine (11 mg/kg) can be given in combination to facilitate restraint.[6, 7] High doses of meperidine may cause muscle tensions, convulsions, and death. Other tranquilizers such as chlorpromazine, propyl promazine, and perphenazine may be used.[9, 17] Meperidine is one of the few narcotic analgesics which is not likely to produce excitement in cats. An advantage of most of the injectable ataractics and meperidine is that they may be given simultaneously from the same syringe. Unfortunately, they are irritant to the tissues and the animal must be under control when the injection is made. The intramuscular route is preferred because absorption is more rapid, and less irritation results.

Phencyclidine may be used to immobilize large cats or act as a basal anesthetic. Following the intramuscular injection of 1.1 to 2.2 mg/kg, ataxia catatonia and sedation and immobilization are produced. Muscle spasms and extension of the forelegs may be observed in some animals.[14] Phencyclidine, chlorpromazine, and hyoscine have been employed by means of Cap-Chur gun to immobilize lions in the natural state.[2, 10] The combination of a tranquilizer and phencyclidine will reduce the catatonia produced by phencyclidine alone. One-half of the recommended dose of both is given; this will reduce the generally long duration of action that large doses of phencyclidine have in cats. (See Chapter 13).

Succinylcholine can be used intramuscularly (0.4 mg/kg (20 mg/100 pounds)), the drug takes effect in about 3 to 10 minutes with a duration of 3 to 12 minutes. Larger doses prolong the duration of effect but may cause paralysis of the respiratory muscles. Refrigeration of succinylcholine is necessary in order to prevent loss of potency. Carnivores are apt to protrude their tongues when this drug and phencyclidine are used simultaneously, and thus the lingual vein can easily be used for injecting other drugs. Chlordiazepoxide (55 mg/kg orally) will produce tranquilization in some animals.[17]

GENERAL ANESTHESIA

Preanesthetic agents reduce the required amount of barbiturate for general anesthesia so that light anesthesia with pentobarbital will not result in a prolonged recovery period. When pentobarbital or other short acting agents are used alone, large cats may require 2 to 3 days to recover. Thiopental or thiamylal alone has a longer duration of action in the large *Felidae* than in other carnivores.

Dosages of pentobarbital, thiopental, thiamylal, and other barbiturates will vary according to the degree of sedation produced by the preanesthetic medication. A range of 11 to 22 mg/kg for these drugs has been used in undomesticated cats. It is advisable that these animals be premedicated and barbiturates given to effect.

Squeeze cages and anesthetization chambers described for bears can also be used in cats. Inhalation anesthesia with endotracheal intubation or a face mask utilizing the rebreathing system has been used in the small and large cats. The induction of anesthesia with an ultrashort acting barbiturate followed by maintenance with an inhalation agent will prevent the prolonged recovery period. Methods which can be used for anesthetization of other domestic animals can be used for the large cats (see Chapter 17).

REFERENCES

1. Bolz, W.: Neuroleptica und potenzierte Narkose speziell bei Zootieren. Proceedings of the Fourth International Symposium on Diseases in Zoo-Animals. Nord. Vet. Med. *14:* (suppl. 1), 17, 1962.
2. Campbell, H., and Harthoorn, A. M.: The capture and anaesthesia of African lion in his natural environment. Vet. Rec. *75:* 275, 1963.

3. Clarke, N. P., Huheey, M. J., and Martin, W. M.: Pentobarbital anesthesia in bears. J. Amer. Vet. Med. Ass. *143:* 47, 1963.
4. Clifford, D. H.: Observations on effect of preanesthetic medication with meperidine and promazine on barbiturate anesthesia in an ocelot and a leopard. J. Amer. Vet. Med. Ass. *133:* 459, 1958.
5. Clifford, D. H., and Fletcher, J.: Construction of a cage to confine, transport and treat bears. Int. Zool. Year Book *3:* 121, 1961.
6. Clifford, D. H., Good, A. L., and Stowe, C. M., Jr.: Observations on the use of ataractic and narcotic preanesthesia and pentobarbital anesthesia in bears. J. Amer. Vet. Med. Ass. *140:* 464, 1962.
7. Clifford, D. H., Stowe, C. M., Jr., and Good, A. L.: Pentobarbital anesthesia in lions with special reference to preanesthetic medication. J. Amer. Vet. Med. Ass. *139:* 111, 1961.
8. Crandall, L. S.: *The Management of Wild Mammals in Captivity.* The University of Chicago Press, Chicago, 1964.
9. Graham-Jones, O.: Tranquillizer and paralytic drugs. An international survey of animal restraint techniques. Int. Zool. Year Book *2:* 300, 1960.
10. Graham-Jones, O.: Restraint and anaesthesia of some captive wild mammals. Vet. Rec. *76:* 1216, 1964.
11. Hall, T. C., Taft, E. B., Baker, W. H., and Aub, J. C.: A preliminary report on the use of Flaxedil to produce paralysis in the whitetailed deer. J. Wildlife Manage. *17:* 516, 1953.
12. Heuschele, W. P.: Immobilization of captive wild animals. Vet. Med. *56:* 348, 1961.
13. Jenkins, J. A., Feurt, S. D., Haynes, F. A., and Crockford, J. A.: A preliminary report on a field method using drugs for capturing deer. Proc. Southeastern Ass. Game and Fish Commissioners Meeting *9:* 41, 1955.
14. Kroll, W. R.: Experiences with Sernylan in zoo animals. Int. Zool. Year Book *4:* 131, 1962.
15. Louw, A. J.: The Use of chlorpromazine hydrochloride ("Largactil-Maybaker") in anaesthesia of a brown bear (*Ursus arctos*) J. South African Vet. Med. Ass. *28:* 261, 1957.
16. Mortelmans, J., and Vercruysse, J.: The use of succinylcholine to restrain captive wild animals. Proceedings of the Fourth International Symposium on Diseases in Zoo-Animals. Nord. Vet. Med. *14:* (suppl. 1), 72, 1962.
17. Smits, G. M.: Some experiments and experiences with neuroleptic and hypnotic drugs on ungulates with special regard to Librium. Proceedings of the Fifth International Symposium on Diseases of Zoo-Animals. Roy. Neth. Ass., Tij. Dierg. *89:* 195, 1964.
18. Thomas, W. D.: Chemical immobilization of wild animals. J. Amer. Vet. Med. Ass. *138:* 263, 1961.

31
The Action and Toxicity of Local Anesthetic Agents

KARL L. GABRIEL

The Nerve Impulse

The nerve cell consists of suspended materials (proteins) and dissolved materials (various metallic ions) all intimately involved in an aqueous environment and enclosed by a membrane. This membrane is considered to be composed of a layer of lipoid material, two molecules thick, the molecules being arranged tail to tail with hydrophilic groups outside, covered by a layer of protein. It is about 100 Å thick and is covered in many instances with a thick myelin sheath.

The membrane is semipermeable, and certain substances can pass into the cell by a process similar to diffusion. In addition, it is selectively permeable to potassium ions and impermeable to sodium ions. In the normal resting nerve cell, the concentration of potassium ions inside the cell is greater than the concentration outside (Fig. 31.1), while the concentrations of sodium and chloride ions inside are less than those outside. This is believed to be brought about by the "sodium pump," which is capable of operating against a considerable chemical potential gradient. Since 2,4-dinitrophenol is known to reduce the ability of this "pump" reversibly, and since 2,4-dinitrophenol is known to interfere with energy-yielding metabolic processes, it is believed that the energy driving the "sodium pump" is derived from adenosine triphosphatase.

The nerve cell membrane is polarized, with the outside being positive with respect to the inside, and a measurable potential difference exists. This potential is considered to arise from the differences between the internal and external concentrations of potassium ions and, to a lesser extent, to differences in sodium ion and chloride ion concentrations. If the membrane is depolarized by applying an electric potential, the cellular permeability to ions is completely altered. Sodium ions now pass into the cell and potassium ions pass out. As the concentration of sodium ions inside the cell increases, the portion of the membrane adjacent to the point of application of the potential becomes positively polarized on the inside. This polarization alters the permeability of the adjacent membrane; the process repeats itself. This polarization and altered permeability is self-perpetuating and spreads along the axon in both directions, away from the point of application of the stimulus. The increased permeability to sodium ions is only transitory, and the original ionic state is restored rapidly.

A negative potential difference between the surface and the inside occurs during stimulation. This is followed by a return to the positive resting potential. While the movement of sodium ions contributes most to the electrical changes observed (Fig. 31.2), this does not completely ac-

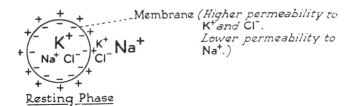

Resting Phase

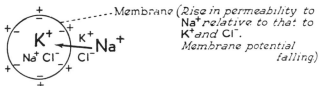

Early Rising Phase of Nerve Action Potential

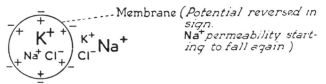

Peak of Action Potential

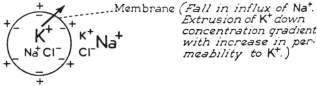

Decline of Action Potential

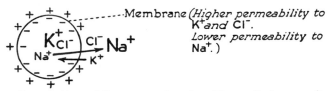

Completion of Return to Resting Phase (Refractory)

FIG. 31.1. The movements of ions which take place across the nerve fiber membrane during the passage of a nerve impulse. The direction of ion movement is shown by *arrows*. Relatively large concentrations of an ion are shown by the use of larger, thicker lettering. For example, the extracellular concentration of sodium is always greater than that in the cells, and the converse is true for potassium. (From *Lewis: Introduction to Pharmacology*, Ed. 3, p. 487. E. and S. Livingstone, Ltd., Edinburgh, 1964.)

count for the size and shape of the action potential. The movements of other cations and anions make a significant contribution.

The movement of ions through the membrane may be brought about by either or both of two mechanisms: by the opening of pores or by the action of enzymes. The movements of ions during the passage of an impulse cannot be adequately accounted for by simple diffusion. The membrane thus appears to contain mechanisms for the active transport of particular ions, but the mechanism by

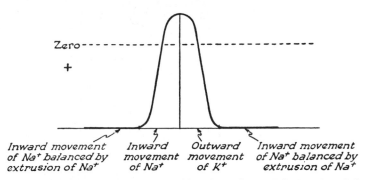

FIG. 31.2. The relationship between movements of ions in and out of the interior of the nerve fiber and the nerve action potential (see Fig. 31.1). (From *Lewis: Introduction to Pharmacology*, Ed. 3, p. 490. E. and S. Livingstone, Ltd., Edinburgh, 1964.)

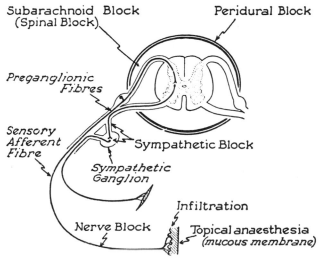

FIG. 31.3. The sites at which local anesthetics are applied and act. (From *Lewis: Introduction to Pharmacology*, Ed. 3, p. 491. E. and S. Livingstone, Ltd., Edinburgh, 1964.)

which the membrane is able to distinguish between potassium and sodium ions is not understood. It may be on a physical basis or it may be entirely enzymatic in nature.

Mechanism of Action of Local Anesthetic Agents

Local anesthetics will prevent passage of the nerve impulse at a) sensory nerve endings, b) ganglionic synapse, c) myoneural junctions, and d) nerve trunks (Fig. 31.3).

Blocking of the reflex arc at the sensory nerve ending can be demonstrated with the strychninized frog preparation. Immersing the frog in a solution of cocaine allows the anesthetic to affect the skin sensory nerve endings. External stimuli will no longer reach the cord, and the hyper-reflexia and the convulsions produced by external stimuli will not appear. The reflex arc is blocked at the sensory nerve endings in the skin.

Blockage at the ganglionic synapse can be demonstrated by perfusing a nerve ganglion with a solution containing procaine HCl and by stimulating the preganglionic fibers. The postganglionic fibers fail to exhibit a stimulatory effect, indicating that the ganglion is blocked. Acetylcholine, which is responsible for the transmission of the nerve impulse from the preganglionic to the postganglionic fibers, is antagonized by procaine.

Blockage at the myoneural junction can be demonstrated with procaine where it blocks the response of acetylcholine in stimulating the contraction of skeletal muscle. Here procaine is acting similarly to curare. The effects of curare and procaine at the myoneural junction are additive.

When local anesthetics are directly applied to the nerve trunk or injected into surrounding tissues, the agent influences the nerve cells by contact with the membrane and cytoplasm. Small nerve fibers which exhibit the greatest surface per unit of volume are affected before the larger fibers. If cocaine is applied to the vagus nerve, the smaller efferent cardiac inhibitory fibers are initially blocked. The larger fibers involved in carrying respiratory impulses are not as quickly affected.

Local anesthetics interfere with nerve conduction in small concentrations, an action which is reversible. The mechanism of the action in producing a discontinuity of the capacity of a nerve to transmit an impulse is not clearly understood.

The typical local anesthetic molecule is both lipophilic and hydrophilic, with the hydrophilic part invariably being an amino group. This amino grouping is believed to be attracted to polar groups in the lipoprotein film of the nerve. This is the membrane containing metallic ions which are responsible for the propagation of nerve impulses. The lipophilic part of the molecule is also anchored to the lipoid phase of the molecule. This disturbs the phase boundary equilibrium and interferes with nerve conduction.

Local anesthetic agents also inhibit the oxidation of glucose, succinate, and ascorbate in brain homogenates, but do not affect anaerobic glycolysis of glucose. Local anesthetics inhibit the oxidation and reduction of cytochrome c. This work on cellular metabolism, together with the work on lipoid adsorption phenomenon, provides a tentative hypothesis for the action of local anesthetics.

The myelin sheath is relatively impermeable to local anesthetics, and the plasmatic membrane appears to contain the target molecules. The local anesthetics raise the threshold at which the nerve will respond to stimulation, thereby blocking conduction. These drugs do not alter the rate of conduction along a nerve fiber once the wave has been initiated.

The un-ionized part of the drug penetrates the nerve membrane although the positive ion form is required for local anesthetic activity within the cell. An acid medium would produce a preponderance of ionic form with a resultant poor penetration of the nerve membrane and poor anesthesia. In a blocked nerve, a rise in intracellular pH would result in an increase in the amount of un-ionized drug and would lead to loss of anesthesia.

The Chemistry of Local Anesthetic Agents

Local anesthetic agents can be divided into two broad categories: a) those which cause local analgesia through the production of cold, usually liquids of low boiling point such as ether, ethyl chloride, methyl chloride, or CO_2 snow; and b) those which have a specific effect on the sensory nerves or their endings, such as the cocaine analogues. Various protoplasmic poisons will also produce local analgesia, but this type of anesthesia is not usually reversible.

The local anesthetic agents which are clinically useful as secondary tertiary amines of relatively weak base strength. They are usually oils or low melting solids which are relatively insoluble in water. The anesthetics related chemically to cocaine are esters of p-aminobenzoic acid in which an alkyl amine has been introduced into the alkyl group.

Absorption and Metabolism

Procaine and certain slightly soluble local anesthetics are poorly absorbed when applied to mucous membranes. Many soluble agents are well absorbed after topical administration.

Procaine has been studied extensively insofar as its metabolism is concerned. It is hydrolyzed by cholinesterase (procaine esterase) but at a much slower rate than is acetylcholine, although procaine has a much greater affinity for the enzyme.

The liver is the most important organ involved in the metabolism of local anesthetics after absorption into the systemic circulation. The toxicity of a local anesthetic agent is determined by the rate of absorption and the rate of destruction by the tissues. Differences in rates of absorption can be modified by using a vasoconstrictor-type drug in the anesthetic solution injected.

Local Anesthetic Agents

COCAINE

Cocaine was first used as a local anesthetic in 1880. It is an ester of benzoic acid which, in addition to exhibiting local effects on sensory nerves, also exerts important systemic effects on the central nervous system and smooth muscle of blood vessels. Cocaine was used as an ophthalmic anesthetic agent for many years. It is known to have an ulcerative effect on the cornea, since cocaine has a local vasoconstrictor action. The local vasoconstrictor action of cocaine may be due to its inhibitory effect on monoamine oxidase enzyme systems, thus preventing the destruction of endogeneous epinephrine. It is too toxic to be used by injection, and it is not effective on intact skin. Therefore, its use was restricted to mucous membrane-type structures.

PROCAINE

Procaine, the first of the synthetic substitutes for cocaine, was introduced in 1905. It remains the most widely used and important local anesthetic agent for injection. Procaine is the diethylaminoethyl ester of p-aminobenzoic acid. It is nonirritant to tissues, acts promptly, and is as effective as cocaine when injected. It does not penetrate well when applied to mucous membranes and so is used by injection only. Procaine is relative nontoxic, being destroyed rapidly by the liver. It disappears rapidly from the blood and is converted into nontoxic end products which are eliminated by the kidneys.

BUTACAINE

Butacaine was introduced for surface anesthesia, especially in the eye, nose, and throat. It is the dibutylaminopropyl ester of p-aminobenzoic acid. It is unsuitable for injection or for spinal anesthesia. It is used principally for ophthalmic anesthesia of short duration.

TETRACAINE

Tetracaine differs from procaine in that one of the amino hydrogens of the aminobenzoate group is replaced by a butyl group, and the two ethyl groups of procaine are replaced by two methyl groups. It resembles procaine in action, but is more efficient when applied to mucous membranes.

LIDOCAINE HYDROCHLORIDE

Lidocaine hydrochloride, U.S.P., a member of the xylidide series, is active as a surface anesthetic as well as an injectable anesthetic agent. It produces a longer duration of anesthesia than does procaine, while having a shorter latency period and being somewhat less toxic at concentrations under 0.5%. The liver is the chief site of biotransformation, and conjugates of lidocaine are found in the urine. Toxic reactions to lidocaine are characterized by extreme depression rather than excitation as with procaine.

MEPIVACAINE HYDROCHLORIDE

Mepivacaine hydrochloride is also a member of the xylidide series and is closely related to lidocaine in potency and toxicity. Similar to lidocaine, it exerts its local anesthetic action most efficiently with the concomitant use of vasoconstrictor agents.

PROPARACAINE HYDROCHLORIDE

Proparacaine hydrochloride differs chemically from procaine in that the amino group on the benzoic acid ester ring is in the meta rather than the para position. Proparacaine is used as a surface anesthetic in ophthalmology, and its potency is somewhat greater than tetracaine.

PHENACAINE HYDROCHLORIDE

Phenacaine hydrochloride, N.F., has as its chief advantage its prompt action. A 1% solution instilled in the eye promptly produces a prolonged local anesthetic effect. It is possibly even more toxic than cocaine on injection, and so its use is limited to surface anesthesia in the eye.

HEXYLCAINE HYDROCHLORIDE

Hexylcaine hydrochloride, N.F., is about equal to cocaine topically, and as an infiltration agent it is more rapid in onset and longer lasting than procaine. It is as toxic as most of the other local anesthetic agents.

DYCLONINE HYDROCHLORIDE

Dyclonine hydrochloride is an organic ketone and does not contain the usual ester or amide linkage typical of the procaine-type agents. Its toxicity is low, and it is said to produce a low incidence of sensitivity reactions. This agent is used only for topical application and is not injected.

PRAMOXINE HYDROCHLORIDE

Pramoxine hydrochloride, N.F., also differs chemically from the benzoate ester procaine type of local anesthetic agent. It is irritating when injected and so is used only on the skin. It is not used in the eye or on the nasal mucosa.

Many other agents have also been and are being employed to produce local anesthesia. Their properties will vary, but in essence they are all modified procaine.

ETHYL ALCOHOL

Ethyl alcohol has been employed as a local anesthetic agent. It has been used in horses as an alternate to performing a neurectomy. It is injected perineurally to produce a degeneration of the nerve trunk, thus blocking the passage of painful stimuli. The effect of the injection of alcohol around a nerve may last for many months. Alcohol injections have been utilized in treating trigeminal neuralgia and severe sciatica in man. The injection of alcohol around a nerve trunk may cause interference with motor activity as well as disrupt the sensory function.

ETHYL CHLORIDE

Ethyl chloride spray is used as a local anesthetic agent in situations requiring very short superficial anesthesia duration. Its use is not without danger since the freezing of the tissues induced by ethyl chloride can become irreversible if the material is applied for too long a period of time.

Adjuvants Used with Injectable Local Anesthetics

EPINEPHRINE

Frequently, epinephrine is added to procaine solutions used for injection anesthesia. Epinephrine will act as a vasoconstrictor and thereby prolong the period of action of the local anesthetic. The vasoconstrictor will also decrease the toxicity of the local anesthetic by delaying absorption and preventing high blood concentration.

HYALURONIDASE

Hyaluronidase, a mucolytic enzyme, hydrolyzes hyaluronic acid and increases diffusion of injected materials. It will promote the absorption and penetration of drugs. It is nontoxic in therapeutic dosages.

Toxicity of Local Anesthetic Agents

The symptoms of toxicity seen with local anesthetic agents are related primarily to stimulation of the central nervous system and consist chiefly of restlessness, muscle tremors, and, finally, clonic convulsions. The period of stimulation is followed by a depressive stage, and death may result from respiratory failure. A barbiturate suitable for intravenous administration may be utilized to control the central nervous system stimulation. This should be accompanied by oxygen administration.

The incidence of toxicity due to local anesthetic agents in domestic animals is low compared to the incidence in humans. When intoxication occurs by slow absorption in humans, the toxic state may be preceded by laughter, confusion, vertigo, and palpitation. The accidental intravenous injection of a local anesthetic agent may cause immediate death of the patient. The extensive application of a local anesthetic agent in solution to traumatized mucous membranes or to the urethra also may be followed by toxic reactions.

In general, toxicity and efficacy are directly related. Toxicity is also related to the dosage and concentration employed. It is best to use as little of the chemical as is feasible for the clinical result sought.

Attributes of a Suitable Local Anesthetic Agent

Attributes of a suitable local anesthetic agent are as follows. a) It is freely soluble in water to produce a solution of suitable concentration and stability. b) It is heat stable, for sterilization. c) It is nearly neutral in pH reaction and produces minimum tissue reaction when injected. d) It has specific effect on sensory nerve endings with a minimal effect on surrounding tissue. e) It is devoid of addictive properties. f) Absorption from site of injection should be poor. This minimizes systemic toxicity and accentuates local anesthetic action. g) Systemic toxicity should be minimal. h) Duration of anesthesia should be capable of being controlled by varying the concentration of the solution. i) Recovery of sensation in the anesthetized area should not be prolonged after completion of surgical procedure. Recovery should leave no tissue damage.

The most important property is minimal systemic toxicity.

32
Epidural Analgesia

ALAN M. KLIDE

This form of regional analgesia has been referred to as epidural, extradural, and peridural, and the effect has been called both analgesia and anesthesia. Anesthesia usually implies a state which has, among its effects, sleep; since sleep is not a direct effect produced by this technique, the term epidural analgesia has greater accuracy.

The effect is the result of injecting local anesthetics into the epidural space, in contrast to spinal analgesia where the drug is injected into the subarachnoid space and mixes with the cerebrospinal fluid (CSF).

Of these two techniques, spinal analgesia is more common in man as contrasted with the almost exclusive use of epidural analgesia in the dog and cat. The reason for this difference is primarily anatomical. In man, the spinal cord ends at about L1, but the subarachnoid space containing CSF extends into the sacrum; therefore, safe lumbar subarachnoid puncture usually is possible over several lumbar spaces. In the dog and cat the distance between the end of the spinal cord and the end of the subarachnoid space may only be one segment, and this terminal portion of the subarachnoid space is usually very small, making it difficult to penetrate safely and consistently.

The usual site of injection is through the lumbosacral intervertebral space, and when placed in this location it is called lumbosacral epidural analgesia. In man, an epidural which is placed through the sacral hiatus, a notch at the caudal end of the sacrum, is designated as caudal analgesia. In dogs and cats, caudal epidural analgesia can be produced by injection at S3-Co1 or Co1-Co2.

History

Cocaine, an alkaloid found in the leaves of the plant *Erythroxylon coca*, was the first local anesthetic used. Memann isolated this alkaloid in 1859 and reported that it produced numbness of the tongue. In 1880, Vasili K. von Anrep wrote a review on cocaine in which he said that the local anesthetic effect of this drug might become important someday.[1] Freud studied cocaine, and in 1884 he successfully treated a morphine addict with it, thereby producing the first modern day cocaine addict. In 1884, Karl Koller clinically demonstrated and reported the use of cocaine as a local anesthetic agent for the eye.[1, 17, 20] Hall and Halsted, in 1883, used cocaine to produce conduction anesthesia, and in 1885 Corning reported on anesthetization of the spinal cord.[13] This was done in one dog and one man; however, it is not clear whether he produced spinal (subarachnoid) or epidural analgesia.[10]

In 1901, two papers appeared independently (one week apart) describing the epidural space and the effects of cocaine injected into this space in dog and man.[8, 22]

Anatomy

For epidural block, the needle is inserted through the lumbosacral intervertebral space. Other lumbar spaces potentially could be used, but it is more difficult to insert a needle into these spots. There also is more danger of inadvertent subarachnoid injection and penetration of the spinal cord. Injection is also possible at the sacrococcygeal or Co1-Co2 spaces, but accurate placement of the needle may be difficult. The chances of subarachnoid injection are less when a puncture is made caudal to the sacrum. If a local anesthetic solution containing epinephrine is accidently placed subcutanously in this area there is a possibility of producing ischemia and gangrene of the tail.

Pertinent bony landmarks are the right and left cranial dorsal iliac spines of the ilium, the spinous process of the seventh lumbar vertebra, and the median sacral crest (Fig. 32.1 and 32.2). Important features to notice in a sagittal section (Fig. 32.3) are (a) the location of the ligamentum flavum, (b) the relative shape of the spinous process of the seventh lumbar vertebra and the median sacral crest, (c) the terminal portions of the spinal cord, and (d) the terminus of the dural sac. The vertebral level at which the cord and the dural sac end is variable in both the dog and cat. In the dog the cord usually ends at L6–7 and the dural sac at L7–S2. In the cat these levels are usually extended caudad one more vertebra.

Site of Action

Several possible sites of action for the production of epidural analgesia have been postulated (Fig. 32.4). It has been shown that India ink and radiopaque dyes injected into the epidural space pass through the intervertebral foramina into the paravertebral space.[5, 6, 16, 23, 24, 25] Thus, it was postulated that epidural analgesia was in fact multiple, bilateral paravertebral nerve blocks due to the passage of the local anesthetic into the paravertebral space. Recent evidence suggests that this does not occur in all cases, especially in the aged where the intervertebral foramina are reduced in size. Epidural injection of radiopaque material in geriatric patients suggests that sometimes the material does not diffuse into the paravertebral spaces.[6] The amount of local anesthetic available for each paravertebral space is too small to account for the spread, intensity, and duration of an epidural injection.[6, 18]

Another possible mechanism is that the local anesthetic in the epidural space crosses the dura and arachnoid and mixes with the CSF and produces a true spinal block. Concentrations of local anesthetics in the cerebrospinal fluid after epidural injection have been measured.[4] The possibility of leakage of drug from the epidural space into the CSF around the sampling needle places doubt on the value of such measurements.[4, 21]

The route by which the local anesthetics reach the CSF has been studied and led to the latest theory of the site of action. In a review, Bromage has concluded

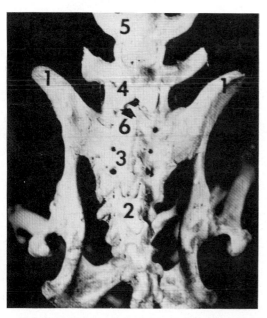

FIG. 32.1. Dorsal view of dog skeleton. *1*, cranial dorsal iliac spine; *2*, first coccygeal vertebra; *3*, sacrum; *4*, seventh lumbar vertebra; *5*, sixth lumbar vertebra; *6*, lumbosacral intervertebral space.

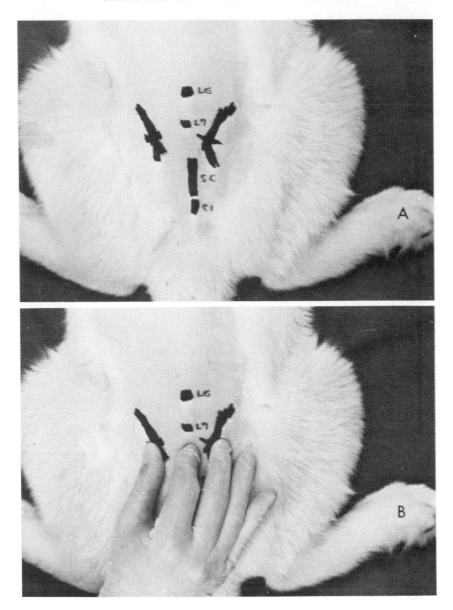

FIG. 32.2. Dorsal view of dog back. *A*, *curved lines* represent wings of the ilium with *crossed lines* showing cranial dorsal iliac spines (*L6, L7, C1*), spinous processes (*SC*), median sacral crest. *B*, position of fingers for locating the lumbosacral intervertebral space. (Courtesy of Klide, A. M., and Soma, L. R.: Epidural analgesia in the dog and cat. J. Amer. Vet. Med. Ass. *153:* 165, 1968.)

that local anesthetics pass rapidly from the epidural space into the cerebrospinal fluid, and that the pathway of movement of local anesthetic solutions is by "preferential diffusion in the region of the dural cuffs, followed by centripetal spread to the cord in the subperineural and subpial spaces."[4] A recent study has shown a differential distribution of labeled lidocaine injected into the subarachnoid space; "uptake of drug was higher in the grey matter than in the white matter of the

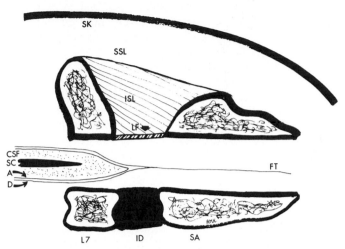

FIG. 32.3. Schematic representation of midsagittal section of lumbosacral area. *SK*, skin; *SSL*, supraspinous ligament; *ISL*, interspinous ligament; *LF*, ligamentum flavum; *CSF*, cerebrospinal fluid; *SC*, spinal cord; *A*, arachnoid; *D*, dura mater; *FT*, filum terminale; *L7*, seventh lumbar vertebra; *ID*, intervertebral disc; *SA*, sacrum. Notice the difference in shape between the spinous process of L7 and the median sacral crest. (Courtesy of Klide, A. M., and Soma, L. R.: Epidural analgesia in the dog and cat. J. Amer. Vet. Med. Ass. *153:* 165, 1968.)

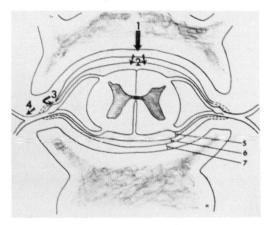

FIG. 32.4. Schematic cross-section of the spinal cord and adjacent structures. *1*, injection of a local anesthetic into the epidural space. Possible sites of action: *2*, passage of drug across dura into CSF; *3*, preferential diffusion in the region of the dural cuffs; *4*, paravertebral block; *5*, subarachnoid space (CSF); *6*, dura; *7*, epidural space.

cord, and posterior nerve roots had a higher concentration than the anterior roots."[9]

Physiological Effects

It is generally accepted that small nerve fibers are blocked first and by lower concentrations of a local anesthetic than larger fibers. The usual explanation is that the small fibers have a larger surface to volume ratio than larger fibers, and therefore they can absorb drugs more quickly. It appears that blockade of the small sympathetic nerves occurs first, followed by larger sensory nerves and finally the larger motor nerves. Sequential blockade, however, is only a crude approximation of the actual events.

There is evidence that the effect of nerve fiber diameter on susceptibility to chemical blockade only holds within a group of nerve fibers which conduct impulses by the same mechanism. Even within a group of fibers, for example, myelinated fibers, it may not be the surface to volume ratio which influences the blockade, but the ratio of the magnitude of the current developed at the active node to the amount of current needed to depolarize the membrane of the next node.[19] This ratio is called the "safety factor." Fibers with a "low safety factor" are more susceptible to blockade than those with a higher "safety factor." It is possible for some large motor neurons to be blocked while some smaller fibers remain unaffected. Although it is preferable to use a concentration of local anesthetic which blocks all fibers exposed, the maximum concentration is limited by the volume, the route of injection, toxicity of the local anesthetic, and the condition of the animal.

The extent and direction of change of blood pressure as related to epidural analgesia has not been studied accurately in the dog. The general opinion, at present, is that there is a decrease in blood pressure. Several compensating physiological mechanisms are activated when a partial sympathetic blockade occurs. Generally there is a peripheral vasoconstriction in areas not under the influence of the blockade and an increase in heart rate as a compensating mechanism to maintain cardiac output and blood pressure. As the blockade extends to the sympathic cardioaccelerator nerves, a bradycardia, and not an increase in heart rate, may occur.

The respiratory effects are dependent upon the cranial extent of the blockade. The intercostal nerves are blocked (caudocranially) and complete paralysis of all the intercostal muscles occurs when the block extends to T1. Extension to C5 to C7 will block the phrenic nerves, resulting in paralysis of the diaphragmatic muscles.

There is usually a fall in body temperature due to the peripheral vasodilation in the area of the blockade. The immobility and inability to shiver also contributes to heat loss.

Method and Equipment

The amount and type of restraint necessary depends on the temperament and physical condition of the animal. In lethargic or depressed animals, no sedative drugs are necessary. If chemical depressants are necessary for restraint in the dog, narcotics are preferable, since they provide sedation and analgesia and their effects can be reversed with narcotic antagonists if serious depression occurs. In the cat, the combination of a cyclohexylamine (such as ketamine) with epidural analgesia might be a very useful technique.

Phenothiazine tranquilizers can be used, but they may potentiate any hypotensive effect of disease and/or of the epidural blockade.

The patient may be placed in any one of several positions for placement of the needle (Fig. 32.5), but sternal recumbency is preferred. The major factor in determining the proper position, however, is the dog's or cat's comfort and condition. A large splint on the hind limb, for example, will make the sternal position uncomfortable. Ventroflexing the animal to enlarge the lumbosacral intervertebral space has been recommended,[7, 28] but is rarely necessary in animals and it only adds discomfort and may increase the restraint problem.

The lumbosacral intervertebral space is located as follows (Fig. 32.2). (a) The cranial dorsal iliac spines of the ilium are palpated. (b) The thumb is placed on one, and the third finger placed on the other. (c) The index finger is used to locate the intervertebral spaces on the midline. (d) The lumbosacral space is located a variable distance (depending on the animal) caudal to a line connecting the two spines. Occasionally there is some confusion in differentiating between lumbar space 6 and the lumbosacral space (Fig. 32.3). The spinous processes of the lumbar vertebrae 6 and 7 are prominent and pointed; the median sacral crest is lower, longer, and has several ridges; therefore, by finding the median sacral crest, the proper space can be identified.

The site is prepared by clipping the hair from the area, washing with surgical soap, and applying alcohol. To minimize discomfort when the spinal needle is placed, 2% lidocaine is infiltrated subcutaneously and into the supraspinous and interspinous ligaments.

A sterile epidural pack should contain the following material (Fig. 32.6): (a) small "eye" drape; (b) several 4 by 4 inch gauze sponges; (c) sponge forceps; (d) 2-ml glass syringe; (e) 5-ml glass syringe; (f) an ampule of epinephrine (1:1000); (g) 2 ampules (2 ml) of lidocaine; (h) 22-gauge needle for filling syringe and local infiltra-

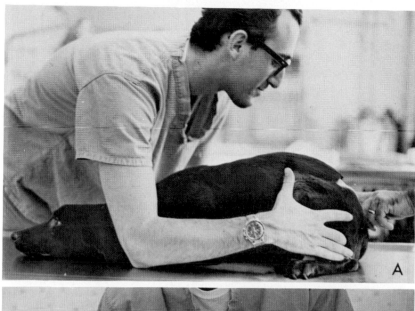

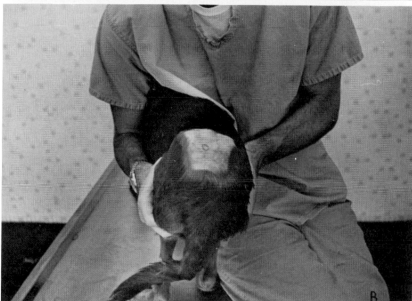

FIG. 32.5. Positions for injection. Sternal (A) on table (B) supported by assistant.

tion; and (i) 2-inch, 20-gauge spinal needle. A pack for larger dogs includes a 10-
ml glass syringe and a 10-ml ampule of
2% lidocaine. Sterile disposable spinal
needles are available, and an appropriate
size needle can be added to the pack
immediately before use. The pack used for
continuous epidural, which will be described in detail below, is similar to the
aforementioned, except that it includes a

17-gauge 3-inch Touhy needle instead of
the standard spinal needle, an 18-inch
medical grade vinyl catheter (0.02-inch
inside diameter, 0.036-inch outside diameter) which will fit through the 17-gauge
Touhy needle, and a 23-gauge dulled needle which fits into the end of the catheter
for injection of the local anesthetic agent.
   For the epidural injection, a short bevel
spinal needle with stylet is preferred to a

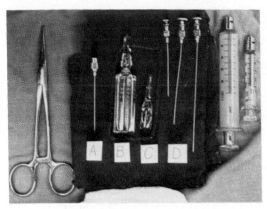

FIG. 32.6. Contents of epidural pack (from *left* to *right*): sponge forceps; *A*, filling needle; *B*, ampule of 2% lidocaine hydrochloride; *C*, ampule of epinephrine, 1:1000; *D*, spinal needles, 20-gauge, 2, 3, and 4 inches; "eye" drape (*under needles*); gauze sponges (at *bottom*); two glass syringes. (Courtesy of Klide, A. M., and Soma, L. R.: Epidural analgesia in the dog and cat. J. Amer. Vet. Med. Ass. *153:* 165, 1968.)

regular hypodermic needle (Fig. 32.7). The short bevel is generally a duller needle and adds some resistance to passage of the needle which aids in the differentiation of structures as the needle approaches the epidural space. If the dural sac is present at the injection site, it is less likely to be punctured by the short bevel needle. Spinal needles are marked on the hub to indicate direction of the bevel by a notch which engages the head of the stylet. The needle used for most dogs and cats is a 2-inch, 20-gauge spinal needle.

NEEDLE PLACEMENT

There are several conflicting reports on the proper angle for insertion of the needle into the epidural space (Fig. 32.8).[2, 7, 11, 12, 26, 28] Inserting the needle perpendicular to the skin and directly on the midline is the most effective and in most cases successful. A lateral, *i.e.*, slightly off midline, approach is possible and can be used, but is more difficult and offers no advantage in the dog and cat. If difficulty is encountered entering the intervertebral space, the needle can be angled slightly in a caudal or cranial direction. After passage through the skin, little resistance is

encountered until the ligamentum flavum is reached. On advancing through this ligament, some resistance is encountered and usually a distinct "pop" is felt when the needle has passed through the ligamentum flavum and entered the epidural space (Fig. 32.3).

Some authors advocate that the needle be advanced until it hits the floor of the vertebral canal and then withdrawn a short distance.[2] This method is not necessary to assure proper placement and should never be done intentionally. As soon as the "pop" is felt, the needle advancement should be stopped and tested to determine if it is in the epidural space. In determining proper needle placement, the needle should be at a reasonable depth, from ½ to 1½ inches in most cases, depending on the size of the dog or cat. The stylet is removed and examined for blood or cerebrospinal fluid. Blood on the stylet is obvious; however, CSF is more difficult to observe. If the stylet is held up to the light and slowly rotated, CSF may appear as small sparkling pinpoints on the stylet. Next observe the hub of the needle for a brief period for appearance of blood or CSF. Aspiration of CSF from a subarachnoid puncture in this area is difficult, so it is important to observe the needle, and if the needle has been placed into the subarachnoid space, the CSF will rise slowly, especially if the animal is in lateral recumbency. After observing the hub, the needle should be aspirated. If no blood or CSF is seen, the fingers are placed over the skin on either side of the

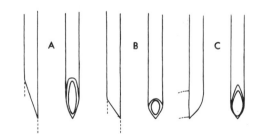

FIG. 32.7. Schematic showing lateral view and bevel of needles. *Dotted lines* indicate direction of catheter exiting from bevel; *A*, normal hypodermic needle; *B*, spinal needle; *C*, Touhy needle.

needle and 1 to 2 ml of air injected. Crepitus in the subcutaneous tissues may be detected if the needle is improperly placed. There should be no resistance to the injection of air or the local anesthetic agent (Figs. 32.9 and 32.10). Before beginning, all the syringes to be used should be tested to assure that the plunger functions and to determine how much resistance is inherent in the syringe.

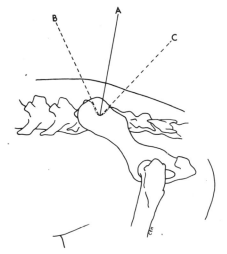

FIG. 32.8. Schematic of ilium and vertebrae showing possible needle angles. *A*, usual; *B* and *C*, alternative positions if difficulty is encountered.

The knowledge of the direction of the bevel is very important, for this will direct the flow of the local anesthetic in the epidural space. In most cases it is directed cranial; however, if a perineal block is intended and it is desirous to limit the cranial level of the blockade, the bevel should be directed caudal. A larger volume of drug can be injected without the danger of a high block, thereby prolonging the perineal block. Directing the bevel of the needle laterally will usually produce a more solid block on that side.

The rate of injection will also vary the cranial extent of the block and a spotty, more cranial block of shorter duration will be obtained with a rapid injection. A rapid injection also increases cerebrospinal fluid pressure causing discomfort. A slow injection produces a more caudally located block. If the dog is in lateral recumbency, a one-sided (lower side) blockade can occur.

CONTINUOUS EPIDURAL ANALGESIA

For procedures which require a long period of time or for those which the exact duration of surgery is unknown, continuous epidural analgesia, a modification of the "single shot" epidural technique, is

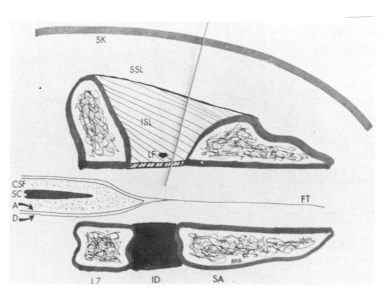

FIG. 32.9. Schematic showing proper needle position (see Fig. 32.3 for definition of abbreviations).

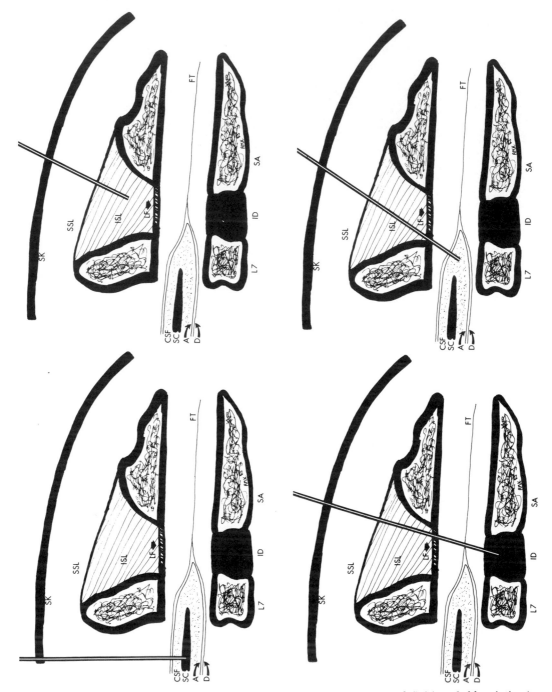

FIG. 32.10. Schematic showing improper needle placements (see Fig. 32.3 for definition of abbreviations).

indicated. A larger needle is placed in the epidural space and serves as a guide through which a catheter is passed. The needle is then withdrawn, but the catheter left in place, and local anesthetics can now be injected through the catheter as often as necessary.

Any spinal needle of sufficient diameter to allow the passage of a catheter can be used; however, a Touhy needle offers some advantages. It is similar to the standard spinal needle except that the distal end opens at an angle to the shaft (Fig. 32.7). The angulation facilitates the passage of a catheter into the epidural space and more accurately controls its direction. The needle is placed into the epidural space as was described above for the spinal needle. After the stylet has been removed and the proper location of the needle verified, the catheter is placed into the epidural space before injecting the local anesthetic. As the catheter is slowly passed into the needle, it may be mechanically impeded at the distal end of the needle at the point of angulation. A slight increase in pressure is enough to overcome this slight resistance; if it is not, the needle may have to be repositioned so the angle made by the skin and needle on

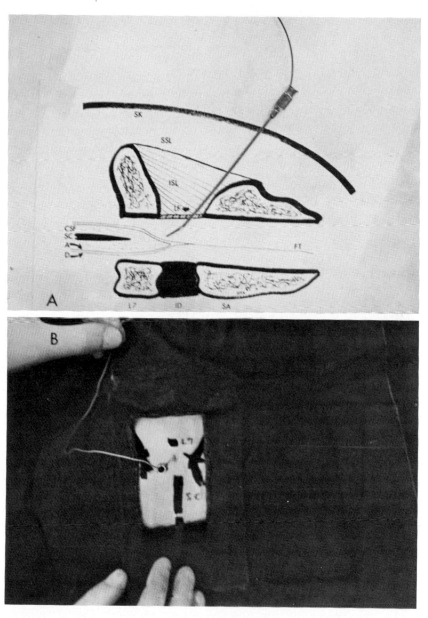

FIG. 32.11. Touhy needle and catheter. A, schematic; B, dorsal view of dog back.

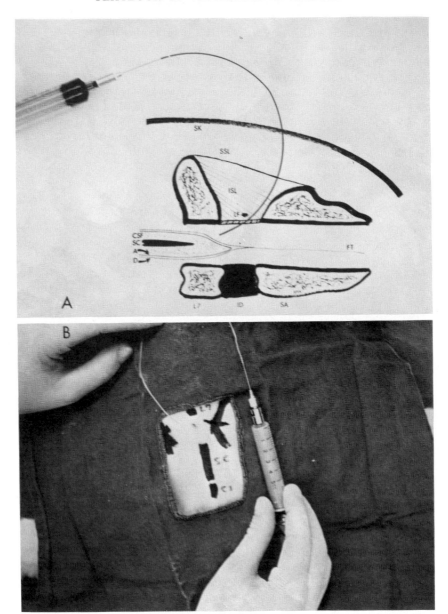

FIG. 32.12. Touhy needle and catheter in final position. *A*, schematic; *B*, dorsal view of dog back.

the bevel side is more obtuse. Only about ½ to 1 inch of catheter should be inserted into the epidural space (Fig. 32.11). To prevent cutting the catheter, *never* pull it back through the needle point. The needle is carefully removed by advancing the catheter slightly as the needle is withdrawn.

A blunt 23-gauge needle is inserted into the end of the catheter for the injection of the local anesthetic (Fig. 32.12). The catheter is taped in place along the patient's back, positioning the needle in such a manner that it can be easily reached after the animal is draped. Injections can be made as often as necessary. Usually one-half of the initial dose of lidocaine (with epinephrine) is added every hour. If the administration of additional doses is anticipated before the actual need arises, a

TABLE 32.1
ONSET AND DURATION OF EPIDURAL ANALGESIA FOR SOME LOCAL
ANESTHETICS

Agent	Concentration	Epinephrine	Onset	Duration
	%		*min*	*hr*
Lidocaine	2	Not added	3-12	1
		Added	3-12	1½
Mepivacaine	2	Not added	3-12	1
		Added	3-12	1½
Tetracaine	0.25	Added	10-30	4
Lidocaine	2	Added	3-12	3
and tetracaine	0.2			

more constant level of blockade will be maintained, less drug will be necessary, and fluctuations in the level of the block will not occur.

LOCAL ANESTHETIC AND DOSE

Many local anesthetics are used for epidural analgesia. The most common are lidocaine, mepivacaine, and tetracaine (Table 32.1). Tetracaine is the longest acting of these and could be used in those cases where a long surgical procedure is anticipated, or in which the duration cannot be accurately determined, or where the continuous method cannot be used. The onset of analgesia is longest with tetracaine. A combination which will have a rapid onset and a long duration is tetracaine with lidocaine or mepivacaine. The most convenient way to mix these drugs is as follows. A 20-mg ampule of tetracaine crystals is added to the standard pack of a 10-ml ampule of 2% lidocaine and 1-ml ampule of 1:1000 epinephrine. The dead space or 0.05 ml of epinephrine is drawn into the 10-ml syringe, followed by the lidocaine solution. This mixture is added to the tetracaine crystals to dissolve them. Withdraw this solution and then draw up the remainder of the 10 ml of lidocaine. The solution now contains 2% lidocaine, 0.2% tetracaine, and approximately 1:200,000 epinephrine. The drugs used for epidural analgesia should be in "single use," preservative free ampules. The local anesthetics should be heat stable so that they can be autoclaved in the epidural pack. A drug in common use is 2% lidocaine which has proven to be stable, safe, and reliable. An advantageous property of lidocaine which has not been found in other local anesthetics is that it produced a significant degree of sedation after absorption from the epidural space.

The onset of epidural block with lidocaine is relatively rapid (3 to 12 minutes), and the duration of action (45 to 90 minutes) is suitable for most surgical procedures. The total time of blockade depends on the concentration of the anesthetic, the rate of injection, the initial level of blockade, the age and condition of the patient, and whether or not a vasoconstrictor is added to the solution.

Epinephrine is added to the anesthetic solution in order to decrease the rate of absorption of the local anesthetic and thus decreasing the chance of toxic blood levels, increase the duration of the blockade, and produce a more rapid onset with a more even distribution of the anesthetic. Lidocaine or other local anesthetics which have been packaged with epinephrine should not be used. The lidocaine-epinephrine combination must be acidic for preservation of the dilute epinephrine. A basic solution increases the rapidity of development of the block. Epinephrine should be added to the local anesthetic just before use. This is done by drawing up a small amount of epinephrine (1:1000) into a syringe, and then flushing it out. The epinephrine that remains in the dead space of the syringe will approximate a 1:200,000 dilution when the lidocaine is drawn into the syringe. This 1: 200,000 concentration has been shown to affect the absorption of lidocaine from the epidural space.[3] Multiple dose vials containing preservatives should not be used for epidural analgesia.

The accurate determination of a suitable dose of drug is one of the greatest difficulties of epidural analgesia. Several tables and rates have been published, but these serve only as guides.[7, 11, 28] There are many factors which will affect the level of analgesia, so that great care must be used when using different dose range tables. The clinician must develop judgment regarding doses and levels in various size dogs and cats, and each patient must be evaluated as to its condition and the site of surgery.

Doses for an "average" dog have been estimated. Lidocaine (2%), 1 ml/10 lb of body weight, will produce a sensory block as far cranially as L1, 1 ml/7.5 lb will block cranially to T5 in a healthy, relatively lean, middle aged dog. For most abdominal surgery, a midthoracic block (T5) is necessary. For surgery of the hind limbs, a block as far cranially as the thoracolumbar junction is adequate; however, the level of analgesia soon begins to recede caudally so that only brief procedures can be done. If more time is needed, then either a continuous technique must be used or a higher initial level must be achieved with a single shot technique. For perineal surgery, 1 ml/10 lb of body weight with the bevel of the needle pointed caudally is adequate in most cases.

FACTORS INFLUENCING LEVEL OF ANALGESIA

There are a great many factors which affect the cranial level of analgesia. The epidural space can be visualized as a tube, sealed at both ends, with a bilateral series of holes representing the intervertebral foramina. When a liquid (local anesthetic) in injected at one end, it will move toward the other end, leaking out of the holes in the tube as it goes. If the fluid is injected too slowly, it may run out as fast as it goes in, and the fluid will not advance very far in the tube. When fluid is injected rapidly it will advance far in the tube before much of it can leak out. It can be seen that the rate of injection will affect the level of an epidural block. The more rapid the rate of injection, the more cranial in extent will be the analgesia, but the block may be spotty, *i.e.*, irregular in distribution and of shorter duration.

The volume of drug injected is probably the greatest single factor affecting the level of block. A larger volume produces a more extensive block cranially. Using the previous model it can be seen that if fluid is injected at a constant rate, it will advance further down the tube as a larger volume is injected. Drug mass (total number of milligrams) also influences the cranial extent of the block; higher concentration produces a higher block. Figure 32.13 shows the relationship between volume and mass in the same dog. The injection of 2 ml of a 0.2% solution of tetracaine produced a block to L1; injection of the same volume, *i.e.*, 2 ml of a 1.0% solution produced a block to T5, thus showing that of two solutions with the same volume, the one with the higher mass (20 mg) produced a more cranial block. When 10 ml of 0.2% tetracaine is injected, the

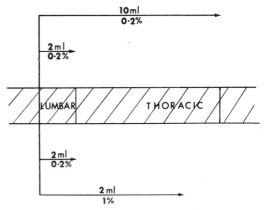

Fig. 32.13. Mass versus volume. The *upper section* compares the levels achieved with different volumes but the same concentration. The *lower half* compares the level when the volume is kept constant and the mass varied. The *upper* and the *lower sections* compare different volumes and concentration, but the same mass.

block extends to T1. This shows that in two solutions having the same mass but different volumes, the larger volume will produce a more cranial block.

Another important factor is the direction of the needle bevel. It directs the flow of the anesthetic agent and can be used effectively in creating cranial, caudal, or unilateral blocks. The size of the epidural space will also influence the extent of the block.

Using the tubular model, it can be understood that if a space-occupying material were inserted into the tube, less fluid would have to be injected for the fluid to reach a desired point. In the patient, the material could be fat or distension of the vertebral venous sinuses. In older dogs, a more cranial block and one of longer duration generally occurs because of smaller intervertebral foramina. This decrease in size is thought to be due to progressive fibrosis. Referring to the model, if the holes are smaller, the fluid will run out at a slower rate and the level achieved by the initial injection will extend further.

Position (gravity) can affect the ultimate level of blockade to a slight degree. If the animal is tilted head down at the time of injection or right afterwards, the level achieved may be slightly (one segment) more than anticipated. This effect may be useful in a situation where a one-sided block is appearing. By placing the animal on the unblocked side, it may be possible to produce a bilateral block.

The effect of pregnancy or any other large mass in the abdomen on the extent of analgesia is not known with certainty in the dog. The basic premise is that caudal vena cava compression causes congestion of the vertebral venous sinuses and thereby decreases the size of the epidural space. Experimental work in the dog has shown that acute complete caval obstruction causes a dye column in the epidural space to be fragmented with cranial advancement.[14, 15]

A complete lack of blockade is usually due to a misplaced needle. It can occur with a continuous technique if the catheter has passed out through an interverte- bral foramen or if it has been pulled out as the needle was removed. A one-sided block is more likely to occur when the injection is made with the dog or cat on its side, especially if the drug is injected too slowly. It can also occur if the patient is rolled onto its side too soon after injection. Another possible cause of a one-sided block is presence of a midline membrane or adhesions. Insufficient extent of blockade can result from an inadequate volume of anesthetic agent, low concentration, slow injection, improper bevel direction, or receding extent of analgesia during a prolonged procedure.

Complications

Toxic levels of local anesthetics can occur from inadvertent injection into a vertebral venous sinus or from rapid absorption of an excessive amount of local anesthetic injected into the epidural space. Signs of mild toxicity are tremors, vomiting, or both. The tremors must be differentiated from shivering due to a fall in body temperature. Shivering occurs in all areas of the body not blocked, is coarse in appearance, and may appear or increase in intensity with inspiration. The tremors of toxicity are very fine and may be difficult to see. They occur in variable areas of the body and do not vary with respiration. Such conditions usually do not require treatment. More severe reactions such as convulsions usually respond to small intravenous doses of ultrashort acting barbiturates (e.g., thiopental and thiamylal). If not, succinylcholine chloride can be given to produce complete muscle paralysis, and the patient can be intubated and ventilated.

If some or all of the intercostal nerves are blocked by the epidural drug, adequate ventilation is generally maintained by a more vigorous use of the diaphragm.[27] This may not be necessarily true in a fat dog or cat placed on its back or with severe respiratory depression from other drugs or disease. Blockade as far cranially as the phrenic nerves (C5 to C7) is needed to produce complete respiratory paralysis.

If hypoventilation or apnea occurs, ventilatory support should be initiated.

As analgesia extends cranially, more of the sympathetic nervous system will be blocked and variable amounts of hypotension may occur. If hypotension occurs, treatment depends on the severity. Should cardiovascular collapse occur, the patient is placed in a slight head down tilt to enhance venous return, ventilated with oxygen, and given intravenous fluids rapidly. Vasopressors such as norepinephrine or methoxamine to sustain blood pressure should be given only if peripheral pulses are not palpable. The vigor of treatment will be determined by the severity of the collapse and the response to each preceding treatment. Hypovolemic, anemic patients and those in shock should be watched closely and supported in any way necessary to maintain adequate cardiovascular function.

Shivering of the unparalyzed portions will occur if the patient's body temperature falls. This is more likely in smaller dogs and cats in air-conditioned rooms on metal operating tables. The patients should be insulated from the table and room air; if necessary, a source of external heat should be provided.

Indications

The decision to use epidural analgesia will depend on the medical problems of the patient, its temperament, the clinican's experience with epidural analgesia, and the duration of the surgical procedure. Theoretically, the technique can be used for any surgical procedure caudal to the diaphragm; however, it is more suited to some procedures and circumstances than others. Some pre-existing conditions which might warrant epidural analgesia are pulmonary, liver, or kidney disease. Epidural analgesia is useful in conjunction with extremely painful procedures such as orthopedic, rectal, or perineal surgery, because it seems to produce noticeable postoperative relief from pain. This technique is the preferred method of analgesia for cesarean section. It is useful in cases where profound muscle relaxation is required, especially if other anesthetic techniques for producing this are not available.

The use of epidural analgesia for patients with anemias, hypovolemia, or in shock is controversial. Because of the recent changes in the treatment of shock (the use of vasodilator therapy), epidural analgesia should not be discarded as a possible method of handling those shock cases which require surgery.

Epidural analgesia had been used successfully for critically ill animals; however, it must be stressed that this technique is not a panacea, and severely ill animals or animals which are depressed severely with other drugs must be watched carefully and adequate supportive therapy instituted as needed.

The advantages of epidural analgesia are (a) minimal expense, (b) relative simplicity, (c) excellent muscle relaxation, (d) rapid recovery, (e) minimal effect on respiration, (f) good postoperative analgesia, and (g) minimum effect on most organ systems. The disadvantages are (a) possible complications as stated above, (b) restraint in some animals, and (c) unfamiliarity with the method. There are very few absolute rules in the practice of anesthesia. Each case and method of anesthesia has to be evaluated on its own merit and experience of the clinician. Epidural analgesia should probably be avoided in vertebral column deformities, spinal or peripheral neural disease, local lumbosacral infection, septicemia, and abnormality of the clotting mechanism.

Epidural Analgesia for Farm Animals

The range of uses for epidural analgesia is more limited in farm species because many become very distressed when their hind legs are paralyzed. Safety to the animal and those handling it can be a problem if excitement occurs. The greatest use for this technique in the equine and bovine is for procedures which can be done with a block which does not impair motor activity of the hind limbs. This limits the technique to procedures involving the tail, anus, vulva, perineum, and some obstetrical manipulations.

The spinal cord and dural sac in the horse, cow, pig, and sheep end within the sacral portion of the vertebral canal. Lumbosacral injection carries several risks in these species which caudal injection does not. The risk of lacerating the spinal cord exists if the animal moves at the time of puncture. The location of the lumbosacral space is somewhat difficult in the horse and pig and easier in the cow and the sheep. Lumbosacral injection is more likely to produce a motor block of the hind limbs than caudal injection, and in these four species, the possibility of a subarachnoid injection is great with a lumbosacral puncture.

The techniques, equipment, and principles are the same as described above for the small animals, except the needles may have to be longer with a larger diameter, the volume injected is different, and the response by the species has to be taken into account.

SHEEP

Epidural analgesia can be produced by either placing the needle through the lumbosacral space or between coccygeal vertebrae. The lumbosacral space is located the same way as in a dog; however, when this approach is used there is a good chance for subarachnoid puncture. Popping of the needle through the interarcuate ligament should be done slowly and the needle advancement stopped as soon as it occurs.

The operator should anticipate that the sheep will move at this time unless it is too depressed by disease or drugs. If subarachnoid puncture does occur, the same dose of local anesthetic can be injected as for epidural analgesia. This equality of dose for spinal and epidural analgesia is very different from that in man and dog. In the latter species, the dose necessary for epidural analgesia is much greater than that for spinal analgesia. If subarachnoid puncture does occur, great effort must be taken to stabilize the needle so that it does not transect or hemisect the spinal cord. Indicators may be used to try to identify the epidural space and to help avoid subarachnoid puncture. One example of this is the Macintosh needle. This is essentially a spinal needle in which a spring-loaded plunger replaces the stylet. When the needle is pushed through tissue, the plunger is pushed against the spring and protrudes from the hub of the needle. As soon as the epidural space is entered there is no pressure on the plunger, the spring advances it, and it disappears from the hub of the needle. The local anesthetic drugs used and their concentrations are the same as the dog. If hypotension occurs, it should be treated as described for small animals. A dose from which to start calculating the final dose is 1 ml of 2% lidocaine for each 7.0 kg of body weight for a midthoracic block. The factors influencing the final dose are described in the previous section on small animals. For a block of longer duration, 20 mg of sterile tetracaine powder is reconstituted with 10 ml of 2% lidocaine, and 6 to 8 ml is injected. This dose is suggested for sheep between 45 and 60 kg. The filling of the dead space of the 10-ml syringe with 1:1000 solution of epinephrine will extend the block from 4 to 5 hours to 6 to 8 hours.

PIG

Lumbosacral epidural analgesia has been used in pigs, but the location of landmarks in larger pigs can be difficult. In pigs it has been recommended to use a point on the midline 13 to 15 cm in front of the base of the tail; however, this does not hold in larger pigs (over 100 lb).[12, 28] For larger pigs, the tuber coxae is located on a vertical line drawn from the fold of the flank. The lumbosacral space is located on the midline 2.5 to 5 cm caudal to a line connecting the tubera coxae. The needle size used varies with the size of the pig; 8.75 cm is used for a pig up to 75 kg, and 15 cm is used for pigs greater than 75 kg. The dose is about 1 ml/5 kg to 1 ml/10 kg of 2% lidocaine for a hind leg block; the greater dose in small pigs, the small dose in large pigs.

CATTLE

Epidural analgesia is generally administered caudal to the sacrum between the coccygeal vertebrae for procedures which can be done with a sensory block. Lumbar segmental epidural analgesia can be used to produce analgesia of either flank without paralyzing the hind limbs.[12] This could be used for rumenotomies and cesarian sections. The needle is inserted through the intervertebral space between the first and second lumbar vertebrae. The needle may be inserted on either side of the spinous process of the second lumbar vertebra at its anterior edge, which is usually ½ to ¾ inch caudal to the anterior edge of the transverse process of the second lumbar vertebra. A skin wheal should be used and then a small skin incision made or a large gauge needle used in the skin through which a spinal needle is passed. The spinal needle should be advanced at an angle of about 10° from the midline. When the needle passes through the ligamentum flavum the animal will respond. This is true in all species even when local analgesics are injected. The entrance into the subarachnoid space is possible, so the needle should be checked for cerebrospinal fluid before the injection of the local anesthetic. Care must be taken not to push the needle into the spinal cord. The dose usually varies between 5 and 10 ml of 2% lidocaine.

The more common technique is injecting the local anesthetic caudal to the sacrum for procedures involving the vagina and rectum. The first moveable articulation is usually the one between the first two coccygeal vertebrae and is located by lifting and lowering of the tail. There also is often depression of the skin at this site. The needle is inserted on the midline. The dose in adult cattle varies between 5 and 10 ml of 2% lidocaine. For anesthesia of the hind limbs and abdominal wall, 30 to 80 ml of 2% xylocaine is used. Care must be taken to prevent severe abduction of the hind limbs. If the animal becomes excited, it should be sedated with a tranquilizer or chloral hydrate. If hypotension occurs it should be treated.

HORSE

It is possible to produce lumbosacral epidural or spinal analgesia in this species but is rarely done. These animals become extremely upset when their hind limbs are paralyzed. The commonly used epidural technique in the horse is caudal analgesia, using the same site as described in cattle, i.e., between the first two coccygeal vertebrae. The needle may be placed perpendicular to the vertebrae canal or at an angle of 30° from it. Five to 10 ml of 2% lidocaine is used in adult horses.

REFERENCES

1. Von Anrep, Vasili K.: Pflueger Arch. Ges. Physiol. 21: 38, 1880.
1a. Bloom, J. N.: On the use of cocaine for producing anesthesia on the eye. Lancet 2: 990, 1884.
2. Bone, J. K., and Peck, J. G.: Epidural anesthesia in dogs. J. Amer. Vet. Med. Ass. 128: 236, 1956.
3. Braid, D. P., and Scott, D. B.: Effect of adrenaline on the systemic absorption of local anesthetic drugs. Acta Anaesth. Scand. (supple. XXIII), 10: 334, 1966.
4. Bromage, P. R.: Physiology and pharmacology of epidural analgesia. Anesthesiology 28: 592, 1967.
5. Bromage, P. R.: Epidural Analgesia. E. S. Livingstone, Ltd., Edinburgh, 1954.
6. Bromage, P. R.: Spread of analgesic solutions in the epidural space and their site of action: a statistical study. Brit. J. Anaesth. 34: 161, 1962.
7. Brook, G. B.: Spinal epidural anesthesia in the domestic animals. Epidural anesthesia in the dog. Vet. Rec. 15: 665, 1935.
8. Cathelin, M. F.: Une nouvelle voie d'injection rachidienne. Methode des injections epidurales par le procede du canan sacre. Application a l'homme. C. R. Séances Soc. Biol. 53: 452, 1901.
9. Cohen, E. N.: Distribution of local anesthetics agents in the neuraxis of the dog. Anesthesiology 29: 1002, 1968.
10. Corning, J. L.: Spinal anesthesia and local anesthesia of the cord. New York J. Med. 42: 483, 1885.
11. Frank, E. R.: Regional anesthesia in the dog and cat. J. Amer. Vet. Med. Ass. 25: 336, 1928.
12. Hall, L. W.: Wright's Veterinary Anesthesia and Analgesia, 6th ed. The Williams & Wilkins Company, Baltimore, 1966.
13. Hall, R. J.: Hypochlorate of cocaine. New York J. Med. 40: 643, 1884.
14. Hehre, F. W., Yules, R. B., and Hipona, F. A.: Continuous lumbar peridural anesthesia in obstetrics. 3. Attempts to produce spread of

contrast media by acute vena cava obstruction in dogs. Anesth. Analg. (Cleveland) *45:* 551, 1966.

15. Kalas, D. B., Sinfield, R. M., and Hehre, F. W.: Continuous lumbar peridural anesthesia in obstetrics. 4. Comparison of the number of segments blocked in pregnant and non-pregnant subjects. Anesth. Analg. (Cleveland) *45:* 848, 1966.

16. Klide, A. M., Steinberg, S. A., and Pond, M. J.: Epiduralograms in the dog: the uses and advantages of the diagnostic procedure. J. Amer. Vet. Radiol. Soc. *8:* 39, 1967.

17. Koller, K.: On the use of cocaine for producing anesthesia on the eye. Wien Med. Blatt. *43:* 1352, 1884.

18. Lund, P. C.: *Peridural Analgesia and Anesthesia.* Charles C Thomas, Publisher, Springfield, Ill., 1966.

19. Nathan, P. W., and Sears, T. A.: The susceptibility of nerve fibers to analgesics. Anaesthesia *18:* 467, 1963.

20. Noyes, H.: Med. Rec. *26:* 417, 1884.

21. Saker, G., and Schroeder, G.: Grundlagen der Periduralanaesthetic. I. Durchlassigkeit der Dura. Anaesthetist *3:* 259, 1954.

22. Sicard, J. A.: Les injections medicamenteuses extra-durales par voie sacrococcygienne. C. R. Séances Soc. Biol. *53:* 396, 1901.

23. Sicard, J. A., and Cestan, R.: Etude de la traversee meningoradiculaire au niveau du trou de conjugaison le nerf du conjugaison. Bull. Soc. Med. Hop. Paris *21:* 715, 1904.

24. Sicard J. A., and Forestier, J.: Radiographic method of exploration of epidural space using Lipiodol. Rev. Neurol. *28:* 1264, 1954.

25. Sicard, J. A., and Forestier, J.: Roentgenologic exploration of the central nervous system with iodised oil (lipiodol). Arch. Neurol. Psychiat. *16:* 421, 1926.

26. Smiley, H. D.: Some further experiments with lumbar anesthesia in canines. J. Amer. Vet. Med. Ass. *33:* 560, 1932.

27. Ward, R. J., Bonica, J. J., Freund, F. G., Aka, A. T., Danziger, F., and Englesson, W.: Epidural and subarachnoid anesthesia—cardiovascular and respiratory effects. J. Amer. Vet. Med. Ass. *191:* 275, 1965.

28. Westhues, M., and Fritsch, R.: *Animal Anesthesia*—Local Anesthesia, 1st ed. (English), J. B. Lippincott Company, Philadelphia, 1964.

33
Regional Analgesia in Large Animals

LOREN H. EVANS

The method of regional analgesia comprises the infiltration of a local analgesic solution around sensory nerves. This regional method of anesthesia can include the infiltration around a specific nerve or group of nerves, multiple injections along an incisional line, and commonly "U," "L," or ring blocks surrounding the surgical area. Regional analgesia also includes epidural and spinal form of anesthesia.

The skin, after cleansing, is tensed, and a small gauge needle attached to a syringe containing a local anesthetic is quickly injected to desensitize the skin. In the larger species, approximately 1 to 2 ml of solution are injected, producing a small weal through which the needle is passed for infiltration of a specific area. When creating a block by multiple injections, the needle is always injected into a previously blocked area and the weal advanced. An area can also be blocked by subcutaneous infiltration from a single weal. A long needle is inserted through the skin weal and slowly advanced subcutaneously. The solution can be injected either when advancing or withdrawing the needle. This method is generally used for infiltration under a small mass.

For abdominal surgery or incisions into deeper muscle masses, subcutaneous infiltration is insufficient. Deeper infiltration is necessary after the cutaneous desensitization is completed. The surgeon may prefer to locally infiltrate muscle prior to its incision. It is important that the peritoneum be included.

In the following discussions, 2% lidocaine is the local anesthetic, preferred because of its potency, stability, and diffusibility.

Head

A review of the anatomy of the nerves and the location of their foramen is advantageous before attempting nerve blocks of the head. The ideal block is produced when the anesthetic solution is deposited at the foramen where the nerves emerge or enter. The deeper the foramen the more difficult the technique becomes. Care should be taken not to injure major vessels located near the nerves. The length of the needle required for regional analgesia of the head in the horse and cow will vary from 1 to 6 inches (2.5 to 15 cm). The 18- to 20-gauge needle is most practical for the deeper blocks.

ANATOMY

The three branches of the trigeminal nerve (ophthalmic, maxillary, and mandibular) supply most of the head with sensory fibers. They supply the cutaneous areas of the forehead, eyes, nose, and lips, as well as the mucous membranes of the head with the exception of the lining of the guttural pouch, pharynx, and larynx. All roots of the teeth are innervated by two of the three branches; the lowers by the mandibular and the uppers by the infraorbital off the maxillary nerve. Of the three branches, the maxillary and the ophthalmic are purely sensory, while the mandibular branch has both sensory and motor fibers. The cutaneous areas supplied by the branches of the trigeminal nerve are quite similar in the bovine and the equine with the exception of the horn and the skin around its base. Also, there is a difference between the cow and goat. In the cow this area is supplied by the cornual nerve, while in the goat the infratrochlear and the cornual supply the horn and surrounding skin. There is also a difference in the site of emergence of the maxillary nerve from the cranium in the horse and the cow. In the horse the maxillary nerve passes through the foramen rotundum, while in the cow it leaves the cranium close together with the ophthalmic nerve through the foramen orbito-rotundum. In the cow, the frontal nerve, which is a branch off the ophthalmic, does not pass through the supraorbital foramen as it does in the horse but runs dorsally over the margin of the bony orbit to supply sensation to the upper eyelid and skin of the forehead. The three branches of the ophthalmic nerve are lacrimal, frontal, and nasociliaris. The lacrimal nerve supplies the lacrimal gland, the upper eyelid, and skin above the temporal angle of the orbit. The zygomatic branch of the lacrimal supplies the skin and connective tissue in the temporal area. The frontal nerve, also termed the supraorbital, crosses first within and then outside the periorbita to emerge through the supraorbital foramen and ramifies in the skin of the forehead and the middle portion of the upper eyelid. The nasociliary nerve, also called the palpebronasal, divides into two branches, the ethmoidal and infratrochlear. The ethmoidal supplies the dorsal nasal mucosa, anterior half of the frontal sinus, dorsal half of the nasal septum, and adjacent roof of the nasal cavity. The infratrochlear runs forward within the orbit to the medial can-

thus and ramifies in the skin of this region. It also supplies the third eyelid, conjunctiva, and lacrimal organs.

ANESTHESIA OF THE EYE IN THE HORSE

A method for anesthetizing the eyeball, conjunctiva, most of eyelids, and adjacent skin by directly blocking the ophthalmic nerve has been described[3] (Figs. 33.1 and 33.2). The needle is inserted at an angle of 40° to the vertical in a medioventral and somewhat caudal direction at a point *behind* the supraorbital or zygomatic process of the frontal bone at the level of the supraorbital foramen. A 4- to 5-inch (10 to

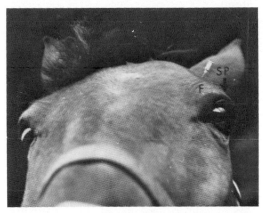

FIG. 33.1. A 5-inch 18-gauge needle is inserted 40° off the vertical just posterior to the bony edge of the orbit and in line with the supraorbital foramen (*F*). Supraorbital process (*SP*).

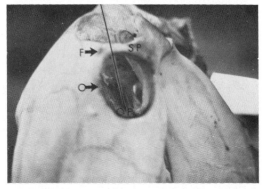

FIG. 33.2. When properly positioned, the needle should rest at the orbital foramen (*OF*); supraorbital foramen (*F*); medial edge of orbit (*O*); supraorbital process (*SP*).

12½ cm) needle is needed to reach the orbital foramen. A minimum deposit of 20 ml of anesthetic solution is then made. A nerve block at this site will get all three branches of the ophthalmic—lacrimal, frontal, and nasociliaris. However, the auriculopalpebral nerve block must be made to stop all sensation to the lids. By blocking the ophthalmic nerve, the eyeball, conjunctiva, eyelids, and skin of the forehead become desensitized. The ocular musculature is also paralyzed because the oculomotor, the trochlear, and the abducent nerves either emerge through the orbital foramen or, in the case of the trochlear, immediately above the orbital foramen.

A second method suggested is to enter the lateral canthus of the eye with a 5-inch needle (12.5 cm), directing it toward the opposite temporal mandibular joint to a depth of about 2½ to 4 inches (6¼ to 10 cm).[3] At least 20 ml of solution of anesthesic should be deposited.

It is difficult to use the two techniques mentioned due to location of the orbital foramen. A review of the anatomy of this area shows the ethmoidal and optic foramina to be located directly above the foramen orbitale. The thin vertical pterygoid crest separates the alar canal from the previously mentioned foramina, and also offers a landing point for the needle when attempting to find the foramen orbitale.

Retrobulbar injections have been successfully used. To use this method, the eyelids must first be anesthetized with a local infiltration, then a slightly curved 4- to 5-inch needle (10 to 12½ cm) is directed behind the eyeball, and several small deposits of the anesthetic solution are made. This forces the eyeball to bulge from the socket.

Lightenstern[15] recommends that a needle 4 inches (10 cm) long be inserted ¾ inch (1.5 cm) behind the middle of the supraorbital process and directed toward the last upper premolar tooth on the opposite side. Twenty to thirty milliliters of anesthetic solution is deposited after the needle has penetrated the orbit. This feels much like "penetrating a drum skin." This technique will only anesthetize the eyeball. The eye-

lids and surrounding skin have to be locally infiltrated. Similar results are claimed by directing the needle from the medial or lateral orbital margins.

ANESTHESIA OF THE EYE IN THE BOVINE, GOAT, AND SHEEP

The innervation of the ruminant's eye is quite complex, with 6 of the 12 cranial nerves involved. The optic nerve containing special sensory fibers of sight has a sheath composed of extensions of the meninges of the brain and includes continuations of the subdural and subarachnoid spaces. This accounts for the bad effects and fatalities which result when the anesthetic can also be deposited directly into the subdural and subarachnoid spaces, reaching the vital centers in the medulla oblongata, by entering the ethmoidal foramen when approaching the area from the side.[29] The ideal area to block the eye and its associated structures is just anterior to the foramen orbitoruncum where the oculomotor, trochlear, abducent, ophthalmic, and maxillary nerves emerge. Peterson[18] describes a technique (Fig. 33.3) for reaching this site by using a 4.5-inch (11¼ cm) 18-gauge needle which has been slightly curved. Under aseptic conditions insert a short 16-gauge needle through the skin in the depression just posterior to the point where the supraorbital process meets

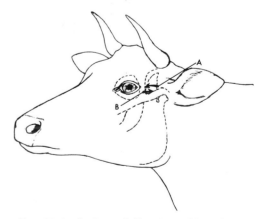

FIG. 33.3. *A*, site and direction to block deep and superficial structures of the eye; *B*, site and direction to block remaining sensation to eyelids—auriculopalpebral nerve.

the zygomatic arch. A small amount of anesthetic is deposited. Withdraw this needle and insert the 4½-inch curved needle with the concavity of the curvature of the needle directed posteriorly and with the hub of the needle held at a point slightly higher than the point of insertion. Insert the needle until it hits the coronoid process of the mandible (1½ to 2½ cm). Work the point of the needle off the anterior border of the process, and, by holding the hub slightly above the horizontal plane, insert the point until it hits the bony plate forming the floor of the pterygopalatine fossa. The depth of insertion will vary from 3 to 4 inches (7½ to 10 cm), depending on the size, sex, and breed of the animal. Fifteen milliliters of solution should be deposited. With this technique it is almost impossible to deposit the anesthetic into the subdural and subarachnoid spaces, as the pterygoid crest forms a shelf protecting the optic foramen. Also, if the hub of the needle is kept above the horizontal plane, it is not possible to enter the ethmoidal foramen.

There may still be considerable twitching of the eyelids due to the fact that the auriculopalpebral branch of the facial nerve has both motor and sensory fibers going to the eyelid. This nerve can be blocked when withdrawing the needle so that its point lies just beneath the skin. Then direct the needle posteriorly in the superficial fascia lateral to the zygomatic arch for a distance of 2 to 3 inches (5 to 7½ cm), infiltrating the tissue with the anesthetic solution as the needle is inserted.

Retrobulbar infiltration is the same as described for the horse. First, block the skin and eyelids around the eye, and then use a slightly curved needle to deposit the anesthetic just behind the eyeball. It is possible to enter the optic foramen from this approach, so do not insert the needle too far posteriorly in the bony orbit.

ANESTHESIA OF THE HORN IN THE BOVINE

The horns of cattle are supplied with sensory fibers through the cornual nerve, which is a branch off the lacrimal, one of the three branches of the ophthalmic nerve.

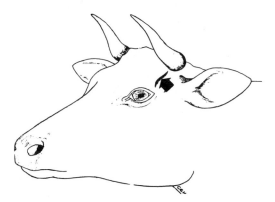

FIG. 33.4. The site for anesthetizing the bovine horn.

The cornual nerve passes through the periorbital tissue dorsally and then runs along the lateral border of the frontal crest to the base of the horn. The nerve becomes more superficial as it gets close to the base of the horn. The block is most easily performed at a site in the upper third between the lateral canthus of the eye and the horn base. A short 16-gauge needle is inserted just under the skin and the lateral edge of the frontal bone. Some have recommended a site closer to the horn base where the nerve is more superficial.[7, 30] The block is made 1 to 1¼ inches (2 to 3 cm) in front of the horn where the nerve lies 7 to 10 mm below the skin. The site is located by palpating the lateral edge of the frontal bone (Fig. 33.4). Too deep an injection should be avoided. In older cows and bulls, skin sensation may be supplied from the first cervical nerve, thereby requiring a deposit of anesthetic just posterior to the base of the horn.

ANESTHESIA OF THE HORN IN THE CAPRINE

The goat has two cornual nerves supplying its horns both with sensory fibers. The cornual, a branch of the lacrimal, is blocked the same as in the cow. It supplies the lateral, anterior lateral, and the posterior lateral horn base and adjacent skin. The medial, anterior medial, and posterior medial portions are supplied by a cornual nerve, a branch off the infratrochlear nerve. This nerve is one of the two branches which come off the nasociliaris, a branch of the ophthalmic nerve. At the

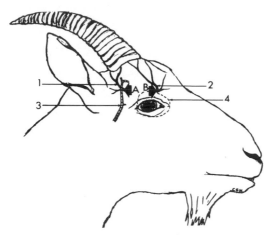

FIG. 33.5. There are two sites (*A* and *B*) for anesthetizing the goat's horn. *1*, cornual branch of lacrimal nerve; *2*, cornual branch of infratrochlear nerve; *3*, superficial temporal artery; *4*, outline of bony orbit. (After Vitums.[27])

notched dorsal medial wall of the orbit, the nerve can be felt as a flat structure which will slip beneath the finger. The nerve is blocked through the skin with a 1-inch 20-gauge needle at the osseous orbital margin directly over the nerve (Fig. 33.5).

ANESTHESIA OF THE MANDIBLE IN THE HORSE AND COW

The complete mandible, teeth, and lower lip will become anesthetized by blocking the mandibular nerve as it enters the mandibular foramen on the medial side of the mandible. Several methods have been given to block this site, but the one given by Bemis,[1, 2] with some modifications,[6, 8] is the easiest and most successful. The mandibular foramen is located by drawing an imaginary line along the occlusal surface of the teeth and a vertical line from the lateral canthus of the eye. Where these two lines intersect is the foramen, which lies on the medial side of the mandible. A 6-inch (15 cm) 18-gauge needle is inserted from the lower angle of the jaw and directed vertically along the medial aspect of the mandible to the mandibular foramen.

The required depth should first be established by measuring on the needle the distance from the point of insertion to the point where the lines mentioned above

cross. A deposit of 15 to 20 ml of anesthetic solution should be made (Fig. 33.6). Even though the mandibular nerve is blocked, all the skin or cutaneous area over the jaw is not anesthetized because of the innervation coming from the superficial temporal nerve, which is derived from the maxillary and the facial nerves.

ANESTHESIA OF THE SKIN OF THE CHEEK IN THE HORSE AND COW

The superficial temporal nerve can be blocked in the horse as it bends around outside the vertical portion of the ramus of the mandible below the mandibular joint. This will desensitize the skin over the facial crest and cheek to the corner of the mouth. Insert the needle ½ to 1 inch below the temporal mandibular joint, directly over the prominent posterior border of the vertical portion of the ramus. The 2-inch (5 cm) needle is inserted to contact bone at the posterior margin and under the subfascia; 10 ml of anesthetic is deposited.

ANESTHESIA OF THE LOWER LIP IN THE HORSE AND COW

To achieve anesthesia of the lower lip, the mental nerve coming from the mental foramen is blocked. Unfortunately, depositing the anesthetic at this site will not desensitize the incisors. To desensitize the incisors, the mandibular nerve must be blocked either at the mandibular foramen,

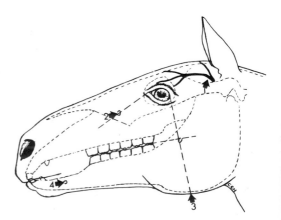

FIG. 33.6. Site and direction for common nerve blocks of the horse's head. *1*, auriculopalpebra; *2*, infraorbital; *3*, mandibular; *4*, mental foramen.

or a small needle can be passed up the canal from the mental foramen. To do this a 2½ inch (6¼ cm) fine needle is inserted about ½ to 1 inch in front of the mental foramen and parallel to the mandible. The skin should be stretched forward to aid in palpation and passage of the needle. The needle is inserted as far as possible into the very narrow canal, injecting anesthetic as the needle is inserted. Due to the size of the canal, the anesthetic does not diffuse far, which limits the certainty of the block. Usually, the incisors are blocked, and the cheek teeth have been reported blocked as far back as the first molar. The mental foramen is easily found by palpating on the lateral sides of the mandible about 1 inch posterior to the commissures of the lips. A depression is detected by pushing upward the round tendon of the depressor labii inferioris muscle. Usually, the horse resents the pressure applied to the nerve. A 20-gauge 1- to 1½-inch needle (2½ cm) is adequate to deposit the anesthetic at the foramen, or up into the canal if the needle is slightly bent so that the concave part is toward the lateral side (Fig. 33.6).

ANESTHESIA OF THE UPPER LIP, NOSE, AND UPPER JAW IN THE HORSE AND COW

Depending on the area to become desensitized, the clinician has several choices of sites to block. The maxillary nerve, which is purely sensory, is the mother nerve from which the other nerves continue. Infiltration of the infraorbital nerve at its entry into the upper jaw at the maxillary foramen has been described.[1] To inject the anesthetic over the nerve, a 4½-inch (11 cm) needle is inserted at a point about 1 inch below the lateral canthus of the eye. This point is below the facial crest, and the needle is inserted where it will not injure the transverse facial vessels. The average depth of the foramen is about 3 inches (7½ cm). The needle is directed in a medial anterior direction until it strikes the perpendicular portion of the palatine bone close to the maxillary foramen. The point of the needle should be moved around until it strikes the nerve. When this point is reached the horse will jerk his head. If the needle strikes the internal maxillary artery or vein, which are below the nerve, the point of the needle should be directed higher. Ten milliliters of anesthetic should be deposited at the site.

In the cow, the same nerve can be blocked by using the method described for the Peterson nerve block (Fig. 33.3). All the upper teeth, the gums, the upper lip, and skin will be anesthetized.

Tosco described a technique where the horse's maxillary nerve is blocked as it emerges from the foramen rotundum located just below the foramen orbitale.[24, 28] He suggests this site to avoid danger of infiltrating an anesthetic within the pterygopalatine fossa and hitting or damaging the vena reflexa and buccal vein.

The site is located on the aboral surface of the zygomatic process of the frontal bone, close to the external frontal crest and about 1 cm anterior to the point where the temporalis muscle runs deeply. This site is approximately 5 inches (12.5 cm) medial to the mandibular joint. A needle 4¾ inches (12 cm) long is inserted here at right angles to the frontal bone and inclined about 20° medially to a depth about 1½ times the diameter of the orbit. This distance should first be measured and the needle marked accordingly. Ten milliliters of an anesthetic solution is injected. As a safeguard against vasopuncture, a short beveled needle should be used.

BLOCKING THE INFRAORBITAL NERVE AT THE INFRAORBITAL FORAMEN AND IN THE CANAL

The nostril, upper lip, gums, and incisors can be effectively anesthetized by blocking the infraorbital nerve as it emerges from the infraorbital foramen. The flat levator nasolabialis muscle and the oval levator labii superioris cover the foramen. The landmarks to find the foramen are the nasomaxillary notch and the distal end of the facial crest. Midway between these two points and 1½ inches (3.7 cm) above the imaginary line, the foramen can be felt by pushing the oval shaped levator labii superioris proprius muscle forward (Fig. 33.6). A 20-gauge 1-inch needle (2⅕ cm) can be

used to deposit 10 ml of the anesthetic solution at the foramen. Some horses will
jerk back when the needle is inserted in
the nerve; therefore, the needle should be
fixed in place before the syringe is attached
to it. A twitch usually offers the best restraint when placing the needle. The area
desensitized is the skin of the lip, nostril,
and face on that side up to the foramen.

The bony roof of the nasal cavity and
related skin almost to the medial canthus
of the eye, the upper lip, the incisors, and
back to the first and second molars can be
anesthetized by inserting the needle into
the infraorbital canal. This is done by reflecting the muscle upward and starting
the needle ¾ inch (2 cm) in front of the
foramen. It is necessary to pass the needle
at least 1 inch (2.5 cm) into the canal to
deposit 5 ml of solution.

ANESTHESIA OF THE FOREHEAD AND UPPER EYELID IN THE HORSE AND COW

The frontal nerve, which is a branch of
the ophthalmic, emerges through the supraorbital foramen. The foramen is felt as
a small depression midway across the supraorbital process on a vertical line running upwards from the medial angle of the
eye. A 20-guage 1-inch (2.5 cm) needle is
used to deposit 5 ml of anesthetic solution.
In the bovine, the frontal nerve does not
emerge from the supraorbital foramen but
sends several fibers out of the orbit and up
along the supraorbital process. To block
this nerve which supplies the upper eyelid
and skin of the forehead, it is necessary to
start the injection a little above the medial
canthus and spread it laterally along the
supraorbital process toward the temporal
region.

THE AURICULOPALPEBRAL NERVE BLOCK IN THE HORSE AND COW

The auriculopalpebral nerve is a mixed
nerve supplying innervation to the circular
muscles of the eye and the orbicularis oculi.
Blocking this nerve does not anesthetize
the eyelids, but it does stop voluntary closure of the eyelids. This block has been
suggested to relieve the spasms of the eyelids following an eye injury.[22] The course of

the nerve differs in the horse and cow. In
the horse (Fig. 33.6), the nerve runs
obliquely medially to the zygomatic process
of the zygomatic arch to end near the
medial canthus of the eye where it joins
with terminal branches of the ophthalmic
and goes to the circular muscle of the eye,
while in the cow (Fig. 33.3), it runs immediately over the facial crest past and below
the eye and gives off its branches on the
way.

To block the auriculopalpebral nerve in
the horse, use a 20-gauge 1-inch (2.5 cm)
needle. The site is about 1 inch (2.5 cm)
below the highest point of the dorsal border
of the zygomatic arch. The needle is inserted until it contacts bone and then is
pushed along the bone until the point almost reaches the border of the zygomatic
arch. Five milliliters of solution are injected subfascially. Good results can be
obtained by depositing 5 ml of solution in a
fan-shaped manner subfascially into the
depression where the caudal border of the
ramus of the mandible and the zygomatic
arch meet. This depression is felt just anterior to the base of the ear. The needle is
inserted into the depression at the ventral
edge of the vertical or temporal portion of
the zygomatic arch and directed upward to
a position caudal to the highest point of the
arch.

In cattle, the injection site is directly
anterior to the base of the auricular musculature at the aboral end of the zygomatic
arch. The needle is inserted obliquely and
dorsally to contact the bone and is pushed
forward until its point lies at the dorsal
border of the zygomatic arch. Ten milliliters of solution should be injected subfascially.

Front Leg of the Horse

ANATOMY

Regional analgesia can be achieved either by intra-articular, intrabursal, of peri-
neural injections.[2, 4, 5, 10, 11, 12, 30] The nerve
supply to the foreleg of the horse is quite
constant, and in the lower leg the nerves
are easily palpated. The sensory innervation of the leg below the elbow joint is from

the medial, ulnar, the cutaneous branch of the musculocutaneous, the cutaneous branch of the radial, and the cutaneous antibrachii dorsalis, which emerges below or through the lateral head of the triceps and ramifies on the dorsal lateral surface of the forearm as far distal as the carpus. The musculocutaneous nerve divides to give off two branches; one goes to the brachialis muscle, and the other is cutaneous. This cutaneous branch (the medial cutaneous antebrachial nerve) can be felt cranial to the cephalic vein, proximal to the junction of the cephalic and accessory cephalic veins, near the medial border of the extensor carpi radialis. This nerve supplies the medial surface of the forearm and the dorsomedial surfaces of the carpus, metacarpus, and as far distal as the fetlock. In the region of the elbow, the ulnar gives off a branch (the cutaneous antibrachii caudalis) which supplies the skin of the medial and volar aspects of the upper foreleg. Near the level of the accessory carpal bone the ulnar divides into two terminal branches, a superficial or dorsal branch, and a deep or volar branch. The dorsal branch perforates the deep fascia between the tendons of the ulnaris lateralis and flexor carpi ulnaris and ramifies in the skin over the dorsal lateral surface of the carpus, metacarpus, and the upper part of the fetlock. The nerve cannot be traced distally this far without the dissecting microscope. It is this dorsal branch of the ulnar that accounts for the sensation found over the dorsal aspect of the fetlock when the deep and superficial volar (metacarpal) nerves

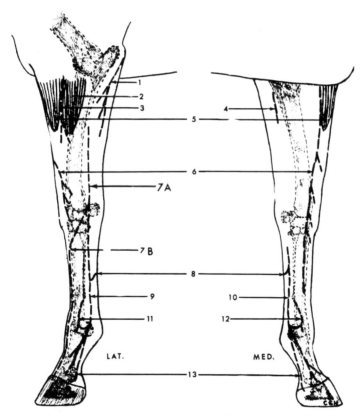

FIG. 33.7. Nerve distribution of horse's left front leg. *1*, caudal cutaneous antebrachial nerve; *2*, long digital extensor muscle; *3*, a terminal branch of radial nerve; *4*, median nerve; *5*, extensor carpi radialis muscle; *6*, cutaneous antibrachii dorsalis—branch from radial nerve; *7A*, ulnar nerve; *7B*, dorsal branch of ulnar nerve; *8*, anastomosing branch from medial to lateral; *9*, lateral superficial volar (metacarpal) nerve; *10*, medial superficial volar (metacarpal) nerve; *11* and *12*, deep volar (metacarpal) nerve; *13*, posterior digital nerve.

are blocked. The deep or volar branch of the ulnar joins the lateral branch of the median to form the lateral superficial volar (metacarpal) nerve. The lateral volar (metacarpal) nerve sends off a branch high in the metacarpus that divides and descends on both sides of the leg between the suspensory ligament and the third metacarpal bones. They emerge at the distal end of splint bones MC II and MC IV as the deep volar (metacarpal) nerves which supply the dorsal part of the fetlock, and anastomose with branches of the superficial volar (metacarpal) nerves (Fig. 33.7).

The median nerve descends on the medial side of the elbow joint under the very dense deep fascia in the furrow between the radius and the anterior border of the flexor carpi radialis muscle. It usually lies with the median vein or on the vein.

The medial superficial volar (metacarpal) nerve which arises from the medial terminal branch of the median nerve arises at a variable distance above the carpus and descends in the carpal canal along the medial border of the superficial flexor tendon under the deep fascia, and in the proximal third of the lower leg becomes

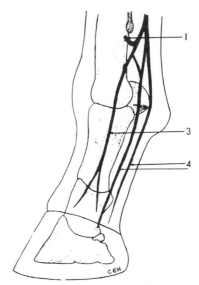

Fig. 33.9. Uncommon nerve distribution to the horse's fetlock. 1, deep volar (metacarpal) nerve; 2, superficial volar (metacarpal) nerve; 3, dorsal digital nerve; 4, two posterior digital nerves.

superficial. In the middle of the lower leg, or metacarpus, it gives off a large anastomotic branch which winds obliquely over the flexor tendons and joins the lateral superficial volar (metacarpal) nerve. At a variable distance near the fetlock, the nerve divides into two or more branches making up the digital nerves. The dorsal digital nerve ramifies in the skin and the corium of the hoof on the dorsal face of the digit. The volar or posterior digital nerve descends behind the digital artery on the border of the deep flexor tendon and innervates the posterior part of the hoof, frog, sole, navicular bone, and posterior part of the third phalanx. Below the dorsal branch there are several small twigs and some fairly good sized branches that descend with the posterior digital nerve and cross to anastomose in a variable manner with the dorsal branch. The areas innervated by these small branches are not well defined and are usually the cause for skin sensation following a posterior digital neurectomy (Figs. 33.8 and 33.9).

With the exception of the anastomotic branch in the middle of the metacarpus, the lateral superficial volar (metacarpal) nerve has the same termination on the lat-

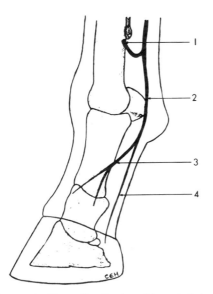

Fig. 33.8. Nerve distribution of horse's fetlock. 1, deep volar (metacarpal) nerve; 2, superficial volar (metacarpal) nerve; 3, dorsal digital nerve; 4, posterior digital nerve.

eral side of the leg and foot as that described for the medial superficial volar (metacarpal) nerve.

MEDIAN NERVE BLOCK

The nerve and artery can be palpated through the thin posterior superficial pectoral muscle on the medial side of the elbow joint. The nerve is blocked at the ventral limit of this muscle of approximately 5 inches (12.5 cm) below the pectoral muscles. A 20-gauge 1½-inch (3.75 cm) needle is inserted through the very dense deep fascia in the furrow between the radius and the anterior border of the flexor carpi radialis muscle. The nerve lies posterior to the radius on the large vein and in association with the median artery. Inserting the needle in an oblique direction helps to direct it under the fascia without entering the vein. At least 10 ml of anesthetic should be deposited.

ULNAR NERVE BLOCK

This nerve is blocked 4 to 6 inches (10 to 15 cm) above the accessory carpal bone near the level of the chestnut in the groove between the ulnaris lateralis and the flexor carpi ulnaris muscles. This groove can be detected by lightly running the finger over the prescribed area. A 1-inch (2.5 cm) 20-gauge needle will easily reach the nerve. Deposit 10 ml of anesthetic under the deep fascia that covers the nerve, artery, and vein. If a bleb or weal appears during the injection of the anesthetic, the point of the needle is not deep enough. The point of the needle must be just under the tight fascia. A depth of ¾ to 1 inch is maximum.

CUTANEOUS BRANCH OF THE MUSCULOCUTANEOUS NERVE BLOCK

This is the medial cutaneous antebrachial nerve. It is best blocked where the nerve lies on the surface of the radius halfway between the elbow and carpus immediately in front of the cephalic vein. Another landmark is a approximately 5 inches (12.5 cm) above the chestnut on the medial side of the leg. The needle should be inserted under the skin and directed upward along the radius in the direction of the nerve. Ten milliliters of local anesthetic should be spread in this area.

CUTANEOUS BRANCH OF THE RADIAL NERVE

The cutaneous branch of the radial nerve is called the lateral cutaneous antebrachial, and as described above supplies sensory fibers to the skin on the lateral surface of the forearm as far distal as the carpus. It emerges from the distal border of the lateral head of the triceps muscle. It is blocked by the subcutaneous infiltration of local anesthetic in the area of its emergence over the lateral and dorsal aspects of the forearm. The cutaneous areas of analgesia after local injections of the nerves have been described[4] (Fig. 33.10).

METACARPAL VOLAR NERVE BLOCKS

A high superficial (metacarpal) volar block is done 4 inches below the carpus above the anastomotic branch running from the medial to lateral volar nerve. The injection is made by using a 20-gauge 1-inch (2.5 cm) needle. The skin is raised by pinching it between the thumb and finger, and the point of the needle is placed below the fascia just anterior to the deep flexor tendon.

A low superficial (metacarpal) volar block is made in the groove just dorsal to the fetlock and sesamoid bones. The leg can be left on the ground or it can be held by an assistant while the 20- or 25-gauge 1-inch needle is used to deposit the anesthetic just under the skin directly over the nerve, which is easily felt just in front of the deep flexor tendon. A weal or bleb should form when the anesthetic is deposited.

Although a medial and lateral superficial volar (metacarpal) nerve block will anesthetize most of the digit, it will not affect the dorsal branch of the ulnar which supplies the dorsolateral surface of the fetlock, pastern, and coronet. In addition, the deep volar metacarpal nerves which arise from the lateral volar (metacarpal) nerve high in the metacarpus are not affected by a volar nerve block. The deep volar (metacarpal) nerves emerge at the distal end of the splint bones to supply the dorsal part of the

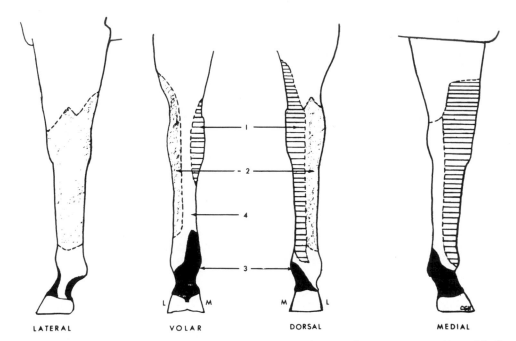

LATERAL   VOLAR   DORSAL   MEDIAL

Fig. 33.10. Cutaneous innervation of the left front horse's leg by musculocutaneous nerve (*1, straight lines*), ulnar nerve (*2, light shade*), or median nerve (*3, black shade*). *4,* all three nerves may aid in supplying (no shade). (After Bolz.[5])

fetlock and to anastomose with the dorsal branches of the digital nerves. To completely anesthetize the fetlock, pastern, and foot, the following five nerves must be blocked: (a) lateral superficial volar metacarpal; (b) lateral deep volar metacarpal; (c) dorsal branch of the ulnar; (d) medial superficial volar metacarpal; and (e) medial deep volar metacarpal.

A sesamoidan block is done just under the skin as the superficial volar metacarpal nerve passes over the abaxial surface of the sesamoid bone. The digital nerve is easily felt and controlled. This allows the clinician to deposit the anesthetic directly on the nerve. A 25-gauge ⅝-inch (1.0 cm) needle is ideal for this block. This block has limited value, since it may not block the entire foot unless a large volume is deposited, simultaneously blocking the dorsal branch going to the foot. If the block is done with 1 to 2 ml of solution, it offers little more than a posterior digital nerve block, depending on the division and location of the dorsal branches (Figs. 33.8 and 33.9).

A posterior digital block is done just below the enlargement of the fetlock joint in the triangular area formed by the head of the first phalanx, the edge of the flexor tendon, and the first phalanx proper. The clinician flexes the leg, holding it by the pastern with one hand. By using the thumb or finger, the nerve is held firm and a small needle is inserted. The nerve lies just under the superficial fascia which allows a weal to form when the anesthetic is deposited. Three milliliters of solution are used to obtain good analgesia of the heel, frog, sole, wings of the third phalanx, and the navicular area. For diagnostic purposes, it is best not to block in the above described triangle because of the spreading of the anesthetic over to the dorsal or intermediate nerves. Blocking the dorsal nerves will confuse the results of the block. To avoid this, insert the needle just proximal to the lateral cartilages along side of the deep flexor tendon which will be 2 to 2.5 (5 to 6 cm) inches lower than first described. The nerve can be felt more easily there than further up in the pastern.

INTRA-ARTICULAR INJECTIONS

The Shoulder Joint. The injection site is at the cranial border of the tendon of the infraspinatus muscle, 2 cm above the lateral tuberosity of the humerus.[3] Here, the tendon, approximately 2.5 cm in thickness, can be felt as a band. A long needle is inserted horizontally for a distance of 2 to 4 inches (5 to 10 cm), until the point hits the bone or until synovia appears, which rarely happens. This is a large joint and will require at least 10 to 20 ml of anesthetic solution.

The joint can also be entered between the fissure of the anterior and posterior part of the lateral tuberosity of the humerus.[25] The needle is directed backwards and inwards in a horizontal plane. A slight tremor can be felt when the needle pierces the joint capsule. The horse should be allowed to walk after the injection to circulate the anesthetic. The joint should be anesthetized in 5 to 10 minutes. The same landmarks are used for the bovine (Fig. 33.11).

The Elbow Joint. To enter the elbow joint, first locate the lateral tuberosity of the radius 4 inches (10 cm) below the olecranon in the middle of the lateral surface of the foreleg. One to one and one-half inches (2 to 3 cm) above this prominence is the similarly shaped lateral epicondyle of the humerus. Between these two prominences is the lateral collateral ligament which is easily identified. The needle is inserted in the distal third along the cranial border of this ligament in an oblique and inward direction for a depth of 2 inches (4.5 cm) or until synovia appears. The point of the needle should be inserted just under the margin of the lateral condyle of the humerus, which can be palpated (Fig. 33.11).

If the needle is inserted behind the ligament, the anesthetic will be injected into the communicating bursa under the ulnaris lateralis. Ten milliliters of solution should be deposited as soon as synovia is aspirated.

The Bovine Elbow Joint. The elbow joint in the cow can be reached by injecting the local anesthetic at the cranial border of the lateral collateral ligament as in the horse. Another method for anesthetizing the elbow joint of the cow is to enter the pouch of the joint which extends into the olecranon fossa.[28] The lateral epicondyle of the humerus is found 2.5 inches (6.5 cm) distal and 4 inches (6 cm) cranial to the olecranon. At the midpoint of a line joining the epicondyle to the olecranon, the needle is inserted obliquely forward and downward into the angle between the humerus and the olecranon to a depth of about 4 inches (10 cm) or until synovia fluid is released.

The Carpal Joints. The carpus is made up of three joints of which the radial carpal joint is the largest and does not communicate with the lower joints. The intercarpal joint communicates with the carpal metacarpal joint between the third and fourth carpal bones, therefore eliminating the

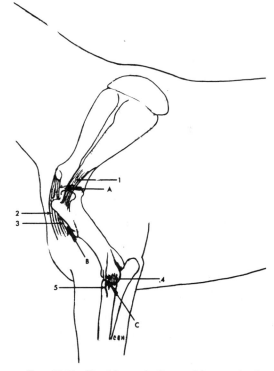

FIG. 33.11. Shoulder and elbow of horse. *A*, site to enter shoulder joint; *B*, site and direction to enter bicipital bursa; *C*, site to enter elbow joint. *1*, tendon of infraspinatus muscle; *2*, biceps brachii muscle; *3*, bicipital bursa; *4*, lateral collateral ligament of elbow; *5*, lateral tuberosity of radius.

need to enter both joints. With the leg flexed the joints are readily defined. A 20- or 22-gauge 1-inch (2.5 cm) needle is inserted on either side of the tendon of the extensor carpi radialis until synovia appears. If the joint is overdistended, synovia fluid should be withdrawn in another syringe before depositing up to 10 ml of solution.

The Fetlock Joint. This joint is most easily entered through the cul-de-sac of the joint capsule. With the leg in the standing position, the cul-de-sac of the fetlock joint can be felt in the triangular space formed by the third metacarpus, the sesamoid bone, and the suspensory ligament. A 20- to 22-gauge needle 1 inch (2.5 cm) long is inserted at right angles to the skin. If synovia does not appear, redirect the needle slightly downward and in. Five to seven milliliters of solution can be injected, depending on the degree of distension of the joint by the synovial fluid.

The Pastern Joint (Proximal Interphalangeal). The site of injection is located by first finding the medial and lateral epicondyles at the distal end of the first phalanx. One inch (2.5 cm) proximal to the epicondyles and ¾ inch (2 cm) from the midline, a 20- to 22-gauge 1- to 1½-inch (2.5 cm) needle is inserted through the skin obliquely in a medial and downward direction until the point lies on the bone in the midline below the extensor tendon. Five milliliters of anesthetic are deposited.

The Pedal (Coffin or Distal Interphalangeal) Joint. The site for injection lies ½ inch (1.2 cm) above the coronary band and ¾ inch (1.8 cm) medial or lateral to the midline. The foot is flexed, opening the interphalangeal joint, which facilitates entering the proximal compartment of the joint capsule. The proximal portion of the capsule extends upward onto the second phalanx. The needle is directed downwards, medially, and backwards for a depth of 1 to 1.5 inches (2.5 to 3.7 cm) under the extensor tendon until it enters the proximal sac of the joint capsule. Injection should be made slowly, as considerable pressure is built up when 10 ml of anesthetic is deposited. The anesthetic will diffuse among the distal sesamoid (navicular) bone.[3] This limits the use of this block for diagnosing osteoarthritic changes in the distal interphalangeal joint (low ringbone) from podotrochleitis (navicular disease).

Intertuberal or Bicipital Bursa. To block the bicipital bursa a 2- to 2½-inch (6.25 cm) 18-gauge needle is inserted at the level of the proximal end of the deltoid tuberosity, which is easily identified on the lateral aspect of the radius 6 inches (15 cm) below the point of the shoulder. The needle is directed obliquely upward between the deltoid tuberosity and the lateral edge of the biceps brachii tendon until synovial fluid appears. At least 10 ml of anesthetic should be injected.

Carpal Sheath. This synovial sheath can be entered either from its proximal end or distal limits. Either way it is difficult if the sheath is not distended with fluid. The point of entry is just above the accessory carpal bone between the tendons of the lateral digital extensor and the lateral flexor of the carpus. The distal approach is made by holding the leg in a flexed position. The needle is inserted in the angle between the suspensory ligament and the deep flexor tendon in the lateral proximal third of the metacarpus. The needle is directed horizontally along the dorsal border of the deep flexor tendon to a depth of less than 1 inch (1 to 2 cm).

Digital Sheath (Sheath of Flexor Tendons). If the digital sheath is filled with synovia fluid it can be entered from the proximal end. The deep flexor tendon should be grasped with one hand while the needle is inserted horizontally 2 inches (5 cm) above the sesamoid bones. Synovia will appear when the needle enters the sheath. A normal sheath should be entered distally to the fetlock joint in the triangular space bordered by the upper part of the proximal digital annular ligament, the proximal sesamoid bone, and the flexor tendons. The site is easily palpable, and entry is simple.[25]

Regional Analgesia of the Bovine Front Foot

The nerve supply to the foot of the bovine is more complex than the horse. Each digit has four nerves: two axial and two

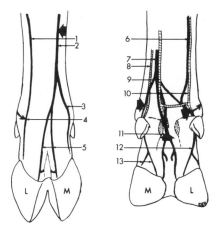

FIG. 33.12. Nerve supply to right front foot of a bovine. *Heavy arrows* mark sites for nerve blocks. *1,* dorsal branch of ulnar nerve; *2,* dorsal metacarpal—branch of radial nerve (both nerves are blocked from same site); *3,* abaxial dorsal digital nerve of third digit; *4,* abaxial dorsal digital nerve of fourth digit; *5,* axial dorsal digital nerves; *6,* volar branch of ulnar nerve; *7,* volar branch of median nerve; *8,* medial deep volar metacarpal artery; *9,* medial superficial volar metacarpal artery; *10,* lateral deep volar metacarpal artery; *11,* axial volar nerves; *12,* abaxial volar nerve to fourth digit; *13,* abaxial volar digital nerve of third digit.

abaxial. The digital nerves are branches, or continuations, of the radial, ulnar, and median nerves. Several methods have been advocated using either four or five injections to completely anesthetize the foot. A method using four injection sites has been described[19] (Fig. 33.12).

THE DORSAL METACARPAL NERVE

This nerve is a branch of the radial nerve and lies on the dorsal surface of the metacarpal bone medial to the extensor tendon. At the junction of the proximal and middle thirds, it is possible to feel the nerve roll beneath the finger. A ½-inch 22-gauge needle (1.25 cm) is used at this site. This will desensitize the dorsal surface of the foot.

THE ABAXIAL DORSAL

This nerve, the dorsal branch of the ulnar, and the abaxial volar, a branch of the median, can be blocked with one injection. The site for this injection is 1 inch (2.5 cm) above the fetlock joint on the lateral side

between the suspensory ligament and the flexor tendons. The abaxial dorsal nerves cross the fetlock in close association with the abaxial volar nerves, contrary to textbook illustrations.

THE AXIAL VOLAR DIGITAL

These nerves are branches of the median nerve and lie in a groove at the bifurcation of the flexor tendons. To block these nerves, inject 5 ml of anesthetic ½ to 1 inch (2.5 cm) proximal to the dew claws on the volar midline.

THE ABAXIAL VOLAR

This nerve of the third digit is the medial branch of the median nerve and is blocked 1 inch (2.5 cm) proximal to the fetlock joint in the groove formed by the suspensory ligament and the flexor tendons.

To block the medial digit, inject at Points *1, 3,* and *4* (Fig. 33.12). To block the lateral digit, inject at Points *1, 2,* and *3* (Fig. 33.12). The median nerve supplies most of the lateral and volar aspects of the leg, and the best site for blocking would be before the median nerve divides (Fig. 33.12). Unfortunately, at this point the nerve is situated deeply to the artery and vein and is not accessible for injection.

Hind Leg

ANATOMY

The terminal branches or the sciatic nerve, tibial and peroneal, innervates most of the hind leg below the stifle. The saphenous nerve, a branch off the femoral, helps supply part of the skin along the medial portion of the upper leg (Fig. 33.13). The tibial nerve (Fig. 33.14, *3*) runs distally between the biceps femoris and semitendinosus muscles to emerge with the recurrent tibial vein medially in front of the Achilles tendon, and is covered by deep fascia of the gaskin. Directly above the hock the nerve divides into medial and lateral branches which later become the medial and lateral superficial plantar (metatarsal) nerves. These descend the rest of the leg on both sides of the deep flexor tendon and divide below the fetlock the same as the volar nerves of the front leg.

The anastomotic branch from the medial to the lateral plantar nerve is more distal than in the front leg, and is absent in some cases.[23]

Before the lateral plantar nerve becomes superficial it gives off a deep branch high in the metatarsus to the suspensory ligament. This branch then divides into two branches: the lateral deep plantar nerve, which supplies the periostium of the metatarsus, and the medial deep plantar nerve, which emerges at the distal end of the medial splint bone and helps supply the laminar corium.[21]

Sensation is therefore supplied by the tibial over all the posterior aspect of the leg. In the middle posterior upper leg the tibial nerve gives off a cutaneous branch called the cutaneous surae which supplies the skin over the lateral and posterior region of the hock as far distal as the chestnut (Fig. 33.14, *4*). Also, at the proximal end of the Achilles tendon, the tibial gives off another cutaneous branch that supplies the posterior medial surface of the hock.

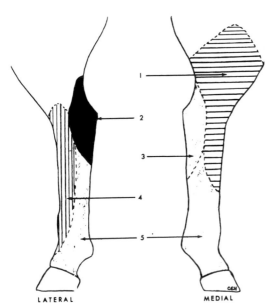

FIG. 33.13. Left rear leg of horse desensitized by blocking saphenous nerve (*1*), caudal cutaneous surae nerve (*2*), cutaneous branch off tibial nerve (*3*), peroneal nerve (*4*), tibial nerve (*5*).

The peroneal, also called the fibular in some texts, becomes superficial over the lateral head of the gastrocnemius muscle to the head of the fibula. The nerve divides in this area into superficial and deep branches. The deep peroneal (Fig. 33.14, *5*) descends between the muscle bellies of the long and lateral digital extensors. It innervates the hock, the flexors of the hock, and the extensors of the digit before dividing into lateral and medial branches called medial and lateral metatarsici dorsales (Fig. 33.14, *8*). These descend on both sides of the long extensor tendon on the dorsal surface of the large metatarsal bone and innervate the periosteum and the skin over both aspects of the dorsal metatarsus. They also supply almost the entire innervation to the fetlock joint and capsule, the dorsal aspect of the pastern, the interphalangeal joints, the center part of the coronary band, and part of the dorsal laminar corium.[17]

From this short review of the innervation to the hind digit, one should note the difference in the areas innervated by the volar nerves as compared to the plantar nerves. Blocking above the level of the sesamoid bones in the hindleg will not provide analgesia of the fetlock capsule or joint as is true when a volar nerve block is made in the front leg. The two superficial plantar (metatarsal) nerves supply most of the sensation to the joints below the fetlock, but not to the same extent as the volar nerves do in the front leg. The branches of the deep peroneal described above still innervate part of the dorsal aspect of these joints as well as the dorsal coronary band and laminar corium.

The saphenous nerve, a branch of the femoral, is found on the medial side of the leg lying in contact with the cranial surface of the saphenous vein, and is distributed with its tributaries below the hock of the medial and dorsal surfaces of the metatarsus as far distal as the fetlock. To block this nerve, an anesthetic must be deposited just under the skin along the saphenous vein. The injection should be made as high as possible or at the area where the sa-

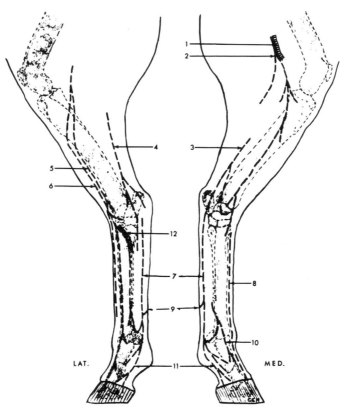

FIG. 33.14. Nerve distribution to the horse's left rear leg. *1*, saphenous vein; *2*, saphenous nerve; *3*, tibial nerve; *4*, caudal cutaneous surae branch off tibial nerve; *5*, deep peronal nerve (see also *8*); *6*, superficial peroneal; *7*, superficial plantar (metatarsal) from tibial; *8*, deep peroneal; *9*, anastomosing branch; *10*, deep plantar (metatarsal) from lateral plantar; *11*, posterior digital; *12*, great metatarsal artery.

phenous vein disappears into the medial thigh.

TIBIAL NERVE BLOCK

This nerve is infiltrated on the medial side of the leg 4 inches (10 cm) above the point of the hock in the groove between the Achilles tendon and the flexor hallucis longus muscle. Palpation of the nerve is easy at this site, especially when the leg is slightly flexed. Insert a 20-gauge 1-inch (2.5 cm) needle obliquely through the fascia, and inject 10 to 20 ml of anesthetic. If a bleb arises, the point of needle is too shallow. The cutaneous branch off the tibial that supplies the medial surface of the hock can be blocked at the same time by infiltrating under the skin during withdrawal of the needle.

The superficial peroneal can be felt through the skin where it lies just under the fascia in the furrow of the long and lateral digital extensors. It supplies the skin on the craniolateral surface of the limb down to the fetlock. This nerve is blocked 4 inches (10 cm) above the tibiotarsal articulation in the furrow described above. The anesthetic must be deposited subfascially and subcutaneously.

DEEP PERONEAL NERVE BLOCK

This nerve can be blocked 4 inches (10 cm) above the tibiotarsal joint and cranial to the septum between the long and lateral digital extensors where the superficial peroneal can be felt subcutaneously. The nerve lies about 1 inch (2.5 cm) below the skin surface and under a deep fascia. The

20-gauge 1-inch (2.5 cm) needle is inserted obliquely and slightly anteriorly. An attempt should be made to stay within the groove between the two muscle bellies until the point penetrates the deep fascia. Ten milliliters of anesthetic are deposited. The superficial peroneal nerve can be blocked at the same time by depositing 5 to 10 ml of solution subcutaneously while withdrawing the needle.

The common peroneal nerve can be blocked where it crosses over the head of the fibula on the lateral side of the leg at the level of the tibial tuberosity. Here, the common nerve has already divided, but both branches can be easily felt as they lie close together. Blocking the nerve here also blocks out all innervation to the extensors of the digit, causing the horse to knuckle over on the pastern. Therefore, this block has limited value when diagnosing a rear leg lameness.

INTRA-ARTICULAR INJECTIONS

Hip Joint (Coxofemoral Joint). To find the site of injection for the hip joint, it is necessary to identify the anterior and posterior parts of the trochanter major. On the center between these two parts and 1 inch dorsally, a needle can be passed into the hip joint. The skin at the injection site should first be anesthetized. A 14-gauge 1.5-inch needle can be used as a trocar so that an 18-gauge 6- to 7-inch (15 to 17 cm) needle can be easily directed into the joint. A 6-inch 2-mm trocar can also be used to prevent the needle from deviating out of line.[25] Ten to twenty milliliters of solution should be injected. If the needle has entered the joint and it is not possible to withdraw synovial fluid, the injection of a few milliliters of air will clear the needle for aspiration.

Stifle Joint. This joint is made up of three separate synovial sacs: the femoropatellar, the medial femorotibial, and the lateral femorotibial. The femoropatellar and the medial femorotibial communicate at the ventral portion of the medial ridge of the femoral trochlea. The lateral femorotibial joint communicates with the femoropatellar in 18 to 25% of the stifles.[9]

There are two sites for entering the femoropatellar joint. One is located on the anterolateral surface of the stifle joint between the lateral and middle patellar ligaments at the ventral margin of the patella, and the other is between the middle and medial patellar ligaments at the ventral margin of the patella. The latter site provides a larger space for injection due to the space between the attachments of the patellar ligaments; however, this site may be somewhat more difficult in fat or heavily muscled horses.

A small area of subcutaneous infiltration over the selected site will aid in directing the needle slowly into the joint. The subcutaneous infiltration over the anterolateral surface of the stifle will anesthetize branches of the lateral cutaneous nerve of the thigh (off the common peroneal nerve) and ventral cutaneous branches of the first lumbar nerve.[21, 23] with the horse bearing full weight on the leg, an 18-gauge, 2-inch (5 cm) needle is inserted through the skin in a horizontal anteroposterior plane under the ventral edge of the patella. Care should be taken not to force the point of the needle into the articular cartilage. If the needle is directed ventrally toward the tibial crest, a mass of adipose tissue will be encountered under the patellar ligaments. Injection in this area will give poor results. Unless there is an excess of synovial effusion, the joint yields only a small amount of synovial fluid.   Due to its size and communication with the medial femorotibial joint, 20 to 40 ml of anesthetic can be injected into this joint.

The site for entering the medial femorotibial joint is between the medial patellar ligament and the medial collateral ligament of the stifle joint. The skin over the area should be infiltrated subcutaneously to anesthetize the cutaneous branches of the common peroneal and the saphenous nerves. An 18-gauge 1½- to 2-inch (3.7 to 5 cm) needle is inserted through the skin just posterior to the medial patellar ligament in a mediolateral horizontal plane and just above the medial condyle of the tibia. The clinician should proceed slowly until the joint cavity has been entered. Should the needle be forced too deeply, the point will pass through the joint cavity and enter the large mass of adipose tissue under the patellar ligament. In view of the fact that this synovial sac communicates with the femoropatellar joint, the need of this approach is little, and it is rarely performed.

The site for entering the lateral femorotibial joint is between the lateral patellar ligament and the lateral collateral ligament of the stifle joint. The skin over the area should first be infiltrated to block out the cutaneous branches of the first and second lumbar nerves. An 18-gauge 1½- to 2-inch (3.71 cm) needle is inserted just posterior to the lateral patellar ligament on a horizontal, slightly posterior, plane. The clinician should proceed slowly until the point of the needle has entered the joint. If the needle is forced too far, it may enter the adipose tissue under the ligament and anterior to the intercondylar groove of the femur. Ten milliliters of anesthetic are deposited in the joint.[26]

ANESTHESIA OF THE HOCK JOINT (TIBIOTARSAL ARTICULATION)

The tibiotarsal articulation is the only joint of the four intertarsal joints that lends itself to intra-articular injection. The best site to enter this joint is on the anteriomedial surface on either side of the saphenous vein. A 20-gauge 1- to 1¼-inch (2.5 to 3 cm) needle can be used, and 10 to 20 ml of anesthetic are injected. Arthrocentesis for the rest of the joints in the hind leg is the same as described for the front leg.

Anesthesia of the Hind Leg for the Bovine

Regional analgesia of the hind foot can be accomplished by four injections using a ½- to 1-inch (2.5 cm) 20- to 22-gauge needle and depositing 5 ml of anesthetic at each site[19] (Fig. 33.15).

Superficial Peroneal Nerve. This nerve is located just below the skin on the dorsal surface of the metatarsal bone at the junction of its middle and proximal thirds. This block should be made before this nerve divides into its three terminal branches. If the block is not made at this

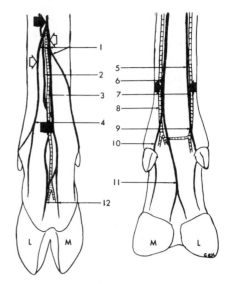

FIG. 33.15. Nerve supply to the right rear foot of a bovine. *Heavy arrows* mark sites for nerve blocks. *1*, three branches from superficial peroneal nerve; *2*, deep peroneal nerve; *3*, deep dorsal metatarsal artery; *4*, abaxial dorsal nerve of fourth digit; *5*, lateral plantar nerve (branch from tibial nerve); *6*, medial plantar nerve (branch from tibial nerve); *7*, lateral superficial plantar metatarsal artery; *8*, med. superficial plantar metatarsal artery; *9*, abaxial plantar nerve of fourth digit; *10*, abaxial plantar nerve of third digit; *11*, axial plantar nerve to third and fourth digits; *12*, axial dorsal nerve to third and fourth digits.

site, but lower, it will be necessary to block on both sides of the dorsal metatarsal vein.

Deep Peroneal Nerve. This nerve is blocked at the junction of the middle and distal thirds of the metatarsus. A 1-inch needle is inserted from the lateral side and is directed medially beneath the extensor tendons so that the point lies on the dorsal surface of the bone. The needle is inserted its full length. The dorsal metatarsal artery lies in the same groove as the nerve, so the syringe should be aspirated prior to injection.

The deep peroneal nerve can also be approached on the dorsal side of the fetlock through the proximal part of the interdigital space. The deep peroneal nerve emerges between the bifurcation of the long extensor tendon at this point as it is joined by the superficial peroneal nerve.

Lateral Plantar Metatarsal Nerve. This nerve is the lateral branch of the tibial nerve and lies between the suspensory ligament and flexor tendons. It is the continuation of the abaxial nerve of the fourth digit. A 1-inch needle is inserted under the fascia covering the nerve at the middle of the metatarsus.

Medial Plantar Metatarsal Nerve. This medial branch of the tibial nerve assumes the same position as the lateral nerve but on the medial side. It divides at the fetlock into the abaxial plantar nerve of the third digit and the two axial plantar digital nerves. Block this nerve by injecting the anesthetic agent at the middle of the metatarsus medial to and between the suspensory ligament and the deep flexor tendons.

Sciatic Nerve Block. The sciatic nerve emerges through the greater sciatic foramen as a broad flat band and passes downward and backward on the lower part of the sacrosciatic ligament. It turns downward in the hollow between the trochanter major of the femur and the tuber ischii. The site for blocking this nerve is a line drawn midway between the trochanter major and the lateral tuber ischii. Multiple injections have to be made in this area due to the width of the nerve. The 6-inch (15 cm) 18-gauge needle is inserted horizontally in a mediocranial direction until it comes in contact with the posterior margin of the acetabulum. Withdraw the needle ¾ to 1 inch (2 to 2.5 cm) and deposit 10 ml of anesthetic. Withdraw the needle and reinsert it 1 inch posteriorly until bone is hit; withdraw the needle the same as before and deposit 10 ml of solution. Repeat this for a total of 4 to 5 injections. A total of 50 to 60 ml of solution should be used. The block will produce complete analgesia, as well as paralysis, of the hind leg with the exception of the anterior thigh, which is supplied by the femoral nerve.

Analgesia of the Perineum

PERINEUM OF THE HORSE

The perineum, the area between the anus and the scrotum, can be anesthetized by blocking the superficial subcutaneous and deep subfascial branches of the perineal nerves as they pass ventrally over the ishial arch. An injection must be made on both sides where an imaginary line 1 inch dorsal to the ischial arch crosses a vertical line 1 inch lateral of the anus. The first injection is made subcutaneously depositing 5 ml of anesthetic; then the needle is inserted dorsally under the fascia for another ½ inch to deposit another 5 ml.[16]

THE INTERNAL PUDENDAL (PUDIC) NERVE BLOCK (BOVINE)

The internal pudendal nerve block was first described by Larson and added to by Habel.[13, 14] The site for the injection is the deepest point of the ischiorectal fossa, which may be filled with fat in heavy beef bulls. To determine the site on these fat animals, the sacrotuberous ligament can be palpated and the site chosen which will allow the needle to pass medial to the sacrotuberous ligament. A bleb of anesthetic is first injected intradermally at the chosen puncture sites using a 26-gauge needle. Next, a short 15-gauge needle is inserted through the skin to serve as a cannula for the 18-gauge 4½-inch (11.5 cm) needle. The left hand is then inserted into the rectum where the internal pudendal nerve can best be located by first palpating the part of the lesser sciatic foramen which extends anterior to the coccygeus muscle. This area gives the impression of a weak spot in the sacrosciatic ligament just dorsal to the anterior part of the lesser sciatic notch. The readily palpable internal pudendal artery also passes through this part of the lesser sciatic foramen. The left hand is moved anteriorly 2 to 3 inches using the sciatic spines as a guide, and the hand is brought back in a caudodorsal direction applying lateral pressure with the fingers against the sacrosciatic ligament. The nerve, aboute the size of an ordinary extension cord, can be felt to slip under the fingertips. It then becomes a simple matter to bring the point of the needle in proximity to the internal pudendal nerve. Deposit 25 ml of solution around the nerve and somewhat cranial to the lesser sciatic foramen. Then 10 to 15 ml of anesthetic is deposited caudal and dorsal to the original injection in an attempt to block the middle hemorrhoidal nerve which carries sympathetic fibers to the retractor penis muscle. It takes at least 30 minutes for this block to work. In blocking heavy beef bulls, a 5-inch (12.5 cm) 17-gauge needle going through a short 12-gauge needle should be used.

To insure complete anesthesia of the perineum and penis or vulva, the ventral branch of the pudendal nerve should also be blocked.[13, 14] This can be anesthetized by blocking the nerve from the same approach. The nerve can be palpated by feeling ventral to reach the surface of the obturator internus just inside the lesser sciatic foramen. The internal pudendal artery lies next to the nerve. Ten to fifteen milliliters of solution should be deposited at this site. With the advent of tranquilizers, there is a limited need for this nerve block.

Anesthesia for Castration of the Horse

The spermatic cord and testicle are innervated by the internal spermatic sympathetic plexus, and the blood supply is from the internal spermatic artery. The tunica vaginalis of the cord, the testicle, the cremaster muscle, and the skin of the scrotum are innervated by the external spermatic, ilioinguinal, and iliohypogastric nerves. It is not possible to block all of these nerves individually.

With the horse in the standing or cast position, infiltrate a total of 10 ml of solution in the cutaneous area on either side and parallel with the medium raphe. Anesthetic solution is injected as the skin is pulled onto the needle. If the horse is standing, the operator works from the left side. The testicle is grasped with the left hand near the penis and the spermatic cord between the thumb and the finger. A 20-gauge 1-inch (2.5 cm) needle attached to the syringe is directed into the spermatic cord as high as possible. The cord can be felt distending when the anesthetic is being deposited. Care should be taken not to inject into a blood vessel. The anesthetic should be deposited in more than one area in the cord, but without withdrawing the needle through the skin. A total of 10 ml of anesthetic should be used for each cord. To block the opposite cord, insert the needle through the cord being held by the thumb and index finger. The onset of anesthesia can be determined by the paralysis of the cremaster muscle. The testicle does not retract when handled.

Another method of producing regional analgesia for castration in all animals can be produced by the intratesticular route. The anesthetic solution quickly passes from the center of the testicle up the spermatic cord via the lymph vessels.[20] The impregnated vessels will then anesthetize the spermatic cord. The bulk of the injection is carried into the blood stream by the lymphatic system, so systemic toxicity is possible. The following dosages are recommended: horse, 20 ml in each testicle; bull, 5 to 25 ml in both testicles; boar, 5 to 15 ml in each testicle; sheep and goats, 2 to 10 ml in each testicle. A subcutaneous infiltration of the skin incision must be made.

REFERENCES

1. Bemis, H. E.: Local anesthesia in animal dentistry. J. Amer. Vet. Med. Ass. 51: 188, 1917.
2. Bemis, H. E., Guard, W. F., and Covault, C. H.: Anesthesia general and local. J. Amer. Vet. Med. Ass. 64: 413, 1924.
3. Berge, E., and Westhues, M.: Veterinary Operative Surgery, 1st English ed. Medical Book Company, Copenhagen, Denmark, 1966.
4. Bolz, W.: Contribution to the local anesthesia of the forelimb of the horse below the carpal joint. Berlin. Munchen. Tieraerztl. Wschr. 44: 769, 1928. Abstract in Vet. Rec. 12: 588, 1932.
5. Bolz, W., and Grebe, W.: Experiments for the determination of the areas of anesthesia after local injections of the nerves of the foot in the horse. Tieraerztl. Rdsch: 38: 101, 1932. Cited in Vet. Rec. 12: 588, 1932.
6. Bressou, C., and Siliza, S.: Contribution a l'étude de l'anesthésie dentaire chez le cheval et chez le chien. Rec. Med. Vet. Ecole Alfort 107: 129, 1931.
7. Browne, T. G.: Local anesthesia (nerve-blocking) for dehorning of cattle. Vet. Rec. 48: 1178, 1936.
8. Dykstra, R. R.: Local anesthesia in veterinary surgery. Vet. Med. 23: 60, 1928.
9. Ellenberger, W., and Baum, H.: Handbuch der vergleichenden Anatomie der Haustiere, 15 Auflage. August Hirschwald, Berlin, 1921. Cited in Van Pelt.[26]

10. Frank, E. R.: *Veterinary Surgery*, 2nd ed. Burgess Publishing Company, Minneapolis, 1955.
11. Gabel, A. A., and Jones, E. W.: *General and Local Anesthesia in Equine Medicine and Surgery*, 1st ed., p. 63. American Veterinary Publications, Inc., Santa Barbara, Calif., 1963.
12. Getty, R., Sowa, J. A., and Lundvall, R. L.: Local anesthesia and applied anatomy as related to nerve blocks in horses. J. Amer. Vet. Med. Ass. *128:* 583, 1956.
13. Habel, R. E.: A source of error in the bovine pudendal nerve block. J. Amer. Vet. Med. Ass. *128:* 16, 1956.
14. Larson, L. L.: The internal pudendal (pudic) nerve block for anesthesia of the penis and relaxation of the retractor penis muscle. J. Amer. Vet. Med. Ass. *123:* 18, 1953.
15. Lightenstern, G.: Die Verwendung von Tropakain in der tierärztlichen Chirurgie mit besonderer Berücksichtigung hinsichtlich seiner Verwendbarkeit in der Augapfel-infiltration beim Pferde. Berlin. Munchen. Tieraerztl. Wschr. *55:* 337, 1911.
16. Magda, J. J.: Lokalanasthesie bei Operationen am mannlichen Perineum bei Pferden. Veterineriya *25:* 34, 1948. Cited in Westhues and Fritsch.[28]
17. Nilsson, S. A.: Vidrag til Kannedomen om fotenus innervation hos häst. (English summary) Skand. Vet. Tidskr. *38:* 401, 1948.
18. Peterson, D. R.: Nerve block of the eye and associated structures. J. Amer. Vet. Med. Ass. *118:* 145, 1951.
19. Raker, C. W.: Regional anesthesia of the bovine foot. J. Amer. Vet. Med. Ass. *128:* 238, 1956.
20. Reiger, H.:   Die testikulare Injektion. Berlin. Munchen. Tieraerztl. Wschr. *67:* 107, 1954.
21. Rooney, J. R.: *Guide to the Dissection of the Horse*, 3rd ed. J. W. Edwards, Publishers, Inc., Ann Arbor, 1956.
22. Rubin, L. F.: Auriculopalpebral nerve block as an adjunct to the diagnosis and treatment of ocular inflammation in the horse. J. Amer. Vet. Med. Ass. *144:* 1387, 1964.
23. Sissons, S., and Grossman, J. D.: *The Anatomy of the Domestic Animals*, 4th ed. W. B. Saunders Company, Philadelphia, 1956.
24. Tosco, G.: L'anestesia alta de nervo mascellare negli equidi. Nuovo Ercolani *40:* 1, 1935. Cited by Westhues and Fritsch.[28]
25. Tufvesson, G.: *Local Anesthesia in Veterinary Medicine*. Astra International, Division of AB Astra, Sodertalje, Sweden, 1963.
26. Van Pelt, R. W.: Intra-articular injections of the equine stifle for therapeutic and diagnostic purposes. J. Amer. Vet. Med. Ass. *147:* 490, 1965.
27. Vitums, A.: Nerve and arterial blood supply to the horns of the goat with reference to the sites of anesthesia for dehorning. J. Amer. Vet. Med. Ass. *125:* 284, 1954.
28. Westhues, M., and Fritsch, R.: *Animal Anesthesia*, 1st English ed., p. 56. J. B. Lippincott Company, Philadelphia, 1964.
29. Worthman, R. P.: Lecture notes and personal communication from surgical anatomy, Washington State University, 1960.
30. Wright, J. G.: *Veterinary Anesthesia*, 1st ed., p. 18. Alexander Eger, Inc., Chicago, 1941.

34
Analgesia of the Eye

LIONEL F. RUBIN AND KIRK N. GELATT

Topical Analgesic Agents

A large number of agents are available which are capable of producing topical corneal and conjunctival analgesia. Most of these are surface-active agents and are not intended for parenteral administration. The few drops applied topically for routine clinical purposes rarely cause systemic problems, although absorption is extremely rapid (Fig. 34.1).

Agents for topical analgesia should have the following characteristics: (a) ability to penetrate epithelial barriers; (b) adequate duration of effect; (c) the absence of secondary effects (such as mydriasis); (d) systemic toxicity; (e) minimal tissue irritation; and (f) to a minor extent in veterinary medicine, freedom from allergenicity. Repeated application of topical anesthetics can produce epithelial erosions of the cornea, infiltration of cells into the stroma, and delayed healing[16] (Table 34.1). With the continued use of topical analgesia, the blink reflex is impaired. Exposure keratitis and foreign body penetration may follow, complicating the presence of induced corneal erosions. The insensitive cornea is especially prone to various forms of trauma due to impaired protective reflexes.

The deleterious effects of topical agents may be the result of toxic effects on the corneal nerves.[3] Ointments are less likely to produce these deleterious changes than anesthetic collyria.[49] It is unwise to prescribe any topical analgesic agents for un-limited topical use because of the danger of retardation of healing and damage to normal corneal epithelium. Restricted application, limited to no more than four times daily, is probably not dangerous. Repeated instillations can produce tachyphylaxis, and the effectiveness of local application is markedly diminished.[3, 4]

All topical anesthetics rapidly penetrate corneal and conjunctival epithelial linings; therefore, the inability of procaine to penetrate the epithelium precludes its topical use. Addition of vasoconstrictors does not retard absorption through mucous membranes; therefore, there is no rationale for adding epinephrine or its analogues to topical ocular anesthetic agents.[10]

The duration of effect of topical anesthetics varies with the species (Table 34.2), agent, and amount instilled. In general, several instillations of topical agents over a short time will prolong analgesia significantly. For example, a single instillation of proparacaine produces 10 to 15 minutes of corneal analgesia while repeated applications may produce a topical effect for over 2 hours.

Topical analgesia can be used clinically for examination procedures, including palpation of the conjunctival fornices, removal of corneal and conjunctival foreign bodies, surgical removal of the glands of the third eyelid, chemical cauterization of the cornea and conjunctiva, tonometry, β-ray therapy, insertion of a lid speculum, suture removal, and, in some instances, for relief of blepharospasm secondary to corneal damage. Topical anesthetic agents should not be used when attempting to obtain bacterial cultures from infected eyes, since most commercial topical anesthetic agents in multidose vials contain preservatives.

Tetracaine in 0.5% solutions and cocaine in 2.5% solutions have been shown to inhibit growth of *Pseudomonas aeruginosa*, *Candida albicans*, and *Staphylococcus albus* (coagulase-negative). Benoxinate (0.4% solution) inhibits growth of the latter two organisms, but does not inhibit growth of the former. Proparacaine (0.5%) fails to inhibit growth of any of the three test organisms.[25]

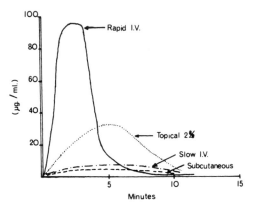

FIG. 34.1. Blood levels in dogs after administration of 30 mg of tetracaine by different routes. *I.V.*, intravenous. (Modified from Adriani.[1])

The standard compound to which drugs for topical analgesia are compared is cocaine (Fig. 34.2). This was first used for topical ocular analgesia in 1884 by Koller. Cocaine has been largely supplanted as an ocular agent by synthetic substitutes which avoid the disadvantages inherent in the use of cocaine, *i.e.*, production of epithelial erosions[11] and sympathomimetic action (not seen in the horse).[38] In veterinary medicine, the value of cocaine is its ability to inhibit the amine oxidase enzymes which destroy norepinephrine. Its norepinephrine-preserving action is useful in diagnosing preganglionic lesions in sympathetic denervation of the iris. Instillation of 4% cocaine solution into the eye of dogs or cats with Horner's syndrome will produce mild dilation of the pupil if the abnormality has occurred in the preganglionic pathway. The indirect mydriatic effect of cocaine in normal dogs is not clinically evident.[45]

Tetracaine is generally administered as a 0.5% solution. Instillation of tetracaine is followed by a transitory stinging sensation, but the subsequent analgesia is of sufficient depth to allow tonometry in dogs within 1 minute. For more manipulative procedures such as suture removal from the cornea, several instillations are necessary. Repeated and prolonged administration induces the usual corneal toxicity.[17]

TABLE 34.1

*Healing of puncture wounds in rat corneal epithelium after instillation of 1 drop of anesthetic every 15 minutes for 3 hours**

Drug	Concentration	No Healing	Healing	Partial Healing
	%		X	
Control				
Cocaine	4.0	X		
Butacaine (Butyn)	2.0	X		
Benoxinate (Dorsocaine)	0.4	X		
Phenacaine (holocaine)	1.0	X		
Dibucaine (Nupercain)	0.1	X		
Proparacaine (Ophthaine)	0.5	X		
Piperocaine (Metycaine)	2.0		X	
Lidocaine (Xylocaine)	2.0		X	
Tetracaine	0.5			X

* From Marr *et al.*[37]

TABLE 34.2

*Duration of corneal anesthesia after instillation of 1% anesthetic solution**

Compound	Guinea Pigs	Rabbits
	min	*min*
Tetracaine	52	
Butacaine	40	30
Hexylcaine	19	19
Cocaine	18	30
Neothesin	16	5
Procaine	0	0

* From Beyer et al.[7]

Systemic toxic reactions to tetracaine have not been reported in animals. The authors have observed an instance in which instillation of 0.5% tetracaine was followed by the rapid development of conjunctival chemosis and erythema which persisted for about 1 hour. This occurred in all of a group of 30 young beagle dogs. The reaction could not be avoided by preliminary instillation of antihistamines or vasoconstrictors.

Proparacaine has been advocated as an excellent topical anesthetic because of lack of signs of irritation following instillation.[15, 35] A single drop produces corneal analgesia lasting 10 to 15 minutes, while repeated instillations may produce analgesia for over 2 hours. Proparacaine causes less corneal punctate epithelial damage than tetracaine. Linn and Vey[31] state that there is no significant difference in duration and intensity of anesthesia among solutions of 0.5% tetracaine, 0.4% benoxinate, and 0.5% proparacaine. While highly recommended, a disadvantage of commercial proparacaine solutions is that they must be refrigerated. In the authors' experience, proparacaine produces no initial signs of irritation after instillation of non-refrigerated solutions; unfortunately, animals do resent instillation of a cold solution which is an inconvenience in clinical practice.

Benoxinate (0.4%) is identical with proparacaine (0.5%) in time of onset, intensity, and duration of analgesia. It causes less irritation and less punctate epithelial damage than tetracaine.[46] The anesthetic effect of a single instillation lasts no more than 15 minutes.

Butacaine (2%) produces adequate corneal analgesia after several instillations. Butacaine must be stored in amber bottles to prevent deterioration by light. Butacaine produces more epithelial pitting and conjunctival engorgement than cocaine.[11]

Piperocaine (2%) and lidocaine (2%) do not inhibit corneal epithelial regeneration.[37] Instillation is followed by signs of irritation. Westhues and Fritsch[52] state that a 6% lidocaine solution is equivalent in topical anesthetic effect to 1% tetracaine.

Dyclonine (0.5%) produces corneal analgesia lasting about 1 hour in rabbits. It may be used topically in concentrations up to 2%, although high concentrations (10%) produce corneal opacification. In addition to its analgesic properties, dyclonine is both fungicidal and bacteriocidal, and commercial preparations are stated to be self-sterilizing.

Other topical anesthetics for corneal instillation are hexylcaine,[7] cornecaine, eucaine B, holocaine, dicain,[18] sovcain,[39] and dibucain.

It must be emphasized that anesthetic compounds should not be used in the eye unless specifically recommended for ocular usage. The authors have observed corneal anesthesia lasting at least 7 days after topical administration of a benzocaine-containing compound.

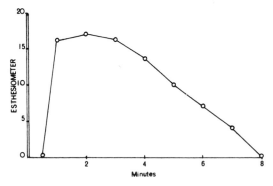

FIG. 34.2. Duration and onset of corneal anesthesia as measured by von Frey hairs after instillation of 1 drop of 2% cocaine. (From Bellows.[5])

Akinesia of the Eyelids

Akinesia of the eyelids is produced by local infiltration of the motor components of the facial nerve that innervate the orbicularis oculi muscles. Topical analgesia combined with regional nerve infiltration is necessary if the eyelids are to be traumatized. In dogs, akinesia of the eyelids is useful for temporary relief of spastic entropion and superficial irritation of the cornea. It is also a useful adjunct in the examination and treatment of the eye in large animals. Akinesia produced by regional nerve block, combined with topical analgesia, is useful for administering bulbar subconjunctival injections in large animals.

Two methods have been suggested for regional infiltration to produce akinesia of the eyelids in the dog (Fig. 34.3).

a. Palpate the border of the orbit, insert the needle about 2 cm lateral to the lateral canthus, and inject a small amount of anesthetic. Introduce the needle until the point strikes bone, then move it along the surface of the bone ½ cm from the upper orbital margin, infiltrating the tissues along the path of the needle. Proceed in the same way along the lower orbital border.[51]

b. Insert the needle subfascially over the midpoint of the posterior third of the zygomatic arch directly over its dorsal border

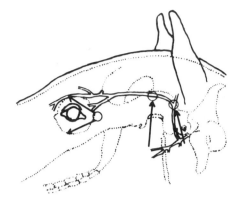

FIG. 34.4. Location of the auriculopalpebral nerve in the horse. *Arrows* indicate alternate sides of injection for inducing akinesia of the lids.

and direct it toward the middle of the forehead. Inject 5 ml of 2% procaine.

Akinesia is evidenced by narrowing of the palpebral fissure, drooping of the upper eyelid, and eversion of the lower lid. There is no interference with the animal's ability to rotate or retract the globe. The nictitating membrane will still protrude, but this can be overcome by a retrobulbar block and infiltration of the medial canthus with a local anesthetic agent.

In the horse, akinesia with eyelid analgesia may be obtained by a field block around the orbital rim, but in horses which have painful ocular diseases, injections close to the irritated eye may be hazardous. Production of akinesia by infiltration at a site distant from the eye is more desirable (Fig. 34.4).

In the horse, the auriculopalpebral nerve may be blocked[44] by infiltrating the local anesthetic agent in a fan-like manner subfascially in the depression just caudal to the posterior ramus of the mandible at the ventral edge of the temporal portion of the zygomatic arch. The needle is directed upward just caudal to the highest point of the arch. Complete akinesia may not occur, since occasionally small motor branches to the eyelids may accompany the main trunk of the facial nerve and approach the eyelids from the facial crest area. Care should be exercised to avoid injections into the rostral auricular artery and vein when using this technique.

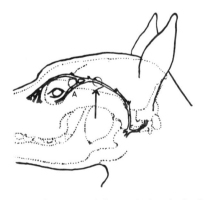

FIG. 34.3. Location of the auriculopalpebral nerve in the dog. The *circle* marked *A* indicates the site for producing akinesia as recommended by Uberreiter. The nerve may also be blocked by injecting more caudad, the direction of injection corresponding to the *arrow*.

An alternate method is to insert the needle 3 cm ventral to the highest point of the dorsal border of the zygomatic arch. The needle is directed obliquely and dorsally to contact bone and is advanced along the bone until the tip is just below the border of the zygomatic arch.

In cattle, the auriculopalpebral nerve is blocked just anterior to the base of the auricular muscles[36] (Fig. 34.5). The needle is inserted obliquely caudad and dorsally until it contacts the bone. The needle is advanced until the point is located at the dorsal border of the zygomatic arch. Approximately 10 ml of 2% procaine are necessary to produce adequate anesthesia.

Regional Analgesia (Anesthesia) of the Eyelids

In some instances, lesions of the eyelids can be removed under regional analgesia which obviates the need for complete ocular analgesia. Occasionally a more specific frontal nerve blockade may be useful for upper eyelid tumors instead of regional infiltration only.

The upper eyelid of the horse can be locally anesthetized by injecting a local anesthetic agent equivalent to 2 to 5 ml of 4% procaine into the supraorbital foramen anesthetizing the supraorbital nerve. The foramen is situated on a line drawn vertically and dorsally from the medial canthus. The supraorbital foramen is palpable as a small depression midway across the supra-

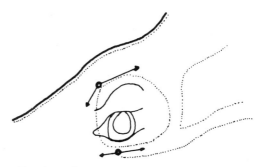

FIG. 34.6. Injection sites for local anesthesia of the eyelids in cattle. *Circles* indicate site of insertion of the hypodermic needle. (After Schreiber.[48])

orbital process.[8] A 20-gauge needle is inserted to a depth of 2 cm and the local anesthetic agent injected. This block is useful in the removal of small tumors of the upper lid and, in conjunction with topical conjunctival anesthesia, for the repair of minor lid lacerations.

Blockade of the frontal nerve in cattle is accomplished by field-type block.[48] The needle is inserted slightly dorsal to the medial canthus and directed laterally along the supraorbital process (Fig. 34.6). At least 10 ml of 4% procaine are infiltrated as the needle is advanced.

Anesthesia of the eyelids in the dog is accomplished by field block infiltrating in the area of the orbital rim.

Regional Analgesia of the Eye

Retrobulbar anesthesia can be used for ocular and orbital surgery, but its efficiency varies among the species due to anatomical differences and placement of the nerve block. In cattle, retrobulbar anesthesia is satisfactory; it is less so in the horse and dog. In the horse, retrobulbar analgesia does not prevent nystagmus associated with chloral hydrate narcosis, so that ocular surgery under these conditions is difficult. If slight proptosis of the eye is desired for surgery, the retrobulbar injection of saline is sufficient in small animals under general anesthesia. One advantage of retrobulbar analgesia is that intraocular pressure tends to decrease (Fig. 34.7). This drop is enhanced by digital massage (Fig. 34.8).

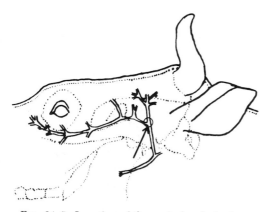

FIG. 34.5. Location of the auriculopalpebral nerve in the cow. *Arrow* indicates site of injection for inducing akinesia. (After Maksimovic.[36])

Anesthesia of the eye and orbit is achieved by blocking the ophthalmic division of the trigeminal nerve. Because of their proximity to the foramen carrying the ophthalmic nerve, the abducens, oculomotor, and trochlear nerves are usually paralyzed, thus producing akinesia of the globe. Ideally the retrobulbar anesthetics must be deposited near the orbitorotundum foramen or orbital fissure in order to block these nerves. The retrobulbar block incorporates the parasympathetic innervation to the iris sphincter, and mydriasis follows. If pupillary constriction is desired, as in intraocular surgery, direct acting parasympathomimetic agents (acetylcholine or pilocarpine) must be used. The anticholinesterase miotics have no effect.

Injections of local anesthetics into the retrobulbar space occasionally result in undesirable side effects. These include optic nerve damage, injections into the optic nerve meninges, and penetration of the globe. If the orbital venous sinuses or veins are damaged, the resulting orbital hemorrhage may be sufficient to exert considerable pressure on the globe. In dogs, the injection of excessive amounts of fluid in the retrobulbar space may produce a degree of chemosis and subconjunctival accumulation of the injected fluid. The globe will be placed under external pressure, and in the dog, cat, and horse, in which scleral rigidity is lacking, retrobulbar fluids may induce vitreous prolapse

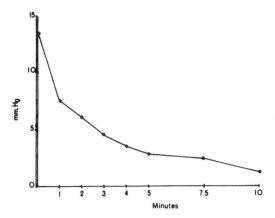

FIG. 34.8. Average drop in intraocular pressure in man following retrobulbar analgesia and digital pressure on the globe. (From Kirsch.[24])

during intraocular surgery. Infiltration of local anesthetics into the retrobulbar space should be used cautiously for the surgical repair of descemetocoele or iris prolapse, since the weakened cornea provides little impediment to extrusion of ocular contents.

HORSE

The ophthalmic nerve, along with the nerves to the extraocular muscles, can be blocked at the orbital fissures. In Berge's method[6] for injection at the orbital fissure, the needle is inserted at a point behind the zygomatic process of the frontal bone at the level of the supraorbital foramen. The needle is inclined 40° to the vertical and is directed medioventrally and somewhat caudally. In another method,[33] the orbital fissure is reached by inserting the needle through the previously anesthetized conjunctiva at the lateral canthus. The needle is directed toward the mandibular joint of the opposite side until bone is felt. Fifteen to thirty milliliters of 2% procaine should be injected starting at a depth of about 6 cm.* Occasionally hemorrhage will accompany the injections at the orbital fissure, necessitating cancellation of surgery. To avoid this contingency, an ocular sensory block of the globe can be produced. This

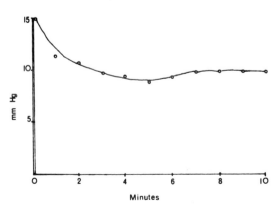

FIG. 34.7. Intraocular pressure measurements after retrobulbar injection of local anesthetic. (From Everett et al.[14])

---

* Magda[33] states that this will be effective in the dog using 8 to 15 ml of 2% procaine.

block is produced by inserting a 10-cm needle 1.5 cm behind the middle of the supraorbital process and directing it toward the opposite upper last premolar.[29] Puncture of the somewhat taut fascia of the muscle cone can be felt. At least 20 ml of 2% procaine are required. As an alternative to the latter method, the retrobulbar area can be approached through the medial or lateral orbital margin.[21]

DOG

For retrobulbar analgesia, an 8-cm 20-gauge needle is inserted through the skin at the lateral canthus or through anesthetized conjunctiva and is pushed past the globe toward the opposite mandibular joint. Three to eight milliliters of 2% procaine are injected when the needle hits bone. Blockage of the maxillary nerve may also occur.

In Barth's method (Fig. 34.9), a 5- to 8-cm needle is inserted just below the zygomatic process at the level of the lateral canthus.[2] The point of the needle is 0.5 cm in front of the anterior border of the vertical portion of the ramus of the mandible. The needle is pushed medially to the ramus caudally and slightly dorsally so that it reaches the orbital fissure. This block tends

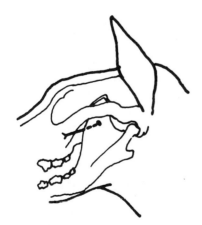

FIG. 34.9. Infiltration of the ocular nerves at the orbital fissure in the dog. The needle is inserted ventral to the zygomatic process at the level of the lateral canthus. The needle passes medial to the ramus of the mandible, slightly caudal and dorsal to meet the ocular nerves at the orbital fissure. (After Barth.[2])

to obviate the danger of accidental puncture of the globe.

Dietz's method utilizes a special needle 5 cm long curved to conform to the roof of the orbit, entering the conjunctival sac at the vertical meridian and injecting 1 to 3 ml of 2% procaine.[12] Anesthesia lasts an hour.

RABBIT

The needle is inserted at the dorsal border of the zygomatic arch midway between its anterior and posterior ends. The needle is directed caudomedially for 25 mm, bringing it close to the orbitorotundum foramen. It is important to avoid penetration of the orbital venous sinus and the nearby internal maxillary artery.[47]

CATTLE

Several nerve blocks for producing anesthesia of the globe are available. Their usefulness depends on individual practice, but all are practical.

In Peterson's block, after the skin is anesthetized at the point where the supraorbital process meets the zygomatic arch, a 4½-inch 18-gauge needle, having an arc of curvature corresponding to a circle of 10-inch radius, is inserted with the concavity posteriorly and with the hub of the needle slightly higher than the point of insertion.[41] It is inserted until the needle strikes the coronoid process of the mandible. By working the point of the needle off the anterior border of the process and inserting it downward until it hits the floor of the pterygopalatine fossa, the area of the orbitorotundum foramen will be at the point. Insert 15 cc of solution after withdrawing on the plunger to be sure the internal maxillary artery has not been entered. The pterygoid crest forms a protective shelf around the subdural and subarachnoid spaces of the optic nerve.

An auriculopalpebral block can be placed at the same time by withdrawing the needle until it lies subcutaneously, then directing it posteriorly in the fascia lateral to the zygomatic arch for 2 to 3 inches, infiltrating anesthesia along the way. This will produce akinesia of the lids.

Schreiber's method of approach through the conjunctiva (Fig. 34.10) involves inserting the needle about 1.5 cm lateral to the inner canthus at the lower eyelid through the previously anesthetized conjunctiva.[48] The point of the needle is pushed below the globe toward the base of the horn at the opposite side. After crossing the bony floor of the orbit, the needle is directed about 15° more ventrally to a depth of about 10.5 cm, and 15 to 20 ml of 2% procaine are injected. The distance of insertion is critical as the approach to the foramen is direct and there is the potential danger of entering the brain.

Another method of Schreiber (Fig. 34.10) involves insertion of a curved 18-cm needle through the anesthetized conjunctiva at the level of the middle of the supraorbital process, directing the needle past the globe toward the opposite horn, and curving it along the dorsal orbital wall downwards until the base of the orbit is contacted at a depth of 12 to 13 cm.[48] Thirty milliliters of 2% procaine are injected.

The foramen may also be reached through insertion of the needle through the temporal fossa. The needle is inserted behind the base of the supraorbital process of the frontal bone and pushed ventromedially (inclined to the nose) at an angle of

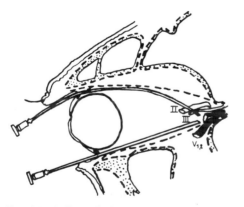

FIG. 34.10. Lateral view of left orbit showing conjunctival approach for producing anesthesia of the bovine eye. *II*, optic nerve; *III*, oculomotor nerve; $V_{1,2}$, ophthalmic and maxillary branches of the trigeminal nerve. (After Schreiber.[48])

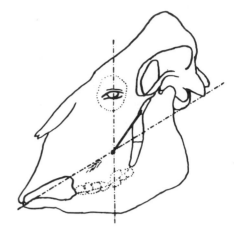

FIG. 34.11. Landmarks and direction of insertion of needle for anesthesia of the globe in the cow. (After Hare.[19])

40° to the supraorbital process to a depth of 10 cm where 15 to 30 ml of 2% procaine are injected.

In Hare's block (Fig. 34.11), the point of insertion is a line drawn through the facial tuberosity parallel to the frontal surface of the skull meeting a perpendicular line drawn through the middle of the eyes *when the head is held in natural position*.[19] If the width of the head (measured across the frontal bones between the dorsal margin of the bony orbits) exceeds 8½ inches, the point of insertion is on the perpendicular line at the levels of the alveolar border of the maxilla.

An injection makes the skin insensitive. A 1½-inch 16-gauge needle used for the skin injection is then directed mesiad as far as the maxilla, infiltrating the tissues along the path of the needle. The short needle is withdrawn and is replaced with a 7-inch (or 8-inch if the head width exceeds 8½ inches) 14-gauge needle. This is directed mesiad until it strikes the maxilla. It is then passed caudad along the surface of the bone until it can be pushed further caudomesiad over the surface of the maxillary tuberosity ventral to the zygomatic process of the malar bone, as far as the medial wall of the pterygopalatine fossa (6 to 8 inches).

From its point of entry the needle should be directed towards the base of the opposite horn. Fifteen milliliters of anesthetic are injected.

Characteristically, as it enters the periorbita, the eyelids become half closed and flicker in response to further passage of the needle. The reflex closing of the eyelids must be obtained before depositing anesthesia. A reflex movement of the head merely indicates a nerve (probably the maxillary) is being stimulated.

The eyelids are immobilized by blocking the auriculopalpebral nerve where it crosses the notch in the zygomatic arch at the level of the temporomandibular joint. Both of these are palpable.

After injection of the periorbita, the head should be elevated so that the anesthetic solution will gravitate towards the apex of the sac. Hare believes this to be easier than Peterson's block becuase a straight needle is used and is directed toward a palpable bony landmark.

This block is similar to Schreiber's, except that the point of insertion of the needle is located further rostrad, thus lessening the chance of damaging the buccinator nerve and vein. The likelihood of reaching the optic nerve and making an inadvertent injection into the optic nerve sheaths is also reduced, because the ventral border of the zygomatic process of the malar bone prevents it from being directed as far dorsad as the optic foramen.

Effects of Anesthetics and Preanesthetics on Intraocular Pressure

Most general anesthetics decrease intraocular pressure;[28] the decrease is directly related to the depth of anesthesia (Fig. 34.12). The ocular hypotension probably results from relaxation of extraocular muscle tone and an increase in the facility of aqueous outflow,[26] although decreased aqueous production may contribute to the drop in some instances. Digital pressure exerted on the globe may enhance the drop in intraocular pressure. Respiratory difficulties and other conditions which can produce an increased venous pressure may produce a moderate and prolonged rise in intraocular pressure. Paraldehyde produces

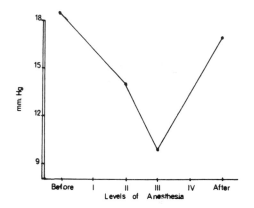

FIG. 34.12. Fall in intraocular pressure of man during administration of halothane anesthesia. (From data of Magora and Collins.[34])

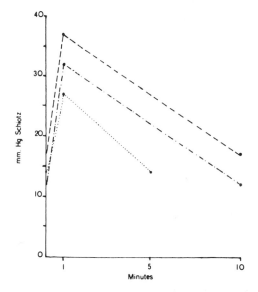

FIG. 34.13. Effect of intravenous administration of succinylcholine in three dogs lightly anesthetized with thiamylal sodium.

no decrease in intraocular pressure in either normal or glaucomatous animals.[34, 47]

Tranquilizers also decrease intraocular pressure.[20, 40, 43] The ocular hypotension induced by chlorpromazine is accompanied by a compensatory decrease in facility of aqueous outflow that may be sympatholytic in nature. Chlorpromazine-induced ocular hypotension may last up to 7 hours. In most animals, miosis is present, but an interesting paradoxical mydriasis has been observed with the use of chlorpromazine in cats.[40]

In contrast to ocular hypotension resulting from the use of anesthetic agents, succinylcholine chloride, even when used in conjunction with light anesthesia, produces a transient, but significant, elevation in intraocular pressure in animals[29, 30, 32] (Fig. 34.13).[50] Because of this rise, it is unwise to administer succinylcholine in animals in which the cornea has been perforated or is likely to become so with increased intraocular pressure.

After administration of succinylcholine, the extraocular muscles contract in a tetanic fashion, apparently exerting sufficient tension on the globe to produce a rise in manometrically-determined intraocular pressure. Section of the extraocular muscles will prevent such a rise.[32] In cats administered succinylcholine, the eyes assume a superolateral divergent position.[30] When succinylcholine chloride is to be used, it should be administered well in advance of the corneoscleral incision.

Although it has been shown that normal eye reflexes persist through curare akinesia,[22] curare combined with thiamylal sodium has been used with no apparent adverse effect for dogs[9] undergoing lens extraction, and in rabbits the intraocular pressure was shown to decrease.[23]

REFERENCES

1. Adriani, J., and Campbell, D.: Fatalities following topical application of local anesthetics to mucous membranes. J. A. M. A. *162:* 1527, 1956.
2. Barth, P.: Die Leitungsanästhesie am Kopf des Hundes. Dissertation. Zurich, 1948. Cited by Überreiter.[51]
3. Behrendt, T.: Experimental study of corneal lesions. Amer. J. Ophthal. *41:* 99, 1956.
4. Behrendt, T.: Experimental secondary effects of topical anesthesia of the cornea. Amer. J. Ophthal. *44:* 74, 1951.
5. Bellows, J. G.: Surface anesthesia in ophthalmology. Arch. Ophthal. (Chicago) *12:* 824, 1934.
6. Berge, E.: Indikation und Technik des kunstlichen Ankyloblepharons unter Berücksichtigung der Operations am Bulbus. Berlin. Tieraerztl. Wschr. *43:* 509, 1927.
7. Beyer, K. H., Latven, A. R., Freyburger, W. A., and Parker, M. P.: A comparative study of the activity and toxicity of hexylcaine (1-cyclohexylamino-2-prophylbenzoate): a new local anesthetic agent. J. Pharmacol. Exp. Ther. *93:* 388, 1948.
8. Bolz, W.: Ein weiterer Beitrag zur Leitunganästhesie am Kopf des Pferdes. Berlin. Munchen. Tieraerztl. Wschr. *46:* 529, 1930.
9. Brinker, W. O.: Use of surital sodium and curare in small animal surgery. North Amer. Vet. *32:* 832, 1951.
10. Campbell, D., and Adriani, J.: Absorption of local anesthetics. J. A. M. A. *168:* 873, 1958.
11. Coles, H. W., and Rose, C. L.: Irritation as produced on the rabbit's cornea by local anesthetics. J. Lab. Clin. Med. *15:* 239, 1930.
12. Dietz, O.: Eine retro-bulbare Anästhesie beim Hund zur Erzeugung einer Mydriasis. Berlin. Munchen. Tieraerztl. Wschr. *15:* 235, 1954.
13. Everett, W., Vey, E., and Finlay, J.: Duration of oculomotor akinesia of injectable anesthetics. Trans. Amer. Acad. Ophthal. Otolaryng. *65:* 308, 1961.
14. Everett, W. G., Vey, E. K., and Veenis, C. Y.: Factors in reducing ocular tension prior to intraocular surgery. Trans. Amer. Acad. Ophthal. Otolaryng. *63:* 286, 1959.
15. Formston, C.: Ophthaine (proparacaine hydrochloride)—A local anesthetic for ophthalmic surgery. Vet. Rec. *76:* 385, 1964.
16. Friedenwald, J. S., and Buschke, W.: Influence of some experimental variables on epithelial movements in healing of corneal wounds. J. Cell. Physiol. *23:* 95, 1944.
17. Gunderson, T., and Liebman, S. D.: Effect of local anesthetics on regeneration of corneal epithelium. Arch. Ophthal. (Chicago) *31:* 29, 1944.
18. Gurjanova, M. P.: Dicain und seine Verwendung in der Veterinärophthalmologie. Veterinariya *3:* 1941. Cited by Magda.[33]
19. Hare, W. C. D.: A regional method for the complete anaesthetization and immobilization of the bovine eye and its associated structures. Canad. J. Comp. Med. *21:* 228, 1957.
20. Havener, W. H.: *Ocular Pharmacology,* p. 38. The C. V. Mosby Company, St. Louis, 1966.
21. Jakob, H.: *Tierärztliche Augenheilkunde.* R. Schötz, Berlin, 1920.
22. Jones, L. M.: Some effects of curare upon domestic animals. North Amer. Vet. *31:* 731, 1950.
23. Kirby, D. B.: Use of curare in cataract surgery. Arch. Ophthal. (Chicago) *43:* 678, 1950.
24. Kirsch, R. E.: Further studies on the use of digital pressure in cataract surgery. Arch. Ophthal. (Chicago) *58:* 641, 1957.
25. Kleinfeld, J., and Ellis, P. P.: Effects of topical anesthetics on growth of microorganisms. Arch. Ophthal. (Chicago) *76:* 712, 1966.
26. Kornblueth, W., Aladjemoff, L., Magora, F., and Gabbay, A.: Influence of general anesthesia on intraocular pressure in man. Arch. Ophthal. (Chicago) *61:* 84, 1959.
27. Kornblueth, W., Jampolsky, A., Tamler, E., and Marg, E.: Contraction of the ocularotatory muscles and intraocular pressure. Amer. J. Ophthal. *49:* 1381, 1960.

28. Leopold, I. H., and Keates, E.: Drugs used in the treatment of glaucoma. II. Clin. Pharmacol. Ther. 6: 262, 1965.

29. Lichtenstern, G.: Die Verwendung von Tropakokain in der tierärztlichen Chirurgie mit besonderer Berücksichtigung hinsichtlich seiner Verwendbarkeit in der Augapfel-infiltration beim Pferde. Munchen. Tieraerztl. Wschr. 55: 337, 1911.

30. Lincoff, H. A., Ellis, C. H., DeVoe, A. G., De Beer, E. J., Impastato, D. J., Berg, S., Orkin, L, and Magda, H.: The effect of succinylcholine on intraocular pressure. Amer. J. Ophthal. 40: 501, 1955.

31. Linn, J., and Vey, E. K.: Topical anesthesia in ophthalmology. Amer. J. Ophthal. 40: 697, 1955.

32. Macri, F. J., and Grimes, P. A.: The effects of succinylcholine on the extraocular striate muscles and on the intraocular pressure. Amer. J. Ophthal. 44: 221, 1957.

33. Magda, I. I.: Lokalanaesthesie, p. 63. VEB Gustav Fischer Verlag, Jena, 1960.

34. Magora, F., and Collins, V.: The influence of general anesthetic agents on intraocular pressure in man. Arch. Ophthal. (Chicago) 66: 806, 1961.

35. Magrane, W. G.: Investigational use of ophthaine as a local anesthetic in ophthalmology. North Amer. Vet. 34: 568, 1953.

36. Maksimovic, B.: Akinese des M. orbicularis palpebrum bei Rindern. Vet. Arh. 20: 75, 1950.

37. Marr, W. G., Wood, R., Stenterfit, L., and Sigelman, S.: Effect of topical anesthetics. Amer. J. Ophthal. 43: 606, 1957.

38. Nicolas, E.: Veterinary and Comparative Ophthalmology, p. 541. (Translated by H. Gray.) H. W. Brown, London, 1929.

39. Pantjuschew, N. A.: Die Verwendung des Sovcains für die Oberflachenanästhesie in der Veterinärophthalmologie. Veterinariya 4: 1951. Cited by Magda.[33]

40. Paul, S. D., and Leopold, I. H.: The effect of chlorpromazine (thorazine) on intraocular pressure in experimental animals. Amer. J. Ophthal. 42: 107, 1956.

41. Peterson, D. R.: Nerve block of the eye and associated structures. J. Amer. Vet. Med. Ass. 118: 145, 1951.

42. Prince, J. H.: The Rabbit in Eye Research, p. 618. Charles C Thomas, Publisher, Springfield, Ill., 1964.

43. Rehak, S., Skranc, O., and Juran, J.: Effect of chlorpromazine on the flow of aqueous through the eye in experimental animals. Acta Ophthal. (Kobenhavn) 40: 535, 1962.

44. Rubin, L. F.: Auriculopalpebral nerve block as an adjunct to the diagnosis and treatment of ocular inflammation in the horse. J. Amer. Vet. Med. Ass. 144: 1387, 1964.

45. Rubin, L. F., and Wolfes, R. L.: Mydriatics for canine ophthalmoscopy. J. Amer. Vet. Med. Ass. 140: 137, 1962.

46. Schlegel, H. E., Jr., and Swan, K. C.: Benoxinate (Dorsocaine) for rapid corneal anesthesia. Arch. Ophthal. (Chicato) 51: 663, 1954.

47. Schmerl, E., and Steinberg, B.: Role of Diencephalon in regulating ocular tension. Amer. J. Ophthal. 31: 155, 1948.

48. Schreiber, J.: Die anatomische Grundlagen der Leitungsanästhesie beim Rind. I. Die Leitungsanästhesie der Kopfnerven. Wien. Tieraerztl. Mschr. 42: 129, 1955.

49. Smelzer, G. K., and Ozanics, V.: Effect of chemotherapeutic agents on cell division and healing of corneal burns and abrasions in rat. Amer. J. Ophthal. 27: 1063, 1944.

50. Stone, H., and Prijot, E.: Effect of a barbiturate and paraldehyde on aqueous humor dynamics in rabbits. Arch. Ophthal. (Chicago) 54: 834, 1955.

51. Überreiter, O.: Zur Technik der Augenoperationen beim Hunde. Arch. Wiss. Prakt. Tierheilk. 74: 235, 1937.

52. Westhues, M., and Fritsch, R.: Local anesthesia. In Animal Anesthesia, p. 23, Oliver and Boyd, Edinburgh, 1964.

35

Cardiac Resuscitation

W. D. TAVERNOR

Cardiac arrest is an emergency that may occur at any time during surgery. Although the incidence of this condition is not great, in some instances it may be a terminal event in a hopeless case; however, in most cases, the condition is reversible and survival can be expected if prompt and efficient treatment is given.[9] The most important factor in the treatment of the condition is the speed with which restorative measures are rendered. A delay of more than 3 to 4 minutes from the time of arrest may result in irreversible brain damage due to cerebral anoxia, or, at best, damage that is reversible only after a prolonged recuperative period.

The first person to employ direct cardiac massage was Schiff in 1874, who, while investigating the cause of death in dogs due to the administration of chloroform and ether, advocated a technique of direct cardiac massage to restore the heart beat.[15] The first recorded successful cardiac massage in man was in 1902.[17] In animals, the dog and cat lend themselves most readily to this treatment, and the management of this condition in these species has been described by a number of authors.[7, 18, 20]

Etiology of Cardiac Arrest

There are many factors which predispose to the occurrence of cardiac arrest (Table 35.1). Apart from the general physical state of the patient, underlying myocardial and/or pulmonary disease may contribute to the onset of the condition by limiting the contractile power, or oxygenating power, of the heart and lungs.

The major precipitating cause of cardiac arrest is myocardial hypoxia resulting from respiratory insufficiency and/or reduced coronary blood flow. Reduction in arterial oxygen tensions may result from several causes, the most common of which are (a) impairment or blockage of the airway; (b) use of an anesthetic mixture containing too little oxygen; (c) inadequate respiratory exchange resulting from depression of the respiratory control mechanisms by drugs; (d) insufficient pulmonary ventilation during controlled respiration; and (e) reduction in the oxygen-carrying power of the blood due to anemia or blood loss.

There are two main forms of cardiac failure, ventricular fibrillation and ventricular asystole. The latter is by far the most common condition and the one that is most likely to be met by the clinician.

Ventricular Asystole

Asystole can result from myocardial anoxia or from vagal stimulation in the presence of anoxia. Disease conditions of the chest such as pneumothorax, pulmonary hemorrhage, or the presence of diaphragmatic hernia are predisposing factors.

Depth of anesthesia is a contributory factor, respiratory or myocardial depression by preanesthetic or anesthetic agents being probably one of the most common

TABLE 35.1
Conditions contributing to cardiac insufficiency or arrest

1. Anesthetic overdose
   A. Absolute, excessive amount administered per unit of body weight
   B. Relative, excessive amount administered due to modifications in the tolerance of the animal to the drug, *e.g.*, hypovolemia, shock, anemia, myocardial disease, emaciation, chronic disease, preanesthetic medication
2. Changes in vascular volume
   Usually acute changes due to hemorrhage or fluid loss during or following surgery
3. Changes in the vascular bed
   Vasodilation of vascular bed due to sympatholytic action of anesthetic agents, epidural analgesia, or adrenergic drugs
4. Reflex mechanisms
   Vasovagal reflex. Tracheal manipulation; contact with thoracic vagus nerve; manipulation of pulmonary hilus; pressure in region of carotid sinus; ocular pressure; traction on viscera
5. Obstruction of venous return
   Compression of vena cava due to abdominal distension or other cause. Mechanical interference with heart action; compression of thoracic great vessels; excessive positive pressure ventilation
6. Hypoxia
   Due to inadequate or obstructed airway; administration of low oxygen tension; inadequate ventilation resulting from poor positioning, compression of chest, obesity, muscular weakness
7. Existing disease conditions of the thorax
   Myocardial disease; pneumothorax; pulmonary edema; pulmonary hemorrhage; diaphragmatic hernia
8. Acute cardiac tamponade
   Hemorrhage within the pericardial sac causing cardiac compression and reduction of diastolic filling
9. Air embolism
   Escape of air into a vein during rapid whole blood administration with an air-pressurized system
10. Hypothermia
11. Severe electrolyte imbalance
    Primary imbalance of potassium, sodium, and calcium is of particular concern during blood transfusions, digitalis therapy, or in cases or uremia
12. Drug effects
    Including premedicant and anesthetic drugs, particularly those that produce respiratory depression
13. Hypercarbia
    This will predispose to an increased incidence of cardiac arrhythmias

causes. Barbiturate drugs, although not depressant toward the myocardium, may depress the respiratory center and produce hypoxia. Gross overdose of anesthetic is less frequently a cause.

Ventricular Fibrillation

Fibrillation usually results from direct myocardial stimulation in the presence of anoxia and/or hypercarbia. General anesthetics can further predispose the heart to ventricular fibrillation. Investigation of the "sensitizing" effect of general anesthetics on the heart of the dog, and subsequent stimulation with epinephrine, showed that the most pronounced effect was produced by trichlorethylene followed by ethyl chloride, cyclopropane, and chloroform, in that order.[11] In some cases, sudden failure of the heart may be related to a triad of anoxia, hypercarbia, and the general anesthetic. This may be linked to an overaction of the sympathetic or parasympathetic nervous system or an imbalance between them.[6] Fibrillation may result from stimulation of the myocardium when cardiac massage is carried out for the treatment of asystole.

Prophylactic Measures

It is obvious that preanesthetic examination of the patient, including cardiac examination, is important. Maintenance of a clear airway during anesthesia is essential, and this is best achieved by the use of a cuffed endotracheal tube, even if anesthesia is to be induced and maintained by a nonvolatile agent. Adoption of intubation as a routine procedure in any anesthetic technique is to be strongly recommended. This is particularly important in the case of brachycephalic breeds. In obstructive conditions of the esophagus, any dilated part of the esophagus should be emptied to prevent subsequent regurgitation during anesthesia. An anesthetic mixture should always contain an adequate amount of oxygen, and in no case should this drop below 20%.

During surgery, hemorrhage should be controlled immediately and replacement therapy applied if significant blood loss occurs. Atropine should be given as part of the preanesthetic medication to control salivation and bronchial secretions, and sedative drugs should be administered to insure a quiet induction. Excitement and excessive struggling can lead to the sudden release of catecholamines (epinephrine) which may prove lethal to a patient with existing cardiovascular or pulmonary disease. Good anesthetic practice will reduce the incidence of cardiac arrest to minimal proportions.

Diagnosis of Cardiac Arrest

The diagnosis of cardiac failure is only too obvious 5 minutes after it has occurred; but, by this time, irreversible central nervous system changes may already have taken place. It may not be immediately realized that the heart has stopped in an animal that is under the influence of a relaxant drug and that is receiving positive pressure ventilation.

The most obvious feature of cardiac arrest is absence of the peripheral pulse, but in veterinary practice this may be difficult to detect. An electronic pulse monitor can be used, but other diagnostic features are cessation of voluntary respiration, dilation of the pupil, absence of a detectable heart beat on auscultation, and cyanosis. In the veterinary patient, one of the earliest warnings of cardiac insufficiency is respiratory arrest followed by dilation of the pupil.

Treatment of Cardiac Arrest

Cardiac massage must commence within 1 to 2 minutes of arrest. If hypoxia has been present for some time before the final arrest of the heart, severe neurological and myocardial damage may result from even shorter periods of ischemia. The successful treatment of cardiac arrest has been recorded in the pig following 5 minutes of hypoxia,[8] and in the dog following hypoxia in exess of 5 minutes, although in the latter case vision was still impaired 9 days later.

The actions to be taken may vary according to the species of animal and the circumstances in which the operator is working, but the general precedence of action is listed as follows: (a) Lower the head. (b) Stop the administration of anesthetic, make sure the airway is clear, and ventilate with oxygen. (c) Apply cardiac massage either externally (closed chest massage), internally via the thorax (open chest massage), or via the diaphragm if the abdomen is open. (d) If no contraction or fibrillation is seen, 10% calcium chloride or 0.1% epinephrine may be administered into the ventricle. (e) Rapidly administer fluids or blood to aid venous return and assist diastolic filling. (f) Add vasopressor to intravenous drip to produce peripheral vasoconstriction to aid venous return and increase peripheral resistance. (g) If fibrillation occurs, 1% procaine or lidocaine hydrochloride may be administered into the ventricle, or electrical defibrillation employed. (h) Add sodium bicarbonate to intravenous drip to counteract the metabolic acidosis occurring during the period of arrest. (i) Apply electrocardiograph leads if such equipment is available. (j) Subsequent treatment is given to maintain circulation and to prevent cerebral edema.

By immediately lowering the head and raising the hind limbs, venous return is augmented; this aids diastolic filling. Administration of anesthetic agent should be stopped and artificial respiration started with oxygen. Simultaneous external cardiac massage should be started. Thoracotomy may have to be performed in some cases.

When a volatile anesthetic agent is being administered through an endotracheal tube, it is relatively easy to continually flush the anesthetic agent from the lungs with oxygen while administering artificial respiration. Ventilation may be carried out by manual pressure on a rebreathing bag or by supplying oxygen to the endotracheal tube via a "T" piece. Alternate closure and opening of the open end of the "T" piece with a finger will produce alternate inflation and deflation of the lungs. If an endotracheal tube is not already in place, intubation of the trachea should be carried out immediately. Any obstruction of the airway in the form of blood or mucus must be removed by swab or suction, rapidly followed by intubation of the trachea. The importance of quickly establishing artificial respiration with oxygen and initiating cardiac massage cannot be overemphasized. Carbon dioxide must be effectively eliminated, since accumulation will contribute to the already existing metabolic acidosis, further lowering pH.

An important consideration in cardiac massage, whether it be external (closed chest) or internal (open chest) massage, is adequate venous return and diastolic filling. The value of the rapid intravenous administration of fluids or whole blood to increase the circulating volume and thus aid venous return is obvious. This can be more readily appreciated during direct cardiac massage when it is possible to palpate diastolic filling. This supportive therapy should be put into effect as soon as possible after ventilation and massage have been instigated.

The addition of vasopressor drugs to the intravenous fluid will also aid venous return by producing peripheral vasoconstriction. It must be emphasized that for the administered drugs to be of value, blood must be circulated by cardiac massage.

In small animals where the abdomen is already open, the heart may be massaged with the tips of the fingers through the intact diaphragm.[16] It is not possible to give completely effective compression in this way, and it must only be considered as a temporary measure while other preparations are made for indirect or direct cardiac massage.

In the dog and cat, external (closed chest) cardiac massage may be carried out through the intact chest wall.[13] The dog is placed on its back with a sandbag against the right chest wall and is then allowed to rest on the sandbag halfway between the supine and lateral positions. Rhythmic downward pressure is applied with the hands to the left chest in the area of the costochondral junction at the rate of 60 to 80 compressions/minute. If application of pressure is made too far caudally, there is a danger of rupture of the liver. It is, of course, impossible to assess the response to the massage when applied to the intact chest, and the effectiveness of the treatment can only be determined by the detection of a femoral pulse and by the contraction of the pupils. It is also difficult to determine the presence of ventricular fibrillation unless an electrocardiograph is available. If fibrillation is detected, the only effective treatment is to apply an electrical defibrillator. This may be applied externally with the electrodes positioned over the manubrium sterni and the left precordial region over the apex of the heart.

A comparison of indirect and direct cardiac massage in dogs following induction of ventricular fibrillation showed that aortic pressures and carotid blood flow were slightly higher using the direct method, but 1 minute after circulation had been restored, the carotid flow was higher following the use of indirect rather than direct massage. It was concluded that the results obtained by the two methods were comparable.[14]

In the larger domesticated animals, external massage is much less practicable, the difficulty increasing with increase in size. It has been suggested that in horses and cattle, sharp blows to the left chest wall may stimulate the heart in the early stages of arrest. This method of treatment has not been supported by factual evidence.

Direct cardiac massage through a thoracotomy incision should be started if indirect massage fails. The advantages of a thoracic approach are direct access to the heart to facilitate massage, the ability to open the pericardium, and the ease with which drugs may be accurately injected into the heart cavities or electrical defibrillation carried out. No time should be wasted in preparation of the site. Figure 35.1 shows the relationship of the heart to the chest wall and diaphragm in the dog, the site of incision being between the sixth and seventh ribs on the left side. Only a knife is needed, and although a rib spreader is useful, it is not essential. In the larger animals, however, some device to spread the ribs apart may be needed. In cases of difficulty the costal cartilages should be cut.

The heart should first of all be inspected for evidence of ventricular fibrillation. Although there is no need to open the pericardium at first, it may be subsequently opened from base to apex to allow full inspection and to enable more effective massage to be carried out. If the heart is fibrillating, the treatment described later should be applied.

If the heart is in a state of asystole, massage should be commenced immediately. This should be given by steady pressure with the palmar surfaces of the fingers (not the finger tips) to the ventricles, against the intraventricular septum. In large animals this pressure should be applied with the palms of both hands. Care should be taken not to angle the heart upwards or the great veins may be occluded. The pressure must be firm, and adequate time should be allowed for the ventricles to refill. Sixty compressions per minute are recommended for the dog.[4] Reduction of the rate to 40/minute shows a marked decrease in cardiac output, while there is no appreciable increase in output when the rate is above 80/minute. The rate of massage is largely governed by the venous return. The more satisfactory the venous return the greater should be the rate of compression. Rapid massage is very tiring and cannot be sustained without relief, particularly in large animals. It must also be remembered that the myocardium is more easily damaged by rapid massage.

Adequate circulation may be maintained by effective cardiac massage in small animals. Systolic pressures of 50 to 70 mm Hg during cardiac massage have been recorded

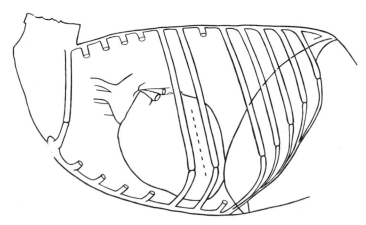

DOG DIAGRAMMATIC VIEW OF LEFT THORAX

FIG. 35.1. Diagram showing relationship of the heart to the chest wall and diaphragm. The *dotted line* indicates the site of thoracotomy.

TABLE 35.2
Suggested drugs for emergency box

Drug	Concentration	Route of Administration*	Dose Range (Small Animals)
Levarterenol bitartrate, U.S.P. (noradrenaline, B.P.)	0.02%	I/C	0.5-1 ml
Levarterenol bitartrate, U.S.P. (noradrenaline, B.P.)	0.2%	I/V	1-2 ml/250 ml of fluid, to effect
Epinephrine HCl, U.S.P. (adrenaline, B.P.)	0.1%	I/C	Dilute to 0.01%, 0.5-1 ml
Isoproterenol HCl, U.S.P. (isoprenaline, B.P.)	0.02%	I/V	0.1-1 ml
Methoxamine HCl, U.S.P.	10 mg/ml	I/V or I/M	0.2 mg/kg (1 mg/10 lb)
Atropine sulfate, U.S.P., B.P.	0.05%	I/V or I/M	0.25-1.5 ml
Lidocaine HCl, U.S.P. (lignocaine, B.P.)	10 mg/ml	I/V	1-4 mg/kg (0.5-2 mg/lb), to effect
Potassium chloride	4%	I/C	5 ml
Sodium bicarbonate	44.6 mEq/50 ml	I/V I/C	50-100 ml/250 ml of fluid 5-20 ml
Calcium chloride	10%	I/C	1-2 ml
Calcium gluconate, U.S.P., B.P.	100 mg/ml	I/V	2-5 ml
Doxapram HCl, U.S.P.	20 mg/ml	I/V	1.0 g/kg (0.5 g/lb)
Levallorphan tartrate, U.S.P., B.P.	1 mg/ml	I/V	0.5 mg
Hydrocortisone, U.S.P., B.P.		I/V	25-100 mg
Aminophylline, U.S.P., B.P.	10%	I/V	4 mg/kg (2 mg/lb), slowly
Ouabain, U.S.P.	0.025 mg/ml	I/V	0.02-0.03 mg/kg (0.01-0.015 mg/lb)
Mannitol hexanitrate, U.S.P., B.P.	250 mg/ml	I/V	0.5-1 g/kg (250-500 mg/lb)
Tripelennamine HCl, U.S.P.	20 mg/ml	I/V or I/M	1.0 mg/kg (0.5 mg/lb)

* I/V, intravenous; I/C intracardiac; I/M, intramuscular.

in man,[2] but whether this could be maintained in large animals such as the horse and cow is doubtful.

It may be advantageous to increase the supply of blood to the coronary arteries and brain by compression of the abdominal aorta.[19] A similar effect may be obtained by clamping the thoracic aorta just below the origin of the left subclavian artery. If massage is to be continued for periods in excess of 20 minutes, these clamps should be released for a short period to reduce the danger of permanent damage to the liver or kidneys.

Occasional beats may occur after a minute or so of cardiac massage, and these should be assisted by massage. In no case should the chest be closed until effective heart action has been observed for 5 to 10 minutes. Cardiac stimulants should not be injected directly into the heart until myocardial color and tone have improved. If no effective beat is seen, the ventricles should be inspected again for signs of fibrillation. If these immediate measures do not lead to the return of a spontaneous heart beat, then the use of drugs must be considered. In many cases, a flabby and dilated heart may persist despite 5 or 6 minutes of massage. This heart is more likely to need pharmacological help than one in which tone and color have improved.

As already stated, no stimulants should be administered until the coronary flow has been restored and the heart muscle oxygenated by a combination of pulmonary ventilation and cardiac massage. The commonly used drugs are calcium chloride, and epinephrine or norepinephrine. These agents not only increase cardiac tone and prolong systole, but they also increase excitability. Anoxia tends to potentiate cardiac excitability, and the risk of ventricular fibrillation is increased when these drugs are given to a poorly oxygenated myocardium.

Epinephrine is probably the drug that will be most readily available, but it is more likely to produce fibrillation than norepinephrine or calcium chloride. In dogs, a dose of 0.1 to 0.5 ml of a 0.1% solution of epinephrine may be injected into the left ventricular cavity. A dilute solution of norepinephrine (levarterenol) for cardiac injection is available, and is recommended. Calcium chloride should be administered in a similar manner using a 10% solution

and a dose of 1 to 2 ml for dogs. Increased doses should be given to larger animals, and the administration of these drugs may be repeated at 5-minute intervals. The use of these agents should be restricted as they may cause fibrillation, and their value is only secondary to the methods of treatment already described. Drugs which should be available for emergency use are listed (Table 35.2). Atropine can be used when an effective but extremely slow beat is present. This vagotonic effect is not uncommon following arrest, and in most cases it can be counteracted by the intravenous administration of atropine.

Intravenous sodium bicarbonate has been found beneficial in cardiac resuscitation in combating the acidosis created by circulatory arrest. An increase in hydrogen

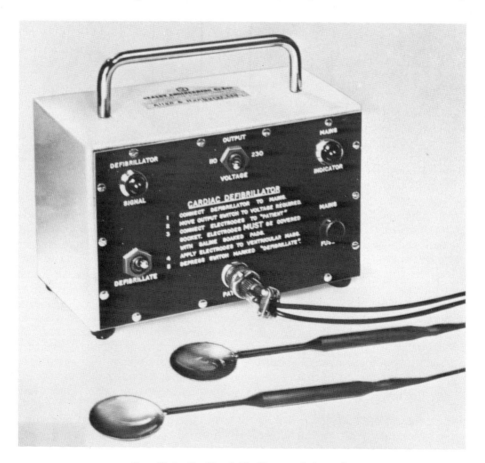

FIG. 35.2. Cardiac defibrillator and electrodes.

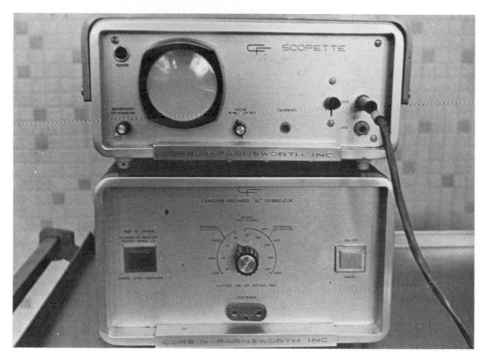

FIG. 35.3. Direct current defibrillator with internal and external capabilities.

ion concentration will depress myocardial function and may contribute to the further demise of a poorly responsive heart.

In some cases, the heart will be seen to be fibrillating on inspection. Fibrillation may also occur after cardiac massage or the administration of drugs. Massage alone may be sufficient to restart a fibrillating ventricle, but in many cases some form of defibrillation is necessary. The simplest method of defibrillation available to the practitioner is by the intravenous or in-traventricular injection of 2% lidocaine hydrochloride or 1% procaine hydrochloride. An initial dose of 1 to 2 mg/kg is used and increased as needed. Local anesthetics depress cardiac contraction and excitability while prolonging the refractory period of the muscle. The blood levels of both drugs are very rapidly reduced, and, in many cases, the ventricle may return to a state of fibrillation. If further massage fails to stop fibrillation, lidocaine may be given by an intravenous drip. Lidocaine as compared to procaine is probably the drug of choice for the chemical treatment of ventricular

fibrillation or other cardiac arrhythmias. In the dog, lidocaine produces less hypotension than procaine.

As an alternative, in the dog, 5.0 ml of a 4% solution of potassium chloride may be injected into the ventricle. Potassium reduces cardiac contraction and prolongs diastole, but it is much more slowly destroyed than lidocaine or procaine, and the depression produced by the dose required to stop fibrillation may be so great that it is difficult to re-establish a spontaneous beat. In such a case, its administration should be followed by the injection of 10% calcium chloride solution in order to restore cardiac tone.

The most satisfactory method of treating ventricular fibrillation is by electrical defibrillation. A simple electrical defibrillator (Fig. 35.2) consists of a transformer which will provide a current of 2 amp at either 110 (adequate for the dog) or 230 volts for periods of 0.1 second; such defibrillators have been described for use in dogs.[1] Direct current (capacitor discharge) defibrillators are also available and are generally considered to be more effective for defibrillating the heart.[10] Most direct current defibrillators have the capability of varying the voltage applied and are capable of internal or external defibrillation (Fig. 35.3).

In internal defibrillation, the current is applied by two spoon-shaped electrodes, and greater contact with the ventricles can be produced by wrapping the electrodes with saline-moistened gauze, thereby assuring an even distribution of current.

External defibrillation has been successful in man[12] and animals,[10] and its experimental use was reported in sheep as early as 1936.[3] External defibrillation can be employed in the resuscitation of the veterinary patient but is of little use independent of closed chest cardiac massage. Also, some sort of heart monitor, preferably a direct writing electrocardiograph or visual oscilloscope, must be available to enable the detection of ventricular fibrillation in the closed chest.

After defibrillation has been effected, the pacemaker mechanism of the heart may not be strong enough to establish and maintain a normal rhythm. In such cases, an electrical cardiac pacemaker may be used. The principle of the pacemaker is to superimpose upon the heart a series of voltage pulses to stimulate ventricular contractions and to maintain an effective beat until the intrinsic heart rhythm returns spontaneously. The electrodes of this instrument are applied in a similar manner to those of the defibrillator, and a very small current of short duration must be used to prevent fibrillation.

Once a spontaneous heart beat has been initiated after direct massage, it is important to keep the heart under observation for at least 10 minutes before closing the chest. It is imperative to make sure that the airway is kept clear during the recovery phase and that artificial ventilation is maintained if spontaneous ventilation is inadequate. Postoperative nursing is most important. If the thoracotomy is carried out without preparation of the site or full aseptic precautions, the patient should be given prophylactic antibiotic therapy. Digi-

talization may be necessary in some animals, especially if previous cardiovascular disease is present. It has been suggested that following the successful treatment of cardiac arrest, any cerebral congestion or edema resulting from anoxia should be treated. This can be achieved by the intravenous administration of 50% dextrose solution or mannitol, both drugs being excreted rapidly from the body unchanged. In dogs, an initial dose should be given which may be repeated at 15-minute intervals during the 1st hour of recovery. Unfortunately, the evaluation of the efficacy of this therapy has been difficult.

It will be appreciated that any treatment given in a case of cardiac arrest must be immediate. There is no time for hesitation, and restorative measures must be taken without delay. It is important that the anesthetist should be conversant with the method of treatment that may be adopted within the limits of the facilities and equipment that are available. If restorative drugs are to be used, they should always be present in the operating room, and fresh stock solutions should be maintained. Endotracheal tubes, laryngoscopes, and equipment for artificial ventilation should be readily available.

REFERENCES

1. Booth, N. H., Will, D. H., Moss, L. C., and Swenson, M. J.: An electrical apparatus and its application in defibrillating the heart of the dog. J. Amer. Vet. Med. Ass. *132:* 117, 1958.
2. Deuchar, D. C., and Venner, A.: The blood pressure during cardiac massage in man. Brit. Med. J. *2:* 134, 1953.
3. Ferris, L., King, B. G., Spencer, P. W., and Williams, H. B.: Effect of electrical shock on the heart. Electr. Eng. *55:* 498, 1936.
4. Hepps, S. A., and Kissen, A. T.: Measurement of cardiac output in dogs during cardiac massage. Amer. J. Surg. *100:* 64, 1960.
5. Hoerlein, B. F.: Cardiac resuscitation in a dog with cardiac arrest. J. Amer. Vet. Med. Ass. *127:* 210, 1955.
6. Keating, V.: *Anesthetic Accidents*, p. 44. Lloyd-Luke, London, 1961.
7. Kling, J. M., Hahn, A. W., and Horne, R. D.: Cardiac arrest in canine practice. Can. J. Comp. Med. *25:* 157, 1961.
8. Konrad, R. M., Schmitz, T., and Tarbiat, S.: Erfolgreiche Behandlung eines Herzstillstandes und seiner zerebralen Folgen bei einen Larfer-

schwein nach 5 Minuten dauernder Hypoxie. Tieraerztl. Umsch. *16:* 104, 1961.

9. Lancet (editorial): Cardiac arrest. *2:* 438, 1953.

10. Lown, B., Neuman, J., Amarasingham, R., and Beckovits, B.: Comparison of alternating current with direct current electroshock across the closed chest. Amer. J. Cardiol. *10:* 223, 1962.

11. Morris, L. E., Noltensmeyer, M. H., and White, J. M.: Epinephrine induced cardiac irregularities in the dog during anesthesia with trichloroethylene, cyclopropane, ethyl chloride and chloroform. Anesthesiology *14:* 153, 1953.

12. Oram, S., Davies, J. P. H., Weinbren, I., Taggart, P., and Kitchen, L. D.: Conversion of atrial fibrillation to sinus rhythm by direct current shock. Lancet *2:* 159, 1963.

13. Ott, B. S.: Closed chest cardiac resuscitation. Small Anim. Clin. *2:* 572, 1962.

14. Redding, J. S., and Cozine, R. A.: A comparison of open chest and closed chest cardiac massage in dogs. Anesthesiology *22:* 280, 1961.

15. Schiff, M.: *Recueil des Memoires Physiologiques*, pg 3, Centre de recherches et d'orientation, Lausanne, 1874.

16. Spreull, J. S. A., and Singleton, W. B.: Cardiac massage. J. Small Anim. Pract. *1:* 210, 1961.

17. Starling, E. A., and Lane, W. A.: Report to the Society of Anaesthetists. Lancet *2:* Part 2, 1397, 1902.

18. Tavernor, W. D.: The management of cardiac arrest in the dog. Advances Small Anim. Pract. *3:* 158, 1962.

19. Vetten, K. B., Wilson, V. H., Crawshaw, G. R., and Nicholson, J. C.: Experimental studies in cardiac massage with special reference to aortic occlusion. Brit. J. Anaesth. *27:* 2, 1955.

20. Walker, R. G., and Rex, M. A. E.: Cardiac arrest and its treatment. Vet. Rec. *70:* 667, 1958.

36
Respiratory Failure and Resuscitation

RHEA J. WHITE

Respiratory failure, for the purposes of this discussion, will be defined as the inability to maintain normal blood gases at rest. The term respiratory insufficiency applies to the animal with normal blood gases at rest, but with a greater than normal tendency to develop respiratory failure following mild stress or exertion. This animal cannot fully engage in the normal activities of healthy animals, although slight degrees of impairment may not be readily noticeable. In other words, the animal with respiratory insufficiency lacks normal respiratory reserve. The onset of respiratory failure may follow a period of respiratory insufficiency in an animal suddenly stressed beyond the limits of his respiratory reserve or in a previously normal animal subjected to illness or trauma. It may be so acute that it can become life-threatening in a matter of minutes. Regardless of etiology, survival of a patient in respiratory failure depends on the degree of blood gas abnormality that results, the interval of time before effective treatment is established, and the amount of damage to the cardiovascular and central nervous systems.

Severely embarrassed or arrested respiration constitutes a medical emergency of the greatest urgency. This point cannot be overemphasized. The immediate control of respiratory failure takes precedence over all other emergency care. The treatment of shock, internal hemorrhage, poisoning, or drug overdose is important but secondary to the establishment of an airway and ventilation in the asphyxiated or apneic animal. Regardless of the original insult, successful respiratory and cardiovascular resuscitation depends on the rapid establishment of an adequate oxygen supply to the body.

Unnecessary delay in the initiation of ventilatory support, while other measures such as cardiac monitoring or fluid therapy receive attention, is a common error in the emergency treatment of the acutely ill or traumatized animal. If the animal is not breathing when first seen, no time should be wasted checking for heart sounds or peripheral pulses. In the clinical situation, respiratory arrest almost always precedes cardiac arrest, and seconds wasted auscultating the chest only increase the likelihood of cardiac arrest from anoxia. This is not meant to imply that circulatory support is unimportant, but to emphasize that circulation of unoxygenated blood is of no avail to the patient.

Etiology and Diagnosis of Respiratory Failure

The processes leading to respiratory failure may be considered under two main categories: (a) ventilatory failure (characterized by hypoxemia and hypercarbia), where the amount of gas moved in and out of the lungs is inadequate; and (b) hypoxemic failure (hypoxemia with normocarbia), where normal oxygen exchange does not occur in spite of adequate ventilation and normal elimination of carbon dioxide (Table 36.1). Since carbon dioxide elimination is impaired only by ventilatory failure, reduced oxygen tension during hypoxemic failure can occur in the presence of a normal arterial carbon dioxide tension. In an animal breathing room air, hypercarbia only occurs in association with hypoxemia.[19] This relationship does not hold true in the animal breathing enriched concentrations of oxygen. Hypercarbia can be a serious complication of oxygen therapy or inhalation anesthesia. Respiratory failure may have a single cause, but frequently several factors exist which contribute to the condition. Ventilatory and hypoxemic failure frequently coexist, and the occurrence of one may predispose to the other. Various chronic conditions common to small animals predispose these animals to episodes of respiratory failure (Table 36.2). Many of these animals may appear clinically normal despite some degree of pulmonary insufficiency.

A confirmation of respiratory insufficiency or failure requires the measurement of arterial oxygen and carbon dioxide tensions and pH. Although this is the ideal situation, these measurements are rarely, if ever, available to the small animal clinician when emergency treatment is necessary. The problem may be compounded by the difficulty in performing an arterial puncture in small dogs and cats. Therefore, clinical evaluation of the patient must form the basis for diagnosis and treatment. While this precludes a confirmed diagnosis, the prevention or treatment of potentially fatal respiratory failure can frequently be accomplished.

It should be emphasized that oxygenation should never be judged adequate simply because cyanosis cannot be detected. Cyanosis is usually an inadequate means for the diagnosis of respiratory failure: first, because it can be misleading —its presence or absence not necessarily indicating the degree of arterial oxygen saturation; and second, cyanosis is a late sign not clinically apparent until very low oxygen tensions in the range of 40 to 55 mm Hg have occurred. The blue color of cyanosis is caused by reduced hemoglobin and may be observed in unpigmented mucous membranes, particularly the tongue and gums in small animals. The interpretation of cyanosis depends on available light, ability of the observer to distinguish between red and blue, hematocrit, and circulatory state of the patient. A very anemic animal may be hypoxic without cyanosis, and an animal with a high hematocrit may have sufficient reduced hemoglobin to appear cyanotic in spite of adequate arterial oxygenation. Cyanosis may also appear as a response to cold when peripheral circulatory constriction traps red blood cells in the capillaries of the mucous membranes.[5]

VENTILATORY FAILURE

Ventilatory failure is probably the most frequent cause of acute respiratory failure encountered by the small animal clinician. It is usually easier to diagnose than hypoxemic failure and almost always more amenable to definitive treatment.[5] Therefore, observation of the animal's ventilation is the first criterion used for diagnosis.

Respiration should be observed for changes in depth, rate, and effort. Depth is evaluated by observation of the expansion of the chest or by direct measurement. Rate is influenced by many factors, and in mammals, normal respiratory rate varies inversely with body weight. Rate must be correlated with depth in order to determine respiratory exchange. The terms hypoventilation and hyperventilation by definition refer to an abnormally high or low arterial carbon dioxide tension. However, in the clinical evaluation of ventilation, they are used to indicate an apparent decrease or increase in ventilatory rate, depth, or both. Dyspnea refers to a subjective feeling of breathlessness by the patient, but, in veterinary medicine, it is defined as labored breathing or a noticeable

TABLE 36.1
Causes of respiratory failure

Ventilatory Failure

1. Depression of the respiratory center
   A. Injury to the brain
      1. Trauma
      2. Hypoxia
      3. Infection
      4. Increased intracranial pressure
   B. Drug overdose
      1. Narcotics
      2. Barbiturates
      3. Inhalation anesthetics
2. Weakness paralysis or spasm of respiratory muscles
   A. Muscle relaxants
   B. Convulsions
   C. High level of epidural anesthesia
   D. Organophosphate poisoning
3. Decrease in bellows action of chest or expansion of lung
   A. Thoracic trauma
      1. Pneumothorax
      2. Diaphragmatic hernia
      3. Hemothorax
      4. Diffuse trauma
   B. Space-occupying lesions in the thorax
      1. Tumors
      2. Fluid
   C. Obesity
   D. Pain
      1. Traumatic
      2. Incisional
   E. Body bandages
   F. Abdominal distension
      1. Pregnancy
      2. Ascites
      3. Obesity
   G. Excessive restraint
   H. Positions
      1. Dorsal recumbency
      2. Head down position
4. Upper airway obstruction
   A. Soft tissue
      1. Tongue
      2. Pharynx
      3. Soft palate
   B. Foreign body
      1. Secretions
      2. Blood
      3. Vomitus
      4. Tumors
   C. Brachycephalic dog
      1. Stenotic nares
      2. Elongated soft palate
      3. Eversion of lateral ventricles
      4. Laryngeal collapse

TABLE 36.1 (*Continued*)

   D. Collapsing trachea syndrome
   E. Laryngospasm
      1. Cats
      2. Subhuman primates
   F. Restraint

Hypoxemic Failure

1. Ventilation perfusion abnormalities
   A. Alveoli underventilated and overventilated—increased oxygen requirement
      1. Contusions of lung
      2. Accumulation of secretions
      3. Chronic diffuse obstructive pulmonary disease
      4. Shock
   B. Alveoli totally unperfused—increased ventilatory requirement
      1. Hypotension—shock
      2. Hypovolemia
2. Right to left shunt
   A. Alveoli totally unventilated
      1. Atelectasis
         a. Shock
         b. Postoperative complications
      2. Consolidation
      3. Pulmonary edema
   B. Congenital heart defects
3. Impaired diffusion at alveolar capillary membrane
   A. Pulmonary edema

TABLE 36.2
Chronic conditions predisposing to respiratory failure

1. Chronic respiratory disease
   A. Bronchitis—obstructive
   B. Bronchiectasis—obstructive
   C. Emphysema—obstructive
   D. Pneumonia—atelectasis, congestion
2. Space-occupying lesions in the thorax
   A. Neoplasm
   B. Fluid—pyothorax, chilothorax
3. Obesity
   A. Increased resistance of chest wall
   B. Atelectasis
4. Brachycephalic dogs
   A. Stenotic nares
   B. Elongated soft palate
   C. Collapse of larynx
   D. Eversion of lateral ventricles
5. Collapsing trachea syndrome

increase in ventilatory effort. There are many causes of dyspnea which are not necessarily associated with respiratory failure.

The nonrespiratory factors that can influence ventilation such as reflexes from internal organs, pain, and excitement must be considered when assessing ventilation.[19] Panting characterized by rapid, shallow, open mouth breathing is the normal response to a high body temperature, and often in the dog, a response to potent narcotics. Panting should be differentiated from hyperventilation, which is characterized by both deep and rapid ventilatory effort. The extremes in ventilation, that is, complete apnea or intense respiratory effort, are immediately obvious. Slight or gradual changes may be difficult to evaluate, but they can be equally as hazardous. The depressed animal with borderline hypoventilation breathing room air may slip gradually into increasingly severe degrees of hypoxia with carbon dioxide accumulation leading to further depression. Similarly, the dyspneic animal maintaining adequate ventilatory exchange only with intense effort may succumb to respiratory failure as exhaustion occurs.

Diminished ventilatory effort occurs with depression of the respiratory center or as a result of weakness, paralysis, or spasm of the respiratory muscles (Table 36.1).[5] Various injuries to the brain, including hypoxia, trauma, infections, and increased intracranial pressure may depress the respiratory center. A more common cause is the overdose of depressant drugs, particularly narcotics, barbiturates, and inhalation anesthetics. Failure of the respiratory muscles to function effectively may be due to muscle weakness or interference in nerve transmission centrally in the spinal cord or peripherally in the phrenic or intercostal nerves. Intense muscle spasm as with tetanus or generalized convulsions may seriously interfere with normal respiration. When muscle relaxants are used during anesthesia, residual effects may extend into the postoperative period, also causing muscle weakness. Similarly, epidural anesthesia may extend beyond the desired level, producing weakness or paralysis of respiratory muscles. Organophosphate poisoning causes muscle weakness by means of its anticholinesterase effect, and there has been some concern that animals wearing flea collars containing organophosphates may be more susceptible to the respiratory depressant effects of narcotics and anesthetics (Fig. 36.1).

When ventilatory failure is the result of airway obstruction or a decrease in the bellows action of the chest in the awake animal, increased ventilatory effort is seen until exhaustion occurs (Table 36.1).[5] In the dyspneic animal, movement of the chest wall cannot be equated with ventilatory exchange. Intense ventilatory efforts in the obstructed animal or the animal in great distress from a pneumothorax or diaphragmatic hernia may result in maximal excursion of the chest wall with little or no gas exchange. The animal must always be observed both for ventilatory effort and gas exchange. Gas exchange can be measured with appropriate ventimeters or at least confirmed by feeling the gas exchange from the nose or endotracheal tube.

Airway obstruction may be caused by secretions, vomitus, tumors, or foreign bodies. Soft tissue obstruction may occur in any unconscious or anesthetized animal when muscles in the tongue and walls of the posterior pharynx relax and allow these structures to occlude the airway. Brachycephalic breeds are particularly prone to soft tissue obstruction, especially those having stenotic nares or elongation of the soft palate. The generation of high negative pressures because of obstructed breathing during inspiration in these breeds may result in collapse of the larynx and eversion of the lateral ventricles, increasing further the resistance to respiration.[10] In brachycephalic dogs with very severe airway problems, partial obstruction may also occur in the awake state, particularly after exercise or stress. The collapsing trachea syndrome in toy breeds is another example in which obstruction may be obvious in the awake or unconscious animal. In cats, obstruction due to laryngospasm is occasionally seen during induction of anesthesia. The use of muzzles of gauze or tape tied around the

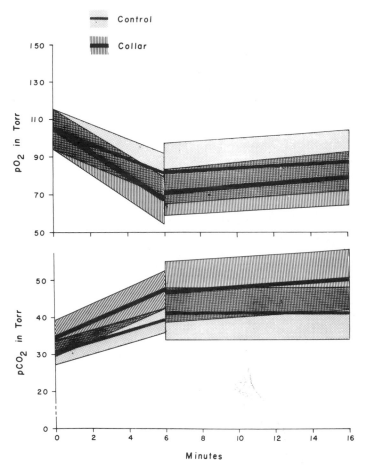

FIG. 36.1. Depressant effects of organophosphate on ventilation after sodium thiopental anesthesia. Each dog served as its own control; thiopental was given prior to and after the placement of a flea collar containing an organophosphate. The respiratory depression is reflected in the lower oxygen tensions and higher carbon dioxide tensions observed in the dogs after they had been wearing flea collars. (Unpublished data courtesy of Dr. Carl Ritter, Department of Pharmacology, School of Veterinary Medicine, University of Pennsylvania, Philadelphia, Pa.)

jaws to keep them closed may cause obstruction by interfering with normal panting. Muzzles can be particularly hazardous in brachycephalic dogs.

Complete airway obstruction is characterized by violent respiratory efforts and choking noises. With partial obstruction of the airway, a respiratory stridor is heard as air is forced around the obstruction. As a general rule, noisy respiration is obstructed respiration. In the diagnosis of obstruction, however, it is very important to realize that in the unconscious animal, obstruction may not be immediately ob-

vious. The ventilatory response to obstruction is depressed and may terminate in respiratory arrest after a brief period of increased ventilatory effort.

Ventilatory failure due to a decrease in the bellows action of the chest or decrease in lung expansion may result from thoracic trauma and the occurrence of diaphragmatic hernia, hemothorax, or pneumothorax. Nontraumatic space-occupying lesions in the chest such as neoplasm, fluid, or enlargement of the heart may have similar effects. Postoperative incisional pain, body bandages, and excessive restraint all tend to restrict movement of the chest walls. Obesity results in a decreased ability to expand the chest and the diaphragm, a problem which is intensified by dorsal recumbency and head down positions. Abdominal distention, regardless of the cause, also interferes with movement of the diaphragm and chest.

In spite of the increased respiratory effort exhibited by the dyspneic animal, a decreased respiratory exchange results. These animals may assume a sitting position and show an increased chest volume on inspiration followed by a forced expiration. Retraction of the respiratory muscles may be evident on inspiration.

HYPOXEMIC FAILURE

Hypoxemic failure is characterized by arterial hypoxemia in the presence of a normal arterial carbon dioxide tension. In this situation ventilation is adequate but oxygen exchange between the alveoli and pulmonary capillaries is not. The causes of hypoxemic failure are (a) ventilation perfusion abnormalities where alveoli are overventilated or underventilated relative to their blood supply, (b) right to left shunting of blood which bypasses functional alveoli and enters the left heart without having been oxygenated, and (c) impaired diffusion at the alveolar capillary membrane (Table 36.1) (see also Chapter 13).

Inequality in ventilation perfusion ratios is the most common form of hypoxemic failure, and its most important cause is chronic diffuse obstructive pulmonary disease. Reduced ventilation perfusion ratios may also occur in animals with normal lungs whenever lower airway obstruction or increased airway resistance develops. Differences in airway resistance throughout the lung result in an unequal distribution of air. Alveoli are therefore overventilated or underventilated in relation to their perfusion. The overventilated alveoli can compensate for underventilated alveoli in the elimination of carbon dioxide, but the nonlinearity of the oxygen dissociation curve prevents this compensation with respect to oxygen exchange. The result is a low oxygen tension in the arterial blood.[19]

Common causes of lower airway obstruction are accumulations of excess secretions, hemorrhage, or edema in the lung. In the depressed animal, secretions may accumulate in the bronchial tree due to suppression of the cough reflex. Similarly, an animal with thoracic trauma may have contusions of the lung resulting in edema and hemorrhage. Therefore, it is obvious that ventilatory failure may predispose the animal to hypoxemic failure. The reverse is also possible. For example, the animal in hypoxemic failure with chronic respiratory disease has a greatly increased susceptibility to the effects of respiratory depressant drugs.

Right to left shunts may cause hypoxemia when congenital heart defects allow blood to pass directly from the right side of the heart to the left, completely bypassing the lungs, or, as an extreme example of ventilation perfusion abnormalities, when totally unventilated alveoli are perfused as in atelectasis, consolidation, or pulmonary edema. Diffuse atelectasis is very common in the postoperative patient and is thought to be initiated by immobility and failure to take deep breaths. Impaired diffusion across the alveolar capillary membrane is usually not a factor in respiratory failure except in pulmonary edema.

Recent evidence has shown that the major cause of death in shock is respiratory failure rather than circulatory failure.[21] Usually hypoxemia precedes a rise in carbon dioxide tension, probably as a result of ventilation perfusion abnormalities and shunting.[22] Physiological dead space is increased leading to hypoxemia and hypercarbia, unless the increased ventilatory requirement can be met by hyperventilation. Consequently, both ventilatory support and oxygen therapy may be urgently needed in cases of severe shock.

Diagnosis of hypoxemic failure can be difficult because ventilation may be adequate even though oxygenation is not. As noted earlier, dangerous levels of hypoxia can exist without obvious cyanosis. Restlessness and anxiety are early signs of hypoxia. The cardiovascular system responds to hypoxia with an increase in heart rate and blood pressure that may be observed until the heart begins to fail from oxygen deprivation. Whenever cardiovascular instability or cardiac arrhythmias occur without obvious reasons, the possibility of hypoxia should be considered. Other signs of hypoxia are nausea and vomiting, dilated pupils, and muscular twitching that may lead to convulsions and death if untreated.

Oxygen administration in mildly elevated concentrations of 30 to 50% to a moderately hypoxic animal will normally relieve the hypoxia, producing a noticeable color change in the mucous membranes. This can be used as a test for hypoxia when a low oxygen tension is suspected. The oxygen administration is not valid, however, when the major cause of hypoxia is right to left shunting.

Treatment

The emergency treatment of respiratory failure, regardless of the etiology, follows basic principles (Table 36.3). The basic steps are as follows. (a) Establish a patent airway. (b) Begin artificial respiration. (c) Supplement the inspired gas with high concentrations of oxygen. Definitive treatment of the cause is secondary to the establishment of a satisfactory airway and initiation of artificial respiration.

AIRWAY MANAGEMENT

Soft tissue obstruction may be corrected by extension of the head and traction on the tongue to pull the soft tissues forward. At the same time, any foreign material in the posterior pharynx that may be occluding the airway should be removed. If considerable airway obstruction persists, the trachea should be intubated. Intubation will relieve the obstruction of a collapsed trachea or that resulting from structural abnormalities in brachycephalic dogs and facilitates the removal of blood, secretions, and vomitus from the airway. Visualization of the airway by laryngoscopy or bronchoscopy is indicated for removal of foreign bodies or secretions and diagnosis of soft tissue abnormalities.

Obstructed animals are frequently presented in acute distress and with intense

TABLE 36.3
Emergency treatment of respiratory failure

1. Establish a patent airway
   A. Extend head, pull tongue forward to relieve soft tissue obstruction
   B. Remove any foreign material occluding the airway
   C. Intubate trachea if obstruction persists
   D. Tracheotomy—indications
      1. Narrowing of laryngeal opening due to edema or tumor
      2. Foreign body lodged within the larynx
      3. Swelling or tumor in the posterior pharynx
      4. Inability to open the jaws
         a. Metastatic invasion of mandibular joint
         b. Improper healing of mandibular fracture
         c. Eosinophilic myositis—atrophy of m a s t i c a t o r y muscles
      5. Facial injuries preventing oral access to airway
      6. Any condition interfering with intubation
2. Initiate artificial respiration
   A. Mouth to mouth—exhaled air
   B. Mouth to endotracheal tube—exhaled air
   C. Bag and mask—room air or oxygen
   D. Bag and endotracheal tube—room air or oxygen
3. Oxygen therapy
   A. Resuscitation of ventilatory failure
   B. Relief of hypoxemic failure—especially when tolerance to hypoxia is decreased
      1) Decreased ability to meet tissue oxygen needs
         a. Low cardiac output or circulatory failure
         b. Reduced oxygen-carrying capacity
            1. Anemia
            2. Carbon monoxide poisoning
      2) Increased tissue oxygen consumption
         a. Increased metabolic rate
            1. Hyperthermia
         b. Increased muscular activity
            1. Convulsions
            2. Dyspnea
            3. Shivering

ventilatory efforts. Conscious animals will normally resist any attempts at intubation, and in unconscious animals chewing and laryngeal reflexes are frequently intact at the time intubation becomes necessary. An injection of an ultrashort acting barbiturate (sodium thiopental) or muscle relaxant (succinylcholine chloride) may be given to facilitate intubation. However, the use of these drugs is not without danger. Cases of cardiac arrest following injection of small amounts of ultrashort acting barbiturates have occurred in this situation, and care must be taken. The arrest may be related to the depressant effect of the barbiturate on an anoxic myocardium. Succinylcholine is probably less depressant to the circulation but should be avoided unless there is assurance that intubation can be performed without delay. Relaxants may be hazardous when the cause of the obstruction is unknown, because after paralysis has occurred, the clinician may discover that intubation is impossible due to swelling or tumor in the pharynx or a foreign body lodged within the larynx.

Awake intubation is the preferred technique whenever possible. The jaws are forced apart by an assistant using a strip of gauze around each jaw. The laryngoscope blade is then placed at the base of the tongue and the soft tissues pulled forward to expose the airway. If time allows, the larynx may be sprayed with a 2% lidocaine solution. Although somewhat lacking in aesthetic appeal, this technique is usually tolerated well by the dog, and can be lifesaving. If awake intubation is not possible, an attempt should be made to relieve the hypoxia with high concentrations of oxygen by mask, before giving thiopental to an obstructed animal.

If intubation cannot be accomplished, an emergency tracheotomy should be performed for relief of obstruction. Indications are given in Table 36.3. An emergency tracheotomy can be performed under local anesthesia, and, in very urgent situations, the trachea should be opened without preparation of the skin or anesthesia.

ARTIFICIAL RESPIRATION

Artificial respiration can be given by a variety of methods depending on the equipment available. Exhaled air contains approximately 16% oxygen and will adequately sustain life in an emergency.

Mouth to mouth respiration can be given to an animal by using one or both hands to seal the jaws and form a channel for blowing air through the nostrils. The head must be extended to open the airway. This method should be effective for most dogs and cats, although it would probably be inadequate in brachycephalic breeds because of soft tissue obstruction. If expansion of the chest is observed, the ventilation is considered adequate. Since the nasal passages may not be patent, it may be necessary to part the lips and blow through the mouth. A bag and mask can also be used for ventilation, although a satisfactory mask fit for intermittent positive pressure ventilation may be difficult to achieve in some animals. An Ambu (Air Shield Inc., Hatboro, Pa.) self-inflating bag, attached either to a mask or endotracheal tube, can be used to deliver air or oxygen in an emergency situation.

The endotracheal tube is the best method for giving intermittent positive pressure ventilation and must be used if ventilation cannot be accomplished by mouth to mouth respiration or by bag and mask. External compression of the chest is of no value in ventilating the lungs. All emergency techniques require the application of intermittent positive pressure to the upper airway. The method used for administering artificial respiration to an apneic animal is of less importance than the speed with which any effective ventilation can be established. This means that immediate mouth to mouth respiration with exhaled air is more beneficial than 100% oxygen delivered by an endotracheal tube 60 seconds later. The high oxygen level cannot compensate for the time elapsed while the equipment was being assembled.

OXYGEN THERAPY

Oxygen therapy is important in the treatment of respiratory failure and essential for the animal in hypoxemic failure. Although animals with ventilatory failure have abnormal levels of both oxygen and carbon dioxide, it is the hypoxia that immediately threatens the animal's life and requires urgent relief. Oxygen therapy is necessary to relieve the hypoxemia of ventilation perfusion abnormalities. It can also be used to improve oxygenation in patients with right to left shunts, although in the event of a large shunt, normal arterial oxygen tensions may not be attained even when pure oxygen is administered.

The occurrence of severe but clinically undetectable levels of hypoxia has been discussed. Various degrees of hypoxia are extremely common in postoperative patients and those having chronic respiratory disease. In the healthy postoperative patient, the cardiovascular and respiratory systems may be able to respond with an increase in function in an attempt to maintain adequate oxygen supply to vital organs. Oxygen therapy is beneficial but not necessarily required, and the oxygen tension returns to its normal level as recovery proceeds. The same degree of hypoxia, however, might be harmful to an old or critically ill animal, or when circulatory compensation for the hypoxia is inadequate.

Any condition that decreases the ability of the body to meet tissue oxygen needs, or increases the metabolic needs of the tissues thereby increasing oxygen consumption, will reduce the tolerance to hypoxia. This includes animals with circulatory failure or low cardiac output as well as those having a decreased oxygen-carrying capacity due to anemia. Oxygen consumption increases when muscular activity is increased due to convulsions, severe dyspnea, or shivering. The violent shivering commonly seen postoperatively can increase oxygen consumption by several hundred percent. This increased oxygen requirement in the immediate postoperative period is occurring during a period of decreased ventilatory capability. Hyperthermia also increases oxygen requirements because of the increased metabolic rate.

Oxygen should be administered by mask or endotracheal tube to any animal suspected of having a potentially harmful degree of hypoxia. A human infant incubator is useful for very small animals; for large dogs, an oxygen tent may be fashioned by running an oxygen line into a cage sealed with polyethylene. In most cases of hypoxemic failure, inhalation of pure oxygen is unnecessary. Inspired oxygen concentrations in the range of 30 to 60% are usually adequate. Oxygen administration by mask is obviously pointless if it evokes strenuous resistance by the animal. Many animals, however, who will not tolerate a snug fitting mask can be oxygenated by using an oversized mask to direct a high flow of oxygen toward the animal's muzzle.

The major complication of oxygen therapy occurs in those animals in which the respiratory response to carbon dioxide is depressed, usually as a result of chronic respiratory disease or depression of the respiratory center by drugs. Respiration is dependent on the hypoxic drive which is depressed by the high concentration of oxygen. The result is hypoventilation or apnea accompanied by carbon dioxide retention. Very high carbon dioxide levels may occur and lead to generalized central nervous system depression.[19]

Respiratory Failure following Thoracic Trauma

Traumatic injuries of the thorax most commonly seen in small animals are penetrating wounds of the chest wall due to bites or blunt trauma caused by automobile accidents or similar crushing injuries. The resulting lesions include pneumothorax (which may be open, closed, or tension), hemothorax, diaphragmatic hernia, and diffuse trauma. The condition of an animal on admission to the hospital following thoracic trauma may vary from minimal to severe distress. In any event, emergency treatment is directed toward the relief or prevention of respiratory failure and circulatory collapse.

PNEUMOTHORAX

Etiology. The admittance of free air into the chest cavity can occur under three circumstances: (a) penetration of the chest wall due to trauma or a surgical procedure; (b) the tearing of the visceral pleura of the lung following the removal of adhesions or rupture of an alveolar bleb; and (c) traumatic pneumothorax following a sudden blow to the chest wall. In the latter type of pneumothorax, there is no actual penetration of the thoracic cavity, and it is due to "closed chest trauma." If a great external force is applied to the thoracic cage in combination with a closed glottis, there will be a sudden rise in intrabronchial pressure. A rupture of alveolar tissue can occur, producing a closed or tension pneumothorax. Alveolar rupture does not necessarily occur at the visceral surface of the lung producing a gross tear, but disruption can occur within the lung parenchyma. The histological appearance of the mediastinum and lungs of cats which have been deliberately overdistended with air has been described.[11] Following alveolar rupture, the escaped air follows the path of least resistance, which is along the sheaths of the larger pulmonary arteries and into the mediastinal space. If the volume of air is large enough, passage will occur bilaterally into the thoracic cavity. Air can dissect along the esophagus and into the peritoneal cavity or subcutaneously into the neck.[2, 11] In most cases, the condition is self-limiting and does not represent a continuous leakage of air as in the case of a tear in the lung pleura or an open chest wound.[20]

During certain surgical or diagnostic procedures, a pneumothorax can occur. Procedures in which iatrogenic pneumothorax can occur are chest wall surgery, spinal disc fenestration of the thoracic vertebrae, surgery in the area of the thoracic inlet, liver biopsy, or excessive intermittent positive pressure ventilation.

Penetration of the chest wall produces an open pneumothorax in which intrathoracic pressure becomes equal to atmospheric. If the defect in the chest wall is large enough to allow air to be sucked into the thorax during inspiration, the lesion is referred to as a sucking wound of the chest. A rupture occurring in the visceral pleura, alveolar tissue, or bronchial tree results in a closed pneumothorax. In some cases, the laceration acts as a one-way valve allowing air to pass into the pleural space during inspiration and preventing its escape during expiration. When intrathoracic pressure becomes greater than atmospheric, the lesion is referred to as a tension pneumothorax.

The admittance of free air into the chest cavity, whether it be by trauma or opening the chest, generally produces in the dog and cat a bilateral pneumothorax (Fig. 36.2). In contrast to man, the mediastinal tissue is scanty and lacks fibrous support. The mediastinal pleura is not fenestrated,[12] but is very thin (especially the postcardial) and can easily rupture, allowing the passage of air from one side to the other. Radiographically, in some cases of pneumothorax, a greater amount of air has been noted on one side or the other. This may be related to the amount of air admitted and the possible fibrous changes in the mediastinum due to disease.

Ventilation during Pneumothorax. When the overlying muscles are removed and the costal pleura is exposed, the movement of the lungs can be seen in contact with the transparent pleura. During normal respiration, the lungs remain in contact with the thoracic wall and, in essence, there is no pleural space, only a potential one. The negative pressure within the thoracic cavity maintains the continuity between lung and thoracic wall. During normal respiration, the negative pressure within the thoracic cavity represents the difference between the elastic and surface tension properties of the lung trying to reduce the lung size and the atmospheric pressure communicating with the alveoli maintaining inflation. The intrapleural pressure is the atmospheric pressure minus the elastic force of the lung.

When air is allowed to enter the chest cavity, the slight film between the costal pleura and lung pleura is broken, and atmospheric pressure acts on the outside of the lung and effects its collapse. As air is introduced into the chest cavity, both lungs can be seen falling away but still undergoing rhythmic expansion and contraction; this, of course, is at a reduced tidal volume. The extent of lung collapse is related to the volume of air introduced.

A volume of air in the chest equal to the functional residual capacity of the lung results in a 30% collapse of the lung. When the volume of air is equal to twice the functional residual capacity, the lung is 60 to 65% collapsed.[8]

The dog has been shown to compensate for a pneumothorax equal to twice the functional residual capacity without great

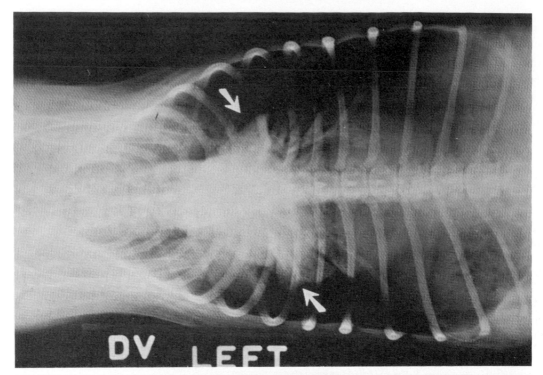

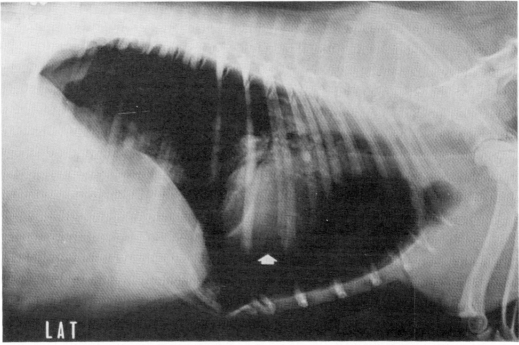

FIG. 36.2. Bilateral pneumothorax and compression atelectasis. *Top*, dorsal ventral view (*DV*); *bottom*, lateral view. Air is present throughout the pleural space, causing collapse of both lungs. In the dorsal ventral view, it is evident that air fills both sides of the thoracic cavity. *Arrows* indicate the borders of the collapsed lung fields. In the lateral view, dorsal displacement of the heart is evident (*arrow*). (all radiographs are courtesy of the Section of Radiology, School of Veterinary Medicine, University of Pennsylvania, Philadelphia, Pa.)

distress.[8] The tolerance to pneumothorax depends on two physiological mechanisms —hyperventilation and increased expansion of the chest wall. Hyperventilation, characterized by an increased respiratory rate and a decreased tidal volume, results in an increased respiratory minute volume. Chest wall expansion is increased by several factors. Separation of the visceral and parietal pleural surfaces by the presence of air in the thoracic cavity releases the thorax from the force tending toward collapse of the chest wall that is normally exerted by the lungs. Therefore, by passive recoil, the chest wall tends to return to its resting position which has a greater than normal volume. Increased inspiratory effort by the animal is another factor that leads to greater expansion of the chest wall. The awake dog with a pneumothorax normally assumes a sitting position, which removes the weight of the abdominal viscera and allows greater descent of the diaphragm.

It should be apparent that failure of compensation for pneumothorax may be precipitated by inappropriate handling and treatment. Ventilatory decompensation may result from positional changes or the use of respiratory depressant drugs.

As the degree of pneumothorax progresses, compensating mechanisms fail and hypoventilation occurs. Respiratory acidosis, hypoxia, decreased pH, and aggravated respiratory distress are the result of a severe pneumothorax.

Circulatory Effects of Pneumothorax. The degree of changes in the circulatory and ventilatory systems depends somewhat on the physical status of the animal, whether under general anesthesia, and the degree of lung collapse. The majority of animal studies have been conducted in the anesthetized dog with a paucity of work in the conscious animal. The creation of partial lung collapse by the injection of air equal to the dog's functional residual capacity (approximately 29.2 ml/kg) not only produced changes in ventilation but a reduction in cardiac output.[13, 17] This rapid reduction in cardiac output has also been noted immediately following thoracotomy.[6] The reported changes in blood pressure following the injection of air or thoracotomy

indicate a great experimental divergence. A slight decrease[3, 17] to a significant reduction[6] has been reported. The variable reported changes in blood pressure are understandable. Different anesthetic agents, the depth of anesthesia, and varying experimental conditions can produce physiological situations whereby the compensating vascular response to a drop in cardiac output varies. For example, sodium thiopental anesthesia produces a reduction in venous tone[4]; because of this, peripheral pooling of blood will augment a condition which in itself will reduce cardiac output. Under thiopental anesthesia there is a lessened peripheral venous constriction in response to a reduction in cardiac output. This venoconstriction as a compensating mechanism in maintaining blood pressure during a fall in cardiac output will be lessened under general anesthesia.

The mechanisms for the reduction of cardiac output have been suggested.[16] The increased pressure on the large but thin thoracic veins effects their partial collapse, producing an increased pulmonary resistance with a reduction in blood flow to the right atrium. This reduction in flow to the right side of the heart is reflected in a reduced left side output. Upon opening the chest or upon admittance of air into the closed pleural cavity, the contiguity between the visceral and parietal pleura is disrupted, allowing the lung to collapse fully. This collapse produces kinking of the pulmonary vessels, in effect a mechanical compression of the pulmonary vasculature.[6] This mechanical compression and the decrease of transmural pressure which tends to maintain the patency of pulmonary capillaries all contribute to an increase in pulmonary vascular resistance and a reduction of blood flow through the lungs.[16] This, and not reduced venous flow to the right heart, may be the major contributor to the reduction in cardiac output. The physiological changes to pneumothorax involve both the respiratory and cardiovascular systems. The most overt change is the clinical manifestation of varying degrees of respiratory distress.

Studies in the conscious dog showed

little change in cardiac output and oxygen saturation when 1.5 to 2 times the functional residual capacity, approximately 50 ml/kg of air, was injected.[9] The conscious dog manifested a greater ability to maintain normal blood gas tensions than the anesthetized dog. This will also vary in the anesthetized dog depending upon the depth of anesthesia and the physical state of the animal.

Management of Pneumothorax. Sucking wounds of the chest and tension pneumothorax are immediately threatening to life due to collapse of the lungs and intense dyspnea. The diagnosis of a sucking wound is readily apparent by the audible sound of air rushing into the chest. The opening in the chest wall should be covered immediately with Vaseline gauze to form an airtight seal and convert the lesion into a closed pneumothorax. This results in considerable relief[1] of the asphyxia which can be rapidly fatal if untreated. The animal with tension pneumothorax is presented in extreme respiratory distress and is cyanotic with an elevated pulse and failing circulation. Intubation and artificial respiration should be initiated at once. The rising intrathoracic pressure is indicated by an increasing resistance to inflation of the lungs. Insertion of a chest tube for evacuation of the air is immediately necessary. When the need for relief is extremely urgent, a large gauge needle and syringe may be used for aspiration, or a needle may be inserted and left open to the air to relieve the tension. A chest tube is then inserted for removal of air.[14]

Closed pneumothorax can usually be treated conservatively following insertion of a chest tube for evacuation of air within the thorax. Occasionally a laceration of the lung will continue to leak air and require surgical intervention for repair or removal of the affected lobe. A defect in the chest wall will, of course, require surgical repair.

THORACIC TRAUMA WITHOUT PNEUMOTHORAX

Diagphragmatic Hernia. Rupture of the diaphragm is not uncommon following trauma in small animals (Fig. 36.3). Moderate to severe respiratory distress is usually noted upon admission to the hospital, although extremely intense dyspnea is rare. Ventilatory support and oxygen therapy should be provided when necessary. The animal should be maintained in an upright position, as recumbency contributes to dyspnea. Auscultation and percussion of the chest will reveal dullness and muffled heart sounds on the affected side. Radiographic examination is necessary and pathognomonic for diagnosis. Surgical repair of the lesion will be required.

Hemothorax. The presence of large quantities of blood in the chest usually indicates rupture of a major vessel or an intercostal vessel. These animals may be dead or in the terminal stages of respiratory failure and hemorrhagic shock upon arrival. Immediate ventilatory and circulatory support are indicated. The diagnosis is confirmed by repeated thoracenteses. Continued blood loss or lack of satisfactory response to ventilatory and circulatory resuscitation are indications for immediate surgical intervention (Fig. 36.4).

Diffuse Trauma. Occasionally an animal is seen following thoracic trauma who exhibits mild to moderate respiratory distress without any observable lesions. Radiographic examination for pneumothorax or diaphragmatic hernia is negative. However, obvious respiratory distress is observed, sometimes with increased expiratory effort. Possible explanations for this condition are contusions or bruising of the lungs associated with local hemorrhage, atelectasis, decreased compliance, and ventilation perfusion abnormalities. The condition is referred to as parenchymal pulmonary hemorrhage and appears radiographically as diffuse areas of increased density (Fig. 36.5). Another factor may be bruising of the chest wall causing pain on inspiration. These animals are kept under observation and cage rest for 48 hours. Conservative treatment is usually adequate and spontaneous recovery occurs.

USE OF DRUGS FOLLOWING THORACIC TRAUMA

Sedative drugs may be harmful following thoracic trauma because of depression of respiration and normal cough reflexes. If

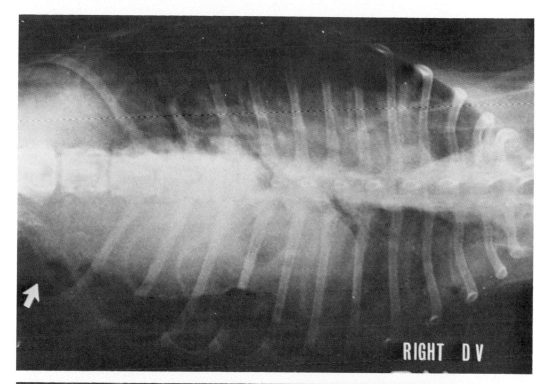

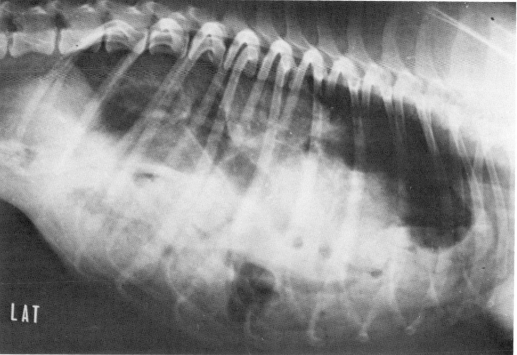

FIG. 36.3. Diaphragmatic hernia. *Top*, dorsal ventral view (*DV*); *bottom*, lateral view. In the dorsal ventral view, the line of the right diaphragm is obliterated (*arrow*), and increased density appears in the right thoracic cavity indicating the presence of abdominal contents. In the lateral view, air-filled lumens of the gastrointestinal tract are visible in the thoracic cavity causing obliteration of the cardiac shadow.

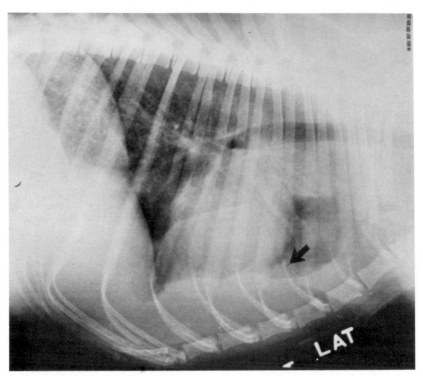

FIG. 36.4. Hemothorax, lateral (*LAT*) view. Fluid density is present in the ventral thorax with dorsal displacement of the heart (*arrow*). The nature of the fluid present in the thoracic cavity cannot be determined by radiography.

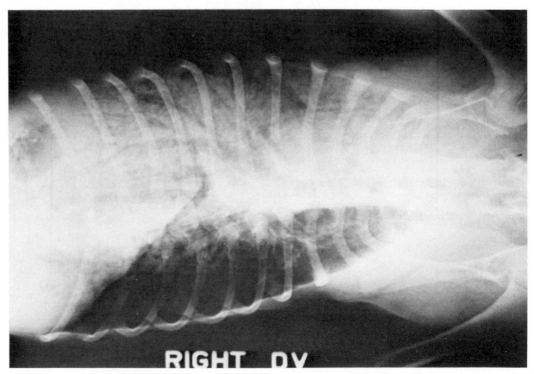

FIG. 36.5. Parenchymal pulmonary hemorrhage, dorsal ventral view (*DV*). Generalized increased density of the left lung is present. This dog had been hit by a car 1 day before the radiograph was taken and exhibited dyspnea.

pain is severe, small doses of meperidine (1 to 2 mg/kg) or morphine (0.5 mg/kg) may be given intramuscularly.

Respiratory Failure in Brachycephalic Breeds

The brachycephalic dog is highly susceptible to upper airway obstruction, especially when the anatomical defect is complicated by stenotic nares or elongation of the soft palate. The high negative pressure produced in the airway during inspiration may result in laryngeal collapse or eversion of the lateral ventricles, thereby intensifying the condition. Some of these animals suffer chronic life-long airway obstruction and, not uncommonly, exhibit dyspnea and cyanosis after minimal stress or excitement. Obstruction of life-threatening proportions can develop very rapidly, making proper airway management critically important in these breeds. Airway complications most commonly occur following induction and recovery from anesthesia, when depressant drugs are used, and as a result of restraint or heat stress.

During induction of anesthesia, obstruction should be anticipated as soon as consciousness is lost. Gas induction by mask is therefore not absolutely contraindicated but is not advised. The method of choice is injection of an ultrashort acting barbiturate followed immediately by intubation of the trachea. If longer acting barbiturates are used instead of gas anesthesia, the trachea should be intubated. This is the only effective means of assuring a patent airway when the animal is unconscious.

Recovery from anesthesia is associated with all the usual postoperative problems which are intensified by the difficulty in maintaining airway patency. The endotracheal tube should be left in place until the animal is nearly conscious. The most severely obstructed animals will require the endotracheal tube in place until they have recovered sufficiently to assume the sternal position. To encourage the dog to tolerate the tube during recovery, the larynx can be sprayed with a local anesthetic (2 to 4% lidocaine). Premature removal of the tube may result in nearly total obstruction with the jaws tightly clenched. If the jaws cannot be pried open, injection of a barbiturate may be necessary for replacement of the tube. Whenever possible, the barbiturate should be preceded by high concentrations of oxygen by mask.

The recovery should be slow and without excitement. This is one situation where sedative drugs are indicated for the brachycephalic dog. Sedation increases the tolerance to the endotracheal tube. Respiratory effort is also reduced, thereby decreasing resistance in the upper airway and preventing laryngeal collapse after removal of the endotracheal tube. Effective sedation is accomplished by small doses of a narcotic and tranquilizer, meperidine (1 to 2 mg/kg), and chlorpromazine (1 to 2 mg/kg). The recovery period is frequently complicated by vomiting in the brachycephalic dog, presumably because the respiratory efforts result in swallowing of large amounts of air. It should be emphasized that close observation of these animals is essential during the postoperative period.

Restraint may be hazardous for these dogs, particularly when a muzzle is used or the animal is grasped around the head or neck. Excessive restraint can result in asphyxia and sudden death. Restraint that interferes with ventilation is useless, because asphyxia causes the animal to struggle more violently. If the dog makes choking sounds or becomes cyanotic, he should be released immediately.

Brachycephalic dogs are especially susceptible to heat stroke, because panting is required for removal of excess body heat. The increased ventilatory requirement results in irritation and swelling of soft tissues of the pharynx and larynx. A viscious cycle develops in which increased body heat causes greater respiratory distress and less efficient heat removal. In warm weather, these animals may be brought to the hospital severely dyspneic and cyanotic. The high body temperature may be overlooked as the cause of the problem, because the respiratory distress draws attention to the respiratory system initially. Emergency treatment consists of oxygen by mask to relieve hypoxia and cold water baths or ice packs to quickly drop the body temperature. Sedation may be helpful by decreasing the inspiratory drive and preventing shivering while the animal is being cooled. Steroids may be helpful in decreasing soft tissue swelling; 50 to 100 mg of hydrocortisone may be given by the intravenous or intramuscular route. The need for careful observation following sedation of brachycephalic dogs cannot be overemphasized.

Respiratory Failure Associated with the Collapsing Trachea Syndrome

The collapsing trachea syndrome is seen in various toy breeds and results in severe airway obstruction in the acute phase. Usually the animal is normal at rest, and respiratory distress occurs following the stress of severe exercise and during the postoperative period. Treatment consists of oxygen by mask and sedation to decrease the inspiratory drive and prevent high negative pressures in the airway which, in turn, increase the tendency toward collapse. The initial 24- to 48-hour period following surgical repair of the tracheal defect is characterized by severe obstruction due to swelling and edema in the trachea. The use of an endotracheal tube is contraindicated at this time because it increases the irritation of the trachea. Treatment during this period consists of oxygen by mask or tent, steroids to reduce inflammation, and low doses of sedatives to diminish the inspiratory drive (meperidine and chlorpromazine).

Postoperative Respiratory Failure

The believe that the surgical patient is out of danger once he is off the table is widespread but highly erroneous. The immediate postoperative period is a critical one for many animals and may be more dangerous than the operation itself. Respiratory failure is the most common postoperative complication and usually results from hypoventilation and atelectasis. Animals with pre-existing pulmonary disease, respiratory disorders, and obesity are most susceptible, although previously healthy animals may also suffer respiratory failure following surgery.

Hypoventilation may result from most of the causes already discussed. These include depression of the respiratory center by drugs; muscle weakness caused by residual effects of muscle relaxants; obstruction due to soft tissue; secretions, blood, or vomitus in the airway; and interference with chest wall movement by pain, body bandages, and obesity.

The diffuse atelectasis that occurs postoperatively is believed to be caused by a lack of deep breathing and coughing by the animal. The result is partial or total collapse of alveoli, ventilation perfusion abnormalities, and hypoxemia.[7] Clinically undetectable hypoxia is known to occur in a large percentage of postoperative patients.

Treatment of postoperative respiratory complications consists of improving ventilation by whatever means are necessary. Oxygen therapy is not necessary in the average postoperative patient because the cardiovascular system compensates for the hypoxia, and the oxygen tension returns to normal spontaneously as recovery occurs. As noted earlier, the old or critically ill animal has less tolerance to hypoxia for a variety of reasons. Hypothermia during surgery followed by violent shivering in the postoperative period is very common in air-conditioned facilities and greatly increases oxygen consumption. Oxygen should be supplemented postoperatively in any animal suspected of having a reduced tolerance to hypoxia or increased oxygen requirements.

Respiratory complications can be minimized by encouraging deep breathing, mobility, and early ambulation in postsurgical patients.[7] Stimulation by paw pinch or vigorous pats on the chest or back will usually cause the animal to take a deep breath. If an animal remains deeply anesthetized in lateral recumbency, he should be turned frequently from side to side. Animals should never be left unattended in the immediate postoperative period. Careful observation is required at least until the animal is alert and able to maintain a sternal position.

Respiratory Failure Resulting from Restraint

Inappropriate restraint as a cause of respiratory failure is important and frequently overlooked. (The problems associated with muzzles and handling of brachycephalic breeds have already been discussed.) Cyanosis is not uncommon in struggling animals being forcibly restrained. Should this occur, the animal must be released immediately. The asphyxiated animal will continue to struggle until his ventilatory distress is relieved or unconsciousness from hypoxia occurs. Collapse and sudden death may occur in exotic animals and sometimes cats being forcibly restrained. This is presumably due to cardiac arrest resulting from hypoxia and catecholamine release.

Use of Drugs in Treatment of Respiratory Failure

ANALEPTICS

Analeptic drugs commonly used by the small animal clinician include pentylenetetrazol, nikethamide, amphetamine, and doxapram hydrochloride. These drugs are not specific antagonists of barbiturates or any other respiratory depressants, nor are they specific stimulants of respiration. They produce generalized central nervous system stimulation. In the depressed or sedated animal, they can produce arousal usually accompanied by an increase in respiratory rate. The effect is usually of short duration. The stimulatory effects may not occur in the presence of severe anoxia, high carbon dioxide tensions, or extremely deep levels of anesthesia. Use of the analeptic drugs is not without danger. Potentially harmful side effects that may occur are excitement, generalized convulsions, poststimulatory depression, and hypotension.

The treatment of barbiturate overdose with analeptics remains controversial.[15] The need for repeated dosages of the stimulant and close observation of the patient as well as the possibility of harmful side effects make the efficacy of this method of treatment questionable. Regular supportive care supplemented by ventilatory support when necessary is probably of greater benefit to the patient. However, stimulant drugs may be beneficial for the animal having a prolonged recovery from pentobarbital anesthesia when respiratory depression is relatively mild and the equipment required for prolonged ventilatory support is not at hand. The routine use of analeptics during normal recovery from inhalation and barbiturate anesthetics is hazardous and unnecessary. Under light planes of anesthesia, an animal may suffer excitement, rigidity of the limbs with opisthotonos, and cardiovascular arrhythmias following injection of stimulants.

Under no circumstances should analeptics be used in the emergency treatment of acute respiratory failure with an apneic patient in immediate danger of death from hypoxia. Use of a stimulant to counteract the effects of an acute overdose of an intravenous injection of barbiturate is to be comdemned. A relative or absolute overdose of barbiturate injected intravenously results in profound respiratory depression and cardiovascular instability. Cardiac arrest may follow immediately. Artificial ventilation must be initiated without delay. If the heart has stopped, cardiopulmonary resuscitation must be initiated. Analeptic drugs are entirely ineffective in this situation.

The analeptic drug of choice is doxapram at a dose range of 1 to 4 mg/kg given slowly intravenously. Stimulation of the respiratory and cardioacceleratory centers in the central nervous system results in an increase in respiratory minute volume and blood pressure. This drug has a high margin of safety, as convulsions ordinarily occur at much higher doses. The transient hypotension that may be seen following intravenous injections of analeptics does not occur with doxapram at the recommended doses.[18]

NARCOTIC ANTAGONISTS

The narcotic antagonists reverse the respiratory, cardiovascular, and sedative effects of narcotics and have no effect on other depressant drugs. Reversal of the narcotic occurs within a few seconds following intravenous injection of the narcotic antagonist. The drugs of choice are levallorphan (1 to 2 mg intravenously) and nalorphine (5 to 10 mg intravenously).

REFERENCES

1. Abreu, A. L. d', Taylor, A. B., and Clarke, D. B.: *Intrathoracic Crises.* Appleton-Century-Crofts, New York, 1968.
2. Baugh, W.: Pneumothorax in the neonate. Brit. J. Anaesth. *36:* 456, 1964.
3. Brecher, G. A.: *Venous Return.* Grune & Stratton, Inc., New York, 1956.
4. Eckstein, J. W., Hamilton, W. K., and McCammond, J. M.: The effect of thiopental on peripheral venous tone. Anesthesiology *22:* 525, 1961.
5. Feldman, S., and Ellis, H.: *Principles of Resuscitation.* F. A. Davis Company, Philadelphia, 1967.
6. Finlayson, J. K., Luria, M. N., and Yu, P. N.: Circulatory effects of thoracotomy and intermittent positive pressure respiration in dogs. Circ. Res. *9:* 862, 1961.
7. Hamilton, W. K.: Postoperative respiratory complications. In *Respiratory Therapy,* edited by P. Safar, chap. 10, p. 262. F. A. Davis, Philadelphia, 1965.
8. Hemingway, A., and Simmons, D. H.: Respiratory response to acute progressive pneumothorax. J. Appl. Physiol. *13:* 165, 1958.
9. Kilburn, K. H.: Cardiorespiratory effects of large pneumothorax in conscious and anesthetized dogs. J. Appl. Physiol. *18:* 279, 1963.
10. Leonard, H. C.: Obstruction of the respiratory tract. In *Current Veterinary Therapy,* 3rd ed. W. B. Saunders Company, Philadelphia, 1968.
11. Macklin, C. C.: Pneumothorax with massive collapse from experimental local over-inflation of the lung substance. Canad. Med. Ass. J. *36:* 414, 1937.
12. Miller, M. E., Christensen, G. C., and Evans, H. E.: *Anatomy of the Dog.* W. B. Saunders Company, Philadelphia, 1965.
13. Moore, R. L., and Cochran, H. W.: The effects of closed pneumothorax, partial occlusion of one primary bronchus, phrenicectomy, and the respiration of nitrogen by one lung on pulmonary expansion and the minute volume of blood flowing through the lungs. J. Thorac. Cardiovasc. Surg. *2:* 468, 1933.
14. Ramsay, B. H.: Surgical emergencies of the chest. In *Management of Medical Emergencies,* edited by J. C. Sharpe and F. W. Marx, Jr., 2nd ed., chap. 24. McGraw-Hill Book Company, New York, 1969.
15. Sharpless, S. K.: Hypnotics and sedatives. In *The Pharmacological Basis of Therapeutics,* edited by L. S. Goodman and A. Gilman, chap. 9, p. 125. The Macmillan Company, New York, 1965.
16. Simmons, D. H., and Hemingway, A.: The pulmonary circulation following pneumothorax and vagotomy in dogs. Circ. Res. *7:* 93, 1959.
17. Simmons, D. H., Hemingway, H., and Ricchiuti, M.: Acute circulating effects of pneumothorax in dogs. J. Appl. Physiol. *12:* 255, 1958.
18. Soma, L. R., and Kenny, R.: Respiratory, cardiovascular, metabolic, and electroencephalographic effects of Doxapram hydrochloride in the dog. Vet. Res. *28:* 191, 1967.
19. Sykes, M. K., McNicol, M. W., and Campbell, E. J. M.: *Respiratory Failure.* F. A. Davis Company, Philadelphia, 1969.
20. Walker, R. G.: Traumatic pneumothorax in small animals. Vet. Rec. *21:* 859, 1959.
21. Weil, M. H., and Shubin, H.: The "VIP" approach to the bedside management of shock. J.A.M.A. *207:* 337, 1969.
22. Wilson, R. F., Kafi, A., Asuncion, Z., and Walt, A. J.: Clinical respiratory failure after shock or trauma. Arch. Surg. (Chicago) *98:* 539, 1969.

37
Shock: Pathogenesis and Treatment

S. G. HERSHEY AND B. M. ALTURA

Since the beginning of this century, when Crile[15] inaugurated the "modern" era of experimental study of the shock syndrome, a large amount of information has been accumulated. Although most studies have been oriented toward developing data which could be interpreted for and applied to the care of the human patient, the dog has been used extensively as an experimental subject. Much of what is known about shock is therefore specifically valid for the dog without having to contend with the uncertainties of interpretations related to actual and potential species differences. It must be emphasized that a complete and accurate description of either the pathogenesis or therapy of the shock syndrome cannot be presented; not so much because of limitations of space, but simply because there is no valid unifying concept of the syndrome which is compatible with all known facts and collective experience either in the dog or man. Despite the wealth of data available, the basic etiology of shock is incompletely understood, as evidenced by the continuing emergence of many concepts and theories of shock. This long history of uncertainty regarding many critical factors in shock has led to considerable confusion and divergent opinions. It should be pointed out first that the study of shock, in its fundamental aspects, involves an extremely complex area and the circulatory and metabolic activities of many tissues. Despite the lack of uniform opinion, a substantial body of valuable information has been developed which is available for effective therapeutic application. The record of clinical experience shows that most subjects in shock are successfully treated and recover completely, provided treatment is prompt and their underlying disease process is compatible with survival.

Enough is already known about the overall cardiovascular dynamics of shock that it might be worthwhile to review these cardiovascular dynamics as a frame of reference prior to discussing current concepts of pathogenesis and present attitudes toward therapy. Such a review serves the important function of allowing for orderly and reasonable assessment of seemingly unrelated and incompletely delineated aspects of both pathogenesis and therapy.

Cardiovascular Dynamics of Shock

Shock is predominantly a cardiovascular disorder which can be initiated by many circumstances: hemorrhage, trauma, sepsis, burns, etc. These initiating factors set in motion a sequence of circulatory changes manifested first by a fall in blood pressure. Hypotension seems to be the event which triggers the overall hemodynamic response,[30] which is functionally organized to correct the hypotension and to prevent its progress. By reflex, this correction is through neurogenic and humoral mechanisms which attempt to readjust the discrepancy between the effective blood volume and the physical capacity of the vascular tree. Peripheral vasoconstriction is the principal vasomotor activity producing this readjustment. Vasoconstriction is accompanied by other corrective changes such as cardiac acceleration, redistribution of blood to more essential tissue areas, and shifting of extravascular body fluids into the intravascular compartment. This readjustment of available blood volume is designed to favor distribution of blood to those tissues which are vital for acute survival (brain, heart, lungs) and to augment the volume of the blood in circulation. The signs of shock and the body's corrective responses to it are simultaneously apparent: hypotension, tachycardia, pallor of the mucous membranes and conjunctivae, increased respiration, decreased cardiac output, oliguria, and depressed sensorium.

This initial sympathetic system response toward insuring acute survival reduces the blood supplied to so-called "less critical tissues" to a level which, in time threatens their metabolic needs and their functional integrity. This happens despite the capacity of such tissues to survive longer than the brain and heart under conditions of ischemic hypoxia and relative anaerobiosis. The cost of maintaining the blood pressure and blood flow to vital areas by persistent vasoconstriction becomes too great if correction is not prompt. The changes generated in ischemic tissues can become incompatible with survival of the whole organism within a matter of hours. Within these ischemic tissues, particularly those in the splanchnic area, products of disturbed metabolism are produced and are permitted to accumulate because of poor circulation. Localized acidosis, high concentrations of normal and abnormal split metabolic products, and electrolyte and fluid imbalance now become critical in the tissue environment.

These local tissue changes, in turn, alter the vasomotor activities of the microcirculation. The pertinent feature of this local situation, in relation to overall circulatory dynamics, is that patterns of peripheral vasomotor activity are changed in the direction of impairment of their co-ordination and efficiency (Fig. 37.1). The small amount of blood which is brought to these tissues is poorly handled from the standpoint of distribution and drainage. Intravascular sequestration and stasis of blood develop and further reduce the volume and rate at which the blood is returned to the heart. Thus, a type of vicious circle develops in which the initial vasoconstrictive readjustment to the hypotension and decreased blood volume results in further embarrassment of venous return and cardiac output—factors which predispose to more severe hypotension and less efficient total circulation.

While this brief account of the general sequence of the circulatory responses to shock by no means completely explains the complexities of the shock disturbance, it does direct attention to several important features. (a) Shock, except in its milder forms, is not a self-limited disorder which the organism can reverse or even hold in abeyance for very long. If untreated, it continues unremittingly to a lethal end. (b) There are certain features which characterize irreversible shock: progressive stagnation of blood in the peripheral vessels, decreased blood and tissue oxygen tensions, rising hematocrit, failure of blood volume expansion and other therapy to sustain the blood pressure, accumulation of vasotoxic materials in the blood, and increased capillary permeability. (c) There is a tissue component which participates significantly in the circulatory derangements in shock. (d) While the circumstances which initiate the syndrome can have their major impact at any level of the circulation (heart, large arteries and veins, small peripheral vessels), the net result is an identical chain of events involving the interaction of the function of small blood vessels with changes in the tissues they supply and drain. As this interaction becomes more firmly established, shock becomes increasingly difficult to treat successfully. It seems reasonable to assume that the nature of

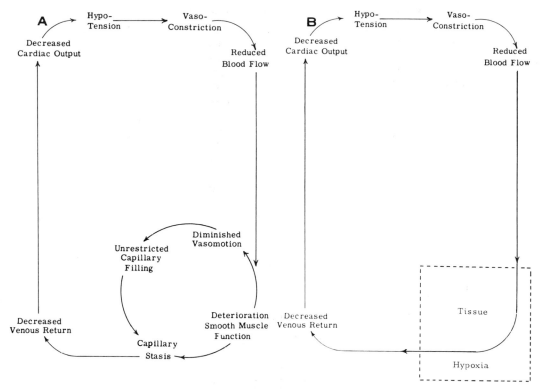

Fig. 37.1. *A*, schema of circulatory events in shock. Peripheral vascular failure follows reduced blood flow to capillary beds (*B*) leading to tissue hypoxia. Peripheral vascular failure includes both a vascular and tissue component. (From Hershey, S. G. (editor): *Shock*, p. 36. Little, Brown and Company, Boston, 1964.)

this interaction between tissues and the microcirculation must contain the answers we seek to the frustrating problem of identifying precisely the complete pathogenesis of shock.

The foregoing list of some of the features characterizing the state of severe shock clearly emphasizes the fact that, as a circulatory disturbance, the syndrome most critically involves the peripheral portion of the circulatory system. In fact, peripheral vascular failure is probably the only valid common denominator in all types of shock and most accurately defines the syndrome.[29] It follows that the improvement of tissue blood flow mediated via the terminal vascular bed is the ultimate target of all forms of antishock therapy. Factors and mechanisms which have been implicated as critical participants in the pathogenesis of the shock syndrome (Table 37.1) represent the bulk of shock research in recent years,

and many of the historical and current theories of shock have emerged from these studies. Data relating to the mechanisms implicated in shock lead to two general conclusions. First, no single concept of shock has been developed where a single mechanism can explain all or even most of the known characteristics of the syndrome. Second, almost all of the pertinent factors involve the hepatointestinal tissue complex or are mediated via hepatointestinal mechanisms. The latter is particularly significant, since there is extensive evidence that the hepatointestinal complex not only represents a critical tissue site in the pathogenesis of the syndrome, but also is prominently involved in the development of peripheral vascular failure in shock.

Pathogenesis of Shock: Current Concepts

For the purposes of review, the various concepts of shock can be grouped together

TABLE 37.1

Some factors and mechanisms
implicated in shock

Decreased regional blood flow, tissue ischemia
Excessive vasoconstriction
Hypersensitivity to catecholamines
Increased capillary permeability—"H" substances
Impaired capillary integrity—serotonin, kinins
Failure of neurohumoral homeostatic mechanisms
Adrenocortical insufficiency
Blood coagulation system alterations
Ferritin (vasodepressor material)—iron release
Breakdown of bacterial defense mechanisms
Bacterial endotoxins
Polysaccharids—endogenous, exogenous
Proteolytic enzymes—purine metabolism
Hydrolytic (lysosomal) enzymes
Antibody depletion—properdin
Reticuloendothelial system depression
Hyperpotassemia—Na-K imbalance
Schwartzman phenomenon (local, general)
Tissue vasoactive products—polypeptides, amines, etc.

on the basis of mechanisms and factors which primarily deal with (a) regional vascular dysfunction and failure of local homeostatic tissue mechanisms; (b) release of and/or altered response of specialized tissues (primarily vascular) to tissue mediator substances, particularly vasoactive humors; (c) the breakdown of endogenous defense mechanisms, especially those related to antibacterial defenses; and (d) a wide variety of toxic or presumably toxic substances of endogenous or exogenous origin. It must be emphasized that the grouping is for the convenience of discussion, and each dysfunction is inter-related.

FAILURE OF LOCAL VASCULAR HOMEOSTATIC
MECHANISMS

The preceding discussion of the cardiovascular dynamics of shock has made it apparent that the peripheral portion of the cardiovascular system is involved in the development of the lethal consequences of the shock syndrome. This distal segment of the circulation (Fig. 37.2) is often referred to as peripheral circulation, capillary circu-

lation, terminal vascular bed, microcirculation or, from a functional viewpoint, the exchange blood vessels. The latter term emphasizes that the most important blood vessels involved in the syndrome are those microscopic in size—the site of tissue-blood exchange of metabolic materials.[62] The functional derangements within the exchange blood vessels affect blood flow in tissues. Shock, therefore, is a peripheral circulatory disorder which impairs tissue homeostasis. The interaction of these two elements, vascular and tissue, as each is affected by the progression of the shock episode, encompasses the most prominent and widely held conceptual view of the pathogenesis of shock, and is referred to as peripheral vascular or microcirculatory insufficiency or failure.

Following the onset of shock, the initial neurogenically mediated vasoconstrictive response of the small blood vessels curtails the volume of blood reaching the tissues.[63] This vasomotor change is compensatory at first and, depending on the duration and intensity of the stress stimulus, can become decompensatory. The initial compensatory response in the microcirculation is somewhat comparable to the compensatory changes in larger systemic vessels (macrocirculation): both aid the readjustment to the imbalance existing between effective vascular volume and vascular capacity. These patterns of increased vasomotor activity (vasomotion) functionally seal off many of the true capillaries and direct the blood through arteriovenous shunts (Fig. 37.2). Increased sensitivity of the peripheral vessels to catecholamines also occurs. The volume of blood entering the vast network of true capillaries is reduced, which facilitates venous return of blood to the heart and thereby aids in the maintainance of cardiac output. If the hypotension is not drastic and the circulating blood volume not critically reduced, tissues can sustain this reduction of tissue perfusion a variable number of hours, depending on the presence of many ancillary factors. If the blood flow through the exchange vessels continues to be markedly reduced, decompensatory vasomotor patterns grad-

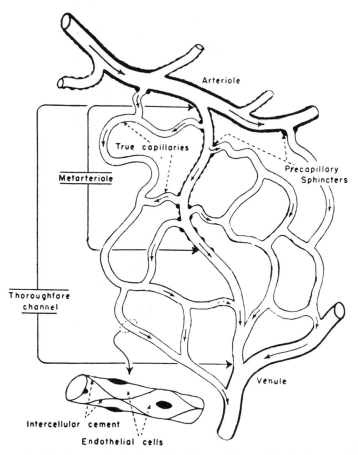

FIG. 37.2. Schematized tracing of a typical module of the capillary bed indicating terminology for different anatomical components. (From Postgrad. Med. *38:* 123, 1965.)

ually replace the pre-existent compensatory responses threatening the maintenance of even minimal metabolic needs. With such interference in oxidative aerobic tissue function, the regulation of the peripheral vascular bed becomes progressively more autonomous and in a direction opposite to its initial responses. This represents an attempt by the local humoral regulatory mechanisms of the microcirculation to counteract tissue hypoxia by increasing its own blood flow. Flow in the microvessels is no longer restricted to thoroughfare channels, because vasomotion of the metarterioles and precapillaries decreases and disappears. The true capillaries, especially the postcapillaries and collecting venules, become overfilled, and stagnation develops because of poor venular outflow. All the muscular vessels in the microcirculation are now hyporeactive to catecholamines. Peripheral circulatory failure is now well advanced. A singular feature of the interaction of the vascular and tissue components of shock is the propagation of an autonomous vicious circle which is ultimately impervious to all known corrective therapy. The net effect is a functional dissociation of the terminal vascular bed from the rest of the circulatory system in terms of total integrated cardiovascular behavior. Circumstances such as the physical status of the animal, the magnitude and nature of the stress, the particular tissue involved in the injury, and the presence of ancillary toxic elements such as infection or deep anesthesia determine the manner and rate at which the initial compensatory response in the microcirculation gives way to decompensation.

These peripheral vascular changes do not uniformly involve all regional vascular beds.[29] For example, the microcirculation in the musculoskeletal structures does not usually develop a decompensatory phase but retains a restricted, ischemic state throughout. Visceral structures show variable vascular changes with the kidneys remaining intensely ischemic. The spleen and adrenals become somewhat congested but still retain sufficient blood flow to sustain their tissue functions. Circulation in the liver and intestine, especially in the dog, is most markedly affected. Progressive severe congestion develops during the refractory phase of shock. Regional differences are probably related to the intrinsic structural and functional organization of the small blood vessels in the different tissues and organs, and particularly to the reactivity of the microvasculature to various vasoactive materials.

ALTERED RESPONSE OF SPECIALIZED TISSUES TO MEDIATOR SUBSTANCES

Local tissue homeostasis is maintained by autonomous humoral regulatory mechanisms of the microcirculation. Local regulation of microcirculatory blood flow is largely dependent upon the liberation of chemical mediators either in the parenchymal tissues in the immediate vicinity of the small blood vessels[2] or possibly in the vascular smooth muscle-endothelial cell complexes.[62] These chemicals modify the vasomotor tone of the muscular components of the capillary bed by directly producing constriction or dilation, thus tempering the local inactivation of blood-borne constrictor or dilator substances, or by altering the reactivity of the microvessels to endogenous humoral stimuli. The fact that biologically active materials with vasotropic effects appear in the tissues and blood during shock, particularly when the animal becomes refractory to therapy, suggests that the final functional deterioration of the cardiovascular system may be due to the specific action of one or more of these biologically active materials.

Many changes could account for the elaboration of such biologically vasoactive materials: (a) tissue hypoxia on a systemic or local level; (b) cellular destruction from ischemia or trauma; (c) altered blood coagulation; (d) activation of proteolytic enzymes; (e) hormonal discharges; (f) changes in local oxidation-reduction systems; and (g) accumulation of cellular metabolic by-products including carbon dioxide and lactic acid.

Ischemic hypoxia of the intestinal tract, for example, can release serotonin (5-hydroxytryptamine), which is present in large quantity in the bowel wall. Serotonin is a humoral regulator of intestinal muscle tonus and possibly of the intestinal mural circulation. In experimental shock in dogs when ischemia of the bowel is present, large amounts of this amine are released into the portal circulation.[8] This amine affects the blood pressure, variably induces either dilation or constriction in different vascular beds, increases capillary permeability, predisposes to thrombus formation, and increases portal vein pressure. In the presence of hypoxia, intestinal barriers are reduced, and the previously contained bacteria or their by-products cross the mucosal wall to enter the circulation. Aerobic and anaerobic bacteria and the toxic components contained in bacterial cells not only undermine homeostatic defense mechanisms, but also have direct undesirable effects on the blood vessels themselves.[20]

The liver is in the direct pathway of the circulatory outflow of the intestine and is subject to the major impact from materials liberated by the hypoxic bowel and is also particularly vulnerable to hypoxia.[49] Although most of the hepatic blood supply is from the portal vein, this vessel supplies only 25% of the liver's oxygen supply. With the marked reduction in intestinal blood flow characteristic of most types of shock, the liver is primarily perfused by blood which may be very low in oxygen content. This is of critical significance, since the liver normally is the most important detoxifying organ. One concept of shock is based on the observation that the hypoxic liver releases an iron-bearing protein, ferritin, into the circulation.[52] Ferritin is a strong vasoinhibitory agent with vasomotor effects remarkably similar in some respects to those observed in the decompensatory phase of shock. Ferritin has been shown to be related to the oxidation of adrenaline. Ferritin is not the specific etiological factor in shock, but it may influence the progression of the syndrome toward irreversibility.

Hypoxia in the ischemic kidney results in the formation of various polypeptides. Angiotensin is a potent vasotropic agent, but its role in the pathogenesis of shock (as opposed to its role in essential hypertension) has not been established. Another such polypeptide called VEM (vasoexcitatory material), originally found in the blood in conjunction with the ferritin sequence, was incorporated into the hepatorcnal concept.[52] VEM is a vasoexcitory substance of renal origin and is present only in the early (compensatory) phase of shock. It cannot be found during the progression toward irreversibility. These findings suggest the existence of the VEM-ferritin systems in the liver and kidney as critical substances with opposite vascular effects as a homeostatic system presumably concerned with regulation of local blood flow.

The adrenal glands also respond characteristically to ischemic hypoxia. Any form of systemic stress results in an almost instantaneous discharge into the circulation of catecholamines from the adrenal medulla and corticosteroids from the cortex.[50] There is no evidence of adrenal exhaustion in shock. The adrenal hormones do alter the responses of all circulatory components, particularly when they are present in higher than normal concentrations. Stress and hypoxia not only activate adrenal responses but also induce an abrupt sympathetic nervous system discharge which can be physiologically significant. This neurogenic reaction involves central nervous system participation and neurohumorally mediated release of a broad assortment of hormones, enzymes, vasoactive amines, and other biochemical substances.[44] These are designed for energy mobilization, permitting the organism as a whole to readjust successfully to the stressful situation. Many of these materials are normally present in the circulation in relatively low concentrations. Excessive concentrations of these highly active biochemicals, particularly when their concentrations are disproportionate in relation to each other, certainly must result in an imbalance in many specific homeostatic mechanisms which may then account for some of the total systemic and regional cardiovascular dysfunction in shock.

Since the activity of so many of the body's homeostatic mechanisms is regulated on the feedback principle, it becomes understandable that the abnormal materials released in shock in turn alter the neurogenic and humoral overactivity which released them.[26] Compounds which have significant vascular effects are: (a) amines such as epinephrine, norepinephrine, histamine, and serotonin; (b) polypeptides such as angiotensin, vasopressin, bradykinin, kallidin, VEM, substance P, and leucotaxin; (c) proteolytic by-products such as globulin, kallikrein, lysosomal enzymes, proteases, and plasmin; (d) tissue metabolites such as adenyl compounds, lactic acid, CO_2, electrolytes (Na, K), polysaccharides, and nucleotides; and (e) miscellaneous substances such as ferritin, acetylcholine, renin, thiols, sulfhydryls, and corticosteroids.

Since Erlanger and Gasser[19] demonstrated that normal dogs developed the typical shock syndrome after prolonged administration of epinephrine, attention has been focused upon the catecholamines epinephrine and norepinephrine as primary factors in the pathogenesis of shock. Excessive vasoconstriction and its direct sequelae continue to be a basic conceptual approach to shock. Many investigations have shown that the pattern of increased and decreased vascular reactivity characteristic of shock is manifested in large measure by altered responses to catecholamines.[66] These materials also have effects on many other tissue elements either directly or by synergistic vasoconstriction. The special role of catecholamines has been strongly supported by many studies which show that adrenergic blocking agents given to animals in shock improve cardiovascular dynamics, regional blood flow, and survival.[43]

As with the catecholamines, the significance of histamine in shock has been considered over the years. This amine lowers blood pressure, dilates small blood vessels, increases capillary permeability, and results in a lethal shock syndrome when administered in large amounts.[17] At one time, primarily from evidence of histological changes noted in the shocked subject, histamine was very seriously proposed as the single etiological substance of shock.[40] Very recently the histamine concept has received renewed impetus based on the postulate that endogenous histamine and catecholamines both act as a balanced dilator and constrictor regulatory mechanism of local blood flow.[48] In shock, presumably, the increased formation of histamine continues for a longer period than the increased secretion of the catecholamines, permitting its eventual domination of the microcirculation. The probable result is dilation and atony of small blood vessels, thus precipitating the onset of peripheral vascular failure. There are, however, serious factual inconsistencies[6, 7] in this relatively theoretical interpretation of the critical place of histamine in shock.

Information recently has become available on the biological effects of a group of polypeptides called kinins, particularly bradykinin. Bradykinin, among its other actions, causes generalized vasodilation, hypotension, and increased capillary permeability. Polypeptides including kinins result from proteolysis,[39] and the possible role of kinins has been postulated on the basis of studies of shock due to acute pancreatitis in which large amounts of proteolytic enzymes are released into the abdominal cavity and blood stream.[56] Kinins have been demonstrated in pancreatic shock and, conversely, proteolytic enzyme inhibitors can protect dogs against this form of shock. Bradykinin itself, however, when injected in large doses into a normal dog, will not produce shock. The participation of the kinins in the pathogenesis of shock remains a possibility, but at present there is insufficient evidence to establish this with reliability.

Another possible shock mechanism related to lysosomal enzyme release recently has been suggested. Lysosomes are subcellular particles containing many hydrolytic enzymes. It is postulated that the confinement of these enzymes within this subcellular structure protects the cell by preventing destructive enzymatic action to its cytoplasm. Cellular death can be the result of stimuli which disrupt their integrity and release their destructive enzymes. Several specific lysosomal enzymes were released from liver cells and could also be found in increased levels in the circulating blood and thoracic duct lymph in animals subjected to several types of experimental shock.[37] Furthermore, when animals were made more tolerant to shock, the levels of these lysosomal enzymes remained normal. While these findings have not been organized into a complete concept of shock pathogenesis, they do direct further attention to the importance of disturbances at a cellular level.

The role of altered tissue responses to metabolites released by the shock process comprises a large but poorly formulated and incomplete set of postulates relative to the pathogenesis of shock. The number of such metabolites which may be implicated is almost limitless. Many have been studied with particular emphasis on their discrete effects on tissue homeostasis and vascular reactivity.[66] None has been definitively shown to account for the irreversible phase of shock. The accumulation of metabolites in blood and tissues generally leads to a metabolic acidosis; unquestionably, the functional components and substances of many of the body's homeostatic mechanisms and organ systems are impaired when the pH of the environment is lowered. However, the question of which, if any, specfic homeostatic mechanism or mechanisms are either primary or contributory to the self-perpetuating shock progression remains unresolved.

BREAKDOWN OF ENDOGENOUS DEFENSE MECHANISMS

It is axiomatic that the organism as a whole is endowed with a large battery of defenses against stressful environmental situations of almost any type or severity, including shock. These defenses undoubtedly have phylogenetic origins reverting to evolutionary adaptation from the emergence of the simplest to the most complex animal species. Such defenses are present in almost all tissue systems of the complex mammalian organism. Extensive studies relating to producing experimental protection against shock have shown a significant relationship between the functional efficiency of certain protective mechanisms and tissue systems and the relative ability to withstand a shock episode.[33] Shock undoubtedly impairs many intrinsic defense mechanisms. A normal animal whose defenses are presumably unimpaired will safely tolerate a stress which is lethal to the animal in shock. The converse is also true in that an animal which has been previously adapted by experimental means will safely tolerate a stress which is highly lethal to a normal subject. In reconciling specific substances or tissue functions with the pathogenesis of shock, we are confronted with a major problem in assessing the importance of individual defense mechanisms. Is the microcirculatory failure the direct consequence of vasotoxic materials or are these materials effectors only because endogenous defense mechanisms are *already* impaired? The answer to this question is fundamental toward solving the problem of the definitive pathogenesis of shock. The question itself is unanswered, a fact which probably explains why so many concepts and theories of shock are continually being proposed. Many of these concepts focus on the primacy of the functional capacity of intrinsic defense mechanisms rather than on the biological effects of specfic materials and factors in the pathogenesis of shock. The body's mechanisms for protection consist of the reticuloendothelial system (RES),[65] the adrenocortical system,[50] the blood coagulation system,[28] and a group of antibacterial defenses[20] such as antibodies, γ-globulins, properdin, etc. Discrete protective functions of each of these adaptive systems frequently overlap into one or more of the other systems and complement each other.

Recticuloendothelial System. The reticuloendothelial system is the largest of the body's defenses, the greatest portion concentrated in the liver. Other RES elements are located in the spleen, lymph nodes, and bone marrow. Individual RES cells migrate continuously through all tissues, body cavities, and along the walls of blood vessels and ducts. The RES is frequently referred to as the "scavenger" or phagocytic system which cleans the blood and tissues of cellular debris and foreign particles, but it also is involved in a multitude of other important regulatory activities.[53] Damage to the liver in shock includes damage to its RES component, the Kupffer cells. Many pathological states such as adrenal insufficiency, severe infection, and shock are accompanied by a hypofunctional or depressed RES. Conditions of stress can hyperactivate the RES.[33]

The RES has been studied during experimental shock.[3, 4, 64] Its phagocytic capacity, measured by the rate at which known amounts of foreign colloids disappear from the blood, is the basis of quantitative evaluation. Experimental studies utilizing both the level of phagocytic capacity and survival rates of animals in shock demonstrate a positive relationship between the two. This relationship holds for various types of experimental shock and for most methods used to induce stimulation or depression of RES activity. On the whole, the experimental data dealing directly and indirectly with the functional state of the RES and the resistance of animals to shock strongly suggest an intimate association between this endogenous defense system and the course of events in shock.

Adrenocortical Systems. Selye[50] demonstrated many years ago that almost any significant stress resulted in an immediate discharge of epinephrine from the medulla and corticosteroids from the cortex. He believed this was an adaptive response providing the readjustment necessary to defend the organism against threatening changes in its environment. Animals with adrenal insufficiency, spontaneously or experimentally induced, succumb very readily to shock episodes which are well tolerated by normal animals. Yet there is no reliable evidence of adrenal exhaustion during shock.[29] Medullary secretion increases early in shock and remains elevated until death. Cortical secretion also is elevated early in shock but is reduced in the later stages of severe stress. Blood levels of these corticosteroids seem to remain high enough for maintenance of normal adrenal dependent organ functions.[55] Participation of the adrenals in shock seems more related to the specific physiological and pharmacological effects of the catecholamines and corticosteroids than through any complex adaptive role the adrenal cortical system may have in total homeostatic balance.

Blood Coagulation System. The changes in the coagulation system of the blood are major factors in the pathogenesis of shock. The alteration of blood coagulation deals with mechanisms which alter the fluid state of the blood, either through byproducts from damaged tissue or by hormones or hormone-like substances released into the circulation. The fluid state of the blood may be changed by factors which permit components of whole blood to leave the intravascular compartment or which induce changes in the components of whole blood itself.

Under normal circumstances, the intact endothelial lining of the blood vessels not only prevents the loss of formed elements from the blood but also serves to retain proper proportions of its fluid and plasma protein components. Normal endothelial surfaces do not stimulate coagulation. It is generally accepted that the coagulation process is initiated by contact of blood components with some intravascular surface (endothelium, blood cell, or platelet membrane) which has been altered physiologically or functionally[25] by several mechanisms including shock. Cells stick to each other and to the endothelial surfaces. Platelets and other formed cellular elements may rupture, releasing their contents and becoming intravascular debris. Enzymes may activate the conversion of fibrinogen to fibrin. The phenomenon of "sludged blood" has been described in several types of experimental shock.[38] Many of the small vessels become blocked by cell aggregates and debris, further curtailing blood flow. The net effect of these changes is widespread intravascular microthrombus

formation.[1, 16, 28] All of the available information indicates that shock and its attendant tissue blood flow favor an environment for bacterial growth. As a result, anticoagulant and fibrinolytic therapy is indicated in management of some types of shock.[47]

Antibacterial Defenses. In early studies of experimental shock, bacterial organisms were cultured from the blood and tissues of animals. This finding suggested that the shock process in some way altered the normal highly effective barriers to bacterial invasion.[20] However, the finding of bacteremia in experimental and clinical shock states was quite inconsistent and has not been confirmed in studies using rigid aseptic methods.[34] This does not preclude the passage into the blood of bacterial toxins. Certainly the intestinal lumen provides a prolific reservoir of bacterial products which must be either retained within the intestine or inactivated by defense mechanisms when small amounts pass into the blood or lymphatics. A recent concept of shock is based on the participation of bacterial endotoxins in the genesis of the irreversible aspects of the syndrome. Fine and co-workers[21] have postulated the bacterial (endotoxin) concept of shock as a breakdown of antibacterial defense mechanisms. They have supported this concept by demonstrating that the manner in which the shocked animal handled endotoxins closely parallels its tolerance to many types of stress. These data also indicate a relationship of bacterial endotoxins to catecholamine sensitivity, peripheral vascular disturbances, RES function, blood coagulation, and many other neurohumoral and cardiovascular homeostatic factors. However, inevitably, as with other earlier concepts, the bacterial concept based on endotoxins as the critical single element in the pathogenesis of shock could not satisfactorily explain many other well documented factors in the evolution of the syndrome.[67]

Among the studies on bacterial mechanisms in shock were many which indicated that the shocked dog, compared with the normal animal, could not clear the blood stream of injected live gram-negative bacteria.[20] These animals also showed decreased amounts of a naturally occurring blood protein, properdin, associated with normal nonspecific antibacterial plasma activity. Properdin studies suggest that the bacterial thesis might be specifically an expression of the disruption of antigen-antibody adaptive defense mechanisms.[45] Plasma properdin levels correlate well with the initiation of shock in experimental animals and also with the course either toward recovery or death.[23]

ENDOGENOUS AND EXOGENOUS TOXINS

It has always been intriguing to consider the possibility of a single toxic substance as being the specific key to the development and progression of the lethal shock syndrome. Toxic material could be of endogenous or exogenous origin, it could be represented by an excessive amount of a material normally present in the body, or it could be an abnormal product of disturbed metabolism. As might be expected, such a "catch-all" interpretation of toxicity has resulted in a group of poorly circumscribed concepts of shock as a toxic entity. It would seem, however, that in irreversible shock, almost any tissue or organ system, if carefully examined, can be found to contain or release substances which are actually or presumably "toxic" to tissues and blood vessels.[59] In addition to toxic factors already mentioned, others include products of intestinal digestion and decomposition, gram-positive bacterial exotoxins, adenosine compounds (adenosine triphosphate, adenosine diphosphate), nonbacterial polysaccharides, ammonia, nucleotides, coenzyme depleters, and cytotoxins. However, the element of toxicity does have a real basis in that the shock process, particularly in the dog, is manifested by marked tissue damage typical of that following exposure to frankly toxic chemicals. Such damage is evident grossly and microscopically in the intestine and liver and undoubtedly underlies the frequent use of the terms "gut" factor and "hepatic" factor in shock. While there is little need to re-emphasize the important role of the hepatointestinal tissue complex in shock, a brief comment relative to concepts of shock is appropriate. Based on hepatointestinal participation in the evolution of the shock syndrome, a sequence of events can be proposed. They include the initial cardiovascular reactions, the onset of microcirculatory insufficiency, and most of the "toxic" substances and tissue mechanisms which can presumably serve to sustain this insufficiency (Fig. 37.3). While this cannot pretend to delineate a unified theory of the pathogenesis of shock (since none really exists), it can offer a dynamic concept of the pathophysiology of the syndrome as a framework into which the multiplicity of shock factors can be fitted quite conveniently.

Treatment of Shock

There is a variety of opinions and principles relative to clinical management of shock. Therefore there is a wide assortment of drugs and other modalities which imply uncertainties as to which course of therapy should be followed in any single case.

The entire spectrum of therapeutic modalities, partially listed in Table 37.2, is only rarely applicable. This somewhat arbitrary approach is based on the point of view that our major concern is with severe shock and that this discussion of therapy should be confined to circumstances of the practitioner's usual role and to the use of dependable measures he can be expected to have at his disposal.

There are, of course, many different kinds of shock (Table 37.3) with different implications, not only as to pathogenesis, but also as to therapy. However, whatever differences and uncertainties exist, the disturbance to be treated is the failure to pump and deliver blood to essential capillary beds. In practical terms, clinically, we are dealing with a situation of too little blood in the arterial system because either the circulating blood volume is reduced, the pumping mechanism is inefficient, or the return of blood to the heart via the venous ystem is inadequate. Except in primary and serious cardiac dysfunction, the intrinsic capabilities of the heart hold up remarkably well. In the presence of a reasonably competent heart and a sustained blood volume, venous return of blood to the heart is adequate to maintain satisfactory overall cardiac function.[60] This

INFLUENCE OF ALTERATIONS OF FUNCTIONS OF LIVER AND BOWEL

ON THE COURSE OF THE SHOCK SYNDROME

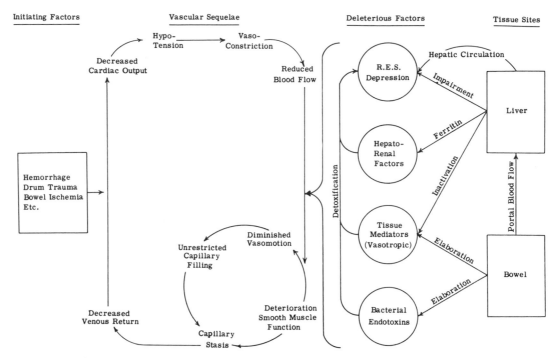

FIG. 37.3. Schema of the pathophysiology of the shock syndrome based on participation of the hepatointestinal tissue complex. (From Hershey, S. G.: Current theories of shock, Anesthesiology *21:* 303, 1960.)

makes it evident that blood volume expansion is the keystone to treating shock. Toxemia and sepsis, which have their major impact on the small peripheral vessels, may be somewhat of an exception to the foregoing statement, but only during early phases of toxemic or septic shock. In severe or protracted shock, a point is eventually reached at which blood volume expansion alone does not re-establish adequate perfusion of the peripheral vessels and maintain an adequate venous return. Blood and fluids infused into the circulation become pooled and do not actively circulate, leading to the classic phenomenon of "bleeding into the capillaries." This occurs because the terminal vascular bed has been damaged by impaired blood flow or toxic materials prior to the institution of blood volume expansion. This indicates that blood volume expansion alone has its limitations, and the management of shock

should also be concerned with the functional integrity of the peripheral circulation and tissue perfusion. Certain drugs and materials, because of some of their special properties, can favorably influence local tissue blood flow and tissue metabolic needs. Unfortunately, the therapeutic armamentarium available to accomplish these needs is rarely entirely dependable. Experience with these agents, however, does not attest to the potency of their corrective actions, their specificity, or complete reliability. The clinician is at a further disadvantage in that the state of local tissue blood flow is not as readily measured as the status of the systemic circulation (blood pressure, pulse, cardiac output, blood volume, hematocrit, etc.). It is therefore vital that therapy must be instituted early, before peripheral vascular failure is sufficiently developed to become refractory or irreversible.

TABLE 37.2

Treatment of shock

Blood volume expansion: whole blood, whole plasma, plasma protein solutions, dextrans, balanced salt solutions, normal saline, etc.

Drugs: vasopressors, vasodilators, corticosteroids, osmotic diuretics, digitalis, heparin, calcium, $NaHCO_3$, antibiotics, etc.

Ventilatory support: oxygen, assisted or controlled respiration, ventilators, etc.

Monitoring: blood pressure, central venous pressure, heart rate, electrocardiogram, hematocrit, temperature, pH, blood gases (O_2, CO_2), urine output, blood clotting, blood volume, cardiac output, ventilation, etc.

Postoperative: supporting and monitoring measures continue.

Miscellaneous: hypothermia, hyperbaric oxygen, warm blood, organic buffers (THAM), anticoagulants, teamwork, details, etc.

TABLE 37.3

Types of shock

Hemorrhagic
Septic—toxic
Radiation
Adrenal
Neurogenic
  Autonomic nervous system
  Central nervous system
Traumatic—wound
Burn—thermal
Anaphylactic
Cardiogenic
  Myocardial infarct
  Cardiac tamponade
  Congestive failure
"Combinations" of above, etc.

In the management of shock, there are a few initial precautions which must be observed. These are listed as follows.

a. Do not delay definitive therapy, surgical or otherwise, to correct the initiating cause. Shock is a progressive entity which, unlike many other disorders, is not self-limited, does not run a predictable or protracted time course, and does not appreciably remain at a fixed, unfluctuating level of severity. The development of irreversibility is time- and intensity-dependent. Management of the shocked animal must be approached with a real sense of urgency. Except in rare situations, operative intervention should not be delayed because of the physical condition of the animal, the need to await the results of laboratory tests, etc. Resuscitation therapy, laboratory evaluation, and corrective surgery should be concurrent and proceed with despatch.[27, 60] Surgery undertaken should be minimal and limited to such operative procedures which are necessary to remove initiating factors, stop hemorrhage, excise infected and devitalized tissues, immobilize fractures, etc.

b. Do not permit unnecessary physical movement of the animal. This implies minimal lifting and transport for purposes of physical examination, x-ray, etc. When movement is necessary, it should be deliberate and gentle. Keep the animal in the horizontal lateral position. A slight head down (10 to 15°) position may be of some benefit, aiding venous return by gravity. The shocked animal's compensatory cardiovascular and respiratory mechanisms are stretched to a precarious balance which is readily upset by stimuli which are of no consequence to a normal animal.

c. Do not administer routine preoperative medication. All narcotics, hypnotics, and analgesics in common use depress cardiovascular and respiratory function. Drugs commonly used as premedication also have many other actions which are undesirable in the stressed organism. The response to pain of the seriously shocked animal is minimal. The severely injured state is accompanied by cerebral depression. If the animal is restless and appears to struggle, the usual cause is hypoxia, which is best treated by giving oxygen and assisting ventilation, not by depressant drugs which further compromise respiration. The high level of circulating catecholamines and dehydration accompanying shock act to minimize secretions. Because of this, belladonna drugs such as atropine and scopolamine can be omitted. Atropine, through its vagolytic effects, may further increase an already accelerated heart rate to a level sufficiently rapid to further compromise cardiac output.

d. Do not subject the animal to deep anesthesia. All anesthetics are inherently toxic drugs differing from each other only as to degree of toxicity. Certainly the lightest level of anesthesia commensurate with the requirements of the surgical procedure should be maintained. Muscle relaxants are clearly superior to increased anesthetic levels to achieve necessary muscular relaxation. In regard to individual anesthetic agents, there is good experimental and clinical evidence to indicate that light levels of nitrous oxide (with at least 35% oxygen), cyclopropane, and halothane are the least deleterious to the shocked animal.[9, 68] Because of the depressed sensorium accompanying shock, analgesic concentrations of anesthetics are usually adequate for the immediate needs. Local analgesia can many times be used effectively. The shocked state is accompanied by a marked increase in response to anesthetics, a fact which must be kept in mind, as use of usual concentrations of anesthetics will readily produce excessive and dangerous levels of narcosis.

BLOOD VOLUME EXPANSION

It can be assumed that all subjects in shock are deficient in effective blood volume. The concept of normovolemic shock does not represent a realistic approach to therapy, even in most cases of septic shock. Loss of blood constituents in shock may not be proportionate to their normal content in whole blood, particularly in regard to relative losses of red cells and plasma. However, in acute shock, these relative losses, in terms of their replacement, are not a significant consideration. The principal consideration is volume replacement and the capabilities and limitations of whatever material is used to maintain volume over a reasonable period of time.

Whole Blood. Whole blood is a good volume expander. However, too vigorous and generous whole blood transfusions given rapidly can be detrimental.[60] Aside from the problems of securing blood for immediate use and the complications associated with detrimental changes in stored blood, there seems to be an inherent relationship between survival and the magnitude of total acute transfusion volume.[13] The sources of hazard in massive transfusions have been the subject of considerable study.[14, 36] There is rarely need to resort to immediate whole blood transfusion to restore circulatory hemodynamics.[60] A single exception is excessive hemorrhage which markedly reduces oxygen-carrying capacity so that the oxygen needs of the brain cannot be met. This becomes a factor when hemoglobin loss is more than 50%. If the blood is circulating and well oxygenated, something less than half the normal hemoglobin level is adequate to supply the needs of the brain. This is demonstrated daily by the pump oxygenators used in open heart surgery primed with nonhemoglobin-containing fluids. Also, subjects after recovery from profound shock very rarely exhibit signs of central nervous system damage from anemic hypoxia.

The use of whole blood in shock is certainly not contraindicated and is of critical importance when frank blood loss exceeds 2% or more of body weight. There is no need for acute replacement of blood loss on a volume for volume ratio. Staying a little "behind" in blood, in the range of 1 to 2% of body weight, is not a therapeutic compromise with maintenance of blood volume or physiological integrity of the peripheral circulation. To the contrary, in shock, a blood volume of low hematocrit and low viscosity has distinct advantages and could be a significant factor in reducing microthrombi and sludge formation.[10] The animal in shock contributes intrinsically to its own blood volume expansion by a process of hemodilution which draws fluids into the intravascular space from generous extravascular stores.[51] This process begins rapidly and can achieve a magnitude equivalent to approximately 15% of the normal circulating blood volume over a period of several hours in the dog. Such hemodilution, however, is not as rapid or as extensive as may often be needed either acutely or even later in the course of shock. This is the basis for the need for and use of whole blood and pharmaceutically available blood volume expanders.

Plasma. In practice, stored whole blood or a donor may not always be at hand at the moment of need, and blood plasma is an ideal expander. When prepared from outdated blood, frozen plasma can be stored for long periods without significant deterioration, making it practical to maintain a supply for emergency use in larger animal care centers. However, if such storage is longer than a few weeks, it does make the final plasma very similar to a solution of albumin in serum which is without blood coagulation proteins and which may be high in potassium content, although it does not appreciably affect its oncotic properties as on expander. With this consideration plus recognition of the fact that the veterinary surgeon cannot easily secure, maintain, or prepare properly processed, viral free, and aged supplies of plasma, it becomes necessary to consider other products for blood volume expansion. Fortunately there are excellent substitutes which are readily available and stable.[27] These are the commercially prepared colloids added to dextrose and water, normal saline, or balanced salt (lactate Ringer's) solutions.

Colloids. Although colloids such as the blood proteins albumin and globulin and dextrans are biological products, it is important to recognize that they are not normal biological materials. To the organism they represent "foreign" substances. Although they are effective expanders, they can be expected to have limitations related to their side effects. Proper use of colloids requires certain considerations. (a) They draw fluids into the active circulation from the tissue spaces which are already depleted by the shock process, a "robbing Peter to pay Paul" situation. Thus, if simultaneous attention is not given to replenishing these extravascular fluids and electrolytes along with expanding intravascular blood volume, the net effect could negate the very purpose of their use, the correction of tissue homeostasis. (b) As foreign materials, they can overwhelm the already taxed phagocytic and detoxification mechanisms of the body. (c) Injudicious use of colloid expanders can lead to uncontrollable hemorrhage and loss of other compensatory functions. Side effects can be prevented by limiting the total dose of colloid used, and tissue hydration can be accomplished by the administration of adequate volumes of intravenous fluid preparations.

Serum albumin (human) is available as a concentrated, sterile, highly stable preparation with 12.5 g/50 ml vial. It requires dilution to 5% concentration (1 vial/250 ml of solution) which is isosmotic with normal plasma. In terms of total dose, its margin of safety is in excess of 5 g/kg of body weight, a dose range (equivalent to 2 liters of infusion in a 20-kg dog) which is usually in excess of that routinely required. Plasma protein fraction is another protein preparation available for therapeutic use. It contains globulin (12%) in addition to albumin (88%) and is already diluted in 0.67% saline as a 5% solution. These protein solutions are probably the best volume expanders available for routine use from a combined viewpoint of practicality, effectiveness, and safety. Concentrated albumin has the advantage of permitting the use of diluents other than saline. This advantage is of some importance if there is need to limit the chloride ion and permit the use of balanced salt solution.

The dextrans are usually termed the best expanders because of overall considerations of their properties, low cost, and availability. They are certainly the best nonprotein colloid expanders in common use.

Dextran 40 has the singular advantage of having specific antiviscosity characteristics which favor its value above other colloids.[10]

There are three principal types of dextran which differ essentially in molecular size and, hence, in oncotic characteristics and capacity to remain within the vascular system. The smaller the molecular size, the more desirable are the antiviscosity properties and the greater are the safe total dose ranges, but the less is the ability to remain confined within the closed circulation without leakage through endothelial capillary surfaces.[24] Dextran preparations having a molecular weight in the 40,000 range are termed low molecular weight dextran (Rheomacrodex). The American dextran has an average molecular weight of 75,000. It has excellent oncotic properties and remains in the circulation to sustain the effects of its oncotic properties on circulating blood volume. Because of the larger molecular size, it loses its antiviscosity properties and, in fact, may increase viscosity, depending on the size distribution within the mixture. The larger molecules also reduce the safe dose level so that predisposition to blood clotting defects and reticuloendothelial system impairment are more apt to develop. British dextran, composed of colloid predominantly in the 150,000 size range, varies in its actions and safety according to the above considerations. All of the dextrans, after very long storage of several years, may lose much of their original oncotic and antiviscosity characteristics.

Rheomacrodex is isosmotic in 5% concentration, but is usually given in isotonic fluids (5% dextrose and water or normal saline) in 10 to 15% solution, a hyperosmotic concentration. It has a wide enough margin of safety in the range of 5 g/kg of body weight, so that the total dose usually required falls well within this safe margin. American dextran, usually administered as a 6 to 10% solution in isotonic fluid, must be used more cautiously if circulatory overload is to be avoided. A total of 500 ml of the 6% solution in the average 20-kg dog should rarely be exceeded.

Crystalloids in aqueous solution have been used in shock as immediate intravenous therapy for many years. These include various isotonic salt solutions and dextrose, singly or in combination. The value of balanced electrolyte solutions, commonly referred to as balanced salt solutions, has gained wide recognition in the management of shock.[41, 51] The basis for this form of fluid therapy derives from documentation of the reactions of the extravascular as well as the intravascular body fluid compartments as these respond to the stress imposed by shock. Since serious blood volume loss results in a signifi-

cant shift of fluid from the interstitial to the intravascular compartment (the phenomenon of spontaneous hemodilution previously described), the extravascular fluid must be replaced. These fluid movements are inevitably accompanied by electrolyte shifts of considerable magnitude, implying that serious electrolyte disturbances go hand in hand with alterations in body water distribution in pathological situations. The physiologically optimal blood volume expansion requires extravascular as well as intravascular fluid and electrolyte replacement. Ringer's or similar electrolyte solutions best satisfy this requirement. When the movement of fluids and electrolytes between compartments is of significant magnitude, it has been suggested that large amounts of chloride anion may seriously hinder favorable fluid redistribution, electrolyte balance, and renal function. Large amounts of sodium are apparently more efficiently handled, and because of this the Ringers'-like balanced salt solution has been modified for chemical use by substituting sodium lactate for much of the sodium chloride (lactated Ringer's solution). More recently, another form of balanced salt solution containing sodium acetate and sodium gluconate in place of lactate has become available.[22] Acetates have the advantage of being metabolized more easily during shock. It is also suggested that the acetate, because of its metabolic course, may be a more effective buffer and a more reliable source of bicarbonate than the lactate. This feature can help counteract the metabolic acidosis generally accepted to be one of the more serious derangements contributing to the progression of the shock syndrome. Balanced salt solutions in large volumes are widely utilized clinically, either alone or with 5% dextrose.

All animals in need of blood volume expansion in shock should receive generous volumes of balanced salt as early as possible. These should be continued along with other expanders. Because of its composition and mobility, these Ringer's solutions are immediately available to the intravascular, interstitial, and intracellular fluid compartments. They serve to replace fluids sequestered in traumatized tissues, to expand directly the circulating blood volume, to permit all of the concomitantly transfused blood to become the effective blood volume, and to decrease the hazard of tissue dehydration. There seems little doubt that lactated Ringer's solution or an equivalent balanced salt reduces the total volume of blood transfusion required to reestablish, stabilize, and sustain satisfactory cardiovascular function.[51] It may frequently eliminate the need for single small transfusions for borderline blood losses which cause modest hypotension and tachycardia. Balanced salt solutions should be administered generously and rapidly since the danger of acute circulatory overload and pulmonary edema is not significant. Most dogs readily tolerate a volume equivalent to 5% of their body weight (50 ml/kg) within a 1- to 2-hour period, the actual volume depending on the severity of the situation and on the character of the animal's response. Approximately 3 to 4 volumes of balanced salt should be administered for each volume of blood required. Following acute resuscitation, all intravenous fluid requirements can be safely and satisfactorily met by continued use of lactated Ringer's, probably in preference to other crystalloid solutions. As with other blood volume expanders, balanced salt solution should not be regarded as a complete substitute for judicious whole blood transfusion. However, these fluids should definitely be considered an ancillary therapy resource of major importance in the management of shock.

Vasoactive Drugs

Vasoactive drugs in shock refer to vasoconstrictor and vasodilator agents, the former exerting a pressor action on blood pressure, the latter inducing some degree of hypotension. Although pressor drugs have long been the bulwark of pharmacological support of circulation, in recent years their value has been seriously questioned. The rationale of the use of vasoactive drugs currently represents one of the most vigorously contested areas in shock therapy.

Many of the demonstrated or inferred undesirable effects of vasopressors are attenuated or reversed by vasodilator drugs, and since the vasodilators also attenuate comparable endogenous, spontaneous vascular reactions to shock, these drugs have been advocated in shock therapy. In considering this aspect of shock therapy, it is difficult to separate the virtues and disadvantages of these diametrically opposite forms of therapy. Despite many categorical and arbitrary attitudes on this subject, the basic position of vasopressors and vasodilators in therapy is quite unresolved.

Enough is known about shock to derive a reasonably valid attitude toward vasoactive drug therapy based on the dynamics of the syndrome. These dynamics clearly spell out the rationale role of vasoconstrictors and vasodilators to be dependent on their net effects on tissue blood flow through the microcirculation. Admittedly, blood flow, blood volume, and blood pathway relationships through the capillary beds are extremely complex. However, in terms of these drugs, we are dealing primarily with their effects on blood pressure and changes in vascular resistance in the periphery—the major factors determining tissue blood flow. All of the mechanisms regulating the level of the blood pressure and the degree of vascular resistance in the three major divisions of the circulatory system—the heart, large vessels, and capillary beds—need not be reviewed here except to indicate that the quality of tissue perfusion at any given moment results from a dynamic balance of the mechanisms regulating pressure with those determining resistance. Blood flow in any given set of vessels is increased as pressure increases or as resistance decreases. Opposite directional changes in pressure and resistance have the reverse effect on flow. The interplay between pressure and resistance changes due to drugs, either dilator or constrictor, is therefore the basic determinant of their value in shock therapy. For example, an increase in peripheral resistance produced by a vasopressor sufficient to negate the influence of increased blood pressure on resultant blood flow is undesirable. Similarly a decrease in resistance in the face of an excessive fall in pressure can be even more acutely disastrous if the hypotension is due to cardiovascular collapse. Since vasopressor drugs in common use increase blood pressure primarily by increasing resistance in most vascular beds, and since vasodilators result in generalized vasodilation with the potential of acute hypotension, a problem arises as to their ultimate influence on cardiovascular hemodynamics and on tissue perfusion.

VASOPRESSOR DRUGS

The basis for evaluating the effects of vasoexcitor pressor agents in shock stems from a very extensive research and clinical experience with the large group of pressor amine drugs of which norepinephrine, phenylephrine, and metaraminol are probably the most commonly used representatives. The polypeptide angiotensin can be considered similar to the amines in its applications in shock. The vasopressor drugs, in principle, can favorably influence tissue perfusion via their actions on the circulatory system. They produce vasoconstriction of the arterioles to raise blood pressure, some have an inotropic effect on the heart to improve cardiac function, and they stimulate the venomotor mechanisms to increase venous return. Unfortunately this principle is not achieved with the pressor drugs in common use.[43] The major indictment of the constrictors is that their potential benefits toward improved overall cardiovascular function and tissue flow are negated by the intense, occlusive type of vasoconstriction at the arteriolar and venular levels. This, despite other favorable cardiovascular actions, results in reduced blood flow to the capillary beds. The resultant tissue ischemia, in time, exaggerates, rather than corrects, the essential shock defect.

It does not follow, as has often been inferred, that pressor drugs have no place in the treatment of shock.[58] They are widely used clinically but, unfortunately, not always wisely. These drugs are no substitute for blood volume expansion and other longer acting corrective measures. They can be used for limited periods to correct or avert acute systemic cardiovascular collapse and, in this way, buy the time necessary to improve cardiovascular function by more compatible means. There is a distinct negative relationship between the duration of pressor therapy and survival. Relatively few subjects on long-term (several days) therapy ultimately survive, even after cardiogenic shock, where these agents still have their widest clinical use. Yet the practitioner should not hesitate to administer a pressor drug *as an immediate measure* to correct serious hypotension from shock. Uncorrected hypotension and its impending hemodynamic collapse can result in death long before the peripheral vascular tissue lesion can progress to an irreversible stage.

When drugs are used to raise blood pressure, they must be administered carefully under constant attention. There is no need to revert blood pressure levels to normal. A range of 10 to 30 mm Hg below initial levels is adequate for acute needs. Pressors are rapidly acting, potent drugs and are best administered well diluted by intravenous drip technique which should be carefully regulated to avoid wide fluctuations in blood pressure. The return of blood pressure to more favorable levels is no indication to relax intense efforts to administer more stable forms of therapy to correct the existing causes of shock. Tachyphylaxis is an inherent property of the pressor amines, and the acidosis accompanying shock further reduces their effectiveness. Unless the underlying need for their temporary use is eliminated, progressively increasing doses of pressors are required to maintain their initial effects on blood pressure. Following prolonged use, hypotension will occur when they are subsequently discontinued. It is well to keep in mind that prolonged administration of large doses of catecholamines to a normal dog will result in a classic type of shock very similar to that following severe hemorrhage.[19]

Studies of vasoactive drugs other than the pressor amines have demonstrated actions which are more selective than those of the catecholamines on the microcirculation.[32] A group of experimental synthetic analogues of the polypeptide posterior pituitary hormones do seem to have promise in the treatment of shock.[5]

VASODILATOR DRUGS

The rationale for advocating vasodilator drugs in shock is based on two related areas of study and experience. Many of the vasomotor responses to stress, while permitting immediate survival of the vital triad of organs—the brain, heart and lungs—accomplish this urgent readjustment at the expense of other organs of less critical importance. With time, if this intense vasoconstriction is sustained because the initiating circumstances remain uncorrected, the relatively deprived organs develop changes which ultimately become incompatible with survival of the organism as a whole. This intrinsic response mediated by the increased release of catecholamines can be of sufficient magnitude to produce tissue ischcmia.[43] Drug-induced vasodilation by adrenergic blockage does increase peripheral blood supply and correct the intrinsic shock response.

The use of pressor drugs to maintain systemic blood pressure has generally proven inadequate to promote other than immediate survival in severe shock unless blood volume expansion and other means of therapy are introduced.

While a number of vasodilator drugs have been evaluated in shock, most experience is based on phenoxybenzamine[43] and chlorpromazine,[31] which are primarily adrenolytic in character, and on thiophanium camsylate,[35] which is ganglionic blocking. Phenoxybenzamine, which is long acting (18 to 36 hours) and still classified as an experimental drug, is by far the most versatile and effective of any of the vasodilators studied and is the basis for this consideration of the place of vasodilator drugs in shock. In addition to its adrenolytic effects, phenoxybenzamine has many other pharmacological properties involving other organs and metabolic functions, implying that the complete profile of the influence of this drug in shock is still incompletely formulated. It is very likely, however, that some of these other properties may be quite significant.

Most of the favorable data with phenoxybenzamine is from studies on dogs in which the drug is administered as pretreatment. The evidence based on its use after the onset of shock is much less extensive and much less uniform.[18] It appears that, to induce its fully beneficial influence, phenoxybenzamine (Dibenzylene) must be present in the tissues for at least several hours. When used in the existing shock situation, there is a substantial incidence of profound hypotension and abrupt cardiovascular collapse. This is particularly true when the full dose of 1 mg/kg is administered fairly rapidly in the presence of a reduced blood volume. Phenoxybenzaamine-induced hypotension cannot be effectively reversed with pressor amines, the actions of which it specifically blocks. However, if the drug is preceded by generous blood volume expansion which is continued during the slow intravenous administration of dibenzyline over a 1-hour period, the incidence of marked hypotension can be quite readily controlled. There is no doubt that following its injection in this manner, the various parameters of cardiovascular function improve impressively, even in situations where these responses have previously been minimal despite vigorous use of all other means of therapy. However, ultimate survival with the use of phenoxybenzamine in existing shock is not nearly as predictable or frequent as when this drug is used before the onset of shock, where its effectiveness is highly predictable and quite remarkable.

CORTICOSTEROIDS

In recent years, it has been accepted that corticosteroids will reduce the severity of reactions in which tissue hypersensitivity from almost any cause may result in injury to cells. Steroids are used very widely in an empirical fashion for numerous conditions involving hypersensitivity reactions.[54] As related to the shock disturbance, several of the numerous pharmacological effects of the corticosteroids seemingly do have discrete and valid purpose: (a) they restore normal patterns of response to catecholamines; (b) they protect tissues from damage by maintaining cell membrane integrity and stabilizing intracellular lysosomes which house hydrolytic and proteolytic enzymes; (c) they increase cardiac output possibly via an inotropic action; and

(d) they may possibly reduce peripheral vascular resistance slightly. In addition, steroids also have a regulatory influence on fluid-electrolyte homeostasis which could be beneficial in various stress situations. Of these pharmacological actions, it is probable that the cellular and cardiovascular inotropic effects represent its major assets in shock.

Steroid therapy in shock is not intended as replacement therapy to correct depressed adrenal cortical function. As mentioned earlier, spontaneous adrenal function is well sustained in shock, resulting in elevated steroid levels. The objective is to expose the tissues to a much higher level of steroids than can normally be secreted by the adrenal gland in either the normal or shocked animals. These "pharmacological" doses, in contradistinction to "physiological" or maintenance doses, are literally enormous considering the brief time interval over which they are given. The steroids should be administered as early in shock as possible and sustained throughout the acute episode. Steroid therapy should rarely exceed 48 hours, as any beneficial effects from its initial use will not likely continue beyond this period. These high doses given over a brief period may be abruptly discontinued without the usual precautions for tapering off the use of steroids, as when they are administered chronically for other medical indications.

While there are many structural analogues and modifications of the steroid molecule available as pharmaceutical preparations, the water-soluble hydrocortisone succinate or phosphate preparations are most suitable. These preparations should be given intravenously by continuous drip or as repeated single doses at intervals. An initial dose of 25 mg for a 15- to 25-kg dog, repeated in 30 minutes to 1 hour and hourly thereafter, should be administered until the animal's response or lack of response is established by clinical signs of improvement (stabilized blood pressure, adequate response to blood volume expansion, etc.). Much larger doses, 50 to 100 mg/kg at shorter intervals during the first 60 to 90 minutes, have been recommended and can be used safely. In fact, for acute administration in stress situations, the steroids seemingly have no significant dose-dependent side effects in these very massive doses. They are also compatible with simultaneous use of most other drugs and agents. Following the onset of clinical improvement or when the corrective surgery is terminated, treatment with steroids is usually continued at a dose level of 50 to 100 mg (15- to 25-kg dog) every 4 to 6 hours until the subject is clearly recovered from shock or it is apparent that the drug is not effective. For this subsequent period of steroid therapy, prednisolone or methyl prednisolone may be substituted for the hydrocortisone and given at one-half the dose range.

It is probably in order to employ hydrocortisone therapy almost routinely in septic shock and also in animals in other types of shock when their pre-existing physical status is poor because of chronic infection debilitation, malnutrition, etc. However, in shock due to other than sepsis, particularly in shock developing during operation, hydrocortisone is usually reserved for animals not responding satisfactorily to more conventional resuscitative measures.

OSMOTIC DIURETICS

In severe shock, there is a reduction in renal blood flow. This reduction in renal perfusion and the accompanying loss of the kidney's autoregulation of its own blood flow lead to oliguria and anuria. The basis of resuscitative therapy is to improve peripheral blood flow to all tissues including the kidneys. Renal function as measured by the formation of satisfactory urine volume and content is aided by nonspecific supportive circulatory measures, some of which can have specific diuretic effects: dextran, alkalizing agents, balanced salt, and vasodilators. However, if the period of renal ischemia is sufficiently intense and prolonged, the damage to the renal tubules and the accumulation of nephrotoxic by-products of injury or transfusion may be extensive enough to lead to the lethal postshock syndrome of tubular necrosis and anuria.[46] To reduce the likelihood of such acute renal failure and to maintain urinary function, many investigators and clinicians recommend that osmotic diuretics be used. Osmotic diuresis can also be initiated following shock states accompanied by significant oliguria or anuria, particularly with a rising blood urea nitrogen. Diuretics which act by suppression of renal tubular function are potentially hazardous in the already impaired nephron, i.e., mercurials and chlorothiazide. Nontoxic crystalloid osmotic diuretics, urea or mannitol, can be used even after severe acute renal ischemic injury without fear of further tubular toxic damage. Mannitol is an inert hexose which is filtered by the glomeruli but is not reabsorbed by the tubules. It creates a high osmotic pressure within the lumen of the renal tubular system and inhibits the reabsorbtion of the glomerular filtrate maintaining tubular irrigation and urine excretion. It is commonly used to establish and maintain adequate urinary output.[46] There is some evidence that mannitol also increases renal blood flow and decreases renal vascular resistance, both of which predispose to improved renal function. Because the diuretic effect of mannitol promotes water loss, it is essential that the animal be well hydrated prior to and during its administration. This drug also creates an obligatory sodium loss which must be balanced by appropriate electrolyte therapy. It should be administered intravenously with an indwelling urethral catheter in place, both to evaluate urinary flow and to prevent overdistension of the bladder. The dose range is variable depending upon the severity and duration of urinary response after the initial onset of mannitol administration. Only the smallest quantity of drug necessary to initiate and maintain reasonably satisfactory urine flow should be used. The initial test dose should be approximately 0.1 g/kg given over a 5- to 10-minute interval administered as a 5 to 20% solution. If the dog responds with a urinary output of approximately 10 ml of urine per hour for the subsequent 2 to 3 hours, the continued use of mannitol is indicated. The average 24-hour total dose may vary from 10 to 50 g in the average 20-kg dog. However, the 50-g dose should rarely be exceeded for fear of increasing organic renal damage, cardiac insufficiency, convulsions, or hyponatremia, all of which are potential complications of large doses of mannitol.

BUFFERS: CORRECTION OF ACIDOSIS

The development of acidosis is a cardinal feature of the shock syndrome. A tissue environment of lower than normal pH creates a broad spectrum of homeostatic alterations involving not only many metabolic and enzymatic activities but also functional changes in virtually every tissue and organ system—cardiac contractility and rhythm, vascular response to catecholamines and other vasoactive mediators, renal and hepatic function, neurohumoral regulation of respiration, etc. Although the specific role of acidosis in the development of irreversibility is not clearly established, it is generally recognized that its correction is logical and deserves attention in the treatment of shock. Most clinicians associate the danger of acidosis principally with its undesirable cardiac effects which can predispose to ventricular fibrillation or cardiac arrest.[57]

The primary etiological source of acidosis is the anaerobic metabolism generated in the tissues by tissue hypoxia. The major acidotic component is a metabolic acidosis which eventually exhausts the body's buffer systems for maintenance of normal blood and tissue pH. Other factors also contribute to the severity of acidosis in shock. Hypoventilation with retention of carbon dioxide is a common consequence of shock and can easily be further aggravated by anesthetic and depressant drugs. Such inadequate carbon dioxide excretion via the lungs leads to a respiratory acidosis which further reduces available buffer base. The fall in body temperature commonly accompanying shock or the hyperthemia frequently seen when infection is present both contribute to metabolic acidosis. Another significant contributor toward acidosis is blood, especially when large quantities are administered with the usual acid citrate dextrose as the anticoagulant. Each 250-ml unit of even freshly banked or prepared blood may have a pH as low as 6.6 and an acid content calculated at 3 to 4 mEq.[36] This acid load can become substantial and important when massive transfusion is required.

The buffers used affect pH changes only in the circulating blood and interstitial space and have no direct effect at the cellular level. It is at this level that the acidotic state is generated and at which the lowered pH probably has its principal impact in the development of irreversibility. Empirically, this form of therapy seems warranted in two general circumstances: (a) where shock is severe and protracted without seeming to respond despite vigorous and apparently adequate resuscitative therapy; and (b) where massive transfusions totaling more than the animal's normal blood volume are required.

For purposes of therapy, sodium bicarbonate is available in stable sterile solution containing 3.75 g (44.6 mEq)/50-ml ampule. One-half of this amount every 45 to 60 minutes can be safely given as a single dose intravenously and should increase bicarbonate blood level significantly. If warranted, several times this dose can be used, as there is little chance for serious alkalosis. Pulmonary excretion of CO_2 can prevent cumulative pH effects. Tris buffer or 2-amino-2-hydroxymethyl-1,3-propanediol (THAM), an organic substance, is another buffer available.[42] It is a hydrogen acceptor which can enter the cell to reduce intracellular hydrogen ions. THAM corrects both intracellular and extracellular pH by forming compounds with carbonic and other acids of metabolic origin. Its action differs from $NaHCO_2$ also in that the salts it forms are excreted by the kidneys so that its buffering effect is independent of alveolar exchange. This drug also produces an osmotic diuresis. THAM is highly alkaline and should be administered slowly intravenously in amounts only sufficient to correct the existing degree of acidosis. Overdose may also cause hyperkalemia and prolonged severe hypoglycemia. Its safe use to secure its full buffering advantages requires electrocardiogram, blood glucose, and serum potassium monitoring.[57] A 0.3 M solution in sterile water (36 g/liter) is recommended as the most satisfactory dilution for the lyophilized powdered form in which THAM is commercially packaged. Specific doses can be calculated correctly only on the basis of laboratory determination of the existing base deficit according to the following empirical formula: milliliters in 0.3 M solution required = body weight (kilograms) $\times$ base deficit (milliequivalents per liter). One of the standard nomograms (Singer and Hastings, Anderson and Engel, etc.) should be used to calculate base deficit from blood gas and pH values. Because of the precision with which THAM must be administered, its use will probably be limited for the present to clinics where needed instrumentation and technical help are available.

VENTILATORY SUPPORT

There is little evidence that the administration of high concentrations of oxygen to the animal in shock significantly improves the chances of ultimate survival. With satisfactory ventilatory exchange, the oxygen content of room air at atmospheric pressure provides adequate hemoglobin saturation of the arterial blood. However, indicating that the need for high concentrations of respired oxygen is not critical should in no way be confused with the critical need for adequate ventilation. Deficient ventilation and its attendant hypo-oxygenation is a serious factor contributing to the unfavorable course of shock.[10] Impaired respiratory function is more common than is generally appreciated and may easily be overlooked in the urgency to deal with other more obvious problems. Decreased ventilation may be due to many factors commonly associated with shock: (a) airway obstruction from secretions, aspirated blood, or gastric contents; (b) splinting of ventilatory muscles from painful incisions or injuries of the chest and abdomen, or from peritonitis; (c) unstable chest from multiple rib fractures; (d) skull and brain injuries which depress the central nervous system; (e) anesthetic and depressant drugs; (f) physical fatigue; (g) bronchospasm; and (h) profound shock itself. All of these conditions and more can produce hypoxia and respiratory acidosis from CO_2 retention which, in turn, will lead to myocardial depression and serious aggravation of any existing metabolic acidosis.

As a first step, the patency of the animal's airway must be determined and reliably established if there is any evidence of impairment. This may require nothing more than positioning of the head, neck, or tongue or clearing the pharynx of any secretions or vomitus. On the other hand, endotracheal intubation or tracheostomy may be required to establish and maintain the airway or to permit adequate cleansing of the tracheobronchial tree. Satisfactory gas exchange may occasionally require relief of pneumothorax or hemothorax or stabilization of a flail chest. In the presence of spontaneous respiration, even though the airway is entirely satisfactory, the development of cyanosis, increasing tachycardia, or agitation suggest the existence of hypoxia from hypoventilation. Even a very mild degree of hypoxia, which is well tolerated by normal animals for surprisingly long intervals, can be deleterious to the animal in shock. It is usual to employ higher than atmospheric oxygen concentrations which increase blood oxygen tensions.

Recently the use of oxygen under greater than atmospheric pressure (hyperbaric oxygen) has been recommended in the treatment of severe shock.[12] This method of oxygen administration increases the oxygen available to the tissues not by increasing the saturation of hemoglobin but by greatly increasing the oxygen dissolved in the plasma. Oxygen supplied at a pressure of 3 atm absolute, when saturated with water vapor, equals 2233 mm Hg. The plasma under this oxygen tension will contain sufficient oxygen to supply the needs of the tissues.

MISCELLANEOUS SUPPORTIVE MEASURES

The clinical practice of observing the clinical course of an animal and performing a variety of measurements and tests with or without the aid of mechanical or electrical instruments is not therapeutic *per se*.

However, such monitoring clearly offers the most important information to guide both the diagnostic evaluation of a case and the best approach to therapy. Routine observations should be done, such as observing color of the mucous membranes, heart rate, blood pressure, body temperature, respiration, urine output, electrocardiogram, and hematocrit. Where more extensive equipment and personnel are available, other parameters such as blood gas analysis, pH determinations, blood coagulability, blood volume, cardiac output, and ventilatory measurements can be undertaken. Most monitoring devices, however, even those which are extremely sophisticated, have been very disappointing in terms of their providing accurate indices either of the progression of the syndrome or of the ultimate outcome. These devices have added only little to the value of the information gained by simple observation of color, blood pressure, heart rate, and urine output. Continuous measurement of the central venous pressure probably provides the best "on-line" information about the animal relative to the severity of the shock and the quality of its response to therapy.[61]

The measurement of central venous pressure (CVP) is technically simple, rapidly accomplished, and accurate. Disposable sterile kits, through which fluid infusion and blood transfusion can be simultaneously accomplished, are commercially available for continuous monitoring of CVP. These kits contain full instructions for proper setting up of CVP measurement. The singular importance of the CVP is based on the fact that clinically, no single aspect of therapy is more essential to survival than the maintenance of an optimal blood volume. Functionally effective blood volume is quite reliably reflected by the level of the CVP except in situations where myocardial insufficiency or increased pulmonary vascular resistance may occur, both in late shock or with pre-existent cardiac or pulmonary disease. When CVP is low (below 6 to 8 cm H_2O), blood volume expansion is indicated. A rising CVP which is sustained at levels up to 8 to 10 cm H_2O

indicates a good response to replacement therapy. Central venous pressures rising to or above approximately 15 cm H_2O indicates either fluid overloading of the circulation or the development of myocardial insufficiency. The latter is almost the only situation in which a rapidly acting digitalis preparation is indicated in shock. When cardiac insufficiency is present in the animal in shock, the CVP can guide the rate and amount of blood and fluid replacement with less danger of overloading the weakened myocardium.

Hypothermia has been recommended by many investigators and clinicians in the management of shock.[11] This subject is considered elsewhere in this text and need not be detailed here. The rationale for its use is based on the reduction in the tissue oxygen requirements of the hypothermic animal. However, clinical and laboratory experience in the use of hypothermia in shock is clearly equivocal and essentially unimpressive. Certainly the cardiovascular and metabolic effects of hypothermia, particularly profound hypothermia, would not seem favorable to the shocked subject. Lowered body temperature does little more than delay the progression of the syndrome, and with rewarming, the sequence is not critically altered. Here, as with hyperbaric oxygenation, the most consistently favorable results have been in cases of septic or bacteremic shock.[11] In this type of shock, mild hypothermia may provide an interval for the effective use of antibiotics.

Any outline of the management of shock would be seriously incomplete if mention were not made of two additional aspects which are important to the successful resuscitation of the seriously shocked animal. Painstaking and constant attention to detail is invariably essential to optimal results. Whatever procedures or drugs are indicated, their use must be accomplished as precisely and completely as possible at the time most appropriate to the indications for their use. One can draw the analogy of comparing the difference between the final result achieved by a fine chef and a poor cook, both of who may use identical ingredients and equipment. Sup-

porting and monitoring measures, so carefully organized during the acute phase of treatment, should continue without relaxation for as long as necessary afterward. Too often, once the tense urgency of the situation has passed, the recently resuscitated and still very sick patient is entrusted to the care of less experienced aides and assistants or placed in a recovery cage only to be "looked in on" from time to time. Practical experience makes it painfully clear that the immediate recovery period, which may last several days, is highly unstable after a serious shock episode.

It has been a relatively simple matter to review the means and basis for treating the animal in shock. However, it is by no means so simple to recapitulate such therapy in a few brief statements and recommendations as a short, all-inclusive guide. In fact, as stated at the outset, such a recipe for clinical care defies practicality and validity except in the most general terms already mentioned. Undoubtedly the best approach to the management of any case must be individualized on the basis of a previously acquired background of theoretical, experimental, and, particularly, practical information. This allows for accurate evaluation of what is happening and for rational and flexible application of combinations of drugs, fluids, and procedures.

REFERENCES

1. Allen, J. G., and Glotzer, D. J.: Acute disseminated intravascular coagulation and fibrinolysis. Arch. Surg. (Chicago) 88: 694, 1964.
2. Altura, B. M.: Evaluation of neurohumoral substances in local regulation of blood flow. Amer. J. Physiol. 212: 1447, 1967.
3. Altura, B. M., and Hershey, S. G.: Use of reticuloendothelial phagocytic function as an index in shock therapy. Bull. N.Y. Acad. Med. 43: 259, 1967.
4. Altura, B. M., and Hershey, S. G.: RES phagocytic function in trauma and adaptation to experimental shock. Amer. J. Physiol. 215: 1414, 1968.
5. Altura, B. M., and Hershey, S. G.: Pharmacology of neurohypophyseal hormones and their synthetic analogues in the terminal vascular bed: structure-activity relationships. Angiology 18: 428, 1967.
6. Altura, B. M., and Zweifach, B. W.: Pharmacologic properties of antihistamines in relation to

vascular reactivity. Amer. J. Physiol. *209:* 550, 1965.

7. Altura, B. M., and Zweifach, B. W.: Endogenous histamine formation and vascular reactivity. Amer. J. Physiol. *212:* 559, 1967.

8. Baez, S., Hershey, S. G., and Rovenstine, E. A.: Vasotropic substances in blood in intestinal ischemia shock. Amer. J. Physiol. *200:* 1245, 1961.

9. Baez, S., and Orkin, L. R.: Microcirculatory effects of anesthesia in shock. In *Shock*, edited by S. G. Hershey, p. 207. Little, Brown and Company, Boston, 1964.

10. Baker, R. J., Shoemaker, W. C., Suzuki, F., Freeark, R. J., and Strohl, E. L.: Low molecular weight dextran in surgical shock. Arch. Surg. (Chicago) *89:* 373, 1964.

11. Blair, E., Cowley, R. A., Mansberger, A. R., and Buxton, R. W.: Physiologic rationale for hypothermia in septic shock. Surg. Forum *13:* 20, 1962.

12. Blair, E., Ollodart, R., Esmond, W. G., Attar, S., and Cowley, R. A.: Effect of hyperbaric oxygenation (OHP) on bacteremic shock. Circulation (suppl.) *29:* 135, 1964.

13. Boyan, C. P., and Howland, W. S.: Problems related to massive blood transfusions. Anesth. Analg. (Cleveland) *41:* 497, 1962.

14. Boyan, C. P., and Howland, W. S.: Cardiac arrest and the temperature of bank blood. J. A. M. A. *183:* 58, 1963.

15. Crile, G. W.: *An Experimental Approach into Surgical Shock*. J. B. Lippincott Company, Philadelphia, 1899.

16. Crowell, J. W., and Read, W. L.: In-vivo coagulation—a probable cause of irreversible shock. Amer. J. Physiol. *183:* 565, 1955.

17. Dale, H. H.: Conditions which are conducive to the production of shock by histamine. Brit. J. Exp. Path. *1:* 103, 1920.

18. Eckenhoff, J. E., and Cooperman, L. H.: The clinical application of phenoxybenzamine in shock and vasoconstrictive states. Surg. Gynec. Obstet. *121:* 483, 1965.

19. Erlanger, J., and Gasser, H. S.: Studies in secondary traumatic shock; circulatory failure due to adrenaline. Amer. J. Physiol. *49:* 345, 1919.

20. Fine, J.: *The Bacterial Factor in Traumatic Shock*. Charles C Thomas, Publisher, Springfield, Ill., 1954.

21. Fine, J., Frank, E. D., Ravin, H. A., Rutenburg, S. H., and Schweinberg, F. B.: The bacterial factor in traumatic shock. New Eng. J. Med. *260:* 214, 1959.

22. Fox, C. L., Jr., Winfield, J. M., Slobody, L. B., Swindler, C. M., and Lattimer, J. K.: Electrolyte solution approximating plasma concentrations. J. A. M. A. *148:* 827, 1952.

23. Frank, E. D., Fine, J., and Pillemer, L.: Serum properdin levels in hemorrhagic shock. Proc. Soc. Exp. Biol. Med. *89:* 223, 1955.

24. Gelin, L. E., and Shoemaker, W. C.: Hepatic blood flow and microcirculatory alterations induced by dextrans of high and low viscosity. Surgery *49:* 713, 1961.

25. Guest, M. M.: Circulatory effects of blood clotting, fibrinolysis, and related hemostatic processes. In *Handbook of Physiology*, edited by W. F. Hamilton and P. Dow, Section 2: Circulation, vol. III, p. 2209. The Williams & Wilkins Company, Baltimore, 1965.

26. Guyton, A. C., and Crowell, J. W.: Cardiac deterioration in shock. 1. Its progressive nature. In *Shock*, edited by S. G. Hershey, p. 1. Little, Brown and Company, Boston, 1964.

27. Hamit, H. F.: Current trends of therapy and research in shock. Surg. Gynec. Obstet. *120:* 835, 1965.

28. Hardaway, R. M., Brune, W. N., Geever, E. F., Burns, J. W., and Mock, H. P.: Studies on the role of intravascular coagulation in irreversible hemorrhagic shock. Ann. Surg. *155:* 241, 1962.

29. Hershey, S. G.: Current theories of shock. Anesthesiology *21:* 303, 1960.

30. Hershey, S. G.: Dynamics of peripheral vascular collapse in shock. In *Shock*, edited by S. G. Hershey, p. 27. Little, Brown and Company, Boston, 1964.

31. Hershey, S. G., Guccione, I., and Zweifach, B. W.: Beneficial action of pretreatment with chlorpromazine on survival following graded hemorrhage in the rat. Surg. Gynec. Obstet. *101:* 431, 1955.

32. Hershey, S. G., Mazzia, V. D. B., Altura, B. M., and Gyure, L.: Effects of vasopressors on the microcirculation and on survival in hemorrhagic shock. Anesthesiology *26:* 179, 1965.

33. Hershey, S. G., and Zweifach, B. W.: Adaptation: the key to the problem in shock. Canad. Anaesth. Soc. J. *8:* 529, 1961.

34. Hershey, S. G., Zweifach, B. W., and Antopol, W.: Factors associated with protection against experimental shock. Anesthesiology *17:* 265, 1956.

35. Hopkins, R. W., and Simeone, F. A.: Tremethaphan camsylate in hemorrhagic shock. Arch. Surg. (Chicago) *89:* 365, 1964.

36. Howland, W. S., Schweizer, O., and Boyan, P.: The effect of buffering on the mortality of massive blood replacement. Surg. Gynec. Obstet. *121:* 77, 1965.

37. Janoff, A.: Alterations in lysosomes (intracellular enzymes) during shock; effects of preconditioning (tolerance) and protective drugs. In *Shock*, edited by S. G. Hershey, p. 93. Little, Brown and Company, Boston, 1964.

38. Knisely, M. H.: An annotated bibliography on sludged blood. Postgrad. Med. *10:* 15, 1951.

39. Lewis, G. P.: Active polypeptides derived from plasma proteins. Physiol. Rev. *40:* 647, 1960.

40. Moon, V. H.: *Shock and Related Capillary Phenomena*. Oxford University Press, New York, 1938.

41. Moyer, C. A., Margraf, H. W., and Monafo, W. W., Jr.: Burn shock and extravascular sodium deficiency-treatment with Ringer's solution

with lactate. Arch. Surg. (Chicago) *90:* 799, 1965.

42. Nahas, G. G.: The pharmacology of tris(hydroxymethyl)aminomethane (THAM). Pharmacol. Rev. *14:* 447, 1962.

43. Nickerson, M.: Vasoconstriction and vasodilation in shock. In *Shock*, edited by S. G. Hershey, p. 227. Little, Brown and Company, Boston, 1964.

44. Page, I. H.: Some neurohumoral and endocrine aspects of shock. Fed. Proc. *20:* (suppl. 9) 75, 1961.

45. Pillemer, L., Blum, L., Lepow, I. H., Ross, O. A., Todd, E. W., and Wordlaw, A. C.: The properdin system and immunity. I. Demonstration and isolation of a new serum protein properdin, and its role in immune phenomena. Science *120:* 279, 1954.

46. Powers, S. R., Jr.: Relation of acute tubular necrosis to shock and the effect of mannitol. Amer. J. Surg. *110:* 330, 1965.

47. Salzman, E. W., and Britten, A.: *Hemorrhage and Thrombosis. A Practical Clinical Guide*, p. 114. Little, Brown and Company, Boston, 1965.

48. Schayer, R. W.: Evidence that induced histamine is an intrinsic regulator of the microcirculatory system. Amer. J. Physiol. *202:* 66, 1962.

49. Selkurt, E. E.: Role of liver and toxic factors in shock. In *Shock*, edited by S. G. Hershey, p. 43. Little, Brown and Company, Boston, 1964.

50. Selye, H.: *The Physiology and Pathology of Exposure to Stress*. Acta Inc., Montreal, Medical Publishers, 1950.

51. Shires, T., Coln, D., Carrico, J., and Lightfoot, S.: Fluid therapy in hemorrhagic shock. Arch. Surg. (Chicago) *88:* 688, 1964.

52. Shorr, E., Zweifach, B. W., Furchgott, R. F., and Baez, S.: Hepato-renal factors in circulatory homeostasis. IV. Tissue origins of the vasotropic principles, VEM and VDM, which appear during evolution of hemorrhagic and tourniquet shock. Circulation *3:* 43, 1951.

53. Smith, J. J.: The role of the reticuloendothelial system in shock. In *Shock and Hypotension*, edited by L. C. Mills and J. H. Moyer, p. 327. Grune & Stratton, Inc., New York, 1965.

54. Spink, W. W.: Adrenocortical steroids in management of selected patients with infectious diseases. Ann. Intern. Med. *53:* 1, 1960.

55. Swingle, W. W., and Reminton, J. W.: The role of the adrenal cortex in physiological processes. Physiol. Rev. *24:* 89, 1944.

56. Thal, A. P., and Sardesai, U. M.: Shock and the circulating polypeptides. Amer. J. Surg. *110:* 308, 1965.

57. Thrower, W. B., Darby, T. D., and Aldinger, E. E.: Acid-base derangements and myocardial contractility; effects as a complication of shock. Arch. Surg. (Chicago) *82:* 1961.

58. Weil, M. H.: Current concepts on the management of shock. Circulation *16:* 1097, 1957.

59. Wiggers, C. J.: *Physiology of Shock*, p. 380. Oxford University Press, London, 1950.

60. Wilson, J. N.: The management of acute circulatory failure. Surg. Clin. N. Amer. *43:* 469, 1963.

61. Wilson, J. N., Grow, J. B., Demong, C. V., Prevedel, A. E., and Owens, J. D.: Central venous pressure in optimal blood volume maintenance. Arch. Surg. (Chicago) *85:* 563, 1962.

62. Zweifach, B. W.: *Functional Behavior of the Microcirculation*, p. 13. Charles C Thomas, Publisher, Springfield, Ill., 1961.

63. Zweifach, B. W.: Microcirculatory derangements as a basis for the lethal manifestations of experimental shock. Brit. J. Anaesth. *30:* 466, 1958.

64. Zweifach, B. W.: The contribution of the reticuloendothelial system to the development of tolerance to experimental shock. Ann. N.Y. Acad. Sci. *88:* 203, 1960.

65. Zweifach, B. W.: Relation of the reticulo-endothelial system to natural and acquired resistance in shock. In *Shock*, edited by S. G. Hershey, p. 113. Little, Brown and Company, Boston, 1964.

66. Zweifach, B. W.: Tissue mediators in the genesis of experimental shock. J. A. M. A. *181:* 866, 1962.

67. Zweifach, B. W.: Hemorrhagic shock in germ free rats. Ann. N.Y. Acad. Sci. *78:* 315, 1959.

68. Zweifach, B. W., Hershey, S. G., Rovenstine, E. A., Lee, R. E., and Chambers, R.: Anesthetic agents as factors in circulatory reactions induced by hemorrhage. Surgery *18:* 48, 1945.

38
Hypothermia

EMIL BLAIR

In the homeothermic mammals, low body temperature can be produced by deliberate induction of hypothermia under controlled circumstances or can result from so-called "accidental" conditions. In 1862, cold narcosis (25 C) of degree sufficient to permit surgery was demonstrated by Walther.[13] This was confirmed and extended by Bakamat'ev in 1902, who observed that a state of poikilothermy could be produced in warm blooded hypothermic animals.[1] During the next 40 years, which has been called "the golden era of physiology," hypothermia served as a tool for the study of basic biological mechanisms. Modern emphasis on hypothermia in the homeotherm is largely the result of its potential in therapy of human ills, especially in cardiovascular surgery. In the 1940's and early 1950's, a number of workers demonstrated that during hypothermia the circulation could be stopped for prolonged periods of time.[3]

Accidental cooling must have existed from the time that the homeotherm emerged from the more primitive poikilothermic species. The unintentional drop of body temperature in the homeotherm can occur following prolonged exposure to a cold environment or due to direct injury or impairment of the thermoregulating mechanism. A common occurrence in animals is the reduction of body temperature as a result of pharmacological depression of thermoregulation, especially by general anesthetics.

Hypothermia is defined in homeotherms as the reduction of body temperature below 35 C. Confusion exists concerning the exact state of hypothermia because of a variety of definitions, the modifying influences of anesthetics, and the quantitative alteration of effects at different temperature levels. Artificial hibernation, a term popular in Europe, is not applicable to the homeothermic animal. Only a hibernator which normally hibernates in the winter can be induced into artificial hibernation during the summer. Artificially induced hibernation in the hibernator is not identical with the physiological state which normally occurs in the winter. Suspended animation has incited popular fancy because of its potentials in space exploration and in prolongation of life. With the current state of knowledge of hypothermia, the attainment of this condition is not possible, except in a restricted regional sense. The production of the poikilothermic state in a homeotherm is perhaps the nearest simulation to the conditions which exist in a natural poikilotherm. This does not mimic completely the reactions of the natural poikilotherm to changing environmental temperatures.

Induced cooling does not yield a true naked state of hypothermia. The thermoregulatory mechanisms usually must be suppressed by anesthetic agents. Since general anesthetics and related drugs exert specific alterations not unlike those seen with hypothermia, a more appropriate term would be "modified hypothermia." In accidental cooling, true hypothermia may exist. Physiologically, this is a stress or fatigue type of hypothermia, and in the higher homeotherms usually is fatal.

Classification of Hypothermia

The range of hypothermia which can be induced in the warm blooded animal with surivival is anywhere from 35 to near 0 C. Since physiological changes occur during progressive cooling, it becomes necessary to speak in terms not just of hypothermia, but of a particular level. The deeper the temperature, the greater the risk; the greater the cooling, the more exacting the control of homeostasis that is required. Also, the permissible hypothermic time is inversely proportional to the depth of cooling and directly related to the level of homeothermic development in a given species.

The depression of organ function generally is exponential within the range of 35 to 20 C. Beyond this level, continued reduction in organ activity is dictated by inert mass physical laws during surface cooling and perfusion rate during extracorporeal cooling. A classification based upon degree of physiological change (Levels I to VI) appears in Figure 38.1. The augmented level (32 C) is manifested by increased central nervous reactivity which does not occur under deep anesthesia. Homeostasis is unimpaired. At the next level, moderate hypothermia (30 to 28 C), homeostasis is unimpaired, but ventilation is depressed.

Metabolic requirements are about 50% of normal.

The next level, moderately deep hypothermia (25 C), represents the first significant departure from normal. Homeostatic mechanisms are compromised, and hypotension, ventilatory depression, and inhibition of reflexes occur. At this level control of ventilation and circulation is essential, and the hazard of ventricular fibrillation exists. Deep hypothermia (20 C) is characterized by marked restriction of homeostatic mechanisms with extracorporeal circulation necessary as a rule. There is serious depression of the central nervous system and its regulatory mechanisms at this level with a complete abolition of many of these systems during the profound level (10 C). Profound hypothermia may be maintained only by extracorporeal circulation. Perfusion is continued above and beyond the anticipated metabolic needs, based upon calculated oxygen requirements. Supercooling (below 0 C) has been achieved experimentally but reanimation is extremely difficult.

The levels for use of clinical hypothermia include the augmented and the moderate. The augmented level may be employed without resorting to special support of the animal. The moderate level of 30 to 28 C is the most commonly used for surgical procedures. These levels are permissible only in the operating room and under rigid control. The other levels of hypothermia have been generally abandoned except for profound hypothermia, which is currently under investigation in neurosurgical problems. Research procedures utilize all levels of hypothermia including supercooling. It is emphasized that beyond the augmented level of cooling, control ventilation by artificial means is absolutely essential.

Temperature Regulation

The homeothermic or warm blooded animal maintains the body temperature within rather narrow limits regardless of environmental change. The regulation is precise and is affected by a complex neurohumoral mechanism. Homeothermy does

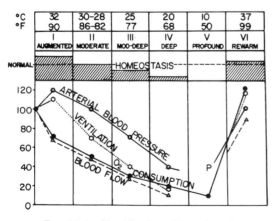

FIG. 38.1. Classification of hypothermia.

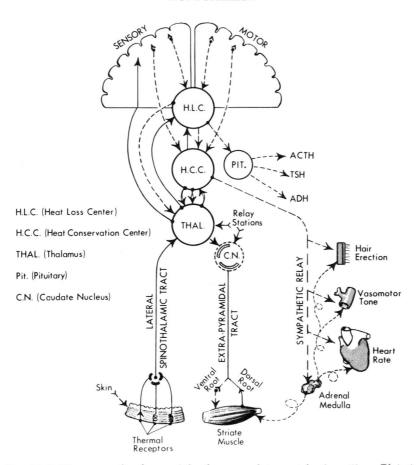

FIG. 38.2. Diagrammatic scheme of the thermoregulatory mechanism. (From Blair.[4])

not imply absolute control in the strictest sense, since rats and mice react to temperature change in a quantitatively different fashion, tolerating cold far better than monkeys, dogs, or cats.

Thermostatic regulation is accomplished by a negative feedback type receptor-effector module operating through a complex integrating system, capable of instantaneously controlled graded response. A diagrammatic scheme of the circuits is shown in Figure 38.2. Signals are sparked from receptors* in the skin, mucous membrane, and from detectors in the hypothalamus.[10]

* Peripheral receptors conventionally are termed Krause (cold) or Ruffini (warm). It is preferable not to consider these as divided groups of distinct structures, since the only differences between them is quantitative.

Cooling stimulates the peripheral receptors maximally, while fewer are activated by a warming environment. Changes in thermal gradients are the key to activation of receptor circuits rather than absolute temperatures. The central detectors are activated by temperature changes of blood perfusing the hypothalamus. Thus the thermoregulating machinery may be set into motion by local or central stimuli. Signals are integrated at all levels of the central nervous system, with rough adjustments below the cervical spinal cord level and finer changes by the reticular formation in the brain. The hypothalamus is the main coordinating mechanism with two anatomically delineated sectors. A heat dissipation center is located in the anterior preoptic and supraoptic nuclei, and a heat production and conservation center is located in the posterolateral area. All thermoregulatory effectors are initiated and controlled by the central nervous system through reciprocal inhibition and facilitation in a quantitative graded fashion.

The effectors are divided into physical and chemical components, the physical being the more important.[5] Signals from the surface thermoreceptors and the central thermodetectors induce thermal panting when there is danger of overheating. In the dog, cortical mechanisms also contribute to panting when the environmental temperature rises. Cutaneous blood flow is altered to accelerate heat loss and is in response to local factors. This constitutes a significant aspect of the physical segment of temperature regulation. The increase in cutaneous blood flow is accompanied by converse changes in striated muscles and in other organs. Increased salivation and piloerection similarly constitute local responses which may be further augmented by central signals. Shivering, consisting of phasic skeletal muscle contractions, does not participate in the normal regulation of temperature and is called into play only when there is a serious danger of a fall in deep body temperature. Active thermogenesis of a significant magnitude can be induced only from central signals which initiate from detectors in the hypothalamus. It has been demonstrated that local signals also may result in accentuated skeletal muscle activity. A maximal response of skeletal muscular activity will increase oxygen consumption 5-fold.

The chemical or hormonal component is concerned only with heat production. It consists of the adrenal glands, the thyroid gland, and the neuroeffector response. Cooling of the skin results in an elevation of circulating catecholamines, and thyroid activity is accelerated during the period of stress induced by exposure to cold. Body water movements are of particular importance although quantitative analysis has not yet been possible.

External cooling initiated via signals from peripheral receptors produces a reflex vasoconstriction which further lowers skin temperature. A positive feedback system is then developed which theoretically, if carried to excess, results in almost a complete abolition of flow to the skin. This does not occur, since reflex dilation ensues, increasing blood flow to the skin. The net result of this increased flow is an acceleration of heat loss. Cooled peripheral blood transmitted to the hypothalamus results in a reduction of the hypothalamic temperatures, stimulating the central temperature detectors. Suppression of activity at the level of the hypothalamus results in a failure of the thermal effector systems to respond to the cold stress. A decrease in body temperature occurs.

Reduction of central or core temperature from increased latent heat loss takes place by evaporation, convection, radiation, and conduction. In the animal evaporation is accomplished by panting. Convection assumes a significant role during attempts to induce lowering of body temperature by surface contact techniques. This physical activity consists of a transfer of energy by means of air or water molecules which collide with the body surface becoming heated and then transmitting the heat externally to the environment. All mammals have what is known as a private climate which consists of a thin covering of air or water which seems to cling to the skin. In order to assure maximal efficiency of convection, it is necessary to maintain a constant flow of air or water. Cooling with water is more effective than with air, since its specific heat is greater. Heat transfer is diminished by reduction in peripheral blood flow resulting in increased tissue insulation. It is also diminished by the shunting of blood from superficial to deep tissues and by an increase in temperature gradient between the skin and the core.

Heat production is markedly inhibited by hypoxia and hypercarbia. During cold, excessive catecholamine outflow occurs with a preponderance of noradrenaline. This contributes to nonshivering thermogenesis.

It has been demonstrated generally that animals can withstand a fall of 10 C better than a rise of 6 C. Thermoregulatory mechanisms may be affected by a number of situations. If central temperature falls below 28 C, the thermoregulatory mechanisms are impaired, and below 20 C they fail completely. Trauma or any injury to the hypothalamic area results in impairment of thermoregulation. During surgical anesthesia, the body temperature of dogs often drifts to 32 C in an average time of 5 hours (Fig. 38.3).

Anesthesia and Hypothermia

There are essentially four components to anesthesia: (a) loss of consciousness; (b) loss of sensory response; (c) depressing of motor activity; and (d) loss of reflex response.

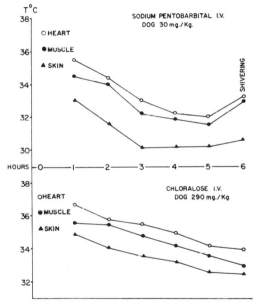

FIG. 38.3. Accidental hypothermia during the course of "normal" anesthesia.

The early phases of cooling stimulate some central nervous system functions, causing an "excitement" state (Table 38.1). This excitement common to cooling and to the early stages of anesthesia becomes more profound with combined anesthesia and hypothermia than with either state alone.[12] This dual modality operates as a positive feedback system and is potentially dangerous because of the failure of recognition of the magnitude of physiological depression. On the other hand, hypothermia permits a greater tolerance to adverse effects of drug intoxication and hypoxia at the deep levels of anesthesia.

General anesthesia is required to depress the thermoregulatory effectors galvanized by cold and to increase skin perfusion. As cooling supervenes and the trembling thermal controls diminish, anesthetic concentrations are decreased. The reduction required must be considered in terms of the physical effects on volatile agents and inactivation of intravenous anesthetic agents at lower temperatures. With declining temperatures volatile gas distribution between air and blood increases,[6] tissue desaturation of volatile agents is slowed, and hepatic conjugation of intravenous drugs is blocked. The net result is a cumulative effect of a given agent.

Table 38.1 shows the general effects of hypothermia and anesthesia at varying temperature levels. In general, the significant depressant effects of anesthetics at normal temperatures bear physiological analogy to those induced by hypothermia at 28 to 25 C. At this level cold narcosis is sufficient for surgical procedures. The combination of anesthesia and hypo-

TABLE 38.1
Relation of anesthesia to hypothermia

Method	Temperature	Consciousness	Reflex	Motor	Sensory
	°C				
Anesthesia	37	Depressed	Depressed	Depressed	Depressed
Hypothermia	37-32	Stimulated or unchanged	Stimulated	Stimulated	Slightly depressed
Hypothermia	28	Depressed	Depressed	Depressed	Depressed
Anesthesia + hypothermia	35-32	Depressed	Depressed	Depressed	Depressed

thermia produces a particular response at a lower level of anesthetic and a more moderate level of hypothermia. The effects of general anesthetics and their relationship to hypothermia with respect to organ function and systems regulation are listed in Table 38.2. All of the anesthetic agents used exert some degree of direct effect upon the central thermoregulation. The reduction of core temperature to 32 C does not depress thermoregulation but stimulates it. Most of the general anesthetics induce skeletal muscle relaxation which contributes to reduction in heat production. Exceptions to this are nitrous oxide, ethylene, and ultrashort acting barbiturates. Urethane is not a good muscle relaxant but in large dosages does impair skeletal muscle tone.

The muscle relaxants are particularly important in the production of hypothermia by the surface technique. The safest are those with a rapid onset and short duration. The agent of choice is succinylcholine chloride, and the least desirable is decamethonium or d-tubocurarine. The rapid fall in plasma level following an injection of a single dose is due to distribution throughout the body fluids and tissues and not to inactivation. For example, about one-half of d-tubocurarine which is injected can be held in extravascular compartments. Coupled with hypothermia, particularly below 28 C, a marked prolongation in recovery occurs with enhancement of dangers of hypoxia because of depressed ventilation. d-Tubocurarine is removed by renal excretion. Succinylcholine, however, is detoxified primarily by enzyme hydrolysis. Impairment is not significantly depressed except below 20 C.

Volatile agents are eliminated by the lungs, and serious effects of hypothermia and anesthesia are not encountered except below 20 to 25 C. However, if ventilation is supported and oxygenation is maintained properly, no significant problem arises. The conventional signs used for delineation of stages of anesthesia once the animal is cooled are entirely unreliable. The depth is usually lower than expected. The anesthetic concentration should be progres-

TABLE 38.2

Principal direct effects* of anesthesia and ancillary agents and relation to hypothermia

Agent	Activity of Organs and Systems								
	Thermo-regula-tion	Cere-bral	Skeletal muscle	Oxygen consump-tion	Skin per-fusion	Respi-ration	Car-diac	Renal	Hepatic
Hypothermia									
35-32 C	E	E	E	D	D	E	N	N	N
30-28 C	D	D	N, D	D	I	D	N	D	D
25 C	D	D	D	D	I	D	D	D	D
Nitrous oxide	D	D	N	N, D	I	N, D	N	N	N
Ethylene	D	D	N	D	I	N, D	N	N	N
Cyclopropane	D	D	D	D	I	D	N	D	N
Ether	D	D	D	D	I	N	D	D	D
Chloroform	D	D	D	D	I	D	D	D	D
Fluothane	D	D	D	D	I	D	D	N	D
Barbiturates									
Long acting	D	D	D	N	I	D	D	N	N, D
Intermediate	D	D	D	N	I	D	D	N	N, D
Short acting	D	D	D	D	I	D	D	N	D
Ultrashort	D	D	N	D	I	D	D	N	D
Urethane	D	D	N	N	N	N	N	N	N
Chloralose	D	D	D	N	I	N	N	N	N

* Surgical anesthesia, no anoxia; E, exicted; N, normal; D, depressed; I, increased.

TABLE 38.3
Accidental hypothermia

Type	Mechanism	Features	Prognosis
Cold exhaustion	TRM* active early, depressed late. Heat loss > heat production.	Yukon syndrome; severe stress; metabolic exhaustion due to marked shivering.	Poor
Trauma	TRM depressed early. Brain stem damage.	Often preceded by hypothermia. No shivering.	Poor
Pharmacological	TRM depressed by anesthetics, opiates, and ataractics. Skeletal muscle depressed by neuromuscular block.	Often not detected. Affects young most often. Recovery from anesthesia prolonged.	Good
Sepsis	TRM depressed. Debility weakens skeletal muscle activity. Reduced flow from shock.	Late in course. Sign of irreversibility.	Poor, unless infection and shock are controlled.

* TRM, thermoregulatory mechanisms.

sively reduced as temperature drops and shivering is controlled with muscle relaxants. Cooling delays the desaturation of tissues when attempting to lighten the anesthetic level. Ventilation should be supported at all times even prior to cooling and during the rewarming period, and intravenous agents should be used in smaller than the estimated dosage.

All agents except urethane and muscle relaxants exert a central effect on thermoregulation. Metabolism is unaffected by phenothiazines and muscle relaxants, but by virtue of inhibition on skeletal muscle activity, oxygen uptake is reduced.

The lytic cocktail, a combination of chlorpromazine, Demerol, and Benadryl, has been used in Europe for the production of hypothermia. There is blockage of the sympathetic nervous system and the suppression of central thermoregulation. The fall in temperature is minimal (2 to 3 C) and standard techniques must be used to obtain deeper levels.

Accidental Hypothermia

Four causes of accidental hypothermia can be considered (Table 38.3): cold exhaustion, trauma, pharmacological agents, and sepsis. Depression of central thermoregulatory mechanisms is common to all. Following exposure to extreme cold, thermoregulatory mechanisms first are active, and finally are depressed as cooling and exhaustion supervenes. Trauma with brain stem damage, resulting in early depression of thermoregulatory mechanisms, may induce hypothermia. Frequently, fall in body temperature is preceded by hyperthermia. The prognosis in both of these groups is poor.

Pharmacological agents, particularly anesthetics, opiates, and ataractics, constitute the most common and easily manageable problems. They produce central depression of the thermoregulatory mechanisms, which will vary somewhat in degree depending upon the drug used. Neuromuscular blocking agents have peripheral effect on skeletal muscles preventing shivering. Newborns are affected much more critically by drug-induced hypothermia than older animals because of relatively immature thermoregulation.

Management of Accidental Cooling

Excessive premedication may directly impair thermoregulation. Since all agents depress the central thermoregulatory mechanisms to some extent, the additive effect of heavy sedation and anesthesia is an important consideration in the selection of drugs. Excessive dosage and prolonged anesthetic periods result in serious depressions of core temperature.

A comfortable environment is essential for both the animal and for the operating team. Air-conditioning with rapid turnover of room air is not contraindicated, but it may produce an environment which will result in lowering of body temperature. The operating table should be equipped with a rewarming pad (electric or circulating fluid type), so that the animal's temperature fall, especially during thoracic and prolonged surgery, can be controlled by the appropriate use of warming.

Anesthesia should be lightened rapidly following surgery to permit recovery of reflexes controlling heat production. Should the hypothermic state persist upon conclusion of the surgical procedure, active rewarming should be instituted. When shivering begins, active rewarming is discontinued. With such agents as barbiturates, the depth of anesthesia cannot be controlled, active rewarming is maintained, and the ventilation is continually supported. Neuromuscular relaxant antagonists should be administered if curare has been used. Following a protracted period of anesthesia and a rather traumatic surgical experience, the animal may lapse into a narcosis after an initial arousal. Such individuals should be kept in a warm environment, and, if not shivering, the animal should be reintubated, ventilated, and actively rewarmed.

The harmful effects of a temperature drop during anesthesia are minimal if the anesthetic period is short, the surgery trivial, and ventilation well maintained during the procedure. If temperature drops are ignored during extensive surgery when major cavities are open, viscera are exposed and cold blood is administered; the excessive cooling that can occur will be additive to the depressant effects of general anesthesia. The primary problems are respiratory acidosis, circulatory insufficiency, and ventricular fibrillation. Cooling potentiates the depressive effects of anesthetics so that the level of anesthesia is deeper than suspected.

A general format for the prevention and management of accidental hypothermia is as follows. (a) Record temperature prior to the induction of anesthesia. (b) Record core temperature during anesthesia. (c) Isolate animal from steel top table by the use of cotton drapes. Place heating pad between cotton drapes, or use a thermostat blanket if excessive temperature drops are anticipated. (d) Begin anesthesia only when everyone is ready. (e) Maintain lightest level of anesthesia compatible with surgical requirements. (f) Intubate and maintain adequate ventilation. (g) When controlling ventilation, avoid excessive hyperventilation. This promotes cooling, especially in cats and small dogs. (h) If the core drops to 36 C, begin rewarming and maintain at 38 to 37 C. (i) Do not suppress shivering unless it impedes the surgical procedure. (j) Keep trauma and blood loss at a minimum. (k) Warm cold blood to body temperature during its infusion, especially in smaller animals and if large amounts are administered. (l) Postsurgically maintain animal in warm environment. (m) Promote rewarming by not suppressing shivering or movement and conserving body heat by the use of blankets. (n) If recovery is prolonged, reintubate the trachea and support ventilation. Actively heat the environment, but avoid direct contact of heating elements with the skin, unless they are maintained at physiological temperatures.

Temperature Gradients

There are three thermal zones in the homeotherm: the superficial zone consisting of skin and subcutaneous tissues; the intermediate zone, which is primarily skeletal muscle; and the core, consisting of the body viscera. The core temperature is usually designated as rectal or as esophageal temperature. The mechanisms in thermoregulation are geared toward the maintenance of the core temperature within narrow limits. Gradients exist between the deeper zones, the superficial zone, and the external environment. The superficial zone temperature is 2 to 4 C lower than core temperatures. This gradient varies considerably depending upon external environmental temperatures; cold induces an increase in temperature differentials and warmth a narrowing of these gradients. Temperature alterations of the superficial zone are primarily a function of the skin and subcutaneous tissue blood flow. In furry animals, piloerection augments those changes. The intermediate zone temperature is somewhere between the superficial and the deep, generally 1 C lower than the core. This temperature also is dictated by blood flow through the muscle masses. The regulating temperature of mammalian homeothermy is the core temperature and in most species is between 37 and 38 C. This is not a constant temperature, but fluctuates from 1 to 2 C depending upon the animal species and upon a given metabolic state. The temperatures of the various zones in the dog are listed in Figure 38.4.

The key to the development of hypothermia, accidental or elective, is the core temperature. To accelerate latent heat loss and cool the core, alterations of the temperatures of the superficial and intermediate zones are required. The inhibition of heat production is also important and is accomplished by controlling active thermogenesis. Thermogenesis is never completely abolished, and as long as there is life, there is some metabolism with heat production.

The body of a warm blooded animal is essentially a heat exchanger in which blood serves as the essential transport mechanism for the conduction of heat. The manner in which thermogradients are altered varies with the method for inducing hypothermia —surface contact or blood stream cooling. Figure 38.5 shows the alterations in temperatures in the dog cooled by the surface exposure method.

During surface cooling, the superficial zone temperature drops precipitously from around 35 C to nearly that of the coolant. The initial cutaneous response to surface cooling is vasoconstriction, which is a local response. This retards core cooling and creates a marked increase in core-superficial zone gradients. Subsequent cutaneous vasodilation results in an increase in blood flow to the cutaneous beds with accelerated heat loss. There is a graded rate of change between the three zones, the superficial zone having the most rapid drop in temperature. Upon removal of the animal from the cold environment, the skin and the skeletal muscle temperatures begin to rise. The core temperature continues to fall. This has been termed the "after-fall," generally averaging 2 C. This drift is the result of a number of factors: rate of cooling, extent of impairment of the central mechanisms, body surface area, lean body mass, vasomotion, ambient temperature, humidity, and the core-skin gradient. As long as a sizeable gradient exists, blood from within is cooled further at the pe-

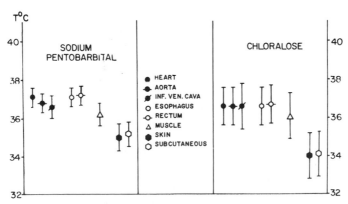

Fig. 38.4. Temperatures of the three zones in the dog. Note the wider variability with chloralose compared to pentobarbital.

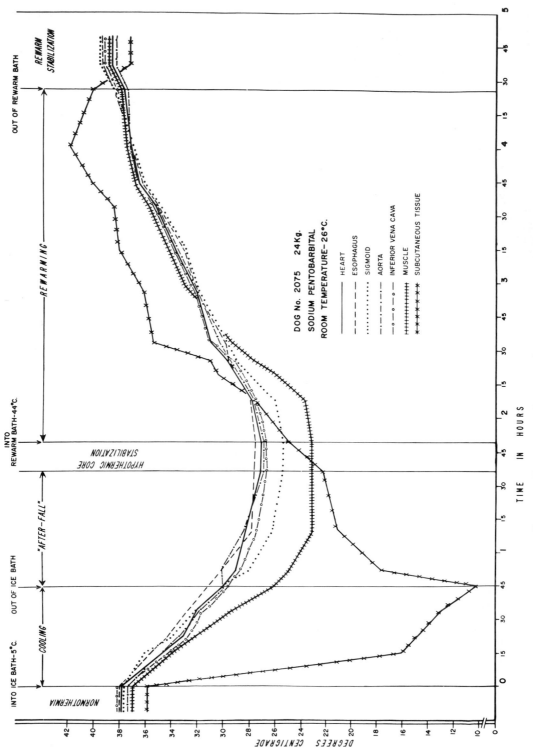

Fig. 38.5. Temperature changes with surface cooling in the dog.

riphery and returns to lower the core temperature. The rate of the "after-fall" slows as skin temperatures rise.

The core temperature becomes stabilized at its lowest point in about 30 minutes, but the superficial and intermediate temperatures continue to rise. Four hours after core stabilization, no appreciable gradient exists between the core and the skin (Fig. 38.6). At this point, the animal enters a state resembling poikilothermy, and the core temperature fluctuates with the environment. Upon rewarming, the reverse happens with a positive gradient developing between the core, the superficial, and intermediate zones. The magnitude of these gradients is less when the rewarming medium is maintained at less than 42 C. This avoids the potentially harmful effects of overheating. The superficial zone first returns to normal temperature and then rises above this point. The result is an increased blood flow to peripheral structures. This occurs at a time when cardiac output is low because of lower core temperatures. The net result of these changes is the development of a circulatory insufficiency which may prove detrimental if allowed to continue too long.

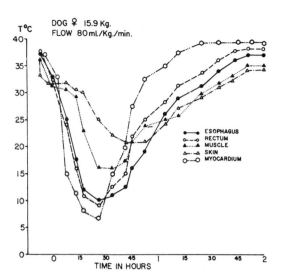

FIG. 38.7. Temperature changes with intravascular cooling. The core becomes cold before the peripheral zones. There are also more sizeable gradients between the various core organs compared with those in surface contact cooling.

At a core temperature of 33 to 32 C, artificial warming is stopped and full resuscitation is achieved by the animal's own heating mechanisms which have become activated at this level.

A different set of circumstances develops when hypothermia and rewarming are induced by intravascular techniques. In this instance, the heart is cooled first and subsequently the muscle and skin. The gradients therefore are reversed. This is illustrated in Figure 38.7. Core temperatures can be rapidly reduced and easily maintained. With this method, the intermediate and superficial zone temperatures cannot be controlled. Core temperatures will rise unless continuously perfused because of the relative warmth of intermediate and superficial zone temperatures. Maintenance of hypothermia, particularly at deeper levels, is permissible for relatively brief periods of time. The rewarming period is prolonged because of the limitation of the temperature of the circulating fluid to 42 C. High temperatures damage red blood cells, which increases hemolysis. When normal core temperatures have been reached, perfusion must be maintained for 15 to 30 minutes to restabilize normal gradients. If

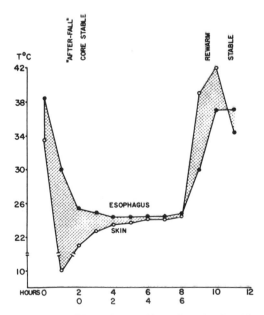

FIG. 38.6. After 4 hours of hypothermia, the skin-core gradient is negligible and the animal enters a state of poikilothermy.

perfusion is stopped when the core reaches its normal temperature, it will drop again due to the colder external zones.

Metabolism

The greatest fall in oxygen uptake occurs between 37 and 30 C. From this point to approximately 22 to 20 C, the fall is approximately exponential. Below this, the rate of decline begins to level considerably. Metabolism continues as long as the animal is alive, regardless of the depth of cooling. The rate of reduction of oxygen uptake varies with the different organs, with the proportionately greater declines taking place in the kidney and the liver. Following stabilization of the animal at a given temperature level, the oxygen uptake does not change significantly for brief periods. Artificial perfusion is required at the deeper levels since the "natural" rate of blood flow reduction is greater than the decrease in oxygen requirement.

Upon rewarming, the oxygen consumption rises progressively with elevation in temperature. The rate and magnitude of the increase of oxygen uptake depends to a significant extent upon the level of narcosis. Generally, anesthesia is lightened in order to hasten recovery of thermoregulation. Oxygen uptake often increases above normal levels, suggesting the repayment of an oxygen debt incurred during hypothermia. Under hypothermia, the respiratory quotient (RQ) declines because of a reduction in carbon dioxide production. At 30 C, RQ decreases from a normal 0.82 to a level of 0.65. Upon rewarming RQ returns to normal.

Carbohydrate metabolism is reduced during hypothermia with a resultant hyperglycemia proportional to the level of cooling. Prolongation of hypothermia or shivering may result in a hypoglycemia. Hexokinase inhibition by cold, failure of transfer across cell membranes, and general reduction in liver function all have some effect on carbohydrate metabolism. Insulin activity is markedly reduced during hypothermia.

Little is known about metabolism of fat and of protein during hypothermia. The administration of glycine delays cooling because of specific dynamic action. Plasma proteins undergo variable changes, but, generally, short term cooling to levels of 25 to 20 C produces no significant alterations. Upon rewarming, there appears to be a tendency toward hypoproteinemia, probably because of trapping of proteins in the capillaries.

Hypokalemia occurs during hypothermia and is related to the level of anesthesia as well as duration and depth of cooling. The potassium decrease persists upon rewarming. The primary reason for reduced blood levels is a retention of K^+ within the cell, not increased urinary excretion. Metabolism of Na^+ is altered at very profound levels of cooling, and hypernatremia may occur. Tissue Na^+ is reduced, and the urinary excretion of Cl^- and of Na^+ is increased. Plasma Ca^{++} and Cl^- levels generally remain relatively unchanged, although a hypocalcemia may develop.

It appears that during hypothermia, particularly at deeper levels, there is a tendency for K^+ to shift into the cell with movement of Na^+ out and loss via the kidneys, resulting in an isosmotic diuresis. The net result is that the cell is well hydrated and overloaded with potassium.

Cardiovascular

During progressive cooling, the heart rate drops (Fig. 38.8), and atrioventricular asynchronism develops until a complete cold block occurs. Eventually, the ventricle ceases all movement, but the atrium continues to contract. If perfusion is adequate, the motionless myocardium retains its normal glistening color. If not, it becomes blue because of anoxia (precisely as in normal temperatures) and shudders into a delicate fibrillation.

Cold-induced bradycardia enhances ventricular efficiency and attains a maximum at 28 C. Myocardial contractility increases progressively, peaking at 28 C. The reduced heart rate parallels the decline in metabolic needs of the heart. Below 28 to 25 C, the direct effects of cold on the pacemaker become more assertive. When temperatures below 28 C are maintained be-

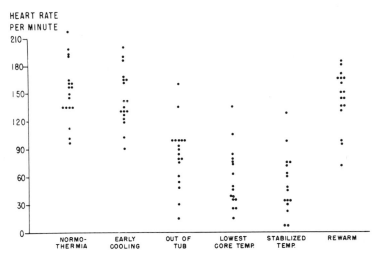

FIG. 38.8. The heart rate falls with cooling, reaching its maximum change coincident with core temperature.

yond 6 hours, heart rate accelerates. Upon rewarming, a tachycardia usually develops, possibly due to (a) temperature "overshoot" and/or (b) "pay-off" of an accumulated oxygen debt. Attempts at altering bradycardia by the use of stimulating drugs or galvanic current should not be attempted.

Electrocardiographic changes are shown in Figure 38.9. The QRS and Q-T become prolonged. The spatial vector for QRS moves from the left lower frontal quadrant to the left lower rear quadrant, gaining in length. The T spatial vector also increases in length and points to the upper right front quadrant. Elevations in the S-T segment are common and U forms may appear, especially if sizeable myocardial temperature gradients exist. The resting membrane potential falls due to alteration in K^+/Na^+ ratio. The length and duration of the ventricular action potential and mechanogram increase (28 C). The P-R interval increases from 0.15 to 0.21 second at 29 C. This is greater than would occur from simple slowing of the heart rate. Auricular fibrillation appears at about 28 C. Atrioventricular (A-V) conduction is progressively depressed until the block is almost complete (15 to 10 C). Premature ventricular beats are frequent, especially below 25 C. The myocardium is more "irritable."

The basis for all these alterations is *cold*. There is no "injury" since perfusion and oxygenation are adequate. Upon rewarming the normal patterns reappear.

Ventricular fibrillation is generally not encountered if the temperature is kept above 28 C. Ventricular fibrillation is a persistent problem at the deeper levels of cooling and is greatly influenced by the anesthetic agent (Table 38.4).

When cyclopropane or pentobarbital is used, the incidence of this cardiac change is 100%. The lowest incidence of ventricular fibrillation occurs when thiopental is used in combination with succinylcholine.

There are two basic etiologies for fibrillation during hypothermia. The first cause and most common is inadequate coronary perfusion, with subsequent anoxia. This is also true at normal temperatures. The second is the effect of cold *per se* and its relationship to the type of anesthesia, temperature depth, and surgical manipulation. A heart above 28 C, if well oxygenated and treated gently, will not fibrillate. When fibrillation does occur, resuscitative measures are conventional: adequate direct massage, oxygenation, and electroshock.

The definite rate of hypothermia in the mechanism of ventricular fibrillation is not clear. The theoretical considerations proposed for the normothermic heart are in

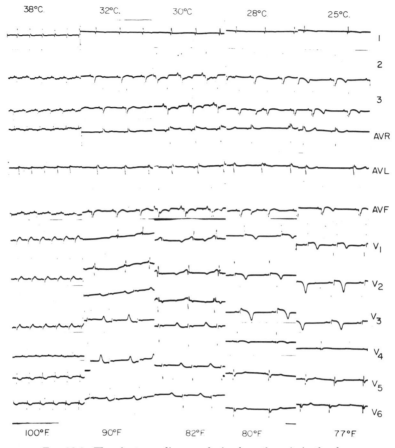

Fig. 38.9. The electrocardiogram during hypothermia in the dog.

order during hypothermia and include modifications of excitatory processes, increased vulnerability, and circus movements. Temperature gradients within the myocardium produce potential differences, presumably disrupting orderly depolarization and recovery. The high incidence of this arrhythmia at the level (25 C) at which homeostasis becomes impaired is not pure coincidence.

Coronary flow remains at a high level because of continued work and oxygen usage relative to the body as a whole (Fig. 38.10); however, oxygen requirements are significantly reduced. The oxygen consumption of the contracting warm heart is 3.9 ml/100 g of tissue/minute. Derangements in electrolyte metabolism occur only at 25 C and below. Intracellular K^+ is reduced. High energy phosphates are unchanged even at these reduced temperatures.

The normal canine heart functions well at 32 to 30 C but fails after a period of 12 hours at 26 to 24 C. There is a progressive decline in output as temperatures decline (Fig. 38.9). Heart rate declines more rapidly than cardiac output, resulting in an increased stroke volume. Below 25 C cardiac output is not adequate, and artificial perfusion is required. Upon rewarming, circulatory failure may occur. This is manifested by hypotension, increased A-V oxygen difference, and lactacidemia. This is more apt to occur if hypothermia below 30 C is prolonged and rewarming is affected too rapidly.

If the anesthetic level is not too deep, the blood pressure may rise at temperatures of 34 to 32 C because of a direct effect of cold on vasculature.[7] Hypotension develops at 25 C due to low output. At this point, the calculated peripheral resistance is high due to reduced flow, vasoconstriction, and increased blood viscosity. Below 15 C, resistance falls due to impairment of vasomotion. Sludging occurs at 30 C and becomes significant below 28 to 25 C.

Circulatory baroceptor reflexes are impaired somewhat at temperatures below 28 C and may be abolished at 20 C.[7] Sympathetic reflexes are affected at a deeper level of cooling, 25 C or lower, markedly impaired at 20 C, and probably abolished below 15 to 10 C.

Hypothermia produces a great variety of changes in blood elements. Generally, these have been considered to be undesirable effects and occur as a rule only in deep hypothermia. The white count is slightly elevated at 32 C, returns at 30 C, and becomes significantly depressed at 28 C, with progressive lowering through 20 C. The red blood cell count is somewhat elevated at 32 C and demonstrates progressive increase throughout all levels of hypothermia. This is accompanied by a significant elevation in hematocrit at temperatures below 28 C. Thrombocytopenia can also occur at this temperature or lower. Clotting mechanisms are not seriously impaired except at 25 C or lower. Below 28 C, increased blood viscosity and sludging occur. The presumed etiology is cellular trapping at the capillary levels. Below 26 C the plasma volume is somewhat reduced, but red cell volume is

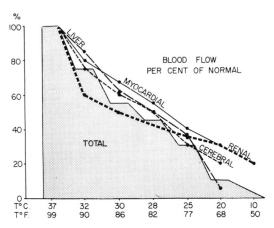

Fig. 38.10. Blood flow changes with hypothermia in the dog. (From Blair.[4])

relatively unaltered. As a rule, all the above changes revert to normal upon rewarming.

Ventilation

Anesthesia exerts a particularly perplexing and profound influence upon ventilatory changes during hypothermia. It is the single most important cause of the wide differences of pulmonary effects observed during cooling. A comparative study of pentobarbital and of chloralose under hypothermia demonstrated a more severe depression with pentobarbital at a given temperature level. In general, there is progressive decrease in ventilatory rate, in minute ventilation, and in tidal volume (Fig. 38.11). The respiratory depression becomes significant at 28 C, and apnea occurs between 22 and 16 C, again depending upon the anesthesia. Hypothermia during light anesthesia induces a reflex stimulation of ventilation resulting in hyperventilation. This is commensurate with the increase in metabolic requirements caused by shivering. Lung volumes are not appreciably altered during hypothermia, while intrapulmonary gas distribution becomes impaired below 30 to 28 C. An index of functional impairment is provided by the ventilation efficiency ration which relates minute ventilation to the time required to excrete a test gas, helium. Insufficiency in ventilation develops at 30 C but

TABLE 38.4
Incidence of ventricular fibrillation under anesthesia and hypothermia

Agents	Temperature	Ventricular Fibrillation
	$^{\circ}C$	%
Cyclopropane	23	100
Ether	21	60
Nitrous oxide	21	50
Pentobarbital	21	100
Pentothal	16	50
Pentothal + succinylcholine	16	22

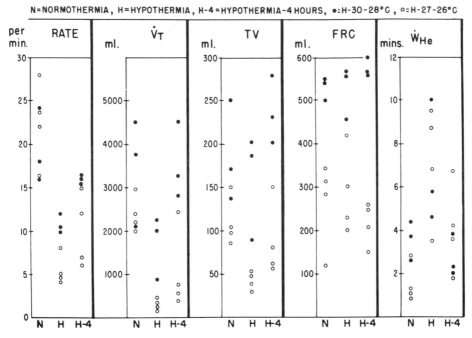

Fig. 38.11. Ventilatory changes with hypothermia in the chloralosed dog. (Reproduced by permission from Blair, E., Esmond, W. G., Attar, S., and Cowley, R. A.: The effect of hypothermia on lung function. Ann. Surgery *160:* 814–823, 1964.)

is significant only below 28 C. As the cooling period is extended, ventilatory efficiency improves. Upon rewarming, all other functions return to normal.

Anatomical and physiological dead space increases below 28 C.[8] At 28 C there is a proportionately greater decline in alveolar ventilation than pulmonary blood flow, such that the ventilation-perfusion ratio is one-half of normal.[9] Lung compliance is unchanged until the temperature level drops below 25 C. Resistance is altered at a somewhat more moderate temperature level, but is only significant at 25 C. Pulmonary diffusing capacity is normal to the level of 25 C.

Reduced ventilation is likely due to three factors: (a) decrease in metabolic need; (b) direct effect on central and peripheral reflex mechanisms; and (c) structural effects. With the progressive decrease in metabolic requirements, there is less need for oxygen and elimination of CO_2. Unfortunately, the decline which occurs is not proportional with the temperature, and, below 28 C, ventilation begins to drop off more rapidly

than the oxygen consumption. This is due to direct cooling of the respiratory centers causing diminished ventilation. As hypothermia is prolonged, ventilation is slightly improved. It appears that the critical level for ventilation is around 28 C.

Pulmonary blood flow is reduced following the general reduction in total blood flow.[4] Pulmonary resistance is increased due to a primary change in the smaller vessels, but below 25 to 20 C the pulmonary resistance drops below normal. At this level of cooling, increase in volume of blood sequestered in the lungs can occur. At progressively lower temperatures, the pulmonary capillary bed becomes filled with blood; sludging occurs and this contributes to pulmonary edema and alveolar hemorrhages.

Gas Solubility and Acid-Base Changes

With progressive hypothermia, there is an increasing alkalinity of the tissue fluid medium. This is profoundly affected by ventilation and internally by the anesthetic agent used.

In the unsupported animal, the pH will rise during hypothermia until core temperature reaches 28 C. At this point acidemia develops (Fig. 38.12). Acid-base imbalance may persist upon rewarming because of disparate distribution of blood flow. If hypothermia has been induced by pump oxygenator techniques, there is usually inadequate perfusion (particularly if the low flow principle is employed) of the skeletal muscles, resulting in hypoxia and lactacidemia. Upon rewarming, the core is warmed, whereas the skeletal muscle tissues remain somewhat cool and the products of anaerobic glycolysis are not adequately metabolized.

Carbon dioxide *per se* is no great problem during hypothermia because of its coefficient of solubility and diffusibility. Buffer base is unchanged unless extracorporeal circulation is used for prolonged periods. Under normothermic conditions, respiratory acidosis is characterized by a rise of plasma K^+, Na^+, and HCO_3^- and by a fall in Cl^- and HPO_4^-. In cold respiratory acidosis, the only change is a fall in K^+. The nature of the acidosis during hypothermia therefore is somewhat different than that observed under normothermic conditions. Nevertheless, the measures for preventing this problem as well as its management are the same.

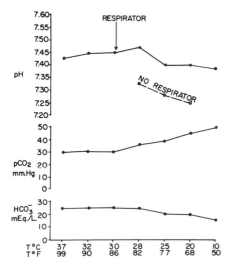

FIG. 38.12. Below 28 C, severe acidosis develops unless a respirator is used.

TABLE 38.5
Safe limits of circulatory arrest during hypothermia

Temperature	Time
°C	min
37	3
30	6
28	8-10
25	12-15
20	20
10	40

The oxygen dissociation curve shifts to left with progressively deeper hypothermia, resulting in increased tenacity with which hemoglobin clings to oxygen. Theoretically, this should be no real problem since the oxygen requirement is reduced. However, should hypothermia be maintained for a prolonged period of time (over an hour), hypoxia may result. As a consequence, measures are recommended which insure release of oxygen by hemoglobin by "reshifting" the curve. These have included the addition of carbon dioxide or dilute hydrochloric acid into the oxygenating chamber.

Central Nervous System

Normally, the brain is approximately 1 C cooler than core temperature. During cooling and rewarming, brain temperature does not alter along with the core. In surface cooling, the brain remains 1 to 2 C warmer than the core, and, with blood stream cooling, the brain may be warmer by as much as 4 to 12 C. This is of critical importance since the brain constitutes the base line or end point of hypoxia during circulatory arrest.

Cerebral oxygen consumption is reduced 6.7% for every degree of fall in temperature, with a linear fall to 25 C, after which the curve of the decline begins to level out.[7] Cerebral blood flow is reduced at about the same rate as oxygen uptake, and there is an increase in cerebral vascular resistance. Cortical vessels begin to constrict at 30 C and lower, and this together with increased blood viscosity and reduced blood flow probably account for the enhanced cerebral vascular resistance. There is little change in the A-V oxygen difference until 10 C is reached; at this point a marked narrowing occurs indicating a reduced oxygen uptake. Following reinstitution of cerebral circulation after 45 to 60 minutes of arrest, a significant A-V oxygen difference develops.

Hypothermia has been propagandized as a magnificent tool because of increasing tolerance to hypoxia. Unfortunately, the criteria for establishing these limits at different temperature levels have been based upon the crude index of life or death. More careful studies of neurological damage have demonstrated that the periods of arrest permissible at a given temperature are somewhat less than those hopefully predicted. Table 38.5 demonstrates the "safe" limits of circulatory arrest at various temperatures. Additional factors affecting "safe" limits of circulatory arrest include age, cardiopulmonary status, and type and depth of anesthesia. In general, the younger animals tolerate periods of vascular occlusion, just as they withstand hypothermia itself, better than adults.

Electroencephalographic (EEG) activity

TABLE 38.6
Routes of anesthetic drug elimination and potential effect of hypothermia

Agent	Route	Hypothermia	Problem	Management
Nitrous oxide	Lung	No effect at 35-30 C. Reduced below 28 C. Increased tissue and fluid solubility.	Conventional signs not reliable. Depth lower than expected. Delayed tissue desaturation. Ileus more pronounced.	Support ventilation always. Reduce agent as temperature drops. Control shivering with succinylcholine. Hyperventilate prior to and during rewarming. Ether or halothane preferred.
Urethane Chloralose Avertin Barbiturates Phenothiazines Morphine Cocaine Procaine Tetracaine Decamethonium	Liver	Little or no effect at 35-30 C. Reduction and conjugation impaired below 25 C.	Cumulative effect during hypothermia, most pronounced on rewarming. Delayed tissue desaturation.	Titration technique. Control shivering with succinylcholine. Always support ventilation.
Avertin Barbiturates Demerol Cocaine Tubocurarine Decamethonium Gallamine Atropine Scopolamine	Kidney	Li tle or no effect at 35-30 C. Below 28 C reduced glomerular filtration rate and impaired tubular function.	Impairment persists 24-30 hours after rewarming. Cumulative effect. Delayed tissue desaturation.	Barbiturates used with great care. All other agents avoided.
Procaine Succinylcholine	Hydrolysis (blood tissue enzymes)	Little or no effect at 35-25 C. Enzyme impairment only in deep and profound hypothermia.	Cumulative effect.	Decrease dosage below 25 C. Support ventilation. Only succinylcholine used.

during hypothermia is modified by general anesthesia. Generally, voltage declines somewhat at 32 C, but serious EEG alterations develop only below this level. Depression is progressive as temperature declines until the EEG becomes silent between 20 and 28 C. Frontal lobe activity persists the longest, with occipital and parietal depression beginning at more moderate levels of cooling. Frontal lobe δ- and θ-activity become intensified at 30 C, with some depression of β- and α-frequencies. θ-Rhythms disappear around 25 C, and the last to go are the slow δ-forms. Rewarming usually results in a reversal of this pattern. Should blood flow be arrested during hypothermia, cessation of all EEG activity takes place within 10 to 30 seconds. When blood flow is reinstituted, some EEG activity reappears within 1 minute but does not return to preocclusion pattern for at least 1 hour.

Miscellaneous

The reduction in oxygen consumption of the kidney compared with other organs is quite precipitous to approximately 30 C; below this the decline becomes more linear. Concomitant with this, blood flow decreases with proportional rise in renovascular resistance. At the deeper levels of hypothermia, the renal blood flow remains comparatively high and is exceeded only by the coronary blood flow. As oxygen utilization is reduced, the A-V difference across the kidney becomes narrower. This is observed at more moderate levels than in other organs, 30 C compared to 20 C. Glomerular filtration is reduced to 80% of normal at 32 C, to 43% at 28 C, and 40% of normal at 25 C. The clearance time of p-aminohippuric acid declines progressively until, at 20 C, there is no evidence of glomerular filtration by this test of excretory activity. The reduction in glomerular filtration rate is not proportional to the reduction in blood pressure. At 30 C with a slight reduction in arterial blood pressure, glomerular filtration rate is reduced to 26%. This as well as other alterations in renal function suggest that metabolic factors probably outweigh the hemodynamic.

The increase in urinary output is probably due to depressed tubular activity resulting in reduced water reabsorption and the production of a cold diuresis. The urinary excretion of Na^+ is increased while that of K^+ is reduced. These changes in electrolyte excretion become significant only below 28 C. Creatine clearance is reduced. Sugar appears in the urine in increasing quantities as the temperature falls. Renal concentration and acidification capabilities are impaired. In contrast to the other organs, body rewarming fails to restore normal kidney function for 24 to 36 hours.

The secretion of endocrine system is markedly altered during hypothermia. Pituitary activity is depressed progressively during hypothermia with complete suppression of corticotropin secretion at 20 C. The adrenals remain responsive to exogenous corticotropin to about 20 C. On the other hand, responsiveness to thyroid stimulating hormone is reduced at a more moderate level of hypothermia. Antidiuretic hormone secretion is reduced and the injection of pituitrin fails to inhibit the increased urinary flow. Epinephrine and norepinephrine secretions are reduced during hypothermia with total abolition around 15 C. Vascular reactivity to exogenous norepinephrine is reduced and the hypothermic heart becomes unusually sensitive to epinephrine. Thyroid activity is reduced beginning at 34 C, as demonstrated by marked inhibition of I^{131} uptake, and is almost totally inhibited at 15 C. The activity of endogenous insulin is markedly reduced.

Liver function is impaired during hypothermia. This is suggested by a 50% reduction in Bromsulphalein uptake occurring at 20 C. At 28 C, the glucose tolerance curve is flattened, suggesting almost complete block of glucose utilization. The most significant effect of hypothermia, particularly with reference to injectable depressants and general anesthetic, is the reduction in detoxifying and conjugating activity of the liver. The half-life of morphine is increased from 3 to 7 minutes to 97 minutes at 24 C. Similar prolongation of barbiturate action occurs.

Pancreatic activity is arrested at a very early level of cooling. Secretions are reduced to 75% of normal at 32 C and totally at 28 C. Enzyme production, however, continues such that on rewarming there is a tremendous release into the blood stream.

Because of this massive release, permanent morphological alterations are the sequelae. Focal necrosis of the myocardium and of the brain have been reported in the human, but rarely in animals. Histochemical alterations of a transient nature have been observed occasionally, such as fat droplets in the heart and depletion of glycogen in the liver and the heart. Within the customarily employed levels of cooling from 32 to 25 C, no morphological or histochemical changes of any real severity have occurred.

One of the most striking observations is ileus. This constitutes the single most common complication from hypothermia. Gastrointestinal tract motility is reduced at 34 C and ceases at 30 C. Gastric secretions are progressively reduced. Blood flow is reduced to such an extent that at 15 C it is only about 10 to 20% of normal.

Impairment of defense mechanisms, particularly those against bacteria, is controversial. Clearance of bacteria (*Escherichia coli* and *Aerobacter aerogenes*) in the blood stream, while perhaps somewhat delayed, is effective at 24 to 20 C. *Staphylococcus aureus* sepsis is relatively unaltered in hypothermic rabbits, but fatal in cooled dogs. The survival period in mixed coliform infections is significantly prolonged in hypothermic (32 to 30 C) dogs. The variety of inocula, study techniques, levels of cooling, and species (in which antibacterial mechanisms are known to differ), all serve to confuse a poorly understood problem. The reticuloendothelial system is not markedly impaired until the temperature level of 27 to 25 C is reached. At this level, activities such as antibody formation are impaired. It is possible that bacterial growth and endotoxin activity at these temperature levels are suppressed so that some sort of balance is probably achieved.

Pharmacology

Drugs have exercised a diverse and confusing role in hypothermia. Elective hypothermia cannot be achieved without the judicious use of pharmacological agents, particularly anesthetics and neuromuscular blocking drugs. On the other hand, anesthetic agents themselves frequently induce unintentional hypothermia which may have undesirable features. Pharmacological agents whose actions are particularly temperature-sensitive would be expected to become modified by cold. The effect of drug action in relationship to hypothermia is concerned with (a) initial induction of cooling, (b) maintenance of hypothermia, and, finally, (c) resuscitation from hypothermia. Induction is at normal temperatures and drug dosages follow essentially standard procedures. Light anesthesia and succinylcholine chloride for control of excessive skeletal activity is the method of choice.

At low temperatures, drug actions are modified by organ perfusion which is reduced as a rule and will vary considerably in its regional distribution depending upon depth and duration of cooling. Low temperatures interfere with deactivation and excretion by depression of the responsible organs and systems (Table 38.6). Return to normal renal and kidney function after rewarming is delayed. The level of hypothermia dictates to a considerable extent problems which may be encountered upon

TABLE 38.7
Effect of hypothermia on drug action

Depressed	Enhanced	No Change
Noradrenaline	Adrenaline	Barbital
Caffeine	Pentothal	Antibiotics
Digitalis	Pentobarbital	Sulfa drugs
Phenobarbital	Chloralose	Metrazol
(LD$_{50}$)		
Angiotensin	Urethane	
Ether	Potassium	
Chloroform	Calcium	
Halothane	Procaine	
Atropine	Cocaine	
	Phenothiazines	
	Ephedrin	
	Morphine	

resuscitation with regard to persistance of or cumulative drug action. Potential difficulty may be anticipated at and below 28 C. In general, those agents whose inactivation depends primarily upon liver detoxification constitute the most serious problems. Inhibition of drug elimination is of serious consequence at deeper levels (below 25 C). Ventilatory activity is depressed below 28 C, and artificial support is essential. If this is maintained, excretion of volatile agents is not a serious problem despite the increase in solubility during hypothermia. Enzyme activity, particularly oxidative, is disturbed to a significant extent only at very deep levels, 20 C or lower.

The modification of drug action at a low temperature is characterized by (a) reduction of effectiveness, (b) enhancement of effectiveness, and (c) no change. These alterations relate to the anticipated reaction for either a normal dosage or toxic dosages under normothermic conditions. The problem of drug toxicity under hypothermia bears additional similarity to anesthesia in that the hypothermic state may inhibit, ignore, or mask a particular drug effect. The influences of hypothermia on a number of commonly used drugs are listed in Table 38.7.

The action of barbiturates in general is enhanced except for sodium barbital; that is, a smaller amount is required to maintain a given level of anesthesia. Duration of anesthesia with sodium hexobarbital at 20 C is increased 2.5 times compared to 30 C. The sleeping time in dogs under sodium pentobarbital is increased 3.25 times at 27C compared to normothermic temperatures. Sodium barbital sleeping time, on the other hand, is not altered. Chloralose and urethane are administered in normal dosages in order to overcome the period of excitability which is augmented at 34 to 32 C. Supplemental dosages are reduced. Halothane is probably the safest anesthetic agent to be used in conjunction with hypothermia since it is volatile and it also produces peripheral vasodilation. Volatile agents recommend themselves highly since they are not metabolized but diffuse in and out according to simple physical laws. Cy-clopropane continues to be a problem because of the hazard of explosion and increased myocardial irritability. Action of local anesthetics is prolonged. Effects of opiates and ataractics are enhanced in therapeutic doses below the level of 30 C. Conversely, toxic dosages of these agents experimentally are better tolerated under deep hypothermia (20 C). The action of atropine is enhanced, and a potential problem exists with the use of atropine during hypothermia. Gradual bradycardia is a natural concomitant of the hypothermic process and should not be tampered with or influenced because of the possible dangers of arrhythmias. Below 25 C parasympathetic activity is depressed, and atropine effect is nullified.[8]

Drugs with major effect upon myocardial activity are of particular significance in the hypothermic state. The action of digitalis glycosides is inhibited by hypothermia. Supplemental dosages are of little value and have proven to be innocuous. The cold heart becomes increasingly tolerant to toxic doses. The myocardium becomes increasingly sensitive to the potassium and calcium ion. The positive inotropic effect of epinephrine is greatly increased, while the pressor effect of norepinephrine is progressively reduced. Hosts of drugs have been recommended as protection against ventricular fibrillation including procaine amide, neostigmine, quinidine, and many others. Too often, pharmacological protection proved quite the reverse, resulting in an unexpected disaster.

Central nervous system stimulants such as strychnine, coramine, and lobeline undergo enhanced activity resulting in increased toxicity during hypothermia. The activity of metrazol is unchanged while that of picrotoxin and caffeine are reduced. Endocrine drugs generally demonstrate reduced action under hypothermia with considerable variation of the degree of inhibition at a given temperature level. Thyroxine activity is affected at a relatively moderate level and its action is almost completely abolished below 25 C. Pituitrin is depressed at 25 C. Corticotropin is impaired at 28 to 25 C. Corticoids are depressed at a fairly moderate level of hypothermia.

The action of antibiotics is unchanged to approximately 25 C. Cancer chemotherapeutic agents are modified significantly at 32 to 30 C such that there is an appreciable increase in tolerance to toxic dosages of nitrogen mustard and cyclophosphoamide.

Phenothiazine drug action is significantly enhanced under hypothermia.

Lethal Limits of Hypothermia

The studies of Bernard and Magendie indicated the lethal limits to be 25 C because of central nervous system damage.[2, 11] These studies were undoubtedly performed with minimal controls over the animal's homeostasis. There is no question that 25 C does represent a significant level physiologically, but it is not the limit of hypothermia. Rigid controls, particularly of circulation and ventilation, are absolutely necessary. There have been numerous studies which have demonstrated that homeothermic mammals can be cooled to as low as 5 or even 0 C and survive, although the mortality rate is quite high. Supercooling has been attempted in mammals including primates with no success in total resuscitation. The determination of the lethal limits rests with animal species and the circumstances under which hypothermia is achieved. The limits are far greater with controlled elective hypothermia than they are with uncontrolled or accidental hypothermia. The tolerance of rodents to hypothermia is far greater than the tolerance of the higher homeothermic mammals such as dogs and primates.

Methods of Producing Hypothermia

To achieve reduction of core temperature, there are two requirements: (a) creation of a cold environment and (b) the disruption of thermoregulation. The primary aim in all techniques is the alteration of the temperature of circulating blood. Whether it remains within the body or is brought to the outside and passed through a heat exchanger, the warm blood must be cooled before hypothermia can be achieved.

Techniques for cooling generally are divided into general hypothermia and regional hypothermia. They are achieved by surface contact or by intravascular techniques (Table 38.8). Surface contact methods have been victimized by extraordinary imagination, but the most satisfactory one is the use of thermostatic blankets since positive control is achieved more satisfactorily. Ice tub immersion is simple and more rapid, but temperature control is difficult. Air cooling has proved useful, but, again, control of the animal is extremely difficult with this technique. Regional cooling is achieved by packing the organ in ice. With this technique, control of the temperature level locally is not possible.

Blood stream cooling is usually accom-

TABLE 38.8
Methods of inducing hypothermia

Type	Technique	Features	Limits
			°C
Surface	Thermostatic blanket	Simple. good control; "after-fall."	28-25
	Ice bath	Simple. fair control; "after-fall."	28-25
	Cold air	Simple. poor control; "after-fall."	28-25
Intravascular	Drew technique Pump oxygenator	Complex. Excellent core control.	None
Regional	Intravascular	Complex. Good control.	None
	Ice cubes	Simple. Poor control.	15-10
	Saline "slush"	Simple. Poor control.	15-10
	Balloons	Complex. Good control.	None

TABLE 38.9

Complications from hypothermia (dog)

Complication	Temperature °C	Accidental or Elective	Incidence	Outcome
Central nervous system				
Brain damage	30-0	A, E*	Occasional. Usually hypoxia; embolic phenomena; direct cold	Death usually
Hindquarter paralysis	30	A, E	Usually after periods of circulatory arrest	Recovery usually
Cardiovascular				
Atrial fibrillation	28-18	A, E	Common	Recovery
Heart block	28-18	A, E	Common	Recovery
Ventricular arrest	37-35	E	Uncontrolled shivering	Recovery with correct resuscitation
	18	E	"Cold arrest"	Recovery
Ventricular fibrillation	28	A, E	Drug- and temperature-dependent	Recovery with correct resuscitation
Myocardial necrosis	15	E	Frostbite Inadequate perfusion	Recovery
Rewarm shock		A, E	Prolonged hypothermia; too rapid rewarm	Recovery
Bleeding	28	A, E	Common	Recovery
Sludging	25	A, E	Common	Recovery
Pulmonary				
Edema	28	A	Uncommon	Death
Insufficiency	28	E	Common	Hypoxia and death
Abdomen				
Ileus	34	A, E	Common	Recovery
Necrosis	0	E	Stomach; fairly common	Recovery usually, occasional death
Metabolic				
Hyperglycemia	30	E	Common	Recovery
Hypoglycemia	28	A	Fairly common	Recovery
Electrolytes	28	A, E	Transient, usually pre-existing	Recovery
Hypoxia	All	A, E	Inadequate ventilation and/or perfusion	Recovery usually; nervous system damage
Respiratory acidosis	28	A, E	Inadequate ventilation	Recovery usually
Metabolic acidosis	15	A, E	Inadequate perfusion	Recovery usually

* A, accidental; E, elective.

plished with a pump oxygenator, employing a heat exchange system. The Drew technique, in which the lungs continue as the oxygenating system, is an alternative method, but the mortality from this has proved to be extremely high. The advantage of blood stream cooling is the exacting control of core temperature and the acquisition of deeper cold levels. Cooling is achieved much more rapidly as is rewarming. The factors which determine the rate of cooling are the size of the animal, temperature of the coolant in the heat exchanger, and the rate of perfusion, of which the latter is important. The most commonly used technique is total bypass in which all the venous blood is shunted through the artificial system and returned via a femoral, iliac, or carotid artery. Venovenous cooling is effective and preferred in some quarters since interarterial cannulation is avoided. A disadvantage of this method is the requirement of a highly qualified team to assure a smooth operation and minimize risk. Heparinization is necessary, and cannulation of the arterial system poses additional hazards. With the introduction of dilution techniques, whole blood is not the problem as it was previously. The equipment must be kept clean, sterile, and uncluttered.

While the core temperature is controlled with the perfusion method, that of the superficial and intermediate zones is not. In order to avoid problems leading to metabolic acidosis during rewarming, thermostatic blankets are advised during the rewarming. These are cooled during induction of core hypothermia and then rewarmed during the resuscitation. This permits more rapid stabilization of thermogradients and avoids the wide discrepancies usually occurring with intravascular techniques. Premature termination of artificial perfusion results in "postpump" temperature drop.

Complications

Complications from hypothermia may be primary or secondary. Primary effects are anticipated from the nature of low temperature itself—ileus and coagulation defects. Secondary types include conventional problems, the occurrence of which may be invited, accelerated, or masked by cold, depending upon depth and character of hypothermia—acidosis and ventricular fibrillation. It is in this group that awareness of physiological alterations is especially important. Table 38.9 lists complications with pertinent associated factors. Central nervous system damage is usually due to hypoxia secondary to inadequate perfusion or embolic phenomena during cardiopulmonary bypass. Necrosis has been found at profound levels from general hypothermia, but in regional cooling of the brain, this apparently does not occur. Arrhythmias are common, directly related to the depth of cooling, and reversible upon resuscitation. Ventricular fibrillation at conventional cold levels results from the same causes as at normal temperatures, with an increased predisposition below 28 C. It occurs infrequently if there is adequate oxygenation and perfusion of the myocardium. Ventricular fibrillation during rewarming from profound hypothermia is a frequent complication, but high flow perfusion will reduce the incidence. During hypothermia, arrest occurs under two circumstances, accelerated reflex activity during a poorly controlled induction and true cold standstill which occurs below 15 C. Coagulation defects, leukopenia, and sludge phenomena are problems only at the deeper temperatures. Pulmonary edema occurs in uncontrolled hypothermia and is usually accidental. Lung-pump syndromes are problems peculiar to extracorporeal circulation. The role of hypothermia not only is probably negligible, but may actually be protective. Ventilatory insufficiency is obviated by recognition of its likelihood below 30 C and institution of conventional supportive measures. Hypoxia may exist at any level of hypothermia. Tissue tolerance to lack of oxygen is relative only, and some degree of perfusion is necessary. Ileus is common and reversible. Massive gastric dilation is a particular threat. Gastrohypothermia below 0 C is causing an alarming increase in necrosis with bleeding and perforation. Rough palpation of the abdomen "cracks" the frozen stomach. Electrolyte imbalance may be fairly common but serious consequences are usually due to pre-existing and uncorrected deficits. Acidosis is due to inadequate ventilation and perfusion. Hypothermia masks this problem since the usual means of detection may be deceptive. Hyperglycemia is common and reversible. Hypoglycemia may be of more serious portent and is prevented by controlling shivering and not cooling starved animals.

The normal, healthy animal, with intelligent controls and recognition of limits, should experience the hypothermic state with little adversity. The older animal with pre-existing organic disease, particularly cardiac, invites greater probabilities of hazards.

REFERENCES

1. Bakamat'ev, V. O.: *The Problem of Acute Hypothermia*. (Translated by R. E. Hammond), Pergamon Press, New York, 1960. Quoted by P. M. Starkov.
2. Bernard, C.: *Leçons sur la Chaleurs Animals*. Balliere, Paris, 1876.
3. Bigelow, W. G., Lindsay, W. K., Harrison, R. G., Gordon, R. A., and Greenwood, W. F.: Hypothermia: its possible role in cardiac surgery: an investigation in dogs at low body temperatures. Ann. Surg. *132:* 849, 1949.
4. Blair, E.: *Clinical Hypothermia*. McGraw-Hill Book Company, New York, 1964.
5. Carlson, L. D.: Temperature. Ann. Rev. Physiol. *24:* 85, 1962.
6. Papper, E. M., and Kitz, R. J. (editors): *Uptake and Distribution of Anesthetic Agents*, p. 5. Blakiston Division, McGraw-Hill Book Company, New York, 1963.
7. Rosomoff, H. L.: The effects of hypothermia on the physiology of the nervous system. Surgery *40:* 328, 1956.
8. Salzano, J., and Hall, F. G.: Influence of vagal blockade on respiratory and circulatory functions in hypothermic dogs. J. Appl. Physiol. *17:* 833, 1962.
9. Severinghaus, J. W., Stupfel, M., and Bradley, A. F.: Alveolar dead space and arterial to end-tidal carbon dioxide differences during hypothermia in dog and man. J. Appl. Physiol. *10:* 349, 1959.
10. Ström, G.: Central nervous regulation of body temperature. In *Handbook of Physiology*, Vol. III: Neurophysiology, p. 1173. American Physiological Society, Washington, D.C., 1960.
11. Varigny, H. de: *Temperature and Life*. Annual Report of the Smithsonian Institute, p. 407. U.S. Government Printing Office, Washington, D.C., 1891.
12. Virtue, R.: Modifying effects of anesthesia on hypothermia. Ann. N.Y. Acad. Sci. *80:* 533, 1959.
13. Walther, A.: Beitrage zur Lehre von der Tierischen Warme. Virchow Arch. Path. Anat. *25:* 414, 1862.

39
Cardiac Arrhythmias During Anesthesia

RHEA J. WHITE

A large percentage of surgical patients have cardiac arrhythmias at some time during anesthesia and surgery.[33] Many arrythmias are transient and may pass unnoticed except in those animals continuously monitored with the electrocardiograph. Although these arrhythmias are not usually an indication of heart disease but rather the effect of various factors directly related to anesthesia and surgery, animals with pre-existing heart disease are more likely to have arrhythmias under anesthesia. Preoperative electrocardiograms are very helpful for proper interpretation of intraoperative changes in cardiac rhythm.

Factors known to influence the development of arrhythmias include the anesthetic agents and ancillary drugs such as atropine, narcotics, muscle relaxants, catecholamines, and digitalis. Other important influences are surgical stimulation, arterial blood gases, arterial pH, arterial blood pressure, body temperature, serum electrolytes, circulatory reflexes, and anxiety during induction. The importance of a calm induction in quiet surroundings is not generally appreciated, and it should be emphasized that fear and struggling during induction may adversely affect both induction and maintenance of anesthesia.[68] The amount of epinephrine released by fear in an animal in some cases is thought to be close to the levels required to initiate ventricular fibrillation in the presence of a myocardial sensitizing anesthetic.[25] Species difference must also be considered when interpreting experimental and clinical data.

Most of the causes of arrhythmias during anesthesia and surgery can be related to stimulation of the autonomic nervous system, with alteration of vagal or sympathetic activity, or to direct effects on the conduction system of the heart.

Electrophysiology and Mechanism of Cardiac Arrhythmias

The mechanism by which cardiac irregularities are produced under anesthesia is not fully understood, but lack of balance in the autonomic nervous system is thought to play a major role. A complete review of the electrophysiology of the heart beat is beyond the scope of this discussion; however, a brief summary of the main points will be presented in order to consider the factors associated with arrhythmias in the surgical patient.

The heart has four physiological properties which enable it to beat independently of nervous control: automaticity, rhythmicity, conductivity, and contractility. Automaticity is the intrinsic ability of the heart to initiate an impulse by means of spontaneous depolarization in certain specialized cardiac cells, the automatic cells or pacemaker cells, that make up the conduction tissue. Automatic cells are found in the sinoatrial node, in certain specialized areas of the atria, in the His bundle, in the right and left bundle branches, and in the Purkinje network which sends extensive peripheral branches throughout the ventricular musculature. It is now believed that the atrioventricular node contains no automatic cells and that ectopic beats commonly referred to as nodal beats or nodal rhythm actually originate in either the His bundel, in the specialized cells between the atrioventricular node and the His bundle, or in the area of the coronary sinus.[28]

Rhythmicity is the rate at which the spontaneous impulse is initiated. Normally the sinoatrial node has the highest rhythmicity and functions as the primary pacemaker of the heart. The normal rhythmicity of the other automatic cells, the latent pacemakers, decreases in order from the specialized automatic cells of the atria to the Purkinje network.

Conductivity is the ability of the impulse to spread through the myocardial syncytium causing depolarization throughout the musculature of the myocardium.

Contractility is a poorly understood phenomenon in which the chemical energy of depolarization is converted to mechanical energy which results in shortening or contraction of the cardiac musculature.

The intrinsic automaticity of the intact heart is modified by the autonomic nervous system through the opposing effects of sympathetic accelerator activity and vagal decelerator activity. Sympathetic innervation is supplied to the entire heart and produces its effect through liberation of the neurotransmitter norepinephrine. However, parasympathetic innervation is confined to the supraventricular area only, i.e., the sinoatrial node and the atria, and liberates the neurotransmitter acetylcholine. Stimuli from various areas including the abdominal and thoracic viscera, the great vessels, the coronary arteries and the corotid sinuses, all pass along afferent pathways in the vagus and sympathetic nerves to the cardiovascular centers of the central nervous system. Efferent fibers carry stimuli from the cardiovascular centers to the heart.[12]

The recent work of Hoffman et al using intracellular micro-electrodes to measure electrical activity in individual cardiac fibers has revealed information on the physiological mechanisms involved in the genesis of cardiac arrhythmias.[27-30] It can be seen that cardiac rhythm is dependent on the initiation of spontaneous depolarization in the automatic cells of the pacemaker to produce an action potential. The action potential causes excitation, i.e., depolarization, in adjacent fibers, and propagation or conduction of the impulse occurs throughout the myocardium. Consequently arrhythmias may result from abnormalities in either automaticity or conduction, or both.

Abnormalities in automaticity result from a change in the rate at which impulses are initiated in the automatic cells or a change in the rate of spontaneous depolarization. Automaticity in the cells of the normal pacemaker may be abnormally depressed or the automaticity in other cells may be unusually increased. In either case the dominant pacemaker activity will switch from the cells with depressed automaticity to the cells with increased automaticity. The result is a change in rate and a downward shift in the pacemaker site, unless the two groups of automatic cells are close together in which case only a change in rate will be apparent on the electrocardiogram, the appearance of the complex remaining the same.

The most important cause of changes in automaticity is the effect of the autonomic nervous system through release of the autonomic mediators, acetylcholine and norepinephrine. Both the sensitivity of automatic cells in various parts of the heart to the neurotransmitters, and the concentrations of the mediators released in different areas of the heart may vary widely, so that the effects of a mediator may be qualitatively and quantitatively variable in different areas of the heart.

Acetylcholine, released by vagal stimulation, decreases the rate of diastolic depolarization in the sinoatrial node and the automatic cells of the atria. Weak vagal tone produces a decrease in the rate of the sinus rhythm. However, the sinoatrial node is more sensitive to acetylcholine than are the other atrial cells. Therefore, stronger vagal tone will cause a downward shift in the pacemaker producing a decrease in heart rate and P wave changes on the electrocardiogram. Very intense vagal tone may completely depress the automatic cells of the sinoatrial node and the atria leading to sinus arrest. Normally this is followed by a downward shift of the pacemaker to the His-Purkinje fibers and is referred to as vagal escape. The lack of sensitivity of the His-Purkinje system of acetylcholine therefore prevents cardiac arrest.

Sympathetic stimulation releases norepinephrine which causes an increase in the rate of diastolic depolarization in all autonomic cells. Again variations in sensitivity to the transmitter among different automatic cells and variations in concentration of the norepinephrine occur in different areas of the heart. Therefore, while sympathetic stimulation may produce only an increase in the rate of sinus rhythm, a downward shift of the pacemaker to the His-Purkinje system may result in the development of ectopic rhythms.

Other factors that decrease the intrinsic rate of automatic cells in addition to acetylcholine include (1) hyperkalemia, (2) hypercalcemia, and (3) hypothermia. Factors that increase the intrinsic rate of autonomic cells in addition to norepinephrine include (1) other catecholamines such as epinephrine and isoproterenol, (2) hypokalemia, (3) hypocalcemia, (4) hyperthermia, (5) hypoxia, (6) hypercapnia, (7) digitalis, especially when associated with hypokalemia, (8) mechanical stretch, and (9) mechanical trauma.

Cardiac arrhythmias may also result from abnormalities in conduction. Normal conduction is dependent on the ability of the action potential of the autonomic cell to cause excitation and initiate depolarization in adjacent fibers so that propagation of the impulse occurs throughout the myocardium. Propagation is affected by (1) the rate of rise of the action potential and (2) the amplitude of the action potential that is produced. A decrease in the rate of rise or amplitude of the action potential interferes with propagation by causing a decrease in conduction velocity which increases the possibility of block.

The most common cause of a decrease in conduction velocity is hyperkalemia. The high level of extracellular potassium decreases both the rate of rise and amplitude of the action potential. The resulting decrease in conduction velocity produces a prolongation of the QRS complex on the electrocardiogram. Very high extracellular potassium values may completely depress excitability in some areas of the heart.

Arrhythmias Common During Anesthesia

Table 39.1 lists a number of arrhythmias frequently seen in the anesthetized patient and the relative hazards involved. Arrhythmias occurring during anesthesia are the same as those observed in the awake animal although the precipitating factors are frequently different. As a general rule, supraventricular arrhythmias with normal heart rates may be considered relatively benign. Ventricular arrhythmias, on the other hand, should always be considered potentially serious.[38] However, unifocal ventricular extrasystoles that occur infrequently or for short periods of time are very common under anesthesia and frequently do not result in serious harm or lead to more serious ventricular abnormalities.

Intense bradycardia should always be viewed with alarm as it may be a sign of impending asystole. Sinus arrest is a rare arrhythmia caused by strong vagal tone in which periods of asystole 3 to 10 seconds in duration are observed. Normally a sinus arrest terminates by spontaneous reversion to a sinus rhythm or by escape of a lower pacemaker, usually by initiation of a nodal rhythm. Should this fail to occur, the heart remains in asystole in a state of complete cardiac arrest.

Supraventricular tachycardia may be well tolerated by the normal heart but may have serious effects for patients with heart disease or hypoxemia. A rapid tachycardia leads to inadequate time for diastolic filling. The result is a decrease in cardiac output and myocardial hypoxia because coronary flow cannot be increased enough to meet the increased oxygen requirements of the rapidly beating heart.[20]

Third degree heart block (complete AV

TABLE 39.1

Arrhythmias commonly occurring during anesthesia

	Benign	Hazardous	Lethal (Cardiac arrest)
Supraventricular	Sinus arrhythmia Sinoatrial block Wandering pacemaker Atrioventricular nodal rhythm First and second degree heart block Atrioventricular dissociation	Sinus Bradycardia Sinus arrest Supraventricular tachycardia Third degree heart block	
Ventricular	Unifocal extrasystoles	Multifocal extrasystoles Tachycardia	Ventricular fibrillation Asystole

block) deserves special mention because of the serious nature of this arrhythmia in relation to general anesthesia. Second degree heart block is common in the horse and in most cases is considered to be a normal physiological response to high vagal tone in the horse at rest. In the dog first degree heart block may occur in a normal heart, although second degree heart block is associated with myocardial disease or with potent vagotonic drugs such as digitalis and morphine. Third degree heart block is considered a sign of serious organic heart disease in all species.[10] It is characterized by a very slow regular pulse and may be associated with fainting spells (Adams-Stokes attack) and pulmonary edema.[11, 17, 18]

The patient with first or second degree heart block and no history of third degree block does not present any serious anesthetic risk as long as care is taken to prevent progression of the conduction defect to complete heart block. However, the patient with third degree heart block is an extremely grave anesthetic risk because of the high incidence of ventricular standstill and cardiac arrest during induction of anesthesia. The anesthetic management of these patients will be discussed in the section on therapy.[22]

Multifocal ventricular extrasystoles and

ventricular tachycardia are hazardous not only because of their deleterious effect on cardiac output and coronary flow but because of the risk of progression to ventricular fibrillation.

Etiology of Arrhythmias During Anesthesia

INHALATIONAL ANESTHETICS

Cyclopropane and certain halogenated hydrocarbon anesthetics sensitize the myocardium to the arrhythmic effects of catecholamines. The term sensitization means that the dose of exogenous catecholamine required to produce a cardiac arrhythmia in the unanesthetized patient is greatly decreased in the presence of the sensitizing anesthetic. Cyclopropane is the agent most likely to cause serious ventricular arrhythmias, presumably because it stimulates the sympathetic nervous system and also sensitizes the myocardium to catecholamines. In the cat ventricular arrhythmias occur under cyclopropane with high levels of carbon dioxide but not during normocarbia.[54] The dog, however, rarely has arrhythmias during cyclopropane unless exogenous catecholamines are infused.[52] Intravenous atropine may also precipitate arrhythmias with cyclopropane.[36] Consequently the injection of either catecholamines or atropine is hazardous and should be avoided during cyclopropane anesthesia.

Halothane is not a central nervous system stimulant but it does sensitize the myocardium. In the cat ventricular arrhythmias are seen with hypercarbia, hypoxia, and sensory stimulation during light levels of halothane.[53] Ventricular arrhythmias usually are not seen in the dog under halothane unless catecholamines are infused.[23, 24] In the horse ventricular arrhythmias have not been reported even with high levels of carbon dioxide under halothane, but they are produced by infusion of epinephrine.[42] Deep levels of halothane produce bradycardia and nodal rhythms in all species. In the cat under deep halothane anesthesia, atrioventricular dissociation has been reported. This effect of deep halothane is believed due to a relative or absolute increase in vagal tone. Intense bradycardia may respond to intravenous atropine although a reduction in anesthetic depth may be a better way of managing bradycardia caused by deep anesthesia.

The subcutaneous infiltration of epinephrine for hemostasis is not without risk during halothane, for ventricular arrhythmias and fibrillation have been reported in man. The safe use of this agent for infiltration of highly vascular areas required careful attention to dose and concentration of the epinephrine solution.[37] The intravenous use of atropine may also be hazardous during halothane anesthesia in those cases where sympathetic nervous activity is indicated by the occurrance of ventricular extrasystoles,[19] or when carbon dioxide retention has occurred.[34]

Diethyl ether stimulates sympathetic activity, but it does not sensitize the myocardium and therefore ventricular arrhythmias are not seen. Various P wave changes are the only alterations that commonly occur during ether anesthesia. The changes in P wave are caused by vagal inhibition of the sinoatrial node and such changes indicate that vagal tone is not completely blocked by ether. Vagal stimulation during ether may be the result of a reflex caused by the inhalation of irritating vapors into the lungs, the so called pulmo-cardiac reflex.[20] Methoxyflurane is a halogenated ether with cardiovascular effects similar to

the effects of halothane, and, pharmacologically, it does not stimulate sympathetic nervous activity. The ability of methoxyflurane to sensitize the myocardium remains controversial. Both the existance and lack of sensitization to epinephrine have been reported in the dog.[6, 13] However, in the clinical situation arrhythmias are ordinarily not seen with methoxyflurane even with high levels of carbon dioxide retension.[8] The use of epinephrine is considered relatively safe during methoxyflurane anesthesia.[4, 51]

It should be noted that much of the data concerning arrhythmias during anesthesia in animals are obtained from laboratory studies rather than from reports of clinical cases. Controlled laboratory studies in healthy animals may not be directly applicable to the clinical situation where seriously ill animals with marked physiological derangements may have to be subjected to anesthesia and surgery.

It can be seen from the discussion of inhalent anesthetics that the cat is more susceptible than the other common domestic animals to anesthetic arrhythmias. The reason for this is uncertain but may be related to a high level of sympathetic tone in this species. The sudden onset of ventricular fibrillation has been observed in healthy cats during induction with inhalational anesthetics for elective surgery. This emphasizes the importance of a calm induction with gentle restraint in order to minimize struggling and excitement in the animal.

PARENTERAL ANESTHETICS

Assuming that adequate ventilation is maintained, cardiac arrhythmias are not observed during barbiturate anesthesia. In some cases the intravenous injection of barbiturates may terminate or prevent ventricular arrhythmias caused by other agents.[54]

Neuroleptanalgesia is a state of analgesia and deep sedation without loss of consciousness produced by the combination of a narcotic and tranquilizer. The common veterinary preparation is Innovar-Vet, a combination of fentanyl and droperidol.

Innovar-Vet is mainly used in the dog although it has also been used in primates, guinea pigs, rabbits, and parakeets. The main effect on cardiac rhythm is a profound bradycardia due to the vagotonic effect of fentanyl. The bradycardia can be prevented or eliminated by atropine.[59, 60] Morphine also produces strong vagal tone that can be abolished with atropine.

ANCILLARY DRUGS

Sympathomimetic drugs are used for one of two reasons during anesthesia, intravenously as vasopressors to control hypotension, and for local infiltration in vascular areas to control hemorrhage. Many anesthesiologists feel that vasopressors are rarely if ever needed during general anesthesia if proper anesthetic levels and adequate fluid replacement are established. The danger involved in the use of epinephrine for local infiltration during halothane anesthesia has already been discussed. As a general rule the epinephrine solution should be diluted 1:100,000 and used in as small amounts as possible. Care should be taken to avoid hypoxia and hypercarbia and the cardiac rhythm closely monitored.

Muscle relaxants which are commonly used in veterinary medicine include succinylcholine, gallamine and, in the horse, guaiacol glycerol ether. Succinylcholine causes vagal stimulation when injected intravenously, especially with repeated doses, and leads to bradycardia and other arrhythmias, although tachycardia is reported in cats.[15] Atropine usually blocks this effect and should be given prior to the use of succinylcholine. Gallamine, on the other hand, like atropine has a vagolytic effect which leads to tachycardia and in some cases ventricular arrhythmias.[67]

Succinylcholine administration in the awake horse leads to tachycardia and ventricular arrhythmias which may terminate in ventricular fibrillation. This is believed due to sympathetic stimulation caused by the fear and pain involved in casting an awake horse with succinylcholine, and by the hypoxia and hypercarbia that occurs during the period of apnea.[62] Induction with guaiacol glycerol ether, a centrally acting muscle relaxant, is characterized by slight changes in cardiac rate, and normal cardiac rhythm.[40] Although some respiratory depression is produced, a period of apnea does not occur. Consequently the risk of serious cardiac arrhythmias and ventricular fibrillation is eliminated.[63]

The use of digitalis during anesthesia and surgery greatly complicates the anesthetic management of cardiac arrhythmias because of the difficulty in defining and maintaining a therapeutic level of digitalis. Digitalis toxicity leads to a great variety of arrhythmias all of which may also be caused by factors not related to digitalis. Intraoperative changes in cardiac rhythm are therefore very difficult to interpret. Furthermore, the patient's tolerance to digitalis may change significantly during anesthesia. It is well known that halothane increases and cyclopropane decreases tolerance to digitalis.[48, 50] Other factors that may decrease tolerance to digitalis include hypokalemia and hypercalcemia.

BLOOD GASES

The relationship between hypercarbia and cardiac rhythm during anesthesia has already been discussed. Since hypercarbia causes sympathetic nervous system stimulation, it is understandable that carbon dioxide retention would increase the likelihood of arrhythmias with those anesthetics that sensitize the myocardium. An elevated carbon dioxide level is also believed to increase the rate of diastolic depolarization by a direct effect on automatic cells.[28] Hypocarbia is usually considered relatively innocuous for the patient and greatly preferable to respiratory acidosis during anesthesia. Most patients in which ventilation is being controlled are hyperventilated to some degree, resulting in hypocarbia. It has been shown that respiratory alkalosis results in a decrease in intracellular hydrogen ion concentration. Consequently, potassium ions enter the cell and the serum potassium level is reduced. The resulting hypokalemia may lead to a variety of arrhythmias. Patients on digitalis are particularly prone to arrhythmias during hypocarbia as the hypokalemia results in digitalis toxicity.[5, 21, 69]

Hypoxia is known to enhance automaticity in the myocardium by increasing the rate of spontaneous depolarization in automatic cells.[28] During severe anoxia in experimental dogs, the first electrocardiographic changes to occur are ST segment elevation and peaked high voltage T waves. Transient atrioventricular dissociation occurs but usually reverts to a sinus rhythm. Supraventricular and ventricular premature beats are common. Within several minutes after circulatory collapse, permanent atrioventricular dissociation occurs. Terminally either ventricular standstill or ventricular fibrillation occurs.[41] It should be noted that reasonably normal electrocardiograph tracings can be seen several minutes after circulatory collapse when effective blood flow has ceased.

During anesthesia various non-specific ST segment and T wave changes may be seen. Although ordinarily associated with myocardial hypoxia, they may result from a variety of other causes.[44] This is especially true during anesthesia and emphasizes the point that the electrocardiogram cannot be depended upon as a warning when serious hypoxia occurs.[14] Significant neurological damage may occur before signs of myocardial hypoxia are revealed by the electrocardiogram.

REFLEXES

Various circulatory reflexes may cause arrhythmias during anesthesia. They are usually vagal reflexes although in some cases may be sympathetic. The afferent stimuli are usually initiated in the thoracic or abdominal viscera, the trachea or pharynx, the corotid sinus, or the extrinsic muscles of the eye. If the efferent pathways are mediated via the sympathetic nerves, the response is hypertension, tachycardia, and arrhythmias. This probably explains some of the arrhythmias associated with intubation of the trachea, although vagal reflexes are probably also initiated by the trachea. If the efferent pathways are mediated via the vagus, hypotension, bradycardia, and arrhythmias occur. The intense bradycardia that may be initiated by pressure on the extrinsic muscles of the eye is a common vagal reflex.[38]

ELECTROLYTES

Serum electrolytes having important effects on cardiac rhythm include potassium and calcium. Hypokalemia causes an increase in the rate of spontaneous depolarization thereby increasing automaticity and the occurrence of ectopic beats. Other effects are an increased membrane potential and retarded repolarization. Decreased T wave amplitude, ST depression, and U waves may be seen on the electrocardiogram. Hyperkalemia results in a decreased rate of spontaneous depolarization and decreased membrane potentials. The effect may be sinoatrial block, atrioventricular block, bradycardia and asystole or ventricular tachycardia and fibrillation. Tall peaked T waves and a shortened QT interval are seen on the electrocardiogram.

Hypocalcemia increases transmembrane threshold therefore increasing cardiac excitability and depressing contraction. Hypercalemia decreases cardiac excitability and increases contraction leading to bradycardia and asystole. The electrocardiogram may have decreased P and T wave amplitudes, a shortened QT interval and a depressed ST segment.[38]

Management of Arrhythmias During Anesthesia

For proper treatment of arrhythmias during anesthesia, the primary emphasis should be directed toward removal of the cause. The first step should be to decrease the anesthetic concentration and ventilate the patient with a high concentration of oxygen. This alone may be sufficient to terminate arrhythmias related to carbon dioxide retention, hypoxemia, and an inappropriate level of anesthetic. If the arrhythmia persists, other measures that should be considered include correction of electrolyte imbalance, adequate replacement of blood and fluids, maintenance of normal body temperature, a change in the anesthetic agent to one less likely to induce arrhythmias, and relief of surgical stimulation which may involve traction on the viscera, pressure on the eye, or manipulation of the heart. In some cases it may be necessary or advisable to terminate the surgical procedure.

Assuming that adequate measures to eliminate the cause of the arrhythmia have been taken, the use of antiarrhythmic drugs during anesthesia should rarely be necessary. In some cases, however, potentially hazardous ventricular arrhythmias may persist in spite of all attempts to improve the anesthetic management. In this situation, the antiarrhythmic drug of choice is lidocaine hydrochloride. The effect of lidocaine in low doses is to depress automaticity, particulary in the cells of the Purkinje network. Its use is contraindicated in the presence of high grade atrioventricular block.[66] At the recommended doses lidocaine has little effect on myocardial contractile force or arterial blood pressure.[26, 49] Lidocaine is given intravenously at a dose range of 0.5 to 1.0 mg/lb. of body weight. The injection should be made slowly and if possible under electrocardiographic control. The injection may be repeated after 10 to 20 minutes if necessary. During thoracotomy when ventricular arrhythmias result from direct stimulation or manipulation of the heart, lidocaine may be used topically by placing a few drops of a 2% solution directly on the myocardium.

The use of adrenergic beta blockers is sometimes advocated for the control of ventricular arrhythmias during anesthesia. Propranolol is the drug commonly used. Beta blockers block the beta adrenergic receptors in the heart that produce cardioacceleration and increased contractile force. Propranolol has been shown to increase the threshold to catecholamine induced arrhythmias during halothane in the cat, horse, and man, and to prevent arrhythmias produced by sympathetic stimulation during halothane.[32, 35, 61] However, the widespread effects of beta blockers on the cardiovascular system impair the ability of this system to respond to stress. Blood pressure and coronary blood flow may be decreased and the ability of the myocardium to respond to catecholamines with an increase in contractile force is depressed. Bronchoconstriction may also occur.[37] In the horse anesthetized with halothane, cardiovascular depression was not reported following propranolol; but during ether anesthesia, hypotension and cardiac arrest occurred.[60] In the dog both cardiovascular depression and lack of it have been reported during halothane and propranolol.[16, 56, 58] It should be noted that these studies involved healthy animals under anesthesia and not subjected to surgical stress. In the anesthetized patient treated with atropine and propranolol, the heart is for all practical purposes denervated because it cannot respond to either vagal or sympathetic stimulation. Consequently the heart cannot increase its rate or contractile force in response to hemorrhage, hypotension, hypoxemia, and the depressant effects of anesthetic agents.[35] Because of the profound effects of beta adrenergic blockade on the cardiovascular system, the use of these agents for the control of ventricular arrhythmias during anesthesia is not recommended.

Atropine is very commonly used both preoperatively and intraoperatively for its vagolytic effect to stimulate cardioacceleration and prevent bradycardia. The intravenous use of atropine to treat the bradycardia associated with deep halothane anesthesia, neuroleptalanalgesia, succinylcholine, and vagal reflexes has been discussed, as well as the danger of precipitating ventricular arrhythmias with atropine during cyclopropane and light halothane anesthesia.

However, it should be emphasized that the vagolytic effect of atropine may be dependent on the dose and rate of administration. Low doses or slow rates of injection may result in an initial slowing of the pulse rate followed by acceleration.[65] This is because the initial effect of atropine is vagotonic due to central stimulation of the vagal nuclei in the medulla. The peripheral parasympatholytic effect is secondary.[1] The effect of atropine during anesthesia may depend on the relative degree of vagal and sympathetic tone produced by the anesthetic, as well as on dose and rate of injection of the atropine.[36] Although atropine or other parasympatholytic drugs are used almost universally for premedication in human patients and by many veterinary practitioners as well, the routine use of these agents prior to general anesthesia has recently been questioned.[2, 31, 47]

The anesthetic management of the animal with complete heart block deserves special mention because of the extremely grave risk associated with anesthesia in this condition, and the high incidence of ventricular standstill which occurs during induction. Ideally a temporary transvenous pacemaker should be placed in the right ventricle of any patient with complete heart block or with a history of third degree block prior to the induction of anesthesia.[38] However, the use of a pacemaker is ordinarily not available to the veterinary practitioner although its clinical use has been reported in the dog and the horse.[11, 64] Assuming that a pacemaker is not at hand, the animal should be premedicated with atropine and the leads of an electrocardioscope applied. An isoproterenol drip may be started prior to induction to increase the ventricular rate or it may be kept ready for use should the ventricular rate become markedly decreased during anesthesia. As an added precaution, a responsible member of the surgical team should be gowned and gloved prior to induction so that thoracotomy and cardiac massage may be performed without delay if asystole occurs. Anesthesia is induced with a small dose of thiopental followed by intubation and maintenance with an inhalent anesthetic and high concentrations of oxygen.[11, 22, 55]

Value of the Electrogram as a Monitor During Anesthesia

The electrocardiograph oscilloscope as well as various cardiac monitors that convert the electrical impulse of the heart into an audible or visual signal are being used in many veterinary hospitals for monitoring of small animal patients during anesthesia.[3, 39, 43] If these instruments are to be used safely, it is of great importance that their limitations as monitors of the anesthetized patient be thoroughly understood. In a variety of situations the electrocardiograph fails to give any indication that the patient is in great distress. These include impending circulatory collapse, irreversible brain damage, anesthetic overdose, uncontrolled hemorrhage, life threatening asphyxia, and the absence of a measurable blood pressure and cardiac output.[7, 9, 45]

The phenomenon of a relatively normal electrocardiogram in a patient who is clinically dead is well known to the experienced anesthesiologist. By clinically dead is meant a patient who is pulseless, with an unobtainable blood pressure, widely dilated pupils, and lack of spontaneous respiration. In this animal, cardiac output has either ceased or is so low that cerebral blood flow is inadequate. It has been shown that a normal sinus rhythm may persist for as long as four to six minutes after cardiac output has ceased.[46, 57]

The mechanism for this phenomenon is poorly understood. But it must be emphasized that the electrocardiogram records only the electrical activity of the heart and is not related to the contractile force. Normally the electrical event, depolarization, is always associated with contraction. Presumably under certain abnormal conditions, depolarization is not followed by contraction, or the contraction is so weak that an effective cardiac output is not produced. This condition is sometimes referred to as electrical dissociation or excitation contraction uncoupling.[46]

During the period of electrical dissociation, cerebral blood flow is interrupted and the brain, which is more susceptible to anoxia than the heart, suffers irreversible damage. This explains why, frequently following cardiac arrest and resuscitation, satisfactory cardiovascular function is restored, but the animal fails to regain consciousness or shows a marked neurological deficit.

The only reliable estimation of adequate cardiac output in the anesthetized animal is based on the vital signs of the patient. Faced with loss of peripheral pulses, absent heart sounds, and widely dilated pupils, the attending veterinarian should initiate cardiac massage and resuscitation without delay, disregarding the electrocardiogram if a normal rhythm is still being recorded. Failure to initiate immediate resuscitation because of excessive reliance on the electrocardiogram may result in the loss of valuable time and greatly decreases the possibility of a successful resuscitation (see Chapters 35, 36).

REFERENCES

1. Adriani, J.: *Current Concepts in Anesthesiology*, Vol. II, C. V. Mosby, St. Louis, 1964. Ch. 11, Atropine—Disturbances in Cardiac Rhythm Following Intravenous Use during Anesthesia.
2. Adriani, J.: Anesthesia problems in small hospitals. Postgraduate Medicine *45:* 116, 1969.
3. Allen, W. V.: Electrocardiographic monitoring of surgical patients. Modern Veterinary Practice *49:* 59, 1968.
4. Arens, J. F.: Methoxyflurane and epinephrine administered simultaneously. Anesth. and Analg. *47:* 39, 1968.
5. Ayres, S. M. and Grace, W. J.: Inappropriate ventilation and hypoxemia as causes of cardiac arrhythmias. Am. J. of Medicine *46:* 495, 1969.
6. Bamforth, B. J., Siebecker, K. L., Kraemer, R and Orth, O. S.: Effect of epinephrine on the dog heart during methoxyflurane anesthesia. Anesthesiology *22:* 169, 1961.
7. Bardens, J. W.: An evaluation of electronic monitoring devices, Small Animal Clinician *3:* 608, 1963.
8. Black, G. W.: A comparison of cardiac rhythm during halothane and methoxyflurane anesthesia at normal and elevated levels of $PaCO_2$. Acta. Anaesth. Scandinav. *11:* 103, 1967.
9. Booth, N. H.: Evaluation of a cardiac monitor. J.A.V.M.A. *140:* 664, 1962.
10. Buchanan, J. W.: Spontaneous arrhythmias and conduction disturbances in domestic animals. Ann. N. Y. Acad. of Sci. *Comparative Cardiology Monograph*, 1965.
11. Buchanan, J. W., Dear, M. G. Pyle, R. L. and Berg, P: Medical and pacemaker therapy of complete heart block and congestive heart failure in a dog. J.A.V.M.A. *152:* 1099, 1968.
12. Burch, G. E. and Winsor, T.: *A Primer of Electrocardiography*, 5th ed. Lea and Febiger, Philadelphia, 1968.
13. Burleigh, B. W., and Green, N. M.: Effect of methoxyflurane on epinephrine-induced ventricular arrhythmias. Canad. Anaesth. Soc. J. *17:* 341, 1970.
14. Cannard, T. H., Dripps, R. D., Helwig, J. Jr. and Zinsser, H. F.: The electrocardiogram during anesthesia and surgery. Anesthesiology *21:* 194, 1960.
15. Conway, C. M.: The cardiovascular actions of suxamethonium in the cat. Brit. J. Anaesth. *33:* 560, 1961.
16. Craythorne, N. W. B. and Huffington, P. E.: Effects of propranolol on the cardiovascular responses to cyclopropane and halothane. Anesthesiology *27:* 580, 1966.
17. Dear, M. G.: Spontaneous reversion of complete A-V block to sinus rhythm in the dog. J. Small Anim. Pract. *11:* 17, 1970.
18. Dear, M. G.: Complete atrioventricular block in the dog: a possible congenital case. J. Small Anim. Pract. *11:* 301, 1970.
19. Evans, F. T. and Gray, T. C.: *General Anesthesia*, Vol. I. Butterworths, Washington, 1965. (Black, G. W. and Dundee, J. W.: Ch. 11. The Pharmacology of Inhalational Anaesthetics.)
20. Evans, F. T. and Gray, T. C.: *General Anesthesia*, Vol. I. Butterworths, Washington 1965. (Johnstone, M.: Ch. 13. The Influence of Anesthesia on the Electrocardiogram.)
21. Flemma, R. J. and Young, W. G.: The metabolic effects of mechanical ventilation and respiratory alkalosis in postoperative patients. Surgery *56:* 36, 1964.
22. Green, N. M.: *Anesthesia for Emergency Surgery*. F. A. Davis, Phila., 1963. (Keats, A. S. and Jackson, L.: Ch. 5. Anesthesia for Emergency Cardiovascular Surgery.)
23. Hall, K. D. and Norris, F. H.: Respiratory and cardiovascular effects of fluothane in dogs. Anesthesiology *19:* 339, 1958.
24. Hall, K. D. and Norris, F. H.: Fluothane sensitization of the dog heart to the action of adrenaline. Anesthesiology *19:* 631, 1958.
25. Hall, L. W.: *Wright's Veterinary Anaesthesia and Analgesia*. Williams and Wilkins, Baltimore, 1966.
26. Harrison, D. C., Sprouce, J. H. and Morrow, A. G.: The antiarrhythmic properties of lidocaine and procaine amide. Clinical and physiologic studies of their cardiovascular effects in man. Circulation *28:* 486, 1963.
27. Hoffman, B. F. and Cranefield, P. F.: *Electrophysiology of the Heart*. McGraw-Hill, New York, 1960.
28. Hoffman, B. F. and Cranefield, P. F.: The physiological basis of cardiac arrhythmias. Am. J. of Medicine *37:* 670, 1964.
29. Hoffman, B. F., Cranefield, P. F. and Wallace, A. G.: Physiological basis of cardiac arrhythmias (I and II), Modern Concepts of Cardiovascular Disease *35:* 103, 1966.
30. Hoffman, B. F.: *Autonomic Control of Cardiac Rhythm*. Bulletin of the New York Academy of Medicine *43:* 1087, 1967.
31. Holt, A. T: Premedication with atropine should not be routine. The Lancet *2:* 984, 1962.
32. Ikezono, E., Yasuda, K. and Hattori, Y.: Effects of propanolol on epinephrine induced arrhythmias during halothane anesthesia in man and cats. Anesthesia & Analgesia *48:* 598, 1969.
33. Jenkins, M. T., ed.: *Common and Uncommon Problems in Anesthesiology*. F. A. Davis Co., Phila., 1968. (Petty, L. D.: Ch. 11. Cardiac Considerations in Anesthesia.)

34. Johnstone, M. and Nisbet, H. I. A.: Ventricular arrhythmia during halothane anaesthesia. Brit. J. Anaesth. *33:* 9, 1961.

35. Johnstone, M.: Propanolol (Inderal) during halothane anesthesia. Brit. J. Anaesth. *38:* 516, 1966.

36. Jones, R. E., Deutsch, S. and Turndorf, H.: Effects of atropine on cardiac rhythm in conscious and anesthetized man. Anesthesiology *22:* 67, 1961.

37. Katz, R. L. and Epstein, R. A.: The interaction of anesthetic agents and adrenergic drugs to produce cardiac arrhythmias. Anesthesiology *29:* 763, 1968.

38. Katz, R. L. and Bigger, J. T.: Cardiac arrhythmias during anesthesia and operation. Anesthesiology *33:* 193, 1970.

39. Kearns, R. J.: A cardiac monitor for canine anesthesia. Modern Veterinary Practice *42:* 41, 1961.

40. Kraft, H.: ECG and narcosis in the horse. Berl. M. Munch. Tierarzt. Wschr. *75:* 165, 1962. (In Catcott, E. J. and Smithcors, J. F.: *Progress in Equine Practice.* American Veterinary Publications, Santa Barbara, California, 1966.)

41. Kristofferson, M. B., Rattenborg, C. C. and Holaday, D. A.: Asphyxial death: the role of acute anoxia, hypercarbia, and acidosis. Anesthesiology *28:* 488, 1967.

42. Lees, P. and Tavernor, W. D.: Influence of halothane and catecholamines on heart rate and rhythm in the horse. Br. J. Pharmac. *39:* 149, 1970.

43. Lumb, W. V.: *Small Animal Anesthesia.* Lea & Febiger, Phila., 1963.

44. Marriott, H. J. L.: *Practical Electrocardiography,* 4th ed. Williams & Wilkins, Baltimore, 1968.

45. Mazzia, V. D. B. and Siegel, H.: Monitors and prevention of death associated with anesthesia. New York State J. of Medicine *63:* 3233, 1963.

46. Mazzia, V. D. B., Ellis, C. H., Siegel, H. and Hershey, S. G.: The electrocardiograph as a monitor of cardiac function in the operating room. J.A.M.A. *198:* 103, 1966.

47. Middleton, M. J., Zitzer, J. M. and Urbach, K. F.: Is atropine always necessary before general anesthesia? Anesthesia & Analgesia *46:* 51, 1967.

48. Morrow, D. H.: Anesthesia and digitalis toxicity. IV: Relationship of digitalis tolerance to catecholamines during cyclopropane or halothane anesthesia. Anesthesia & Analgesia *46:* 675, 1967.

49. Morrow, D. H. and Logic, J. R.: Management of cardiac arrhythmias during anesthesia. Anesthesia & Analgesia *48:* 748, 1969.

50. Morrow, D. H.: Anesthesia and digitalis toxicity. IV: Effects of barbiturates and halothane on digoxin toxicity. Anesthesia & Analgesia *49:* 305, 1970.

51. North, W. C. and Stephen, L. R.: A second look

52. Price, H. L.: *Circulation During Anesthesia and Operation.* Charles C Thomas, Springfield, 1967.

53. Purchase, I. F. H.: Cardiac arrhythmias occurring during halothane anesthesia in cats. Brit. J. Anaesth. *38:* 13, 1966.

54. Robbins, B. H. and Thomas, J. D.: Cyclopropane arrhythmias in the cat: their cause, prevention and correction. Anesthesiology *21:* 169, 1960.

55. Ross, E. D. T.: General anesthesia in complete heart block. Brit. J. Anaesth. *34:* 102, 1962.

56. Rouse, W.: Cardiac effects of propranolol during anesthesia in dogs. Am. J. of Cardiol. *18:* 470, 1966.

57. Sabawala, P., Gunter, R. and Dillon, J. B.: Persistance of electrical activity in the heart after "clinical death". Anesthesiology *18:* 236, 1957.

58. Sharma, P. L.: Effect of propranolol on arterial hypotension induced by halothane in the dog under nitrous oxide anesthesia. Brit. J. Anaesth. *39:* 215, 1967.

59. Soma, L. R. and Shields, D. R.: Neuroleptanalgesia produced by fentanyl and droperidol. J.A.V.M.A. *145:* 897, 1964.

60. Strack, L. E. and Kaplan, H. M.: Fentanyl and droperidol for surgical anesthesia of rabbits. J.A.V.M.A. *153:* 822, 1968.

61. Tavernor, W. D. and Lees, P.: The influence of propranolol on cardiovascular function in conscious and anesthetized horses. Arch. Int. Pharmacodyn. *180:* 89, 1969.

62. Tavernor, W. D. and Lees, P.: The influence of thiopentone and suxamethonium on cardiovascular and respiratory function in the horse. Res. Vet. Sci. *11:* 45, 1970.

63. Tavernor, W. D.: The influence of guaiacol glycerol ether on cardiovascular and respiratory function in the horse. Res. Vet. Sci. *11:* 91, 1970.

64. Taylor, D. H. and Mero, M. A.: The use of an internal pacemaker in a horse with Adams-Stokes syndrome. J.A.V.M.A. *151:* 1172, 1967.

65. Thomas, E. T.: The effect of atropine on the pulse. Anaesthesia *20:* 340, 1965.

66. Vander Ark, C. R. and Reynolds, E. W.: Cellular basis and clinical evaluation of antiarrhythmic therapy. Medical Clinics of North America *53:* 1297, 1969.

67. Walts, L. F. and Prescott, F. S.: The effects of gallamine on cardiac rhythm during general anesthesia. Anesthesia & Analgesia *44:* 265, 1965.

68. Williams, J. G. L. and Jones, J. R.: Psychophysiological responses to anesthesia and operation. J.A.M.A. *203:* 415, 1968.

69. Wright, B. D. and DiGiovanni, A. J.: Respiratory alkalosis, hypokalemia, and repeated ventricular fibrillation associated with mechanical ventilation. Anesthesia & Analgesia *48:* 467, 1969.

at methoxyflurane: four years of experience. Anesthesia & Analgesia *45:* 117, 1966.

40
Euthanasia

DONALD CLIFFORD

Methods which often are considered humane and acceptable for the slaughter of food-producing animals such as use of the poleaxe, firearms, captive bolt, exsanguination, or severance of the spinal cord are generally regarded as unsatisfactory for laboratory animals and pets.[1] A method for euthanasia should fulfill the following criteria. It should (a) be humane or unassociated with pain, fright, or discomfort such as struggling, muscular spasms, emesis, or crying; (b) be safe for attending personnel; (c) be easy to perform; (d) be rapid in action; (e) be economical to use; (f) not produce changes in the tissues which might camouflage findings at necropsy; and (g) be efficient or irreversible. Stunning, for example, should be supplemented by other methods. A final examination should be made to verify the animal's death.

Euthanasia should be performed by trained personnel in a professional manner without soiling the premises or handling the animals in a rough manner. Whenever an animal has sentimental value, it is prudent to have the owner sign a form authorizing euthanasia with or without permission to dispose of the remains. It is, however, unwise to hurry an owner about making such a decision. Advantages and disadvantages of various methods as they apply to (a) small laboratory animals, (b) large laboratory animals and pets, (c) large domestic animals, (d) zoological and feral animals, (e) birds, (f) amphibians, and (g) fish are discussed below.

Small Laboratory Animals

Small numbers of rats, hamsters, guinea pigs, and mice can be quickly euthanatized by placing them in a glass container and exposing them to an overdose of a volatile anesthetic agent such as ether or chloroform. A false bottom made of wire should be provided to prevent the animal from coming in direct contact with the pledgets soaked with ether or chloroform. Halothane and methoxyflurane are effective but are expensive for routine use.

Intraperitoneal administration of pentobarbital is a rapid and effective means of euthanatizing small numbers of rats, hamsters, guinea pigs, and mice. The recommended dose for euthanasia is 3 times the anesthetic dose or 120 to 150 mg/kg.

In experiments where it is undesirable to introduce a chemical agent into the circulation, mice may be euthanatized quickly by placing the thumb and forefinger against the dorsum of the neck and pressing them against a hard surface. Rabbits may be stunned with a sharp blow to the back of the head.

Some studies, *e.g.*, histology of the brain, are benefited by exsanguination or perfusing the animal with a fixative before death. Exsanguination and/or perfusion are easier in anesthetized subjects.

chemicals are to be avoided for other reasons, the means of producing anesthesia is limited to nitrous oxide, carbon dioxide, and electronarcosis. There are numerous specific contraindications for the use of ether or chloroform when lipid studies are being made and for prussic acid, carbon dioxide, or carbon monoxide if the pigments of the blood are being studied. Enzyme studies may be facilitated by plunging the animal into liquid air.[26] Generally; the physical methods, *e.g.*, stunning, cervical disarticulation, pithing, and use of a guillotine are more difficult, less esthetic, time-consuming; and dangerous to attending personnel.

In instances where it is necessary to euthanatize large numbers of rodents, an anesthetization chamber equipped to receive carbon dioxide from a cylinder or hold blocks of sublimated carbon dioxide can be used.[15, 16, 21] Nitrous oxide may be used instead of carbon dioxide but at a much greater cost. Equipment designed to hold various laboratory animals for carbon dioxide euthanasia is available commercially (Carbothanasia, Inc., New York, N.Y.). It should be remembered that carbon dioxide is particularly valuable for euthanasia in studies that may be jeopardized by the presence of chemical agents in the tissues.

Large Laboratory Animals and Pets

Methods that are accepted for euthanatizing small rodents, amphibia, and food-producing animals may meet severe criticism when used in large laboratory animals and pets. For this reason the veterinarian, laboratory investigator, or humane society officer should be concerned that the methods which are used are humane and bring as little discomfort as possible. He should never become calloused or relegate the euthanatizing of animals to untrained personnel.

The intravenous injection of a barbiturate is the most suitable means of euthanatizing pets and large laboratory animals such as dogs, cats, monkeys, and rabbits. Other routes of injection, *e.g.*, intraperitoneal, intrathoracic, and intracardial can also be used. Due to their frequent and effective use for euthanasia, the barbiturates will be discussed first. Other anesthetic agents and techniques that have been used will also be considered.

BARBITURATES

Intravenous, intraperitoneal, intrathoracic, or intracardiac administration of barbiturates, particularly pentobarbital, is undoubtedly one of the most humane and efficient methods of euthanatizing dogs, cats, rabbits, and other medium to large laboratory animals and pets.[5, 14, 23] The fact that this agent is also routinely used as an anesthetic effaces a great psychological barrier to euthanasia, in that the animal simply goes to sleep and dies without any struggling, crying, or evidence of discomfort.

Twice the anesthetic dose (66 mg/kg) of this drug will usually produce death rapidly and easily. An additional amount or at least 3 times the anesthetic dose will insure rapid cardiac arrest in most animals. The heart should be auscultated to make certain that this has occurred. Pentobarbital is the active ingredient of most commercial euthanasia solutions, which contain approximately 200 to 400 mg/ml. The recommended dose is 1 ml for every 2 to 3 kg (4 to 6 lb). Blue dyes are frequently added to identify these solutions. To prevent inadvertent use of these solutions for anesthesia, it is advisable to keep such preparations separate from anesthetic agents. Previously, the principal disadvantage to use of pentobarbital or other barbiturates for euthanasia was their cost. At present, this is not a serious disadvantage since the cost of these preparations has decreased. In some laboratories, unused quantities of pentobarbital which were withdrawn for anesthesia are exhausted into a common multidose bottle for subsequent euthanasia use.

CHLORAL HYDRATE

Chloral hydrate is an effective and inexpensive lethal agent when administered by parenteral routes. Most animals will not consume it voluntarily in drinking water or food. Twenty milliliters of a freshly prepared 10% solution of chloral hydrate are required to euthanatize an animal weighing 2 to 3 kg. The lethal dose of chloral hydrate is approximately 1000 mg/kg.

MAGNESIUM SULFATE

The administration of magnesium sulfate by the intravenous or intracardial route is a common and relatively effective method of euthanatizing laboratory animals.[3, 6, 11] Magnesium sulfate is widely available and is inexpensive. The average dose of a saturated solution (80%) required to euthanatize a 2- to 4-kg animal is approximately 2.5 to 4.0 ml/kg. The injection should be made as rapidly as possible. Sudden movements or excitement may occur prior to collapse, but there is evidence to support the contention that the animal is unperceptive to pain at this time. Immediate autopsy findings are distention of the heart with relaxed cardiac musculature and pulmonary congestion.[4]

CHLOROFORM

Chloroform has been widely used for euthanasia when airtight containers or anesthetization chambers are available.[5, 7, 14] Two to four ounces are sufficient to euthanatize a 2- to 3-kg cat confined in a 12- by 18-inch container for 30 minutes. Chloroform is not a good lethal agent in dogs since it evokes excitement, and large quantities are required to produce euthanasia.

The time required for death, odor of the agent, and, more important, the frenzy and excitement exhibited by some larger animals, particularly if the vapors are increased too rapidly, are reasons for its condemnation.[7, 14]

Intracardial administration of chloroform (5 to 10 ml) causes minimal struggling but the needle must be well positioned in the heart.[11]

ELECTRICAL METHODS (ELECTRICAL STUNNING AND ELECTROCUTION)

There is a great deal of variation in the equipment and methods for causing death by electrical methods.[9, 26] An electrical current of 70 volts with amperage of 0.5 is usually effective for small animals. It is less suitable for cats and rabbits because of increased resistance produced by the passage of electrical current through their long fur, and they usually object to having electrodes placed on them.[6, 14]

A danger of electrical methods, whether they consist of free wires or wires contained in a cabinet, is the possible injury to personnel.[11] Animals urinate, sometimes defecate, and go into rigid spasms, and added shocks may be required to produce death. To those who have witnessed electrocution, some methods do not appear humane and the question has been raised whether the electrical shocks cause an immediate loss of consciousness or allow animals to perceive pain.[8, 20] It has been observed that fear or "apprehension" is present in animals which are located in the same room as others that are being electrocuted.[9] Electrical current can be used to stun so that administration of another agent is facilitated.[12]

Electrocution, like death by exsanguination or decapitation, has the singular advantage of not causing confusing postmortem lesions.[18]

MISCELLANEOUS TECHNIQUES

There are several other methods of euthanasia which are less common and, in most instances, less effective. They may be classified as (a) chemical or parenteral methods in which strychnine, hydrocyanic acid (prussic acid), narcotics, formalin, air, potassium salts, quaternary ammonium chlorides, succinylcholine, or other agents are injected; (b) lethal chambers where exhaust fumes from internal combustion engines, carbon dioxide, nitrogen, or decompression are used; or (c) special physical methods such as use of the captive bolt gun, guillotine, or pithing.

Although used commonly in the past, strychnine does not result in instantaneous death, provokes violent muscular contractions, and cannot be recommended under any conditions.[2, 6, 9, 22] It should be remembered that strychnine is not a central nervous system depressant, but paralyzes the muscles of respiration and thus prevents the animal from vocalizing during the convulsive episodes. In human beings, strychnine poisoning is accompanied by intense pain and presumably this is true for other species.

A 4% solution of hydrocyanic acid (Scheele's acid) has been used for euthanasia.[2, 14] There is an initial increase in respiration and excitement which may occur after injection and, therefore, it should be preceded by a narcotic. Hydrocyanic acid is not a central nervous system depressant, and the death of the animal is by suffocation.[2] This agent is dangerous to attending personnel and is unsuitable for euthanasia.

The administration of opiates produces sedation in dogs, but cats may exhibit signs of central nervous system stimulation as well as vomition and defecation. Large doses are required to produce death, and they are not considered effective lethal agents.[9]

The injection of formalin or other fixing agents is sometimes desired when special staining of tissues is required. These are not initial central nervous system depressants, and the animal should be anesthetized before they are injected.

The injection of air (10 to 15 ml) into the veins has been employed to kill small animals, e.g., cats and rabbits. The principal disadvantage is that it is not a nervous system depressant and some individuals or species (e.g., goats) may tolerate large amounts of air with minimal effect.

Quaternary ammonium chloride, succinylcholine, and nicotine alkaloids have been employed to euthanatize animals, but they have not been used widely in laboratory animals in North America.[10] These drugs produce death by paralyzing the respiratory muscles, and anoxia is the cause of death. Such drugs without prior anesthesia cannot be considered humane methods of euthanasia.

Lethal chambers were used frequently in the past, but with the development of better and cheaper intravenous methods their popularity has declined. Usually, the lethal gas is the exhaust from some internal combustion engine; however, nitrogen, decompression, or volatile anesthetics such as chloroform can be used. Some animals are apprehensive and cry and struggle when placed in chambers, but they have certain advantages when recalcitrant or wild animals are to be euthanatized. The compartmentalization of a truck so that stray animals may be euthanatized by exhaust fumes while the vehicle is in route from one pickup station to another is an ingenious method of utilizing this principle, but it has limited use. When animals are exposed to 3% carbon monoxide, death is painless and almost instantaneous, but the danger to personnel by this method should not be overlooked.[7, 11] In recent years, there has been renewed interest in carbon dioxide as a lethal agent. There are no confusing postmortem changes or chemical agents in the blood and tissues when carbon dioxide is used. Chambers designed for larger laboratory animals are available commercially. Carbon dioxide has been used for narcotizing swine prior to slaughter.

The captive bolt is exceptionally rapid and considered to be humane. Use of the guillotine or exsanguination of anesthetized animals cannot be considered inhumane but usually is not recommended for esthetic reasons. Pithing requires special skill and is best accomplished in anesthetized animals.

Large Domestic Animals

Large domestic animals and zoological species are euthanatized by various techniques depending on their size, circumstances of their confinement, available equipment, and previous experience of personnel. The horse frequently has the same sentimental value as the dog and cat. Thus, euthanasia in this species is approached with more tact and care than in the food-producing animals.

Methods of euthanatizing animals which resemble those used to produce anesthesia for surgical procedures are more tolerable and interpreted to be more humane. One hundred milliliters of a solution containing sodium N-amylethylbarbiturate and butylethylbarbiturate (Lethol) produce rapid collapse with no evidence of pain in horses.[19] Chloral hydrate, 1 g/5 lb, is a suitable means of producing euthanasia in horses. A saturated solution of magnesium sulfate (250 ml for a horse) is less expensive but may result in struggling, excitement, and convulsions. All intravenous drugs used for euthanasia should be in concentrated solutions and injected rapidly.

Electrocution of horses, cows, and other animals may be performed in diagnostic laboratories, veterinary colleges, or other institutions where personnel are experienced with this method and proper facilities are available. Details of the procedure have been discussed by other authors.[14]

Firearms have been used to produce euthanasia in domestic animals. This method is rapid and humane if the bullet is well placed. The brain is damaged and may be unsuitable for postmortem study. The inherent risk to attending personnel and general dislike for this technique, especially in pets, preclude its use other than in rural or unusual situations. The captive bolt pistol can be used when a large number of horses and cattle are to be killed and their meat consumed by animals or humans.

Succinylcholine has been used to immobilize horses and other large animals.[5, 13, 17, 24, 25] Death from overdose of this agent is due to anoxia from paralysis of the respiratory muscles. Thus, it must be compared to suffocation and cannot be recommended.

Preparations which contain other ingredients, e.g., strychnine and nicotine sulfate, as well as succinylcholine have been used in horses. This does not overcome the objection that no central nervous system depressant is contained in this mixture.

Zoological Animals

A common means of euthanatizing apes, bears, lions, and hoofed stock is to first trap them in a squeeze cage or immobilize them with succinylcholine chloride or tranquilizers and then administer an intravenous anesthetic. Smooth and quick acting drugs such as succinylcholine and phencyclidine may have to be used in wild animals with a Cap-Chur gun or bow and arrow. These serve well in a situation when the animal has to be removed quickly and quietly from public view.

The use of firearms should not be disregarded since some zoos are constructed so that it is extremely dangerous and time-consuming to get squeeze cages in the proper position to be used (e.g, in bear or lion grottos), and Cap-Chur guns or other equipment may not be available. Small and large caliber rifles are usually available as well as personnel that know how to use them. Judgment must dictate when and how this means of euthanasia is to be employed.

Oral administration of drugs via the food or water frequently does not result in satisfactory euthanasia. An incoordinated, excited, or severely depressed animal is not a pleasant sight and may be dangerous to other animals and man.

Birds

Dislocation of the cervical vertebrae from the skull is commonly used to euthanatize poultry. The legs are securely grasped with the left hand while the head is grasped and pulled toward the floor. The Burdizzo castrator also can be used for this purpose.[23] Stunning with a sharp blow behind the head followed by decapitation permits birds to be saved for food. Poultry also can be killed by pithing and then severing the major cervical vessels through the mouth. Chicks and small birds may be killed by physical means, exposure to anesthetic or toxic gases, or parenteral injection of barbiturates or other intravenous agents. Canaries and pigeons succumb rapidly when exposed to chloroform.[23]

Amphibians and Reptiles

Amphibians and reptiles are immobilized by cold. Therefore, lowering the temperature of the room or cage and chilling the water will facilitate their capture and restraint. Placing them in a jar with a sponge soaked with ether or chloroform and parenteral injection of an intravenous anesthetic are suitable methods of producing euthanasia. Reptiles require longer exposure to chloroform to produce death than warm blooded species.

Fish

Fish may be euthanatized by adding urethane to the water, pithing, or severing the spinal cord with a scalpel.[23]

REFERENCES

1. Anderson, E. N.: Notes on euthanasia. In *Equine Medicine and Surgery*, p. 44. American Veterinary Publications, Inc., Santa Barbara, Calif., 1963.
2. Anonymous: Euthanasia for cats and dogs. Brit. Vet. J. *1:* 1323, 1937.
3. Aranez, J. B., and Caday, L. B.: Magnesium sulfate for euthanasia in dogs. J. Amer. Vet. Med. Ass. *133:* 213, 1958.
4. Aranez, J. B., and Mendosa, G. O.: Magnesium sulfate for euthanasia in cats. Vet. Rec. *56:* 425, 1961.
5. Belling, T. H., and Booth, N. H.: Studies on the pharmacodynamics of succinylcholine chloride in the horse. J. Amer. Vet. Med. Ass. *126:* 37, 1955.
6. Croft, P. G.: Small animal euthanasia. Vet. Rec. *64:* 274, 1952.
7. Croft, P. G.: Euthanasia. Vet. Rec. Annot. *67:* 42, 1955.
8. Croft, P. G.: Effect of mephenesin alone and in combination with pentobarbitone sodium on consciousness and appreciation of pain. Vet. Rec. *71:* 287, 1959.
9. Dykstra, R. R.: Euthanasia. Vet. Med. *50:* 418, 1955.
10. Eikmeier, H.: Erfahrungen mit einem Präparat zur schmerzlosen Tötung von Kleintieren (T61). Tierärztl. Umsch. *16:* 397, 1961.
11. Gentry, R. F.: Small animal euthanasia. Vet. Med. *40:* 248, 1945.
12. Golledge, C. R.: Application of electricity to euthanasia in dogs and cats. Vet. J. *89:* 312, 1933.
13. Hansson, C. H.: Succinylcholine iodide as a muscular relaxant in veterinary surgery. J. Amer. Vet. Med. Ass. *128:* 287, 1956.
14. Jones, T. C., and Gleiser, C. A.: *Veterinary Necropsy Procedures*. J. B. Lippincott Company, Philadelphia, 1954.
15. Kline, B. E., Peckman, V., and Heist, H. E.: Some aids in the handling of large numbers of mice. Lab. Anim. Care *13:* 84, 1963.
16. Lampman, E. W.: Useful equipment for the animal colony: bedding, bin loader, euthanasia chamber, feed sifter. Lab. Anim. Care *14:* 514, 1964.
17. Pistey, W. R., and Wright, J. F.: Immobilization of captive wild animals. Vet. Med. *54:* 446, 1959.
18. Podgurniak, A.: Obraz Anatomopathologiczny przy Porazenia Pradem Elektrycznym u Zwierzat. Roczn. Nankrol. *68:* 263, 1958. Abstracted in Vet. Bull. *29:* 393, 1958.
19. Roberts, N. C.: Equine euthanasia. J. Amer. Vet. Med. Ass. *129:* 328, 1956.
20. Roberts, T. D. M.: Cortical activity in electrocuted dogs. Vet. Rec. *66:* 561, 1954.
21. Rudolph, H. S.: A small animal euthanasia Chamber. Lab. Anim. Care *13:* 91, 1963.
22. Ryff, J. F.: Euthanasia in small animals. Mich. State Coll. Vet. *5:* 173, 1945.
23. Scott, P. P., Carvalha da Silva, A., and Lloyd-Jacob, M. A.: *The United Federal Animal Workers Handbook on the Care and Management of Laboratory Animals*, 2nd ed., p. 479. Bailliere, Tindall and Cox, London, 1957.
24. Stowe, C. M.: The curariform effect of succinylcholine in the equine and bovine species—a preliminary report. Cornell Vet. *45:* 193, 1955.
25. Thomas, W. D.: Chemical immobilization of wild animals. J. Amer. Vet. Med. Ass. *138:* 263, 1961.
26. Worden A. M., and Lane-Retter, W.: *The UFAW Handbook on the Care and Management of Laboratory Animals*. The Univ. Fed. for Animal Welfare, London, 1957.

41
Anesthetic Records

ALAN M. KLIDE

Accurate recording of clinically observed information can be of great benefit to patients, clinicians, students, and practitioners. The ultimate value to these individuals depends on the forethought given to making the record form, the accuracy and diligence with which the system is maintained, and the adequacy of the information retrieval system. In devising a record system, the following must be kept in mind: (a) the specific function or functions of the system; (b) the personnel responsible for recording; and (c) the personnel utilizing the information. Care must be taken not to produce a system that either will be too complex to handle efficiently or will consume too much time and eventually be discarded. It must be tailored to fit an individual's or group's needs.

Purpose of Record Keeping

Primary reasons for establishing and maintaining a record system is the improvement of patient care, teaching, medical-legal aspects of veterinary medicine, and clinical investigation. Under many clinical situations in veterinary surgery, the general anesthetic is the portion of the overall clinical care most poorly conceived and managed. Often in the critically ill and geriatric patient, the most hazardous segment of time is the anesthetic and immediate postanesthetic period. Total obligation for patient care should begin by careful preanesthetic examination of the patient's record and continue until full re-covery and removal from the recovery area is complete. Occasionally this segment of time may be in excess of 24 hours. Perusal of a previous anesthetic record may reveal past problems which can be avoided. The record may also reveal some problem other than the initial obvious one, and some thought can be given to potential complications and suitable precautions taken to avoid or at least handle the anticipated problems.

During anesthesia, monitoring and recording heart rate, ventilatory rate, and the other signs of anesthesia insures some attention to the patient's vital signs. It must be stressed here that at no time should patient care be neglected for the sake of neat, complete records. A graphic presentation of cardioventilatory parameters allows for anyone to have an instantaneous impression of the state of the animal (Figs. 41.1 and 41.2). It can often display dramatically a developing trend which can be prevented from becoming a catastrophic conclusion. The postanesthetic record provides a record of what is transpiring during the recovery period—information which is important in determining therapy, especially in very ill patients.

The lack of records or poor records, when required to be presented in court, can at best be embarrassing, at worst very expensive in terms of money, time, reputation, and mental unrest. The anesthetic record should be preserved along with other patient records. Requiring students

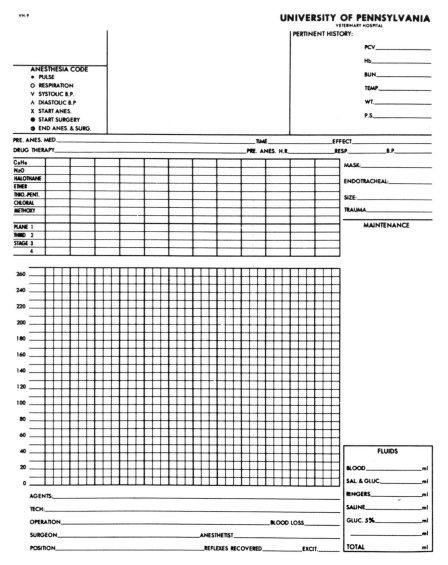

FIG. 41.1. Anesthetic record.

to fill out a detailed anesthetic record will enable them to chronologically observe the anesthetic period and become more aware of the changing events. This is the basis for future course of action on changes which may be a potential danger to the patient. The anesthetic record can provide a source of data for new information or to confirm or deny clinical impressions.

Details of Anesthetic Records

The following is a description of one anesthetic record currently being used (Fig. 41.1), but the arrangement and individual components of the record can be varied as needed to fit local requirements.

IDENTIFICATION

An addressograph plate system is used for identifying any record, request, or report; therefore, space has been provided for it on the anesthetic record. The plate provides the data of admission, date of record, case number, name of client, address, telephone number, species, sex, age, and patient's name (Figs. 41.2 and 41.3).

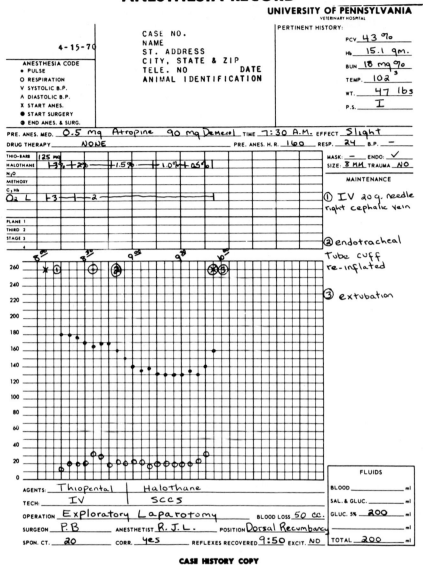

ANESTHESIA RECORD
UNIVERSITY OF PENNSYLVANIA
VETERINARY HOSPITAL

FIG. 41.2 Example of a completed anesthetic record.

PERTINENT HISTORY

This section (*PERTINENT HISTORY*) has space for specifically required information and for pertinent aspects of the history which may influence the course of anesthesia and recovery. The specifics are packed cell volume (*PCV*), hemoglobin (*Hb*), blood urea nitrogen (*BUN*), body temperature (*Temp.*), body weight (*WT*) and physical status (*P.S.*) (see Chapter 20). Other information recorded might be specific cardiovascular problems (*e.g.*, patent ductus) or other disease complications (*e.g.*, Addison's disease).

PREANESTHETIC DRUG INFORMATION

Preanesthetic medication (*PRE. ANES. MED*) is drugs given prior to anesthesia and surgery. The names of the drugs, the total dose, and the time and route of administration are recorded. Drugs which are part of the patient care and are adminis-

4-15-70   CASE NO.
                 NAME
                 ST. ADDRESS
                 CITY, STATE & ZIP
                 TELE. NO   DATE
                 ANIMAL IDENTIFICATION

FIG. 41.3. Addressograph plate for animal identification.

tered prior to anesthesia also should be recorded. The effect (Effect) of depressants is noted on the record as "none," "slight," "moderate," or "marked."

DRUG THERAPY

This category (*DRUG THERAPY*) is for drugs administered for the treatment of a disease state, *e.g.*, cardiac drugs, steroids, insulin, etc. The specific disease state being treated may or may not be related to the surgical problem, but may, in many instances, complicate anesthesia.

PREANESTHETIC HEART RATE, RESPIRATION, AND BLOOD PRESSURE

These parameters (*PRE. ANES. H.R., RESP., B.P.*) are measured just prior to the induction of anesthesia, following the preanesthetic medication. Heart rate and respiratory rate are always measured, but blood pressure is rarely measured.

AIRWAY

There are two spaces which may be checked (*MASK, ENDOTRACHEAL*) to indicate which technique is being used. There is also a block of space to indicate the size of the endotracheal tube (*SIZE*) and also an area for describing the degree of, or lack of, trauma from endotracheal intubation (*TRAUMA*).

ANESTHETIC SECTION

Printed on the record are the most commonly used anesthetics—cyclopropane (C_3H_6), nitrous oxide (N_2O), halothane (*HALOTHANE*), ether (*ETHER*), barbiturates (*THIO.-PENT*), chloral hydrate (*CHLORAL*), methoxyflurane (*METHOXY*), and a blank space in which another agent or flow of oxygen can be recorded. The administration of different

concentrations of agents and the flows of gases can be recorded in this area.

The percentage of concentration of the anesthetic agent and the flow of oxygen or nitrous oxide are recorded numerically. Starting and stopping a drug is indicated by vertical lines in the proper agent column over the time (Fig. 41.2). If the agent is used for a short period of time and is continuously changing, then the two vertical lines are connected and the concentration may or may not be written in. At all other times, the concentration and/or flow is recorded whenever it is changed, and the figures are connected by a horizontal line. When injectable anesthetics are used, the total amount administered each time is recorded.

ANESTHETIC LEVEL

The space designated (*PLANE THIRD STAGE*) is divided into four separate lines (1, 2, 3, 4). These indicate the four traditional planes of 3rd-stage anesthesia, and, as the vital signs are being recorded, the estimate of depth of anesthesia can be recorded. At best this is a very crude estimate, but it does serve a function of categorizing the anesthetic period.

GRAPHIC SECTION

The main graphic section of the record is numbered in the vertical direction from 0 to 260; these may refer either to heart rate, ventilatory rate, or blood pressure. The heavy vertical lines indicate 15-minute, and the light lines, 5-minute intervals. Listed on the record (*ANESTHESIA CODE*) are symbols which are used to indicate heart rate, ventilatory rate, systolic and diastolic blood pressure, start of anesthesia, start of surgery, and end of anesthesia and surgery. Every 5 minutes, the appropriate symbols are used to visualize the vital signs. When something of importance occurs, a number is put on the graph on the time line, and this same number is recorded in the margin of the record (*MAINTENANCE*) and a notation is made of the specific change or event. In the present record, a specific space for indicating correct final sponge count was not included and is presently recorded under maintenance. In subsequent printings this specific space will be included. The use of a sponge count at the beginning and end of a procedure has prevented many potentially embarrassing situations.

FLUIDS

This section (*FLUIDS*) has a list of commonly used intravenous fluids and space for recording the volumes administered. A blank space is also provided for other fluids and a place for the total volume given in the operating room.

AGENTS AND TECHNIQUE

On one line (*AGENTS*) are recorded all drugs given during the anesthetic period, their route, and total dose. The inhalation anesthetic agents used are also noted. The method of delivery or administration (*TECH*) is also indicated, *e.g.*, semiclosed circle, open, nonrebreathing, closed circle, intravenous.

GENERAL OPERATIVE INFORMATION

In this section the name of the procedure or procedures (*OPERATION*) is indicated. The estimated blood loss (*BLOOD LOSS*) is milliliters is recorded, and the operative personnel (*SURGEON*, *ANESTHETIST*) are recorded. The position in which the patient is placed is also noted.

REFLEXES RECOVERED

The reflexes of immediate concern here are the protective airway reflexes. The time at which the patient regains (*REFLEXES RECOVERED*) the ability to swallow, cough, and clear the airway of debris is recorded.

EXCITEMENT

The degree of postanesthetic delirium (*EXCIT.*) is recorded as "slight," "moderate," or "severe."

POSTANESTHETIC PERIOD

On the back of the record is space provided for postanesthetic observations. They include time, heart rate, ventilatory rate, blood pressure, body temperature, and pertinent remarks. There is also space for recording fluids and drugs given in the recovery room. The time of admission to the recovery room, when the patient stands or is reasonably awake, and of discharge from the recovery room is recorded.

Short Form

The record described may be used as a prototype for anyone who wishes this extensive amount of information; however, some hospitals may not have the staff for such an extensive recording system. The following prototype short form is suggested (Fig. 41.4). The heading includes name,

Name: Date of Surgery:	Case No:
Pre-Med. atr mep ms in pz Dose: Route:	Adverse Effects:
Induction: tp ta pb ha my eth Maintenance: tp ta pb ha my eth Technique: iv sccs ccs n/r	
iv drip: No Yes Vol. Site of iv puncture:	Airway: Mask Endo Trauma:
Agent: HR: VR: Time:	
Maintenance: Recovery:	

FIG. 41.4. Short form anesthetic record.

case number, date of surgery, and a section for preanesthetic drugs. A system of circling printed choices can be utilized wherever possible to simplify recording information. For example, the more common preanesthetic drugs can be abbreviated: atropine (atr), meperidine (mep), morphine sulfate (ms), Innovar-Vet (in), and promazine (pz); therefore, all that is necessary is circling the drugs used. The dose and route of administration should also be recorded, and space is provided for recording any adverse effects which result from these drugs.

The next block contains information pertaining to the general anesthetic. Agents commonly used can be printed (tp, thiopental; ta, thiamylal; pb, pentobarbital; ha; halothane; my, methoxyflurane; eth, ether), and all that is necessary is to circle the agent used for induction and the agent used for maintenance of anesthesia. Under technique (Tech.) are listed the commonly used methods, and the appropriate one is circled (iv, intravenous; sccs, semiclosed circle system; ccs, completely closed circle system; n/r, nonrebreathing).

The intravenous section includes information on intravenous therapy, the type, the total volume of fluid, and difficulties encountered.

The airway section is used to indicate whether mask and/or endotracheal tube (endo) was used and the degree of trauma from the intubation: "none," "slight," "moderate," or "marked."

The graphic section is used for the course of anesthesia. Under the appropriate section (Agent, H.R., V.R.) is reported the concentration of the agent being used, the heart rate, and ventilatory rate.

In the maintenance section, any unusual event which occurs during the anesthetic period is recorded, and any problem arising during the recovery period should also be noted.

The Anesthesia Code

This system has been established in an attempt to categorize and store as much information on the anesthetic record as possible. The entire anesthetic vocabulary is mimeographed, and, for each case, a sheet is filled out (Fig. 41.5). The entire code is present on the sheets, and the individual filling out the form extracts information from the anesthetic record and circles all the relevant events. The code is divided basically into preanesthetic and anesthetic information. With this system, the actual case records or the number of cases which fit any vocabulary term or the number of cases which fit in a group comprised of several terms can be recalled. For example, the number of dogs which were anesthetized with halothane in the past 2 years (1,408) can be compared to the number of dogs anesthetized with methoxyflurane (504) and these compared to the total number of dogs anesthetized (2,227).

The Termatrex Data Retrieval System (Jonker Corporation, Gaithersburg, Md.) is the method used by the Data Processing Center, School of Veterinary Medicine, University of Pennsylvania. The basic mechanism by which the system functions is as follows (Fig. 41.6). Each card represents one term of the vocabulary. Holes are punched at a precise position in these cards with the appropriate semiautomatic drill (J301 Data Input Device, Jonker Corporation). The position identifies a case which fits the term in the particular vocabulary used. Up to 10,000 cases can be recorded on each card. To retrieve information, the card representing the characteristic is placed on a calibrated viewer (J52 Reader, Jonker Corporation) and the numbers represented by the punched holes obtained. File cards are kept which convert the numbers obtained to the actual case number; in this manner the actual case record can be retrieved. The number of cases recorded for any characteristic may be obtained in two ways: manually, by placing the card in front of a light and the number of holes counted; or automatically, by using the J500 Scanner (Jonker Corporation). By the use of the scanner, the number of holes are machine-counted. If the information desired is the number of cases which mutually fit several characteristics, the cards

Case# ___ Client ___ Date ___ Anes. ___ Stud ___

1. Species
(B0)- Canine
(B1)- Feline
(B2)- Primate
(B3)- Reptile
(B4)- Avian
(B5)- Rodent
(B6)- Other

2. Weight in Pounds
(B7)- Less than 1
(B8)- 1 to 4
(B9)- 5 to 9
(B10)- 10 to 19
(B11)- 20 to 39
(B12)- 40 to 59
(B13)- 60 to 99
(B14)- more than 100
(B15)- Other

3. Temperament (Prior to medication)
(B16)- Friendly
(B17)- Fearful
(B18)- Difficult to Handle
(B19)- Vicious
(B20)- Not observed

4. Degree of Sedation (Prior to Induction.)
(B21)- No sedation
(B22)- Slight sedation
(B23)- Moderate Sedation
(B24)- Marked Sedation

5. Physical Status
(B25)- I No systemic disturbance
(B26)- II Slight to moderate disturbance
(B27)- III Severe systemic disturbance
(B28)- IV Condition a threat to life
(B29)- Moribund

6. Packed Cell Volume
(B30)- Less than 20
(B31)- 20 to 29
(B32)- 30 to 39
(B33)- 40 to 49
(B34)- more than 50
(B35)- not done

7. Hemoglobin
(B36)- less than 7
(B37)- 7 to 9
(B38)- 10 to 11
(B39)- 12 to 14
(B40)- more than 15
(B41)- Not done

8. Blood Urea Nitrogen
(B42)- Less than 19
(B43)- 20 to 50
(B44)- more than 50
(B45)- Not done

9. Site of Surgery
(B46)- Head, Neck, Eye, Oral
(B47)- intra-thoracic
(B48)- intra-abdominal
(B49)- Rectum, External Genitalia, Anus
(B50)- Caesarean Section
(B51)- Integument (Tumor removal, etc.)
(B52)- Spine
(B53)- Limbs, Orthopedic
(B54)- Limbs, Amputation
(B55)- Other

10. Special Procedures
(B56)- Diagnostic
(B57)- Therapeutic
(B58)- Other

11. Pre-Anesthetic Drugs
(B59)- Demerol 1mg/lb
(B60)- Demerol 2mg/lb
(B61)- Demerol 3mg/lb
(B62)- Demerol more than 3
(B63)- innovar ml/20 lb
(B64)- innovar ml/40 lb
(B65)- innovar, other dose

(B66)- Morphine .5mg/lb
(B67)- Other narcotics
(B68)- Pentobarbital IM
(B69)- Promaine .5mg/lb
(B70)- Promaine 1mg/lb
(B71)- Promaine 2mg/lb
(B72)- Promaine (more than 2)
(B73)- Other tranquilizers
(B74)- Scopolamine
(B75)- Atropine
(B76)- Other

12. Drugs given as part of preanesthetic medication or as preparation for anesthesia and surgery
(B77)- Adrenocorticosteroids
(B78)- Mineralocorticosteroids
(B79)- Anticonvulsants
(B80)- Cardiac Drugs
(B81)- Insulin
(B82)- Diuretics
(B83)- Others

13. Intravenous Barbiturates
(B84)- Thiopental IV
(B85)- Thiamylal IV
(B86)- Pentobarbital IV
(B87)- Other IV

14. Dose mg/lb (of Barbiturates)
(B88)- 1 mg/lb
(B89)- 2 mg/lb
(B90)- 3 mg/lb
(B91)- 4 mg/lb
(B92)- 5 mg/lb
(B93)- 6 mg/lb
(B94)- 7 mg/lb
(B95)- 8 mg/lb
(B96)- 9 mg/lb
(B97)- 10 mg/lb
(B98)- 11 mg/lb
(B99)- 12 mg/lb
(R0)- 13 mg/lb
(R1)- 14 mg/lb
(R2)- 15 mg/lb
(R3)- 16 mg/lb
(R4)- 17 mg/lb
(R5)- 18 mg/lb
(R6)- 19 mg/lb
(R7)- 2C mg/lb

15. Fluid Drugs (Anes.)
(R8)- more than 20 mg/lb
(R9)- Steroids
(R10)- Atropine
(R11)- Cardiac Drugs
(R12)- Insulin
(R13)- Narcotics
(R14)- Pressor-amines
(R15)- Bicarbonate
(R16)- Lactated Ringers
(R17)- Saline or Saline/Dextrose
(R18)- 5% Dextrose
(R19)- Dextran LMW
(R20)- Dextran HMW
(R21)- Blood
(R22)- Plasma
(R23)- Other fluids
(R24)- Other drugs

16. Total fluids ml/lb
(R25)- 0 to 2 ml/lb
(R26)- 3 to 4 ml/lb
(R27)- 5 to 10 ml/lb
(R28)- Greater than 10 ml/lb

17. Heart Rate—Preinduction
(R29)- Less than 50
(R30)- 50 to 99
(R31)- 100 to 149
(R32)- 150 to 199
(R33)- more than 200

18. Respiration Preinduction
(R46)- 0 to 9
(R47)- 10 to 19
(R48)- 20 to 39
(R49)- 40 to 60
(R50)- greater than 50

19. Controlled Ventilation
(R65)- Not used
(R66)- Used during part of anes.
(R67)- Used during all of anes.

20. Intubation
(R68)- Yes
(R69)- No

21. Anesthetic Agents

	Induction	Maintenance
Thio barbiturates	(R70)	(R71)
Halothane	(R72)	(R73)
Halothane N2O	(R74)	(R75)
Methoxyflurane	(R76)	(R77)
Diethyl Ether	(R78)	(R79)
Cyclopropane	(R92)	(R93)
Narcotic - N2O	(R82)	(R83)
N2O ..	(R84)	(R85)
Pentobarbital	(R86)	(R87)
Succinylcholine	(R88)	(R89)
Gallamine	(R90)	(R91)
Local Anesthesia	(R94)	(R95)
Lidocaine I.V.	(G62)	(G63)
Other	(G64)	(G65)

22. Method of Maintenance
(R96)- Epidural analgesia
(R97)- IV
(R98)- Closed Circle
(R99)- Semi-closed circle
(G0)- Pediatric valve (Non rebreathing)
(G1)- Ayers "y" (Non-rebreathing)
(G2)- Mask
(G3)- Open drop
(G4)

23. Anesthesia Time-min.
(G5)- 1 to 14
(G6)- 15 to 29
(G7)- 30 to 59
(G8)- 60 to 120
(G9)- more than 120

24. Blood Pressure
(G10)- Measured
(G11)- Not measured

25. Venus Pressure
(G12)- Measured
(G13)- Not measured

26. EKG
(G14)- Monitored
(G15)- Not monitored

27. Anesthetic Surgical Complications
(G16)- During Anesthesia
(G17)- Post Anesthesia
(G18)- Cardiac Arrest (Resuscitated)
(G19)- Cardiac Arrent (Not resuscitated)
(G20)- Cardia Arrhythmia
(G21)- Normal Cardiac Rhythm abnormal pattern
(G22)- Hemorrhage (During surgery)
(G23)- Blood coagulation defect
(G24)- Hyperthermia
(G25)- Hypothermia
(G26)- Hypotension
(G27)- Blood incompatibility
(G28)- Shock
(G29)- Idiopathic Equicardio respiratory rhythm
(G30)- Inadequate ventilation
(G31)- Improper placement of trach. tube
(G32)- Decrease compliance
(G33)- Respiratory Rate above 50
(G34)- Mechanical Trach. tube problems
(G35)- Insufficient Level of Anes.
(G36)- Infiltrated I.V.
(G37)- Prolonged Apnea
(G38)- Anes. Overdose
(G39)- Laryngospasms
(G40)- Death unexplained
(G41)- Overhydration

(G42)- Vomiting
(G43)- Aspiration
(G44)- Excessive Salivation
(G45)- Injury During Recovery
(G46)- Hemorrhage (postoperative)
(G47)- Other
(G48)- Pulmonary Edema
(G49)- Euthanasia
(R61)- Apnea During Induction
(R63)- Apnea During Maintenance

28. Reflex Recovery
(G51)- In operating room
(G52)- In recovery room

29. Post-anesthetic Delirium
(G53)- none
(G54)- slight
(G55)- severe

30. Post-operative Sedative
(G56)- Narcotics
(G57)- Tranquilizers
(G58)- Both
(G59)- None

31. Personnel Administering Anesthesia
(G60)- Staff
(G61)- Student

Fig. 41 5. Anesthetic code sheet.

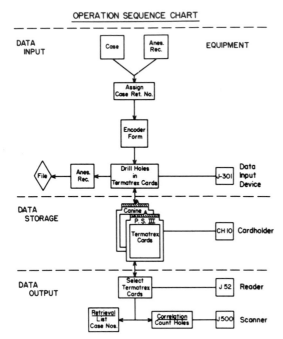

OPERATION SEQUENCE CHART

University of Pennsylvania
School of Veterinary Medicine

DEATH REPORT

Date of Death: Time:
Place of Death (specific)

Date(s) of anesthesia:
    Anesthetist(s):
    Clinician(s):

Clinical Diagnosis:

Clinical Impression of Cause of Death:

Euthanasia: Yes No

Brief Description of Events Surrounding Death

Fig. 41.6. Schematic outline of Termatrex Data Retrieval System.

representing each characteristic are placed upon each other in the scanner and the results counted.

Specific Resuscitative Treatment:

Fig. 41.7. Death report.

Death Reports

Death is a condition which often gets very little attention after the initial repercussions; however, these cases should be studied and reviewed and as much information as possible extracted from them. To try and facilitate this, the Anesthesia Section has a simple death report (Fig. 41.7) which is filled when an anesthetic or an anesthetic-surgical death occurs. These reports are reviewed periodically.

REFERENCES

1. Collins, V. J.: *Principles of Anesthesiology*, chap. 2. Lea & Febiger, Philadelphia, 1966.
2. Dripps, R. D., Eckenhoff, J. E., and Vandam, L. D.: *Introduction to Anesthesia*, 3rd ed., chap. 24. W. B. Saunders Company, Philadelphia. 1967.

Index